Bioethics

Theory and Practice
First Edition

Erick Valdes
George Mason University

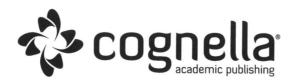

cognella®
academic publishing

Bassim Hamadeh, CEO and Publisher
Michael Simpson, Vice President of Acquisitions
Jamie Giganti, Managing Editor
Jess Busch, Graphic Design Supervisor
Marissa Del Fiero, Acquisitions Editor
Jessica Knott, Senior Project Editor
Luiz Ferreira, Licensing Associate

First published in the United States of America in 2014 by Cognella, Inc.

Trademark Notice: Product or corporate names may be trademarks or registered trademarks, and are used only for identification and explanation without intent to infringe.

Cover images:
Copyright © 2013 by Depositphotos/Tomasz Wyszołmirski.
Copyright © 2012 by Depositphotos/Sergiy Zhukovskyy.

Printed in the United States of America

ISBN: 978-1-62661-695-0 (pbk)/ 978-1-62661-696-7 (br)

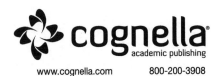

www.cognella.com   800-200-3908

Contents

Part Two: Practice

To Laura Victoria,
for everything you mean to me.

Introduction

Throughout 20th century, diverse fantasies about a world filled with biologically modified humans beings were recurrent in science fiction literature and movies. Those fantasies entertained people by describing incredible societies whose members lived impossible lives and built unique relationships with one another. Nowadays, those stories are no longer fantasies since biotechnology is transforming them into a disturbing reality. Cloning, genetically modified organisms, enhancement, bioinformatics, DNA chips, and bioterrorism, among others do not entertain but at once provoke awe and concern.

At the same time, the biotechnological market proliferates by disfiguring the original meaning and purpose of genetic techniques and bioscientific advances. In this market, the purpose of biotechnology is the production of more biotechnology. Entrepreneurs who fund bioscientific research calculate the eventual earnings of that production, but old economic terminology is insufficient: "risk," "benefit," "profit," "loss," only have an economic connotation and ignore biotechonology's moral implications. Along with this market of biotechnological production other actors come into play: banks that fund biotechnological research; advertising agencies that publicize and present the new products to consumers; web companies that guarantee to globalize new discoveries and to further increase profit. Possible risks that biotechnological techniques may present for the moral, cultural and genetic future of mankind are masked by the spectacle of bioscience's awesome possibility. Are scientists willing to think about these issues? Did they first pause to consider the risks of aerosols for the environment? Did they understand the risks of radioactivity for human beings before atomic energy experimentation? Will scientists think about the possible risks of genetic manipulation?

Biotechnological research is not intrinsically dangerous. Thinking that way would point out a fake dichotomy. However, moral controversies appear when biotechnological research is concreted without adequate precautions and consideration of possible hazards for humans and the environment.

In the same way, when we observe biotechnological development as well as the production and sophistication of genetic techniques with eyes dazzled by the glare of these fascinating new biotechnological powers, we lose objectivity and forget that biotechnology displays two faces: promise and threat.

Technoscientific development and its implications for life as a whole, represent a fundamental milestone in the emergence of bioethics. In fact, bioethics itself may be considered a consequence of biotechnological empowerment and—as such, it must find new ways of questioning the relationship between human beings and technology in an era characterized by the modified scope of human action. Contemporary technology is not only the structural modification of production. It affects and modifies, above all, the quotidian interaction of humans and a world conceived as a technological object free from moral scrutiny.

However, biotechnology acquires an ethical connotation since it is an essentially social phenomenon; that is, it points out an inter-subjective dimension of multifactorial relationships in the public space. For this reason, biotechnology should be addressed from a public policy perspective in which bioethics plays a principal role due to its communicative and pluralist nature.

Biotechnology also raises new challenges to bioethics because there currently is an abyss between what human beings can do and what they can foresee. Hence, biotechnology's achievements entail a new relationship between individuals and current technological possibilities. This is no longer a merely instrumental relationship between subject and object. Being is now technological, supported and strengthened by the manufacturing ability of *homo technicus*. Blind confidence in technical ability to produce implies that biotechnology both allow us to control the world and itself exercises control over us. It is the culmination of our will of power, which implies our own submission to the technoscientific paradigm of contemporary age.

In this sense, the idea of genetic progress is inherent in biotechnology. The balance between human needs and the instruments of their fulfillment is disrupted. Most ends that human beings currently seek—longer and healthier lives, happiness and increased intelligence among others—can only be satisfied by new biotechnological means. Those new means push the proliferation of new needs, and these in turn stimulate the production of other even more sophisticated instruments to meet them. Through this circular relationship, innovation requires that everything theoretically possible be put into practice. Authentic freedom vanishes. Only permanent progress remains, without our discretion and consideration. In this fashion, through advanced biological knowledge, humans can manipulate life and become, themselves, a new object of biotechnology.

By manipulating genetic codes, scientists are able to overcome limitations and frailties of human condition and ultimately control life. Thus, genetic manipulation becomes the most definitive manifestation of rationality, which controls and modifies not only biological life of human beings but also their conceptions, expectations and wishes. Through genetic manipulation our bio-logical dimension turns into a bio-illogical one; that is, life (*bios*) modifies its meaning and logic (*logos*). Genetic codes are altered and our biological axioms are demolished by new paradigms. Biotechnology is revolutionary science since it does not admit perennial axioms. Biotechnological experimentation means functional genetic combinations that pursuit to eliminate random from life. Such a combinations predetermine certain genetic plexuses in order for them to produce a specific genetically ductile biology; namely, susceptible to be modified at will.

The emergence of biotechnology has established revolutionary new pragmatic contexts. Concurrently, a new ethical dimension, fraught with new moral complexities has emerged. Traditional ethics has not been able to address and solve such controversies with a plausible degree of efficacy since it lacks normative elements in tune with current existential conditions. Traditional ethics lacks the norms required to consider biotechnological issues because biotechnology was not yet invented when most traditional ethical systems were formulated.

Specificity and singularity of moral problems, arisen by virtue of biotechnological advancement, call for specific norms, well defined deliberative criteria, and theoretical and procedural guidelines (principles) to give moral content to biotechnological action and, in that way, to carry it out with hope but also with precaution. Bioethics provides deliberative criteria to address the problem of which biotechnology's limits and scopes should be.

The first edition of Tom Beauchamp and James Childress' seminal book, *Principles of Biomedical Ethics* appeared in 1979. This work has been the most universally accepted statement of bioethical principles. The authors consider theories of Ross and Frankena's ethics to identify and define the principles, but it is also possible to find in their work important conceptual antecedents in the thinking of Aristotle, Hume, Kant and Mill, among others. In this sense, the effort of Beauchamp and Childress for creating a dialogue between the two most important branches of Western moral reasoning (teleology and deontology) has been an important contribution to the theoretical deepening of bioethics, as well as a laudable effort to strengthen the basis of the discipline, especially if we consider that both Beauchamp and Childress come from different philosophical conceptions.

The principles of biomedical ethics (respect for autonomy, nonmaleficence, beneficence and justice) received a general acceptance in academic, clinical and scientific circles. They became a kind of reference and guide for rational debate and deliberation on particularly complex cases, and thereby contributed to achieve solutions by promoting reasoning and dialogue among all involved. Those theoretical guidelines are based on our ethical and axiological tradition and emphasize the respect for inalienable individual rights and the observance of unconditional social duties, which had been forgotten in the maelstrom of biotechnological empowerment.

While Beauchamp and Childress' principles are undoubtedly a huge breakthrough for

bioethical deliberation about sensitive issues raised in the heart of science and medicine, they still encounter major difficulties in their application in the practical realm. This situation is originated in several different causes: deficiencies of principles' foundations, logical problems in their definition, ignorance of their limits and scope, procedural and methodological limitations, and an extremely wide variety of interpretations about their meaning and real degree of applicability, among others.

These controversial aspects of Beauchamp and Childress' principlism have brought a considerable array of criticisms which, at the same time, have led the authors to carry out several modifications, redefinitions and extensions to the theoretical and methodological scope of the principles. Basically, the main criticisms are based on what I have called "the problem of principlism" which points out the lack of one or more criteria to rank and balance the principles in order to avoid their practical contradiction. Therefore, the equivalence or theoretical equality of the principles constitutes a problem when they come into play in practice since we do not have any plausible criterion to determine which principle must be imposed on one another and why.

Beauchamp and Childress's book has been an indisputable and undeniable contribution to the study of moral problems inherent to biomedical practice and it has also been an essential material of reference to think about such problems and advance towards their solution. Beauchamp and Childress' attempt is an effort to systematize the approach to moral issues, to provide some rationality to bioethical deliberation, and to integrate argumentation and dialogue in moral reasoning. In this regard, the proposal of these authors tacitly understands bioethics as an intersubjective and dialogical discipline and argues that moral truth is not only present in the individual consciousness but also and very especially in the public space; that is, in the agreement generated through an argumentative and rational encounter of many subjects willing to seek and establish consensus about cross disciplinary issues that affect social harmony and cohesion.

The question for the real degree of applicability of principlism refers to its relationship with the current moral scenario. In fact, an analysis of the status of bioethical principlism should be obligatorily linked with the contemporary moral situation, in which science and technology have reached such a degree of development and success that they seem to be free from moral scrutiny.

Bioethical principlism should, precisely, be a response to the contemporary interpellation of biotechnology and biomedicine, and it should consider, as a fundamental task, the development of foundations and procedures to address new ethical controversies within an intersubjective dialogue and public discussion based on the tacit recognition of our common humanity. In this sense, Jonas' ethics of responsibility, Habermas and Apel's discourse ethics, British analytical pluralism, and Engelhardt's ethics of moral strangers must be taken into consideration to design procedures that can guide moral deliberation.

However, the encounter between traditional ethics and bioethics is undoubtedly problematic. Clarifying possible relationships between philosophical foundations of ethics and bioethics' problems, methods and contents is not an easy task. Ordinary people and even scholars think that bioethics is only the application of certain moral principles and rules on new controversial issues arisen by virtue of biomedical and biotechnological advances. However, bioethical principlism implies a plausible deliberative structure to address moral problems since it has certain features that traditional ethics lacks. First of all, bioethical principlism deals with specific problems that have emerged in professional and social practices as a result of biotechnology and globalization. Secondly, it represents an effort to go beyond the typical divisions of a particular discipline: bioethics is multidisciplinary. And finally, it proposes a dialogical communicative structure that seems to be a direction that could be considered by all

ethics that aspire to be in tune with biomedical and biotechnological empowerment.

The current conditions of existence, dramatically influenced by biotechnological advances, have brought a broad spectrum of moral problems which traditional ethics has not been able to satisfactorily deal with. In this fashion, bioethics constitutes not only a new theoretical perspective to deliberate on complex moral scenarios arisen by virtue of biomedical and biotechnological advances but also and very especially it implies a set of procedural rules to guide decision-making in a completely new ethical arena. However, bioethics has not been exempt from criticism and its principles' epistemological and methodological scope is still profusely discussed.

This book introduces students to the most relevant historical, epistemological, methodological, and practical aspects of bioethics as well as provides theoretical and procedural elements for them to be able to deliberate, in a critical and impartial way, on controversial bioethical issues still unresolved.

Reading

The President's Council of Bioethics, *Beyond Therapy. Biotechnology and the Pursuit of Happiness*, USA, HarperCollins Publishers Inc., 2003: 1–20.

Study Questions

1. What is biotechnology's purpose?
2. What is bioethics' purpose?
3. What are the relationships between bioethics and biotechnology?
4. Why may biotechnological achievements imply bioethical challenges?
5. Are there ethical limits for biomedicine?
6. Can genetic manipulation turn our biological dimension into a bio-illogical one? Why?
7. Why has principlism been a milestone for moral deliberation on biomedical issues?
8. How could you define and explain "the problem of principlism"?

Beyond Therapy: Biotechnology and the Pursuit of Happiness

The President's Council of Bioethics

What is biotechnology for? Why is it developed, used, and esteemed? Toward what ends is it taking us? To raise such questions will very likely strike the reader as strange, for the answers seem so obvious: to feed the hungry, to cure the sick, to relieve the suffering—in a word, to improve the lot of humankind, or, in the memorable words of Francis Bacon, "to relieve man's estate." Stated in such general terms, the obvious answers are of course correct. But they do not tell the whole story, and, when carefully considered, they give rise to some challenging questions, questions that compel us to ask in earnest not only, "What is biotechnology for?" but also, "What should it be for?"

Before reaching these questions, we had better specify what we mean by "biotechnology," for it is a new word for our new age. Though others have given it both narrow and broad definitions,[1] our purpose—for reasons that will become clear—recommends that we work with a very broad meaning: the processes and products (usually of industrial scale) offering the potential to alter and, to a degree, to control the phenomena of life—in plants, in (non-human) animals, and, increasingly, in human beings (the last, our exclusive focus here). Overarching the processes and products it brings forth, biotechnology is also a conceptual and ethical outlook, informed by progressive aspirations. In this sense, it appears as a most recent and vibrant expression of the technological spirit, a desire and disposition rationally to understand, order, predict, and (ultimately) control the events and workings of nature, all pursued for the sake of human benefit.

---

1 These range from "engineering and biological study of relationships between human beings and machines" (Webster's II New Riverside University Dictionary, 1988), to "biological science when applied especially in genetic engineering and recombinant DNA technology" (Merriam-Webster OnLine Dictionary, 2003), to "the use of biological processes to solve problems or make useful products" (Glossary provided by BIO, the Biotechnology Industry Organization, www.bio.org, 2003). In the broader sense of the term that we will follow here, older biotechnologies would include fermentation (used to bake bread and brew beer) and plant and animal hybridization. Newer biotechnologies would include, among others, processes to produce genetically engineered crops, to repair genetic defects using genomic knowledge, to develop new drugs based on knowledge of biochemistry or molecular biology, and to improve biological capacities using nanotechnology. They include also the products obtained by these processes: nucleic acids and proteins, drugs, genetically modified cells, tissues derived from stem cells, biomechanical devices, etc.—in short, any industrially developed, useful agent that can alter the workings of the body or mind

Thus understood, biotechnology is bigger than its processes and products; it is a form of human empowerment. By means of its techniques (for example, recombining genes), instruments (for example, DNA sequencers), and products (for example, new drugs or vaccines), biotechnology empowers us human beings to assume greater control over our lives, diminishing our subjection to disease and misfortune, chance and necessity. The techniques, instruments, and products of biotechnology—like similar technological fruit produced in other technological areas—augment our capacities to act or perform effectively, for many different purposes. Just as the automobile is an instrument that confers enhanced powers of "auto-mobility" (of moving oneself), which powers can then be used for innumerable purposes not defined by the machine itself, so DNA sequencing is a technique that confers powers for genetic screening that can be used for various purposes not determined by the technique; and synthetic growth hormone is a product that confers powers to try to increase height in the short or to augment muscle strength in the old. If we are to understand what biotechnology is for, we shall need to keep our eye more on the new abilities it provides than on the technical instruments and products that make the abilities available to us.[2]

This terminological discussion exposes the first complication regarding the purposes of biotechnology: the fact that means and ends are readily detached from one another. As with all techniques and the powers they place in human hands, the techniques and powers of biotechnology enjoy considerable independence from ties to narrow or specific goals. Biotechnology, like any other technology, is not for anything in particular. Like any other technology, the goals it serves are supplied neither by the techniques themselves nor by the powers they make available, but by their human users. Like any other means, a given biotechnology once developed to serve one purpose is frequently available to serve multiple purposes, including some that were not imagined or even imaginable by those who brought the means into being.

Second, there are several questions regarding the overall goal of biotechnology: improving the lot of humankind. What exactly is it about the lot of humankind that needs or invites improvement? Should we think only of specific, as-yet-untreatable diseases that compromise our well-being, such ailments as juvenile diabetes, cancer, or Alzheimer disease? Should we not also include mental illnesses and infirmities, from retardation to major depression, from memory loss to melancholy, from sexual incontinence to self-contempt? And should we consider in addition those more deep-rooted limitations built into our nature, whether of body or mind, including the harsh facts of decline, decay, and death? What exactly is it about "man's estate" that most calls for relief? Just sickness and suffering, or also such things as nastiness, folly, and despair? Must "improvement" be limited to eliminating these and other evils, or should it also encompass augmenting our share of positive goods—beauty, strength, memory, intelligence, longevity, or happiness itself?

Third, even assuming that we could agree on which aspects of the human condition call for

2 The importance, for assessing biomedical technologies, of the distinction between (1) the techniques and (2) the powers they make available was first developed nearly thirty years ago in a report from the National Research Council/National Academy of Sciences, *Assessing Biomedical Technologies: An Inquiry into the Nature of the Process* (Committee on Life Sciences and Social Policy, National Academy of Sciences, Washington, D.C., 1975). The report recommended (and illustrated by example) that assessment of biomedical technologies concern itself with implications of both the techniques and the perfected powers they provide. (See pages 1 and 9, and the structure of the analysis in each chapter.) We generally prefer the more energetic word "power," with its implication of efficacy, to the more prosaic "capacity" or "ability," but we mean by it nothing ominous or. As we use it, "power" is to be understood as neutral or better, certainly when compared to its opposite, "impotence." At the same time, however, this term invites us to think about power's misuse or abuse; such reminders do not shadow the more quiescent near-synonyms, "capacity" or "ability."

improvement, we would still face difficulties deciding how to judge whether our attempts at improving them really made things better—both for the individuals and for the society. Some of the goals we seek might conflict with each other: longer life might come at the price of less energy; superior performance for some might diminish self-esteem for others. Efforts to moderate human aggression might wind up sapping ambition; interventions aimed at quieting discontent might flatten aspiration. And, unintended consequences aside, it is not easy to say just how much less aggression or discontent would be good for us. Once we go beyond the treatment of disease and the pursuit of health, there seem to be no ready-made or reliable standards of better and worse available to guide our choices.

As this report will demonstrate, these are not idle or merely academic concerns. Indeed, some are already upon us. We now have techniques to test early human embryos for the presence or absence of many genes: shall we use these techniques only to prevent disease or also to try to get us "better" children? We are acquiring techniques for boosting muscle strength and performance: shall we use them only to treat muscular dystrophy and the weak muscles of the elderly or also to enable athletes to attain superior performance? We are gradually learning how to control the biological processes of aging: should we seek only to diminish the bodily and mental infirmities of old age or also to engineer large increases in the maximum human lifespan? We are gaining new techniques for altering mental life, including memory and mood: should we use them only to prevent or treat mental illness or also to blunt painful memories of shameful behavior, transform a melancholic temperament, or ease the sorrows of mourning? Increasingly, these are exactly the kinds of questions that we shall be forced to face as a consequence of new biotechnical powers now and soon to be at our disposal. Increasingly we must ask, "What is biotechnology for?" "What should it be for?"

I. The Golden Age: Enthusiasm and Concern

By all accounts, we have entered upon a golden age for biology, medicine, and biotechnology. With the completion of (the DNA sequencing phase of) the Human Genome Project and the emergence of stem cell research, we can look forward to major insights into human development, normal and abnormal, as well as novel and more precisely selected treatments for human diseases. Advances in neuroscience hold out the promise of powerful new understandings of mental processes and behavior, as well as remedies for devastating mental illnesses. Ingenious nanotechnological devices, implantable into the human body and brain, raise hopes for overcoming blindness and deafness, and, more generally, of enhancing native human capacities of awareness and action. Research on the biology of aging and senescence suggests the possibility of slowing down age-related declines in bodies and minds, and perhaps even expanding the maximum human lifespan. In myriad ways, the discoveries of biologists and the inventions of biotechnologists are steadily increasing our power ever more precisely to intervene into the workings of our bodies and minds and to alter them by rational design.

For the most part, there is great excitement over and enthusiasm for these developments. Even before coming to the practical benefits, we look forward to greatly enriched knowledge of how our minds and bodies work. But it is the promised medical benefits that especially excite our admiration. Vast numbers of people and their families ardently await cures for many devastating diseases and eagerly anticipate relief from much human misery. We will surely welcome, as we have in the past, new technological measures that can bring us healthier bodies, decreased pain and suffering, peace of mind, and longer life.

At the same time, however, the advent of new biotechnical powers is for many people a cause for concern. First, the scientific findings themselves raise challenges to human self-understanding: people wonder, for example, what new knowledge of brain function and behavior will do to our notions of free will and personal moral responsibility, formed before the advent of such knowledge. Second, the prospect of genetic engineering, though welcomed for treatment of inherited genetic diseases, raises for some people fears of eugenics or worries about "designer babies." Psychotropic drugs, though welcomed for treatment of depression or schizophrenia, raise fears of behavior control and worries about diminished autonomy or confused personal identity. Precisely because the new knowledge and the new powers impinge directly upon the human person, and in ways that may affect our very humanity, a certain vague disquiet hovers over the entire enterprise. Notwithstanding the fact that almost everyone, on balance, is on the side of further progress, the new age of biotechnology will bring with it novel, and very likely momentous, challenges.

While its leading benefits and blessings are readily identified, the ethical and social concerns raised by the march of biotechnology are not easily articulated. They go beyond the familiar issues of bioethics, such as informed consent for human subjects of research, equitable access to the fruits of medical research, or, as with embryo research, the morality of the means used to pursue worthy ends. Indeed, they seem to be more directly connected to the ends themselves, to the uses to which biotechnological powers will be put. Generally speaking, these broader concerns attach especially to those uses of biotechnology that go "beyond therapy," beyond the usual domain of medicine and the goals of healing, uses that range from the advantageous to the frivolous to the pernicious. Biotechnologies are already available as instruments of bioterrorism (for example, genetically engineered super-pathogens or drugs that can destroy the immune system or erase memory), as agents of social control (for example, tranquilizers for the unruly or fertility-blockers for the impoverished), and as means to improve or perfect our bodies and minds and those of our children (steroids for

body-building or stimulants for taking exams). In the first two cases, there are concerns about what others might do to us, or what some people, including governments, might do to other people. In the last case, there are concerns about what we might voluntarily do to ourselves or to our society. People worry both that our society might be harmed and that we ourselves might be diminished in ways that could undermine the highest and richest possibilities for human life.

Truth to tell, not everyone who has considered these prospects is worried. On the contrary, some celebrate the perfection-seeking direction in which biotechnology may be taking us. Indeed, some scientists and biotechnologists have not been shy about prophesying a better-than-currently-human world to come, available with the aid of genetic engineering, nanotechnologies, and psychotropic drugs. "At this unique moment in the history of technical achievement," declares a recent report of the National Science Foundation, "improvement of human performance becomes possible," and such improvement, if pursued with vigor, "could achieve a golden age that would be a turning point for human productivity and quality of life."[1] "Future humans—whoever or whatever they may be—will look back on our era as a challenging, difficult, traumatic moment," writes a scientist observing present trends. "They will likely see it as a strange and primitive time when people lived only seventy or eighty years, died of awful diseases, and conceived their children outside a laboratory by a random, unpredictable meeting of sperm and egg."[2] James Watson, co-discoverer of the structure of DNA, put the matter as a simple question: "If we could make better human beings by knowing how to add genes, why shouldn't we?"[3]

Yet the very insouciance of some of these predictions and the confidence that the changes they endorse will make for a better world actually serve to increase public unease. Not everyone cheers a summons to a "post-human" future. Not everyone likes the idea of "remaking Eden" or of "man playing God." Not everyone agrees that this prophesied new world will be better than our own. Some suspect it could rather resemble the humanly diminished world portrayed in Aldous Huxley's novel Brave New World, whose technologically enhanced inhabitants live cheerfully, without disappointment or regret, "enjoying" flat, empty lives devoid of love and longing, filled with only trivial pursuits and shallow attachments.

II. The Case For Public Attention

Despite the disquiet it arouses, the subject of using biomedical technologies for purposes "beyond therapy" has received remarkably little public attention. Given its potential importance, it is arguably the most neglected topic in public bioethics. No previous national bioethics commission has considered the subject, and for understandable reasons. The realm of biotechnology "beyond therapy" is hard to define, a gray zone where judgment is, to say the least, difficult. Compared with more immediate topics in bioethics, the questions raised by efforts to "improve on human nature" seem abstract, remote, and overly philosophical, unfit for public policy; indeed, many bioethicists and intellectuals believe either that there is no such thing as "human nature" or that altering it is not ethically problematic. The concerns raised are complicated and inchoate, hard to formulate in general terms, especially because the differing technologically based powers raise different ethical and social questions: enhancing athletic performance with steroids and genetic selection of embryos for reproduction give rise to different concerns. Analysis often requires distinguishing the primary and immediate uses of a technology (say, mood elevating drugs to treat depression or memory-blunting drugs to prevent post-traumatic stress disorder) from derivative and longer-term uses and implications (the same drugs used as general mood-brighteners or to sanitize memories of shameful or guilty conduct). Speculation about those possible implications, never to be confused with accurate prediction, is

further complicated by the fact that the meaning of any future uses of biotechnology "beyond therapy" will be determined at least as much by the goals and practices of an ever-changing society as by the technologies themselves. Finally, taking up these semi-futuristic prospects may seem a waste of public attention, especially given the more immediate ethical issues that clamor for attention. Some may take us to task for worrying about the excesses and abuses of biotechnology and the dangers of a "brave new world" when, in the present misery-ridden world, millions are dying of AIDS, malaria, and malnutrition, in part owing to the lack of already available biomedical technologies.

Yet despite these genuine difficulties and objections, we believe that it is important to open up this subject for public discussion. For it raises some of the weightiest questions in bioethics. It touches on the ends and goals to be served by the acquisition of biotechnical power, not just on the safety, efficacy, or morality of the means. It bears on the nature and meaning of human freedom and human flourishing. It faces squarely the alleged threat of dehumanization as well as the alleged promise of "super-humanization." It compels attention to what it means to be a human being and to be active as a human being. And it is far from being simply futuristic: current trends make clear how the push "beyond therapy" and "toward perfection and happiness" is already upon us—witness the growing and increasingly acceptable uses of cosmetic surgery, performance-enhancing drugs, and mood- or attention-altering agents.[3] Given the burgeoning research in neuroscience and the ever- expanding biological approaches

---

3 The already widely accepted "beyond therapy" uses of biomedical technologies include: pills for sleep and wakefulness, weight loss, hair growth, and birth control; surgery to remove fat and wrinkles, to shrink thighs, and to enlarge breasts; and procedures to straighten teeth and select the sex of offspring. These practices are already big business. In 2002 Americans spent roughly one billion dollars on drugs used to treat baldness, about ten times the amount spent on scientific research to find a cure for malaria, a disease that afflicts hundreds of millions of people worldwide.

to psychiatric disorders and to all mental states, it seems clear that the expected new discoveries about the workings of the psyche and the biological basis of behavior will surely increase both our ability and our desire to alter and improve them. Decisions we are making today—for instance, what to do about sex selection or genetic selection of embryos, or whether to prescribe behavior-modifying drugs to preschoolers, or how vigorously to try to reverse the processes of senescence—will set the path "beyond therapy" for coming generations. And fair or not, the decisions and choices of the privileged or avant-garde often will pave the way that others later follow, in the process sometimes changing what counts as "normal," often irreversibly.

Taking up this topic is, in fact, responsive to the charge President Bush gave to this Council, formed by executive order "to advise the President on bioethical issues that may emerge as a consequence of advances in biomedical science and technology." Among the specific functions set forth in connection with our mission, the Council was instructed in the first place "to undertake fundamental inquiry into the human and moral significance of developments in biomedical and behavioral science and technology," and then "to explore specific ethical and policy questions related to these developments." Anticipating, as we do, the arrival of technological powers that are likely to affect profoundly the nature, shape, and content of human experience, human character, and human society, we believe that it is highly desirable that we try to articulate as best we can their likely "human and moral significance."

The Council has not only the mandate but also the opportunity to take a more long-range view of these matters. Unlike legislators caught up in the demands of pressing business, we have the luxury of being able carefully and disinterestedly to consider matters before they become hotly contested items for public policy. Unless a national bioethics council takes up this topic, it is unlikely that anyone else in public life will do so. And if we do not prepare ourselves in

advance to think about these matters, we shall be ill prepared to meet the challenges as they arrive and to make wisely the policy decisions they may require.

III. Defining The Topic

Having offered our reasons for taking up the topic, we need next to define it more carefully and to indicate how we mean to approach it. As already suggested, the "beyond therapy" uses of biotechnology on human beings are manifold. We shall not here consider biotechnologies as instruments of bioterrorism or of mass population control. The former topic is highly specialized and tied up with matters of national security, an area beyond our charge and competence. Also, although the practical and political difficulties they raise are enormous, the ethical and social issues are relatively uncomplicated. The main question about bioterrorism is not what to think about it but how to prevent it. And the use of tranquilizing aerosols for crowd control or contraceptive additions to the drinking water, unlikely prospects in liberal democratic societies like our own, raise few issues beyond the familiar one of freedom and coercion.

Much more ethically challenging are those "beyond therapy" uses of biotechnology that would appeal to free and enterprising people, that would require no coercion, and, most crucially, that would satisfy widespread human desires. Sorting out and dealing with the ethical and social issues of such practices will prove vastly more difficult since they will be intimately connected with goals that go with, rather than against, the human grain. For these reasons, we confine our attention to those well-meaning and strictly voluntary uses of biomedical technology through which the user is seeking some improvement or augmentation of his or her own capacities, or, from similar benevolent motives, of those of his or her children. Such use of biotechnical powers to pursue "improvements" or "perfections," whether of body, mind, performance, or sense of well-being, is at once both the most seductive and the most disquieting temptation. It reflects humankind's deep dissatisfaction with natural limits and its ardent desire to overcome them. It also embodies what is genuinely novel and worrisome in the biotechnical revolution, beyond the so-called "life issues" of abortion and embryo destruction, important though these are. What's at issue is not the crude old power to kill the creature made in God's image but the attractive science-based power to remake ourselves after images of our own devising. As a result, it gives unexpected practical urgency to ancient philosophical questions: What is a good life? What is a good community?

IV. Ends and Means

Such a dream of human perfectibility by means of science and technology has, in fact, been present from the start of modern science in the seventeenth century. When René Descartes, in his famous Discourse on Method, set forth the practical purpose for the new science he was founding, he spoke explicitly of our becoming "like masters and owners of nature" and outlined the specific goals such mastery of nature would serve:

> This is desirable not only for the invention of an infinity of artifices which would enable us to enjoy, without any pain, the fruits of the earth and all the commodities to be found there, but also and principally for the conservation of health, which is without doubt the primary good and the foundation of all other goods in this life.

But, as the sequel makes clear, he has more than health in mind:

> For even the mind is so dependent on the temperament and on the disposition of the organs of the body, that if it is possible to find some means that generally renders men more wise and more capable than they have been up to now, I believe that we must seek for it in medicine. ... [W]e could be spared an infinity of diseases, of the body as well as of the mind, and even also perhaps the enfeeblement of old age, if we had enough knowledge of their causes and all the remedies which nature has provided us. (Emphasis added.)[4]

Descartes foresaw a new medicine, unlike any the world had known, that would not only be able effectively to conserve health, but might also improve human bodies and minds beyond what nature herself had granted us: to make us wiser, more capable and competent, and perhaps even impervious to aging and decay—in a word, to make us healthy and happy, indefinitely. Owing to the powers now and soon to be available to us, Descartes's dream no longer seems a mere fantasy.

What exactly are the self-augmenting capabilities that we are talking about? What kinds of technology make them possible? What sorts of ends are they likely to serve? How soon will they be available? They are powers that potentially affect the capacities and activities of the human body; the capacities and activities of the mind or soul; and the shape of the human life cycle, at both ends and in between. We already have powers to prevent fertility and to promote it; to initiate life in the laboratory; to screen our genes, both as adults and as embryos, and to select (or reject) nascent life based on genetic criteria; to insert new genes into various parts of the adult body, and perhaps someday also into gametes and embryos; to enhance muscle performance and endurance; to alter memory, mood, appetite, libido, and attention through psychoactive drugs; to replace body parts with natural organs, mechanical organs, or tissues derived from stem cells, perhaps soon to wire ourselves using computer chips implanted into the body and brain; and, in the foreseeable future, to prolong not just the average but also the maximum human life expectancy. The technologies for altering our native capacities are mainly those of genetic screening and genetic engineering; drugs, especially psychoactive ones; and the ability to replace body parts or to insert novel ones. The availability of some of these capacities, using these techniques, has been demonstrated only with animals; but others are already in use in humans.

It bears emphasis that these powers and technologies have not been and are not being developed for the purpose of producing improved, never mind perfect or post-human, beings. They have been produced largely for the purposes of preventing and curing disease, reversing disabilities, and alleviating suffering. Even the prospect of machine-brain interaction and implanted nanotechnological devices starts with therapeutic efforts to enable the blind to see and the deaf to hear. Yet the "dual use" aspect of most of these powers—encouraged by the ineradicable human urge toward "improvement," exploited by the commercial interests that already see vast market opportunities for nontherapeutic uses, and likely welcomed by many people seeking a competitive edge in their strivings to "get ahead"—means that we must not be lulled to sleep by the fact that the originators of these powers were no friends to Brave New World. Once here, techniques and powers can produce desires where none existed before, and things often go where no one ever intended.

V. The Limitations of The "Therapy Vs.Enhancement" Distinction

Although, as we have indicated, the topic of the biotechnological pursuit of human improvement has not yet made it onto the agenda of public bioethics, it has received a certain amount of attention in academic bioethical circles under the rubric of "enhancement," understood in contradistinction to "therapy."[5] Though we shall ourselves go beyond this distinction, it provides a useful starting place from which to enter the discussion of activities that aim "beyond therapy."[4] "Therapy," on this view as in common understanding, is the use of biotechnical power to treat individuals with known diseases, disabilities, or impairments, in an attempt to restore them to a normal state of health and fitness. "Enhancement," by contrast, is the directed use of biotechnical power to alter, by direct intervention, not disease processes but the "normal" workings of the human body and psyche, to augment or improve their native capacities and performances. Those who introduced this distinction hoped by this means to distinguish between the acceptable and the dubious or unacceptable uses of biomedical technology: therapy is always ethically fine, enhancement is, at least prima facie, ethically suspect. Gene therapy for cystic fibrosis or Prozac for major depression is fine; insertion of genes to enhance intelligence or steroids for Olympic

---

4 Our choice of "Beyond Therapy" as the title for this report is meant to acknowledge that this notion offers a good point of entry: it reflects the medical milieu in which the questions arise; it exposes the untraditional goals of the new uses for biotechnical power; it hints at the open-ended character of what lies "beyond" the goal of healing. Yet for reasons that should become clear, the notion of "beyond therapy" does not seem to us to define the royal road to understanding. For this, one must adopt an outlook not only "beyond therapy" but also "beyond the distinction between therapy and enhancement." One needs to see the topic less in relation to medicine and its purposes, and more in relation to human beings and their purposes.

athletes is, to say the least, questionable. At first glance, the distinction between therapy and enhancement makes good sense. Ordinary experience recognizes the difference between "restoring to normal" and "going beyond the normal." Also, as a practical matter, this distinction seems a useful way to distinguish between the central and obligatory task of medicine (healing the sick) and its marginal and extracurricular practices (for example, Botox injections and other merely cosmetic surgical procedures). Because medicine has, at least traditionally, pursued therapy rather than enhancement, the distinction helps to delimit the proper activities of physicians, understood as healers. And because physicians have been given a more-or-less complete monopoly over the prescription and administration of biotechnology to human beings, the distinction, by seeking to circumscribe the proper goals of medicine, indirectly tries to circumscribe also the legitimate uses of biomedical technology. Accordingly, it also helps us decide about health care costs: health providers and insurance companies have for now bought into the distinction, paying for treatment of disease, but not for enhancements. More fundamentally, the idea of enhancement understood as seeking something "better than well" points to the perfectionist, not to say utopian, aspiration of those who would set out to improve upon human nature in general or their own particular share of it.

But although the distinction between therapy and enhancement is a fitting beginning and useful shorthand for calling attention to the problem (and although we shall from time to time make use of it ourselves), it is finally inadequate to the moral analysis. "Enhancement" is, even as a term, highly problematic. In its most ordinary meaning, it is abstract and imprecise.[5] Moreover, "therapy" and "enhancement" are overlapping

categories: all successful therapies are enhancing, even if not all enhancements enhance by being therapeutic. Even if we take "enhancement" to mean "nontherapeutic enhancement," the term is still ambiguous. When referring to a human function, does enhancing mean making more of it, or making it better? Does it refer to bringing something out more fully, or to altering it qualitatively? In what meaning of the term are both improved memory and selective erasure of memory "enhancements"?

Beyond these largely verbal and conceptual ambiguities, there are difficulties owing to the fact that both "enhancement" and "therapy" are bound up with, and absolutely dependent on, the inherently complicated idea of health and the always-controversial idea of normality. The differences between healthy and sick, fit and unfit, are experientially evident to most people, at least regarding themselves, and so are the differences between sickness and other troubles. When we are bothered by cough and high fever, we suspect that we are sick, and we think of consulting a physician, not a clergyman. By contrast, we think neither of sickness nor of doctors when we are bothered by money problems or worried about the threat of terrorist attacks. But there are notorious difficulties in trying to define "healthy" and "impaired," "normal" and "abnormal" (and hence, "supernormal"), especially in the area of "behavioral" or "psychic" functions and activities. Some psychiatric diagnoses—for example, "dysthymia," "oppositional disorder," or "social anxiety disorder"—are rather vague: what is the difference between extreme shyness and social anxiety? And, on the positive side, mental health shades over into peace of mind, which shades over into contentment, which shades over into happiness. If one follows the famous World Health Organization definition of health as "a state of complete physical, mental and social well-being," almost any intervention aimed at enhancement may be seen as health-promoting, and hence "therapeutic," if it serves to promote

---

5   According to the *Oxford English Dictionary*, "to enhance," means "to raise in degree, heighten, intensify"; "to make to appear greater"; "to raise in price, value, importance, attractiveness, etc." An "enhancement" would designate a quantitative change, an increase in magnitude or degree.

the enhanced individual's mental well-being by making him happier.

Yet even for those using a narrower definition of health, the distinction between therapy and enhancement will prove problematic. While in some cases—for instance, a chronic disease or a serious injury—it is fairly easy to point to a departure from the standard of health, other cases defy simple classification. Most human capacities fall along a continuum, or a "normal distribution" curve, and individuals who find themselves near the lower end of the normal distribution may be considered disadvantaged and therefore unhealthy in comparison with others. But the average may equally regard themselves as disadvantaged with regard to the above average. If one is responding in both cases to perceived disadvantage, on what principle can we call helping someone at the lower end "therapy" and helping someone who is merely average "enhancement"? In which cases of traits distributed "normally" (for example, height or IQ or cheerfulness) does the average also function as a norm, or is the norm itself appropriately subject to alteration?

Further complications arise when we consider causes of conditions that clamor for modification. Is it therapy to give growth hormone to a genetic dwarf, but not to a short fellow who is just unhappy to be short? And if the short are brought up to the average, the average, now having become short, will have precedent for a claim to growth hormone injections. Since more and more scientists believe that all traits of personality have at least a partial biological basis, how will we distinguish the biological "defect" that yields "disease" from the biological condition that yields shyness or melancholy or irascibility?

For these reasons, among others, relying on the distinction between therapy and enhancement to do the work of moral judgment will not succeed. In addition, protracted arguments about whether or not something is or is not an "enhancement" can often get in the way of the proper ethical questions: What are the good and

bad uses of biotechnical power? What makes a use "good," or even just "acceptable"? It does not follow from the fact that a drug is being taken solely to satisfy one's desires—for example, to increase concentration or sexual performance— that its use is objectionable. Conversely, certain interventions to restore functioning wholeness—for example, to enable postmenopausal women to bear children or sixty-year-old men to keep playing professional ice hockey—might well be dubious uses of biotechnical power. The human meaning and moral assessment must be tackled directly; they are unlikely to be settled by the term "enhancement," any more than they are by the nature of the technological intervention itself.

VI. Beyond Natural Limits: Dreams of Perfection and Happiness

Reliance on the therapy-versus-enhancement distinction has one advantage in theory that turns out also to be a further disadvantage in practice. The distinction rests on the assumption that there is a natural human "whole" whose healthy functioning is the goal of therapeutic medicine. It sees medicine, in fact, as thoroughly informed by this idea of health and wholeness, taken as the end of the entire medical art. Medical practice, for the most part and up to the present time, appears to embody this self-understanding of its mission. Yet this observation points to the deepest reason why the distinction between healing and enhancing is, finally, of insufficient ethical, and even less practical, value. For the human being whose wholeness or healing is sought or accomplished by biomedical therapy is finite and frail, medicine or no medicine.

The healthy body declines and its parts wear out. The sound mind slows down and has trouble remembering things. The soul has aspirations beyond what even a healthy body can realize, and it becomes weary from frustration. Even at its fittest, the fatigable and limited human body rarely carries out flawlessly even the ordinary desires of the soul. For this reason (among others), the desires of many human beings—for more, for better, for the unlimited, or even for the merely different—will not be satisfied with the average, nor will they take their bearings from the distinction between normal and abnormal, or even between the healthy and the better-than-healthy.

Joining aspirations to overcome common human limitations are comparable aspirations to overcome individual shortfalls in native endowment. For there is wide variation in the natural gifts with which each of us is endowed: some are born with perfect pitch, others are born tone-deaf; some have flypaper memories, others forget immediately what they have just learned. And as with talents, so too with desires and temperaments: some crave immortal fame, others merely comfortable preservation. Some are sanguine, others phlegmatic, still others bilious or melancholic. When nature dispenses her gifts, some receive only at the end of the line. Yet, one should remember that it is often the most gifted and ambitious who most resent their human limitations: Achilles was willing to destroy everything around him, so little could he stomach that he was but a heel short of immortality.

As a result of these infirmities, particular and universal, human beings have long dreamed of overcoming limitations of body and soul, in particular the limitations of bodily decay, psychic distress, and the frustration of human aspiration. Dreams of human perfection—and the terrible consequences of pursuing it at all costs—are the themes of Greek tragedy, as well as of "The Birth- mark," the Hawthorne short story with which the President's Council on Bioethics began its work. Until now these dreams have been pure fantasies, and those who pursued them came crashing down in disaster. But the stupendous successes over the past century in all areas of technology, and especially in medicine, have revived the ancient dreams of human perfection. Like Achilles, many of the major beneficiaries of modern medicine seem, by and large, neither grateful nor satisfied with the bounties we have received from existing biomedical technologies. We seem, in fact, less content than we are "worried well," perhaps more aware of hidden ills we might be heir to, or more worried about losing the health we have than we are pleased to have it. Curiously, we may even be more afraid of death than our forebears, who lived before modern medicine began successfully to do battle with it. Unconsciously, but clearly as a result of what we have been given, our desires grow fat for still further gifts. And we regard our remaining limitations with less equanimity, to the point that dreams of getting rid of them can be turned into moral imperatives.[6] For these reasons, thanks to biomedical technology, people will be increasingly tempted to try to realize these dreams, at least to some extent: ageless and ever-vigorous bodies, happy (or at least not unhappy) souls, excellent human achievement (with diminished effort or toil), and better endowed and more accomplished children. These dreams have at bottom nothing to do with medicine, other than the fact that it is doctors who will wield the tools that may get them realized. They are, therefore, only accidentally dreams "beyond therapy." They are dreams, in principle and in the limit, of human perfection.

Not everyone interested in the beyond-therapy uses of biotechnology will dream of

---

6 Consider in this connection our attitudes toward organ transplantation. When first introduced into clinical practice some fifty years ago, receiving a life-saving kidney transplant was regarded as a gift, a blessing, a minor miracle, something beyond anything merited or even expected. Today, though the number of such "miracles" increases annually, supply does not equal demand. Expectations have risen to such an extent that people speak and act as if society's failure to meet the need is in fact the cause of death for those who die before they can be transplanted. Who in 1950 could have thought that he was entitled to have his defective and diseased organs replaced? Will people in 2050 think that they are entitled to have any and all their weakened parts replaced, and not just once?

human perfection. Many people are more or less satisfied, at least for now, with their native human capacities, though they might willingly accept assistance that would make them prettier, stronger, or smarter. The pursuit of happiness and self-esteem—the satisfaction of one's personal desires and recognition of one's personal worth—are much more common human aspirations than the self-conscious quest for perfection. Indeed, the desire for happiness and the love of excellence are, at first glance, independent aspirations. Although happiness is arguably fuller and deeper when rooted in excellent activity, the pursuit of happiness is often undertaken without any regard for excellence or virtue. Many people crave only some extra boost on the path to success; many people seek only to feel better about themselves. Although less radical than the quest for "perfection," the quests for happiness, success, and self-esteem, especially in our society, may prove to be more powerful motives for an interest in using biotechnical power for purposes that lie "beyond therapy." Thus, though some visionaries—beginning with Descartes—may dream of using biotechnologies to perfect human nature, and though many of us might welcome biotechnical assistance in improving our native powers of mind and body, many more people will probably turn to it in search of advancement, contentment, and self-satisfaction—for themselves and for their children.

Why should anyone be worried about these prospects? What could be wrong with efforts to improve upon or perfect human nature, to try, with the help of biomedical technology, to gain better children, higher achievements, ageless bodies, or happy souls? What are the sources of our disquiet?

The answers to these questions cannot be given in the abstract. They will depend on a case-by-case analysis, with special attention to the ends pursued and the means used to pursue them. In some cases, disquiet attaches not only to the individual pursuit of a particular goal, but also to the social consequences that would follow if many people did likewise (for example, selecting the sex of offspring, if practiced widely, could greatly alter a society's sex ratio). In other cases, disquiet attaches mainly to the individual practice itself (for example, drugs that would erase or transform one's memories). Speaking in the abstract and merely for the sake of illustration, concerns can and have been raised about the safety of the techniques used and about whether access to the benefits will be fairly distributed. Regarding the use of performance-enhancing techniques, especially in competitive activities, concerns can be raised about unfair advantage and inauthentic performance.

Questions can be raised about coercion, overt and subtle (through peer pressure), should uses of mind-improving drugs become widespread. Other worries include the misuse of society's precious medical resources, the increasing medicalization of human activities, the manipulation of desires, the possible hubris in trying to improve upon human nature, and the consequences for character of getting results "the easy way" through biotechnology, without proper effort or discipline. There is no point here in detailing these further or in indicating additional possible objections. As concerns arise in their appropriate contexts, we shall discuss them further. At the end of this report, we will offer what generalizations seem appropriate. Between now and then, we shall proceed to examine several instances of activities and uses of biotechnical power that look "beyond therapy."

Part One
Theory

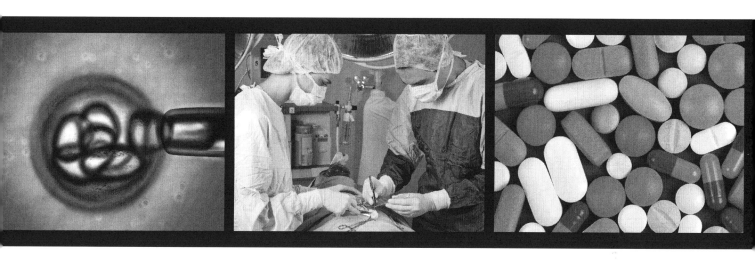

1. Origins of Bioethics

The term "bioethics" was not ushered in with Van Rensselaer Potter's 1970 paper, "Bioethics: The Science of Survival," as many bioethics experts think. In 1927, Fritz Jahr, a German protestant pastor, philosopher and educator published an editorial entitled "Bio-Ethik. Eine Umschau über die ethischen Beziehungen des Menschen zu Tier und Pflanze," ("Bio-Ethics. Reviewing the Ethical Relations of Humans towards Animals and Plants") in the leading German natural science journal *Kosmos*. The origin of the term and concept "bioethics" occurred 43 years before Potter published his famous work. This means that we should consider Potter's ideas a continuation of Jahr's seminal contribution.

Potter never cited Jahr's writings either in his papers or books, and as a result of his silence he has been unfairly considered the creator of bioethics whereas Jahr, who introduced the original idea and also coined the term "bioethics" into philosophical and scientific fields, has been onerously neglected. Between 1927 and 1938, Fritz Jahr published an overwhelming array of papers on bioethics and related topics, such as animal ethics, ecology, public health, and education among others. Unfortunately, his work did not enjoy popularity due to the German political circumstances of those days and the advent of World War II.

It is important to clarify that Jahr's concept of bioethics was far from our current understanding of it, especially procedurally. However, due to his relevant approaches to human-animal-nature relationships, social and sexual ethics, freedom of thought, education, moral law, the duty of self-preservation, and especially because of his bio-ethical Imperative (*bio-ethische Imperativ*), Jahr deserves to be considered the "Father of bioethics." I will try to pay the debt we owe Jahr by showing how valid his ideas still are and stressing his main contributions to contemporary bioethics.

Jahr characterizes bioethics as a fundamental attitude; namely, as an *êthos*, or a way of living. In this sense, bioethics should be developed as part of human character, the affective disposition Aristotle described in *Nicomachean Ethics* when he addressed the concept of *héxis* or *habitude* as Scholastics translated it centuries later. This is important: if Jahr understood bioethics as both a moral principle and a virtue, bioethics should be a theoretically and empirically distinct discipline. Jahr's bioethics has its own identity; it is an independent field of knowledge with unique epistemological and procedural features.

Jahr also redefines traditional moral obligations by extending their scope to all extra-human nature. Thus, human beings' responsibility for their actions leaves the classical anthropocentrism of all previous ethics. This implies a radical reconfiguration of traditional ethical criteria. This premonitory character of Jahr's thought paved the way for the emergence of relevant ideas developed later, such as Jonas's imperative of responsibility and the animal ethics articulated by Singer and Regan, among others. In this regard Jahr implicitly defines bioethics as a secular and pluralistic discipline. In other words, Jahr's bioethics identifies two important features of contemporary bioethical thought. According to Jahr, bioethics requires a new type of moral deliberation to address new moral problems introduced by scientific and technological progress. Also, he understands bioethics as a new normative field to regulate the use of technoscientific advances through public and democratic participation.

Jahr, too, characterizes bioethics as not simply requiring a new deliberative ethical framework but a new set of moral imperatives. Jahr envisioned a global bioethics whose main goal would be to generate the necessary and sufficient conditions for humans to respect all type of life. In order to perform this purpose, Jahr formulates his bioethical imperative: "Respect every living being in principle as an end in itself and treat it, if possible, as such!"

This formulation implies a theoretical and practical extension of Kantian categorical imperative "Act only according to that maxim whereby you can at the same time will that it should become a universal law." Jahr's imperative does not only consider rational beings as subjects or rights but also animals and plants. Thus, the criteria for entities to be respected and considered as an end in themselves is not rationality but life.

At the same time, Jahr borrowed some foundations for his new imperative from the Fifth Commandment "Thou shall not kill." This means that, from a bioethical perspective, to harm any kind of life is not morally allowed.

Also, Jahr added another argument to his imperative: human beings have the right to live but we also have an obligation to live; that is, we must observe an essential duty of self-preservation. Thus, we must care for ourselves by taking responsibility for our actions not only towards others but also towards ourselves. This idea deserves special attention since it stresses the importance of not hurting or harming oneself over seeking pleasure. Therefore, the main idea that underlies this paragraph is nonmaleficence: first and foremost, not doing harm.

Hans-Martin Sass has identified ten features of Jahr's bioethical imperative, considering it as a new: (1) discipline (the bioethical imperative "needs to develop, to educate and to steward personal and collective cultural and moral attitudes and calls for new respect and responsibilities towards all forms of life"); (2) basic virtue ethics ("the bioethical imperative is based on historical and other evidence that 'compassion is an empirical established phenomenon of the human soul'"); (3) Golden Rule principle (as the bioethical imperative implies and stresses moral obligations among human beings and is based on compassion and love, it "cannot allow itself the Kantian luxury of just being formal"); (4) personal health care rule and ethics ("the bioethical imperative includes obligations towards one's own body and soul as a living being"); (5) public health care rule and ethics ("... fulfilling obligations towards oneself is also a duty towards others and towards public health"); (6) global stewardship rule and ethics ("Jahr broadens the 5th commandment into a universal rule and ethics of positively and proactively caring for the health and life of this globe as a part of a living cosmos"); (7) management rule and corporate ethics (the Jahr's "bioethical model of interacting forms of life in a living environment [...] would include social institutions such as those for health care"); (8) terminology rule and terminological ethics ("a clear and precise terminology [...] is a priority and a precondition for clear conceptual and practical work, for communication and for cooperation and for further development"); (9) rule and ethics of differentiation (there must be 'different terms available for different subjects, fields, and issues" since "unclear terminology leads to unclear reasoning and acting; it is an expression of unclear thinking itself"); (10) interaction and integration rule and ethics ("according to Jahr, "animal ethics and social ethics are different fields, but they interact and integrate, bringing different shapes and shades of the Bioethical Imperative"). Finally, and as part of feature (10), Sass affirms that "a new field of geo-ethics is already visible" in Jarhr's bioethical imperative, since his ethics implies not only a personal commitment but also a global responsibility in order to enable "a universal, prudent and reasonable application of the Bioethical Imperative."

The scope of Jahr's ideas is certainly immense and represents the starting point of a new applied ethics concerned with life, health and environment, centered on the idea that both scientific and technological development require new ethics, new moral deliberation, new rules and procedures, and new and clear terminology to address new moral controversies with a higher degree of precision and objectivity.

Beyond Sass's excellent analysis, I think that Jahr's bioethical imperative also implies:

1. The first modern formulation of the non-maleficence principle. Jahr's imperative implies a duty of self-preservation and of not harming others under any circumstance. Jahr starts from an analysis of the Fifth Commandment, dealing with philosophical and religious tradition and elaborating a hermeneutic "of classical old texts of various traditions and cultures" as the foundation of his ideas.
2. An ethics characterized by *phronesis* (practical wisdom) as an intellectual virtue learned through education and integration of cultural and moral attitudes to develop person's character, attitudes and dispositions. Jahr's proposal is stresses a diverse and original rationality with tangible implications. Jahr believes his bioethics can address the new procedural moral challenges presented by advances in science and technology. Jahr realizes the Enlightenment's failure to create a scientific ethics. Neither Kant, with his Categorical Imperative, nor Spinoza, with his geometric ethics, were able to consolidate an ethics like physics or mathematics. However, Jahr knew that to sacrifice rationality is a luxury that ethics cannot afford, and to ignore consequences is equally erroneous. According to Jahr, ethics needs a practical rationality or practical wisdom which considers the consequences of human action as a criterion of moral deliberation. This emphasizes the disciplinary character of Jahr's bioethics.

3. A new ethics that considers both ends and duties as criteria of moral deliberation. We have a duty: to respect all living beings as an end in themselves and treat them as such; but how we carry out this duty is more complex. Thus, Jarh's bioethics represents a combination deontology and teleology because it both outlines duties but also implies the evaluation of consequences. Thereby he does not imply either a tyranny of immovable principles or an abuse of casuistry in moral deliberation.
4. The concept of responsibility as a criterion of deliberation for any ethics. According to Jahr, bioethics is a moral attitude that implies respect and responsibilities towards all living entities. Jahr thinks that it is no longer possible to understand existence if people ignore the possible and unpredictable consequences of human action modified by new science and technology. Thus, Jahr is introducing the concept of responsibility in the ethical discussion long before Hans Jonas did. Also, Jahr is presciently advising us scientific progress, especially in experimental physiology and psychology, and the

need to ethically regulate its power in order to avoid a human tyranny over other living entities:

5. A sympathetic model of ethics which entails a moral and social obligation not only towards other humans but also animals and plants. Humans must extend their moral concerns to the realm of extra-human creatures because all living beings are in constant and reciprocal interaction. Also, human responsibility for animals and plants demonstrates the virtues of respect for life, benevolence, justice and compassion, among others. This point certainly reinforces Jahr's figure as a pioneer of bioethics but also as a precursor of animal and environmental ethics. His imperative also entails an extension of Kantian moral duty by transcending the anthropocentric frontiers of traditional ethics since, according to Jahr, every living entity on the earth is worthy of respect and moral consideration.

6. To recognize all living beings as worthy of respect. Jahr is tacitly talking about extending the human right of dignity to animals and plants. However, I must emphasize that this extension is not absolute. Jahr is not urging us to treat animals and plants as humans. Instead, he thinks that we should respect any kind of life in accordance with its ontological nature. This may be considered as a seminal argument for the concept of *sentience* which Peter Singer addresses in his 1975 book *Animal Liberation*.

7. A public ethics since Jahr not only emphasizes the binding character of nonmaleficence but also its wide scope. The global content of Jahr's bioethics as well as its civic and public character is clear. We are in the presence of a dialogical ethics in which moral truth is not the privilege of an individual consciousness but that of an argumentative community whose decisions might affect the whole of society. This systemic feature of Jahr's bioethics was absolutely visionary regarding the current discipline, and it would be very helpful and useful for its subsequent development if bioethics scholars seriously considered the originality and depth of Jahr's work.

The historical neglect of Jahr's bioethics has been as unfair as it has been unjustifiable. It is practically impossible to find references to Jahr in bioethical literature, even in books authored by bioethicists of recognized prestige and reputation, and it is also difficult to understand why authors of influential books on the history and origins of bioethics completely ignored its real founder.

Jahr's bioethics is not the same as that which we know today. However, his ideas represent the first bioethical guidelines and principals. Indeed, Jahr tacitly includes in his conception of bioethics important principles of autonomy, social justice and nonmaleficence. Therefore, Jahr, beyond being the creator of the term and concept "bioethics," laid the intellectual and theoretical foundations of the discipline. For all these reasons, and due to his brilliant, advanced and precursory thoughts, Jahr deserves a prominent place in the history of bioethics. We should consider that, at least, a moral obligation.

Readings

Jahr, Fritz, "Bio-Ethics: Reviewing the Ethical Relations of Humans Towards Animals and Plants," in Muzur, Amir; Sass, Hans-Martin (Eds.), *Fritz Jahr and the Foundations of Global Bioethics. The Future of Integrative Bioethics*, Germany, LIT Verlag, 2012: **1–5**.

Jahr, Fritz, "Animal Protection and Ethics," in Muzur, Amir; Sass, Hans-Martin (Eds.), *Fritz Jahr and the Foundations of Global Bioethics. The Future of Integrative Bioethics*, Germany, LIT Verlag, 2012: **9–12**.

Jahr, Fritz, "Three Studies on the Fifth Commandment," in Muzur, Amir; Sass, Hans-Martin (Eds.), *Fritz Jahr and the Foundations of Global Bioethics. The Future of Integrative Bioethics*, Germany, LIT Verlag, 2012: **31–35**.

Study Questions

1. Why could we define Jahr's bioethics as an ethics of life?
2. How does Jahr redefine traditional moral obligations?
3. What are the main epistemological and methodological implications of Jahr's bio-ethical imperative?
4. What is the relationship between Jahr's bioethics and practical wisdom?

Bio-Ethics: Reviewing the Ethical Relations of Humans Towards Animals and Plants

Fritz Jahr

The strict distinction between animal and human being [Mensch], dominant in our European culture until the end of the 18th century, cannot be supported anymore. Up to the French Revolution, the heart of the European human being was struggling for a unity of religious, philosophical, and scientific knowledge; but such a unity had to be abandoned under the pressure of more information.

It will always be the credit of modern natural sciences to finally render an unbiased study of the world [Weltgeschehen]. We would not be seekers of truth today, if we would have given up the results of animal experimentation, blood research etc.. On the other hand, we cannot deny that precisely these scientific triumphs of the human spirit have infringed upon the dominant position of the human being in the world in general. Philosophy, formerly prescribing leading ideals for the natural sciences, now has to build her systems on the basis of specific knowledge from the natural sciences,—and it was only a poetic-philosophical [dichterphilosophische] interpretation of Darwin's insight, when Nietzsche considered humans to be a somewhat inferior stage towards a higher stage in evolution, as a 'rope extended between animal and superman [Übermensch].

What resulted from this revolution? First, the fundamental equalization of human being and animal as an object in psychology. Today, it [psychology] does not restrict itself to human beings, but applies the same methods to animals as well; and, as documented by comparative anatomical-zoological research, quite instructive comparisons between human soul and animal soul have been done. Yes, even beginnings of plant psychology are visible,—the most prominent representatives are G. Th. Fechner in the past, R. H. France, Ad. Wagner and the Indian Bose at present, so that modern research in psychology covers all living beings in research. Given these circumstances, it is only logical when R. Eisler speaks of Bio-Psychik (science of the soul of all that lives).

From Bio-Psychik it is only a step to Bio-Ethics, i.e. the assumption of moral obligations not only towards humans, but towards all forms of life. In reality, bio-ethics is not just a discovery of modern times. An especially attractive example from the past is the figure of St. Francis of Assisi (1182-1226) with his great love towards animals, his warm sympathy for all forms of life, centuries before Rousseau's romanticism for the entire nature.

When the unity of the European weltanschauung broke down at the end of the Baroque period, European intellectual life for the first time was able to receive foreign worlds of thought [Gedankenwelten] without prejudice. Already Herder's comprehensive spirit—probably the most sensitive in those days for things to come—expected of humans, based on the image of an all encompassing deity, that they project themselves into each and every creature and sense with it the way it needs. Such a reasoning already reminds us of the Indian philosophy, which by the way of England just had been discovered. But only during the time of Romanticism has India really influenced European intellectual life, and especially in Germany, its most important province. The teaching of reincarnation, as developed in India, has influenced the reasoning of Indian schools of philosophy, especially the school of Sankya. An offspring of this school is the yoga teaching, drawing the most rigorous consequences from those thought processes. The yoga repentant [Jogabüßer] under no circumstances is allowed to live at the cost of co-creatures; above all, he shall under no circumstances kill any animal, and only under certain settings enjoy vegetable foods. He has to wear a veil over his mouth in order not to inhale even a small living being; for the same reason he has to filter drinking water and shall not take a bath. The passion to not harm a living being in the process of self-preservation even leads some Indian repentant to eat horse manure. If in this context Buddha is mentioned, one has to stress that especially this religious leader refused such fanatic self-harm of the school of yoga. Buddha forbade, that food be based on animal products, but fully allows vegetable based foods. How much Buddha himself and his teachings totally believed in re-incarnation of the soul, is very well demonstrated for us Europeans by the collection of Buddhist stories collected by Jatakas, stories ascribed to Buddha and narrating about his early life. He claims that he has lived as a human being before, but also remembers his former lives as an elephant, a gazelle, a crab etc.. Even more beautiful than in Francis of Assisi, these

narratives express the thought, that a human being in essence is related to all creatures.

Such sequences of reasoning caused similar thoughts in European intellectual life, even if not in such a strict version. Theologian Schleiermacher (1768-1834) declared it to be immoral to destroy life and formation [Leben und Gestaltung], as they are, if there is no reasonable cause to do so. Similarly, the philosopher Krause, a contemporary of Schleiermacher, requests to respect each and every living being and not to destroy it without reason. Because, they all, plants and animals, also humans, have similar rights, but not Equal Right, depending on the requirements for reaching their specific destiny. The philosopher Schopenhauer, who claimed as special importance of his ethics as based primarily on the sentiment of compassion, required towards animals as well, openly referred to the Indian intellectual world [Gedankenwelt]. Via Richard Wagner, who was strongly influenced by Schopenhauer and a compassionate animal lover and friend of animal protection, those thoughts have become a common value for a broadest group of people.

Thus, in regard to animals such a rule has become evident, at least as far as needless torture is concerned. With plants it is different, so. For some, it seems at first unreasonable to have certain ethical obligations towards plants. But already [Apostle] Paul directed our compassion towards animals and plants. Comparable are the illuminated sentimental [verklärt stimungsvollen] interpretations in Richard Wagner's 3rd act of 'Parsifal'. In pious devotion, humans at least on Good Friday avoid hurting stalks and flowers in the fields by walking more carefully. But also in the thoughts of plant ethics by a sober philosopher such as Eduard von Hartmann, who passed away 20 years ago, we find similar thoughts. In an article on flower-luxury he describes a cut flower: 'She is an organism deadly hurt, but only her colors not yet destroyed, a head still there, but separated from the torso.— Whenever I see a rose in a glass of water or tied into a bouquet, I cannot fight the unpleasant thought that a human being has murdered a flower life for the sole purpose to enjoy his/her eyes while dying, heartless enough eyes, not to sense an unnatural death under the appearance of life.'

A majority of people naturally is not as sensitive as Ed. von Hartmann. However, everyone knows quite well, that plants are living beings, and that cutting flowers hurts them; but the thought that the flower might sense it, is far away. The concept of a plant-soul so far has not taken hold in us. Additional, we know that flowers also die and dry out, while they are on the plant, and therefore one does not take issue with cutting flowers, in particular when they were cultivated for that specific purpose.

Thus, we start from a totally different point of view than the Indian fanatics, who do not want to hurt any living entity. Also, our regulations by law and police protect specific plants and flowers in certain areas (such as plants in the Alps) are based on totally different assumptions. The police state [Polizeistaat] intends to protect those plants from becoming extinct in those areas, also to be enjoyed by other people in the future. Whenever there are plants abundant, the state does not intervene to protect them as an end in themselves.

Also, our concept of animal protection rests on a decidedly different foundation than the attitude of the Indians. When we read in the novel 'Holy Hate' [Der heilige Hass] by Richard Voss, that a Rodyia-boy, i.e. a member of a despised caste, does even not want to kill a snake, because 'also the snakes are our brothers and sisters', we do not accept such a reasoning; we actually hold it to be our duty to kill harmful animals, if we can. We have our farm animals been killed by the butcher and the harmless prey by the hunter, because we want to eat meat, which in our areas some do not want to do without, while in tropical countries vegetarian food is abundantly available. Our animal protection, thus, has a utilitarian aspect, which is daringly disregarded by the Indians, while we content ourselves with avoidance of unnecessary suffering. Unfortunately, legal regulations against prevention or punishment of those cruelties are not strong enough in all civilized countries [Kulturländern] yet. But, we are on the road of progress and animal protection get more and more support in wider circles, such as no decent human being [anständiger Mensch] will without criticism accept, that a thoughtless lout [Flegel] without any afterthought beheads flowers with a stick while on the hike or that children break flowers only to through them away after a few steps. Our self-education, in this regard, already has made considerable progress, but we have to go further, so that the guiding rule for our actions may be the bio-ethical demand: '*Respect every living being on principle as an end in itself and treat it, if possible, as such!* '

Bio-Ethics, 1927. Bio-Ethik. Eine Umschau über die ethischen Beziehungen des Menschen zu Tier und Pflanze. *Kosmos. Handweiser für Naturfreunde* 1927, 24(1): **2–4.**

Animal Protection and Ethics

Fritz Jahr

Compassion with animals shows up as an empirically given phenomenon of the human soul. This fact has been voiced, among others, by the poet and philosopher Herder in his 'Ideas in History of Humankind' [Ideen zur Geschichte der Menschheit]. The fact, that this phenomenon is more or less present in a normal human soul, is also assumed by the German Penal Code when expressing in paragraph 360(13) that cruelty to animals is a public offense. Exceptions, which of course are there, cannot change the truth of such a psychological observation, similarly as the existence of blind people can be used to argue that the capability of seeing is not an essential part of humans. Such compassion now is the central motive of the idea of animal protection [Tierschutz]. Thus, it does not calculate whether or not one has any benefit from it; e.g. Richard Wagner in an open letter to Ernst von Weber, under the influence of Schopenhauer's 'On the Foundation of Morality' [über das Fundament der Moral], argues: 'Everyone, who reacts indignant when witnessing the suffering of an animal, is motivated solely by compassion, and who works together with others in protecting animals does so similarly only out of compassion, naturally not of calculations of utility by an otherwise unconcerned and determined compassion.'

And if someone does not accept the unconditional nature of Animal Ethics (as one may call it, following Brenzinger, who was the first to publish a scientific Animal Ethics [Tierethik] from an ethical-legal position), one nevertheless may not suppress the question of the relationship between animal protection and ethics, respectively seek to answer such a question. In other words: what are the consequences in our relationships towards our fellow humans when we extend our moral obligations beyond humans towards animals? Don't we have to fear, that we will turn away our awareness from the misery of the latter towards the first? The philosopher Eduard von Hartmann, who, by the way, is not hostile against animals, voices those concerns in his article 'Our Relationship towards Animals' [Unsere Stellung zu den Tieren]. He gives the example of a 'dry old maid', feeding meats and sweets to her pug while letting her employees go hungry. He also finds love towards animal among embittered misanthropes, cold and cruel judges of heretics and bloodthirsty heroes of revolutions. While there are indeed those cases, Hartmann's arguments only target *false* animal love. This kind of false love also may be used towards humans. It is expressed in disgusting pampering, in unjustifiable preferences, in cronyism [Vetternwirtschaft], and unfortunately widely spread otherwise. But if such false love of people is no good argument against ethics, so is occasionally occurring false love of animals no demonstration against the justification of animal protection.

This is the issue: If we have a compassionate heart towards animals, then we will not withhold our compassion and help towards suffering humans. If someone's love is great enough to go beyond the borders of human-only and sees the sanctity even in the most miserable creature, he or she will find this sanctity as well in the most poor and lowest fellow human, will hold it high and will not reduce it to class of society, interest group, one party or what else may be considered. On the other hand, senseless cruelty towards animals is an indication of an unrefined character becoming dangerous towards the human environment as well. Among other thinkers, philosopher Kant expressively has hinted at this fact of highest importance for social ethics, when in 'Metaphysische Anfangsgründe der Tugendlehre' he calls the careful and compassionate treatment of animals a human obligation towards oneself. The word from Count Leo Tolstoi: 'From killing animals to killing humans, it is only one step' might be overly strong; but his position expresses Kant's concept and understanding. This is also the case for R. von Hippel, a jurist, who has collected and organized most of the relevant historical and statistical materials.

But effective and successful animal protection is only possible, when enough knowledge and at least some understanding of nature are present. The reason is, that we only can protect animals in reality, when we are somewhat knowledgeable about their physiological and psychological properties and life conditions. Therefore one of the main goals of the animal protection movement is the promotion of such a kind of knowledge and a better understanding of nature,—awakening, broadening, and deepening it. Such an interest in nature will by itself not limit itself to animals, but on the other side also towards plants and (what is most important in this content) towards humans as well.

If such a goal will only be reached in part, then we can, for sure, expect a positive influence on humans and their way of life, i.e. in the attitude of a normal and healthy naturalness, which has nothing to do with a limitless life of over-excited, unhealthy, and thereby unnatural urges, which quite often wrongly are considered to be natural. The fact that the promotion of knowledge and understanding of nature and of a true love for nature will also have a positive effect on sexual ethics does not need to be demonstrated additionally.

If, indeed, it is true that a correctly understood and executed animal protection works positively on ethics, then it is also true that it has a value in public education and public knowledge; and this may not be underrated at all. On the other hand, everyone, who is active in animal protection, will support as much as possible general ethical activities, which, as already mentioned, cannot ignore or be silent about animal ethics, because this is also indirectly supportive of animal protection.

The fact of a close interrelationship between animal protection and ethics finally is based on the reality that we not only have moral obligations to fellow humans, but also to animals, even to plants—in short: to all forms of life—, so that we can speak about 'Bio-Ethics'.

As such, Bio-Ethics is not just an idea of modern times.—Already Montaigne, a skeptic, was the first Frenchman—so far being the first representative of a modern ethos of sentiment—who dared to reason, that all living beings have entitlement of being treated based on ethical principles: we owe justice towards humans, mildness and compassion towards all other creatures who will have a benefit from it. So he wrote in his 'Essays' in 1588.—Precisely in the same sense, Herder expects from humans to follow the example of a God, who transfigures with sentiment every living entity and is empathetic with it as much as it can feel and need. He expressively includes plants in this.—Highlights are reached by the theologian Schleiermacher and philosopher K. Chr. F. Krause. The first one, in his 'Philosophische

Ethik', declares it to be immoral to destroy life and forms of life, wherever they are, i.e. including animals and plants, without a reasonable cause associated with such an act. The latter, a contemporary of Schleiermacher, requests in his 'Rechtsphilosophie' that every living being be treasured as such and not be destroyed without reason: because they all, plants and animals, also humans, are of equal standing [gleichberechtigt]. But they are not identical, and each only in a way which is a necessary requirement to reach its destination. So we read in Krause's 'Abriss der Philosophie des Rechts'.—A note in the diary of the poet Hebbel reminds us of the intuition of Herder, according to which not only humans, but everything living and moving [was lebt und webt] sees an inscrutable divine light, which one can access only via love.

It must be mentioned in this context that one has tried and still is trying—the longer the more—to support the bioethical thought by biological and biopsychological arguments, and not without success.

At first hand, it might appear utopian to realize such moral obligations towards all living entities. But we may not overlook that such moral obligations towards a living entity in practice are determined by its 'needs' [Bedürfnisse] (Herder), respectively its 'destiny' [Bestimmung] (Krause). So, the needs of animals seem to be lower in quantity and less complicated in content than those of humans. This is even more true for plants, so that practical moral obligations, which are already there towards animals (if not basically, but practically), create less difficulties. Additionally we have to take into account the principle of struggle for life and existence, a principle which in some way also modifies our obligations towards fellow humans, even if we might feel unhappy about it. Our entire life and activity

in politics, in business, in administration, in the laboratory, in the workshop, in the fields is—as Naumann has underlined—in its reasoning and goals not focusing on love in the first place, quite often rather focused on struggle with some sort of fellow competitors. Quite often we don't recognize it, as long as such a struggle is without hate and in an open and legally accepted way. As much as we cannot avoid the struggle with fellow humans, similarly the struggle for survival [Kampf ums Dasein] with other living entities is unavoidable. Nevertheless, neither in the first nor in the second case, we will lose the idea of moral obligations as a principle. The paragraphs of animal protection laws in the penal codes of civilized countries and the activities of animal protection societies give testimony, in which ways animal protection becomes practical. In the field of plant ethics, our intuition will hinder us from killing plants right and left with a cane during a stroll, or from picking flowers only in order to throw them away after a short while, or when we detest the blind acts of destruction by raffian lads breaking the crowns of young trees along the road or in the woods.

From all this follows as guidance for our moral acts the *bio-ethical Imperative: Respect every living being, including animals, as an end in itself, and treat it, if possible, as such!* And if someone does not accept the validity of this principle, as far as it is concerned with animals and plants, then, in repeating what already was said, one nevertheless should follow it in recognition of the moral obligation toward human society in general.

Animal Protection and Ethics, 1928. Tierschutz und Ethik in ihren Beziehungen zueinander. *Ethik. Sexual- und Gesellschaftsethik. Organ des .Ethikbundes'* 1928, 4(6/7): **100–102.**

Three Studies on the Fifth Commandment

Fritz Jahr

How do we do good?—The so called 'Golden Rule' gives answer to this question: Whatever you want the people do to you, the same do to them (Matthews 7:12; Luke 6:31). Kant's 'Categorical Imperative': Act only according to the maxim whereby you can, at the same time, will that it should become a universal law,—this basically means the same.—But are these and similar formulations not only just a formal criterion for 'good' action. The motive, disregarding such a criterion, could just be blatant egoism, a so called contract on reciprocity: Do nothing to me, so that, in return, I will do nothing to you (Schopenhauer hints at this in his 'Grundlage der Moral').

If we are aware that love is the fulfillment of the moral law (Romans 18:10), we indeed are already one step ahead: We know the motive. But we do not yet know the concrete content of the moral law; we don't know what to do or not to do specifically. Here, Schopenhauer, serves as a helping hand: He says that the best, the most concrete specification of the moral act is the sentence: Neminem laede, imo omnes, quantum potes juva! (Don't hurt anyone, but help everyone, as far as you possibly can!)

More than two millennia before Schopenhauer, the 5th commandment already provides such an insight, and, in fact, in a broader perspective than benefit or harm, namely under the perspective of sanctity of life and life's manifestations. Therefore the command: 'You shall not kill!'. We know from Jesus, that the 5th commandment does not only prohibit killing, but prohibits all wrong deeds against others, even the bad word, even the bad thought. This means: He not only forbids the malicious or careless destruction of life, but also everything that, in one way or another, may hamper or trouble life. Luther in his Catechism has made it clear, that the 5th Commandment has to be understood not only in a negative, but as well in a positive way.— Consequently, the 5th commandment is a very good expression of what it means to be morally and practically good.

The Duty of Self-Preservation

When talking about moral duties, normally we mean duties towards other people in the first place. Routinely we do not consider that each person has moral duties towards oneself as well, and that those duties are of immense importance. Christian religion expressively mentions those moral duties of everyone towards oneself. That basically applies to the 5th commandment as well: 'You shall not kill'. In this sense—'You shall not harm or hurt anyone's body or life, rather help and support him/her in all distresses of body and life, wherever you can'[1]—in the first place, meaning the life of our 'neighbor'. In a later consequence, however, it means: in a Christian perspective every human life as such is morally 'sacred'—including one's own life. Preservation of life—and one's own life not excluded—is a duty. And destruction and harm—again, including one's own life—is a moral sin. 'Don't you know, that you are God's temple and that God's spirit dwells in you? You shall keep God's temple sacred and not destroy it.' (following 1. Corinthian 3:16-17)

How should these moral duties, expressed in the 5th commandment towards one's own life, be applied in real life's practice? By not taking one's own life, not shortening it, not harming or endangering it, not weakening one's health by unchastity, excesses in eating and drinking, heavy anger, frivolous foolhardiness and daredevilry, etc.. Particularly important is the protection of sexual virtue and the avoidance of abuse of alcoholic drinks.—As far as the first one is concerned, the judgment of the New Testament is particularly clear: 'If you have loose sex, you sinfully harm your own life' (following 1. Corinthian 6:18). But not only is it a duty to oneself to abstain from fornication, but also avoid anything, which might lead to unchastity: indecent looks, unclean or double talk, dancing, dresses etc.—As far as alcoholism is concerned, the Christian attitude is based on recognizing that 'wine kills many people' (Sirach 31:30), i.e. alcohol endangers life and brings great dangers to health.

Are the duties towards one's own life in conflict with duties towards the neighbor?—That is not necessarily the case. On the contrary: Whoever fulfills the duties towards oneself, avoids many forms of harm to other people. That can be shown in regard to the already mentioned issues of sex and alcohol: Who falls into dependency and unchastity, endangers and weakens oneself physically and spiritually. Venereal diseases threaten as well. Weakness and disease cause the victim to be more and more a burden to the community, harming everyone. If one has offspring, they also are harmed, as they may inherit a weak or sick nature, causing additional burdens and harm to the community. Whoever protects his own life in this regard, he fulfills one's duty also towards the community. Similar with alcohol: Those, who are dependent on consuming alcohol, may eventually expose themselves to severest physical and spiritual dangers. And thus does not only harm oneself, but one's family as well, one's offspring, one's country, and one's race.[2] And again: If one protects oneself in this regard against harm, one does, at the same time, good to one's neighbor, actually to one's entire country.

The Bioethical Imperative

The 5th Commandment admonishes 'Thou shalt not kill'. Now, the term killing always means killing something which is alive. Living entities, however, are not only humans, but animals and plants as well. Because the 5th commandment does not expressively prohibits the killings of humans exclusively, should it not be applied towards animals and plants analogously? But are animals and plants so close to us, that we must recognize and treat them actually as our neighbors?—When we review publications in modern science, we find immediately similar studies of humans and animals as subjects in research, not only in physiology,

---

1 Cf. Luther's explanation of the 5th Commandment, German and Latin

2 Alcohol is 'a mean enemy of our race', cf. the brochure with this title by Wilhelm John, reviewed in no. 2 of 'Ethik'.

but also in psychology. Such equal treatment today is not reserved, as already mentioned, for humans; similar methods are applied in the field of animals, and—as there is a comparative anatomical-zootomic research—similarly very interesting comparisons are made between the human soul and animal soul.[3] Yes, even the beginnings of plant psychology are recognizable—the most well-known among them are G. Th. Fechner[4] in the past, R. H. France,[5] and Ad. Wagner[6] at present—thus modern psychology includes all living beings in its research. Given this, it is only consequent, that E. Eisler,[7] in summarizing, speaks of a Bio-Psychik.

From Bio-Psychik, it is only a small step to Bio-Ethik, i.e. to the assumption of moral duties not only towards humans, but towards all living beings. In fact, bioethics is not a discovery of today. Montaigne[8]—the only early representative of modern ethics of sentiment—already grants all living beings an entitlement of being treated based on moral principles: We owe justice to humans; mildness and mercy towards all living beings, capable of having a benefit from that. Similarly, Herder[9] requires that humans—following the model of God in their sentiments—put themselves into the place of every living being and feel with it, as much as it requires. Those lines of reasoning are continued by the theologian Schleiermacher,[10] who calls it immoral, to destroy life and formation—wherever they are, i.e. including animals and plants—without a reasonable argument for doing so. Therefore

philosopher Krause,[11] a contemporary of Schleiermacher, requests that every living being has to be valued as such and not be destroyed without reason. Because they all, plants and animals like humans, have an equal right; but not totally equal, each only as a precondition to reach its destiny. Schopenhauer[12] in particular refers to the Indian realm of reasoning, stressing compassion as the most important motive of his ethics, and requesting it also for animals. It was Richard Wagner, strongly influenced by Schopenhauer and a passionate animal friend, who made those thoughts commonly known.

As far as animals are concerned, the moral request has become obvious for a long time,[13] at least in that form, not to harm animals without purpose. With plants it is different. However, in regard to new biological and biopsychic knowledge (see above), also regarding the various thoughts mentioned above from Montaigne, Herder, Schleiermacher and Krause, moral duties towards plants become visible. For purely sentimental-poetic argumentation such recognition is nothing new. Think of Goethe, who has Faust call plants his brothers, or of Richard Wagner's Parsival: In pious devotion people, at least on Good Friday, protect weeds and flowers in the meadow by walking carefully, in order not to hurt them. More seriously we have to consider the plant-ethical reflections of a quite matter-of-fact Eduard von Hartmann.[14] In an article on flower luxury he writes about a picked blossom: 'She is a deadly wounded organism, the colors of which are not harmed yet, a still living and smiling head, separated from its stem.—When, however, I put the rose into a glass of water, I cannot help myself but fighting the thought, that man has murdered a flower life, in order to enjoy the dying process

---

3 Among recent publication in animal psychology especially recommendable are: Sommer, Tierpsychologie, Leipzig 1925.—Alverdes, Tierpsychologie, Leipzig 1925.
4 G. Th. Fechner, Nana oder das Seelenleben der Pflanze [1848; 5th ed. 1921]
5 R. H. France, Pflanzenpsychologie als Arbeitshypothese der Pflanzenphysiologie, Stuttgart 1909.
6 Ad. Wagner, Die Vernunft der Pflanze, Dresden 1928.
7 E. Eisler, Das Wirken der Seele, Stuttgart 1908.
8 Montaigne, Essays.
9 Herder, Ideen zur Geschichte der Philosophie der Menschheit.
10 Schleiermacher,   Philosophische   Sittenlehre, Kirchmann 1870.

11 K. Chr. Fr. Krause, Das System der Rechtsphilosophie, Roeder, Leipzig 1874.
12 Schopenhauer, Über das Fundament der Moral.
13 The most comprehensive book in this area still is Bregenzer, Tierethik, Bamberg 1894.
14 Psychological preconditions are discussed in W. von Schnehen, Ed. Von Hartmann und die Pflanzenpsychologie, Stuttgart 1908.

by an eye, heartless enough to not sense the unnatural death under the appearance of life.[15] The requirements of plant ethics, leading to such recognition, are quite clear.

As far as the potential realization of such moral duties to all living beings is concerned, it might seem utopian. But we may not ignore that moral obligations towards a living being related to its 'need' (Herder), respectively to its 'destiny' (Krause). It appears, that needs of animals seem much less in number, and their content less complex than those of people. This applies even more to plants, so that moral obligations to them should produce less complications than those to animals, as they are lower (if not conceptually, so nevertheless practically). Here also comes the principle of struggle for survival into play, a principle which also modifies our moral obligations towards fellow humans at no low scale. Within these limits there always will be enough possibilities for bioethical actions. Paragraphs for animal protection in penal codes of various cultivated nations[16] give guidance in this regard. Confer in particular the new German Reich Animal Law. As far as plant ethics is concerned, we are guided by our sentiment, which will hinder us to pick flowers and then throw them away carelessly shortly thereafter, or to deadhead plants with a walking stick, or when we find it disgusting to recognize the blind destructive impulse of rowdy lads in breaking the heads of small trees along the road. Also, excessive flower luxury—in learning from Ed. von Hartmann—is not morally refined and can be avoided.

In sum, the universal realm of authority of the 5th Commandment is clear and demands application to all forms of life. A transcription of the 5th Commandment results in the Bioethical Imperative: 'Respect every living being in principle as an end in itself and treat it, if possible, as such!'

Three Studies of the Fifth Commandment, 1934. Drei Studien zum 5. Gebot. *Ethik. Sexual- und Gesellschaftsethik.* 1934, 11:183–187.

---

15 Ed. Von Hartmann, Der Blumenluxus, 1885.
16 For the first time, material has been extensively collected and reviewed in R. von Hippel, Die Tierquälerei in der Strafgesetzgebung des In- und Auslandes, Berlin 1891.

2. The Revival of Bioethics

I n 1970, Van Rensselaer Potter published his article "Bioethics, The Science of Survival." In that paper, Potter proposed the name bioethics to define a new epistemological field through which human beings would be able to acquire the "knowledge of how to use knowledge." According to Potter this new wisdom might also be called a "science of survival" since one of the main goals of bioethics should be to improve the quality of life as a whole by promoting the convergence between social sciences and humanities. In this sense, Potter used to say that the term bioethics emphasized "the two most important ingredients in achieving the new wisdom [...]: biological knowledge and human values".

As Potter understood bioethics as a bridge between sciences and humanities, the task of this new discipline was broad. The large scope of bioethics essentially implied its interdisciplinarity, namely, the convergence between sciences and humanities. However, and despite Potter's conception pointed out a complementation between ethics and biology, bioethics should not be considered as a mere junction of both.

What does "a realistic understanding of biological knowledge" mean? Potter neither suggested to abandon traditional science nor to

irrationally embrace a new idea of it. He proposed to cross the boundaries between humanistic and scientific disciplines in order to get a broader vision of human problems arisen by virtue of technological development, and to achieve objective consensus "in terms of the future survival of man and improvement in the quality of life for future generations." In other words, Potter sought, through bioethics, better ways of reexamining scientific premises in order to establish adequate conditions of existence, including individual, social and environmental elements. Therefore, Potter's bioethics attempted to generate wisdom (the knowledge of how to use the knowledge) to reach social good by seeking a realistic knowledge of both human biological nature and biological world.

In 1971, Potter published his book *Bioethics: Bridge to the Future*, in which he insisted on bioethics as a new interdisciplinary knowledge. However, the book is, essentially, a compilation of Potter's articles already appeared in other journals. Most of them did not refer directly to bioethics. Only two addressed the topic: the first article in the book "Bioethics a Science of Survival" (already mentioned), and the last one "Survival as a Goal for Wisdom" in which Potter proposed his bioethical creed.

Nevertheless, and despite the fact that Potter never specifically defined in his book what bioethics was and what its procedures should be, we can find in this two articles several interesting concepts that were quite important for the subsequent development of the discipline: 1) The concept of dangerous knowledge; 2) Human progress and human survival; 3) The obligation towards the future; 4) The control of technology; and 5) The need for an interdisciplinary effort to address new moral controversies arisen in medical and scientific fields.

Potter considered all those issues to redact his bioethical creed which was conceived as a set of moral imperatives with their respective commitments:

1. Belief: *I accept the need for prompt remedial action in a world beset with crises.*
   Commitment: I will work with others to improve the formulation of my beliefs, to evolve additional credos, and to unite in a worldwide movement that will make possible the survival and improved development of the human species in harmony with the natural environment.

2. Belief: *I accept the fact that the future survival and development of mankind, both culturally and biologically, is strongly conditioned by man's present activities and plans.*
   Commitment: I will try to live my own life and to influence the lives of others so as to promote the evolution of a better world for future generations of mankind, and I will try to avoid actions that would jeopardize their future.

3. Belief: *I accept the uniqueness of each individual and his instinctive need to contribute to the betterment of some larger unit of society in a way that is compatible with the long-range needs of society.*
   Commitment: I will try to listen to the reasoned viewpoint of others whether from a minority or a majority, and I will recognize

the role of emotional commitment in producing effective action.

4. Belief: *I accept the inevitability of some human suffering that must result from the natural disorder in biological creatures and in the physical world, but I do not passively accept the suffering that results from man's inhumanity to man.*
   Commitment: I will try to face my own problems with dignity and courage. I will try to assist my fellow men when they are afflicted, and I will work toward the goal of eliminating needless suffering among mankind as a whole.

5. Belief: *I accept the finality of death as a necessary part of life. I affirm my veneration for life, my belief in the brotherhood of men, and my belief that I have an obligation to the future generations of men.*
   Commitment: I will try to live in a way that will benefit the lives of my fellow men now and in time to come and be remembered favorably by those who survive me.

This bioethical creed was conceived as a kind of universal declaration of principles in order to achieve peace, social agreements and conservation of natural resources. Thereby, the main task of bioethics was, according to Potter, to improve the quality of life for all humans. The creed's commitments did not express absolute and eternal imperatives. Potter did know that the whole world was threatened and influenced by very new events, and he also knew that a change in outlook was needed. However, he did not know whether that change would come on time. For this reason, Potter did not consider the creed's commitments as finished products but as moral obligations under "continual reexamination and refinement."

Readings

Potter, Van Rensselaer, "Bioethics: A Science of Survival," in Potter Van Rensselaer, *Bioethics: Bridge to the Future*, New Jersey, Prentice-Hall Inc., 1971: 1–29.

Study Questions

1. Why does Potter define bioethics as a "science of survival"?
2. Why did Potter consider his bioethics as a bridge between sciences and humanities?
3. Can Potter's bioethics be understood as a futuristic ethics? Why?

Bioethics: A Science of Survival

Van Rensselaer Potter

The Cancer Analogy

On December 28, 1954, the American Association for the Advancement of Science held a symposium on "Population Problems," at which Dr. Alan Gregg, vice-president of the Rockefeller Foundation (1951–56), came up with a startling idea: the thought that the human species is to the planet Earth what a cancer is to an individual human being. As a cancer specialist I was aware of the many contributing lines of thought and so was not altogether surprised to note the same idea proposed by another eminent biologist, Professor Norman J. Berrill of McGill University, in his superb book *Man's Emerging Mind.*[1] It was published in 1955, the same year that Gregg's symposium paper appeared in *Science.*[2] The remarks by these two men of science suggest that the effect of an ever-expanding human population on the carrying-capacity of the planet Earth bears examination. We do would well to examine their words.

Earth as Organism

Gregg espoused an idea that was clearly enunciated in 1949 by Aldo Leopold, who referred to "land the collective organism" and stated, "Land, then, is not merely soil; it is a fountain of energy flowing through a circuit of soils, plants, and animals. Food chains are the living channels which conduct energy upward; death and decay return it to the soil."[3] Leopold also anticipated Gregg and Berrill when he remarked, "This almost worldwide display of disorganization in the land seems to be similar to disease in an animal except that it never culminates in complete disorganization or death. The land recovers, but at some reduced level of complexity, and with a reduced carrying capacity for people, plants, and animals" (*Almanac*, 297).

Alan Gregg proposed similar ideas in his aforementioned symposium paper: "If we regard the different forms of plant and animal life in the world as being so closely related to and dependent on one another that they resemble different types of cells in a total organism, then we may, for the sake of a hypothesis, consider the living world as an organism." He went on to say,

What would we think if it became evident that within a very brief period in the history of the world some one type of its forms of life had increased greatly at the expense of other types of life? In short, I suggest, as a way of looking at the population problem, that there are some interesting analogies between the growth of the human population of the world and the increase of cells observable in neoplasms. To say that the world has cancer, and that the cancer cell is man has neither experimental proof nor the validation of predictive accuracy; but I see no reason that instantly forbids such a speculation. ... Cancerous growths demand food; but, so far as I know, they have never been cured by getting it. ... How nearly the slums of our great cities resemble the necrosis of tumors raises the whimsical query: which is the more offensive to decency and beauty, slums or the fetid detritus of a growing tumor? ... If Copernicus helped astronomy by challenging the geocentric interpretation of the universe, might it not help biology to challenge the anthropocentric interpretation of nature?

Norman Berrill was in complete agreement with Leopold and Gregg. In "The Human Crop," chapter 17 of *Man's Emerging Mind*, he discussed the issue at length:

Directly or indirectly there has been a monumental and increasingly extensive conversion of the planet's living potential from the diverse many to the all-consuming one. In terms of our comparison, the virgin prairie with its stable mixture of grasses and flowers has become almost entirely corn, with a few weeds and some blowing dust. All that can be transformed into human protoplasm is being transformed, and anything that stands in the way is pushed against the wall. ... So far as the rest of nature is concerned we are like a cancer whose strange cells multiply without restraint, ruthlessly demanding the nourishment that all of the body has need of. The analogy is not far-fetched for cancer cells no more than whole organisms know when to stop multiplying, and sooner or later the body or the community is starved of support and dies. (209-10)

Berrill saw three possible responses to the problem of overpopulation.

One is that we can increase our resources indefinitely to keep pace with the increasing population, which I have tried to show is impossible. Another is that we employ our collective intelligence and keep our numbers within reasonable bounds, while the third is the pessimistic one that human beings are not intelligent enough as a whole to control their own fertility and will always press hard against the ragged fringe of sustenance ... that always the more fertile or the more prolific human strains or races will outbreed the rest, that population control by any group sooner or later seals its own doom, with those who retain an uncontrollable breeding instinct taking its place. (220-21)

The analogy that sees Earth as an organism with all living species as cells in that organism is not complete in detail because the various species exist by and large by consuming the bodies, living or dead, of other species. In contrast, the cells that form an organism in the human body do not live by consuming other cells in the community, although the total human organism does depend on the intake of plant and animal species as food. Nevertheless, the proliferation of cell types within a human organism is exquisitely regulated by feedback mechanisms of great complexity, and the same can be said for the proliferation of living species on the planet Earth. In either case, when "some one type of its forms of life had increased greatly at the expense of other types of life," to use Gregg's words, we must conclude that the natural feedback mechanisms, evolved over millions of years, have broken down. It becomes clear that in either case the result is brought about by a great excess of births over the number of deaths in a given time interval. If the human species is to survive and prosper, it is essential that we must control not only nuclear armaments but also human fertility and the tendency to crowd out or destroy other forms of life. This statement of "what we must do" is merely an extension of the concluding Leopold Paradigm: "A thing [referring to decent land use] is right when it tends to preserve the integrity, stability, and beauty of the biotic community. It is wrong when it tends to do otherwise" (see chapter 1).

The Issue of Survival

It was perhaps Garrett Hardin more than any other who independently developed the equivalent of the Leopold paradigms and realized that this led directly to the issue of fertility control for the human population. In 1968 he wrote "The Tragedy of the Commons" in which he concluded that "freedom to breed is intolerable."[4] In 1972 he went beyond Leopold when he wrote, "With the flowering of concern for environmental quality and the growth of theory in ecology the time is now ripe, I think, for a concerted attack on the population-environment- quality complex. I think it is almost time to grasp the nettle of population control, which we sometime must, if we are to survive with dignity"[5] With that statement he began what I propose to continue, that is, the adoption of

the criterion of survival as a guide for action, and the discussion of what kind of survival we should advocate.

Like Garrett Hardin, Eugene P. Odum, co-author of *Fundamentals of Ecology*, was concerned with the relation between population and survival. Quoting extensively from Leopold's views on the need to extend ethics to the relation of man to the natural environment, Odum wrote: "We can also present strong scientific and technological reasons for the proposition that such a major extension of the general theory of ethics is now necessary for human survival."[6] Like Gregg and Berrill he noted the cancer analogy: "Growth beyond the optimum becomes cancer. Cancer is an ever-present threat to any mature system and must constantly be guarded against."[7] In proposing "The Emergence of Ecology as a New Integrative Discipline" in 1977,[8] he quoted Alex Novikoff on reductionism and holism: "Equally essential for the purposes of scientific analysis are both the isolation of parts of a whole and their integration into the structure of the whole. ... The consideration of one to the exclusion of the other acts to retard the development of biological and sociological sciences."[9] Odum concluded: "To achieve a truly holistic or ecosystematic approach, not only ecology but other disciplines in the natural, social, and political sciences as well must emerge to new hitherto unrecognized and unresearched levels of thinking and action" ("Emergence of Ecology," 1291), echoing Hardin's plea for "a concerted attack on the population-environment-quality complex."

When Richard Falk of Princeton University wrote *This Endangered Planet: Prospects and Proposals for Human Survival* (1971), he discussed the four dimensions of planetary danger as: (1) the war system; (2) population pressure; (3) insufficiency of resources; and (4) environmental overload. Following Paul Shepard, who in turn had paid tribute to Rachel Carson and Aldo Leopold, Falk reflected Odum's views when he wrote:

Such a posture of concern and position makes of human ecology a kind of ethics of survival. It is a science that relies on careful procedures of inquiry, data collection, and detailed observation as the basis of inference, explanation, and prediction. But it also involves a moral commitment to survival and to the enhancement of the natural habitat of man.[10]

All of the above authors have seen a link between ecology, population pressure, and human survival. They have in general not considered what survival. They have in general not considered what kind of survival, although Hardin spoke of surviving "with dignity" and Berrill visualized humankind always pressing hard against "the ragged fringe of sustenance." Unlike the vast majority of the human species, they are aware that humankind has no guarantee of survival, that survival cannot be assumed.

Survival Cannot Be Assumed

In 1967–70, I was a member of a group of university professors in an Interdisciplinary Studies Committee on the Future of Man. We published a report on the "Purpose and Function of the University," subtitled "University scholars have a major responsibility for survival and quality of life in the future."[11] In this report we stated,

We affirm the views that the survival of civilized man is not something to be taken for granted, that governments throughout the world are experiencing great difficulty in planning for the future while trying to cope with the present, and finally, that the university is one of the institutions that has a major responsibility for the survival

and improvement of life for civilized man.

My book, *Bioethics, Bridge to the Future*,[12] commented on the need for a new synthesis:

Mankind is urgently in need of new wisdom that will provide the "knowledge of how to use knowledge" for man's survival and for improvement in the quality of life. This concept of wisdom as a guide for action—the knowledge of how to use knowledge for the social good—might be called *Science of Survival*, surely the prerequisite to improvement in the quality of life. I take the position that the science of survival must be built on the science of biology and enlarged beyond the traditional boundaries to include the most essential elements of the social sciences and the humanities with emphasis on philosophy in the strict sense, meaning "love of wisdom." A science of survival must be more than science alone, and I therefore propose the term *Bioethics* in order to emphasize the two most important ingredients in achieving the new wisdom that is so desperately needed: biological knowledge and human values.

In this age of specialization we seem to have lost contact with the daily reminders that must have driven home the truth to our ancestors: man cannot live without harvesting plants or killing animals. If plants wither and die and animals fail to reproduce, man will sicken and die and fail to maintain his kind. As individuals we cannot afford to leave our destiny in the hands of scientists, engineers, technologists, and politicians who have forgotten or who never knew these simple truths. In our modern world we have botanists who study plants and zoologists who study animals, but most of them are specialists who do not deal with the ramifications of their limited knowledge. Today we need biologists who respect the fragile web of life and who can broaden their knowledge to include the nature of man and his relation to the biological and physical worlds. We need biologists who can tell us what we can and must do to survive and what we cannot and must not do if we hope to maintain and improve the quality of life during the next three decades. *The fate of the world rests on the integration, preservation, and extension of the knowledge that is possessed by a relatively small number of people who are only just beginning to realize how inadequate their strength, how enormous the task* [italics added]. Every college student owes it to society to learn as much as possible of what these leaders have to offer, to challenge them, to meld biological knowledge with whatever additional ingredient they are able to master, and to become, if their talents are adequate, the new leaders of tomorrow. From such a pooling of knowledge and values may come a new kind of scholar or statesman who has mastered what I have referred to as Bioethics. No individual could possibly master all of the components of this branch of knowledge, just as no one today knows all of zoology or all of chemistry. What is needed is a new discipline to provide models of life styles for people who can communicate with each other and propose and explain the new public policies that could provide a "bridge to the future." The new disciplines will be forged in the heat of today's crisis problems, all of which require some kind of a mix between basic biology, social sciences, and the humanities.

Biology is more than botany and zoology. It is the foundation on which we build *ecology*, which is the relation among plants, animals, man, and the physical environment. Biology includes the science of genetics, which has to do with all aspects of heredity, and physiology, which deals with the function of individuals. For thousands of years men have lived on this earth with no generally disseminated knowledge of their chemical nature. Man's dependence upon his natural environment was widely understood, but Nature's bounty was considered to be limitless and Nature's capacity to recover from exploitation was considered to be ample. Eventually it was realized that man was exploiting the earth to an extent that required the use of more and more science and technology as the richest sources of iron and copper, for example, were used up. From the biological standpoint man has progressively taken over the planet's resources by decreasing the numbers and kinds of other species of life and by increasing only those species that were useful to man, such as wheat, beef cattle, and other consumables. ...

From many uninformed quarters we now hear demands for a moratorium on science, when what we need is more and better science. We need to combine biology with humanistic knowledge from diverse sources and forge a science of survival that will be able to set a system of priorities. We need to start action in the areas where knowledge is already available, and we need to reorient our research effort to get the necessary knowledge if it is not available.

The age-old questions about the nature of man[cf. Trosko][13] and his relation to the world become increasingly important as we approach the remaining three decades in this century, when political decisions made in ignorance of biological knowledge, or in defiance of it, may jeopardize man's future and indeed the future of earth's biological resources for human needs. As individuals we speak of the "instinct for survival," but the sum total of all our individual instincts for survival is not enough to guarantee the survival of the human race in a form that any of us would willingly accept. An *instinct* for survival is not enough. We must develop the *science* of survival, and it must start with a new kind of ethics—bioethics. (1–3)

Having agreed with all those who expressed concern for human survival, and having concluded that ecological bioethics is a key ingredient in attempts to ensure survival, we must now consider what we mean by survival.

The Meaning of Survival

Until recently it has always been assumed that survival of the human species could be taken for granted; the question of whether survival is something to be desired was accordingly not an issue. When Charles Darwin wrote *The Origin of Species* in 1859, he was optimistic about the future of humankind. He wrote in his penultimate paragraph,

As all the living forms of life are the lineal descendants of those which lived long before the Cambrian epoch, we may feel certain that the ordinary succession by generation has never once been broken, and that no cataclysm has desolated the whole world.

Hence we may look with some confidence to a secure future of great length.[14]

In recent years Walter Alvarez and others have produced evidence that Darwin may have been wrong about the possibility of worldwide cataclysms. It appears that the extinction of the dinosaurs 65 million years ago may have been caused by a major impact from an extraterrestrial body, followed by severe climatic changes. Such changes have been recently postulated as a result of the use of nuclear weapons.[15] The danger of producing a "nuclear winter" is now being seriously studied.[16]

With the explosion of the first atomic bomb on July 16, 1945, near Alamogordo, New Mexico, the survival of the human species became a worrisome issue, although many now realize that survival cannot be assumed even in the absence of nuclear war. Jonathan Schell emphasized the ecosystem in relation to nuclear war when he wrote in 1982,

The primary question is not how many people would be irradiated, burned, or crushed to death by the immediate effects of the bombs but how well the ecosphere, regarded as a single living entity, on which all forms of life depend for their continued existence, would hold up. The issue is the habitability of the earth, and it is in this context, not in the context of the direct slaughter of hundreds of millions of people by the local effects, that the question of human survival arises."[17]

He noted that

of all the "modest hopes of human beings," the hope that mankind will survive is the most modest, since it only brings us to the threshold of all other hopes. In entertaining it, we do not yet ask for justice, or for freedom, or for happiness, or for any of the other things that we may want in life. We do not even necessarily ask for our personal survival; we ask only that we be *survived*. We ask for assurance that when we die as individuals, as we know we must, mankind will live on. ... Life without the hope for human survival is a life of despair. (184)

Schell cited Socrates for the principle that the highest good is not life itself—mere survival—but the moral life (130).

This brings us to the question of what we mean by survival. Much has been written on the subject, as seen by book titles alone. We find *Values for Survival* (Mumford 1946)[18] *Road to Survival* (Vogt 1948)[19] *Science and Survival* (Commoner 1966)[20] *The Crisis of Survival* (editors of *The Progressive* 1970)[21] *Exploring New Ethics for Survival* (Hardin 1972)[22] *The Comedy of Survival* (Meeker 1972)[23] *The Tyranny of Survival* (Callahan 1973)[24] and *Challenge to Survival* (Williams 1977).[25] Some of the issues raised by these authors will be considered later in this book. But first we must consider what is meant when the word "survival" is used without qualification.

In contemplating the term "survival" it should be pointed out that survival begins today. None of us knows whether or not we will be alive tomorrow. On the other hand, the possibility of survival for at least some members of the human species may extend into the future for as long as any form of life exists on the planet. But what kind of survival? We can think of the kinds of survival that occur in terms of life-styles and behavior today as well as the kinds of survival that can be projected into the future. We can think of the survival of individuals: our children and grand-children and future generations down through time. But present behavior and future existence in terms of the kinds of survival I shall describe applies not only to individuals but also to tribes, communities, corporations,

and governments. What kinds of survival can be described in the fewest possible categories?

Kinds of Survival

Elsewhere I have proposed that the word "survival," used without a qualifying adjective, is inadequate for discussion in the context of ecological bioethics. I suggested five categories based on qualifying adjectives: mere, miserable, idealistic, irresponsible, and acceptable.[26]

Mere Survival

Mere survival is a term used scornfully by people who dislike talk about survival. Mere survival implies food and shelter but no libraries, no written history, no engineering, no science, no hospitals, no churches, no television, and, presumably, no artificial contraceptives: in other words, a hunting and gathering culture, which incidentally is the only culture that has demonstrated that it can survive for tens of millenia, as in Australia and the Kalahari Desert of southern Africa. In the distant past it may not have been too difficult, but contact with the white man changed all that.[27]

Miserable Survival

A step below mere survival is miserable survival. Some millions of Africans on the verge of starvation, with many actually starving to death, and suffering from widespread malnutrition, diarrhea, respiratory disease and parasitic infestations, and now AIDS, provide a ghastly picture of how miserable survival can be much worse than mere survival. Yet both exist today in many parts of the world, and it is a matter of serious debate as to how much the white man's entry into Africa and disruption of the native cultures has contributed to converting mere survival to present-day miserable survival. In their book *Natural Disasters: Acts of God or Acts of Man?*[28] Lloyd Timberlake, editorial director of the Londonbased group Earthscan, and Anders Wijkman, secretary general of the Swedish Red Cross, said that some disasters, including floods, drought, and famine, are caused more by environmental and resource management than by too much or too little rain, while the effects of natural disasters such as earthquakes, volcanic eruptions, and hurricanes are magnified by unwise human actions. At a press conference in Washington, Timberlake called for refocusing disaster relief which, he said, was often a band-aid on a massive wound.[29] The authors echoed the views of Aldo Leopold in 1933 (see chapter 1) when they said overcultivation, deforestation, and overgrazing tend to reduce the ability of soil to absorb and retain water, making it susceptible to drought and flooding. Population growth and inadequate housing in exposed shantytowns often contribute to larger death tolls from natural disasters, Timberlake said. He noted that in Ethiopia, where famine is threatening millions of people, "the highlands have always been overpopulated and overcultivated."

Idealistic Survival

At the upper end of the spectrum is idealistic survival. I shall not discuss *ideal* survival because that is something we shall never see, and besides, each person has a private notion of what Utopia would be. However, people can have idealistic survival at many economic levels and in many cultures. Idealistic survival would occur when sufficient numbers of people in a society have the economic security, the information, and the ethical concern to become motivated to think personally about Professor Falk's four planetary dangers, and in particular to think about long-term survival and the amelioration of existing

pockets of miserable survival. People cannot agree on the components of ideal survival, but they can universally agree on the undesirability of preventable disease. No culture or religion, primitive or modern, has ever placed a premium on or aspired to starvation, malnutrition, diarrhea, intestinal worms, or other parasitic infestations. So the desirability of eliminating these scourges is something that all can agree upon as a component of idealistic survival.

Smallpox was one of humankind's scourges that decimated populations from time to time, along with typhus, typhoid fever, and many other viral and bacterial infections. But now, international public health efforts have apparently been successful in the total elimination of smallpox from the planet. This was possible because the disease was transmitted from person to person with no intermediate vectors such as mosquitoes, ticks, snails, or other life forms. In the case of smallpox, the last person to have it was prevented from passing it on to anyone else. Idealistic survival would unite people who would seek to eliminate the remaining great miseries that afflict humankind: sexually-transmitted infections, parasitic diseases such as malaria, schistosomiasis and sleeping sickness, intestinal worms of all sorts, and all the other preventable diseases that plague great numbers of the human species.

An example of idealistic survival is the announcement concerning a grant by the MacArthur Foundation for $20 million to fight parasites that cause disease in three billion people around the world. Dr. Jonas Salk, known for his development of a vaccine against polio and now chairman of the foundation's health committee, announced the grant. He said,

> Diseases caused by parasites afflict more than half the world's people. Even when not seriously ill, people who have parasitic disease are chronically sick—weaker, less competent, less productive, and less content than they would be otherwise.[30]

Twelve medical research groups in five states and three foreign nations will participate in the program, which will establish the MacArthur Foundation as the largest private sponsor of parasitology research, according to foundation president John Corbally.

At the same time that we praise the MacArthur Foundation for this example of idealistic survival, we must ask what would be the long-range effects of even partial success of the program on the continent of Africa? Can any program that decreases infant mortality and thereby increases the demands on the ecosystem, without the concomitant educational measures that would protect the ecosystem and promote the idea of zero population growth, be anything but a disaster in the long run? The question is, how bad is a good idea? How can the people of the industrialized nations help the people in the Third World, not with piecemeal efforts or bandaids, as noted by Lloyd Timberlake, but with balanced programs or multi-pronged coordinated programs, when they are unable to control their own unemployment, inflation, environmental pollution, soil erosion, and budget deficits? How can they cope with the dilemma posed by Norman Berrill "that always the more fertile or the more prolific human strains or races will outbreed the rest, that population control by any group sooner or later seals its own doom, with those who retain an uncontrollable breeding instinct taking its place"? The only answer provided by an idealistic survivalist would seem to be that the dissemination of information and motivation for population control, along with public health measures and policies emulating the ethics of Aldo Leopold, is the only sane way to deal with the social dilemma. Both at home and abroad, idealistic survival leads us to Leopold, who said, "An ethic to supplement and guide the economic relation to land presupposes the existence of some mental image of land as a biotic mechanism" (*Almanac*, 214). And at the end of his essay he wrote: "I have purposely presented the land ethic as a product of social evolution ... I think it is a truism that as the ethical frontier advances from the individual to the community, its intellectual content increases" (225). Idealistic survival surely is an interdisciplinary exercise in democracy. It requires that we listen to the views of both the minority and the majority, and that we try to ascertain the facts. For as Leopold concluded in his essay, "The mechanism of operation is the same for any ethic: social approbation for right actions: social disapproval for wrong actions" (225).

Irresponsible Survival

Irresponsible survival, my fourth category, is in a sense the inverse of idealistic survival. Irresponsible survival is doing all the things that run counter to the aspirations of idealistic survivalists. Whereas proponents of idealistic survival seek to promote zero or negative population growth for the immediate future and a healthy ecosystem with concern for future generations, those who are categorized as irresponsible recognize no obligation to the future, proceed entirely in terms of self-interest, have no desire or willingness to control their own reproductive powers or interest in helping others to do so, and do nothing to preserve a healthy ecosystem. Of course, there are few who combine all these characteristics. Among the interesting contemporary phenomena are the organizations that are desperately trying to preserve a healthy ecosystem in terms of beaches, tidal basins, wilderness, wildlife preserves, redwood forests, groundwater, clean air, or other elements in the environment, while ignoring the fact that it is population pressure that underlies all of these problems. A sense of ecological morality will always retreat in the face of economic demands brought about by the growth of local and world populations.

As noted earlier in general terms, irresponsible survival can be discussed in terms of individuals, local communities, corporations, or governments. It can be discussed in terms of agriculture, industry, science and technology, medicine, the military complex, or foreign affairs. Examples are too numerous to be compiled in detail. In the field of agriculture it is irresponsible to use farming practices that accelerate soil erosion, or to use deep-well pumping techniques that progressively lower the water table. According to the 1983 U.S. Geological Survey's National Water Summary, the combined agricultural, industrial, and residential usage exceeds the rate of replenishment in thirty-five of the forty-eight contiguous states.[31] In particular, the states in the Southwest, whose population increased 6–12 percent as a group between 1980 and 1983, have thirty-one percent of U.S. water usage but only 6 percent of the nation's renewable water supply. Water is being "mined" by deeper and deeper wells that must eventually fail to keep pace with demand. State and federal governments are being pressured to implement large-scale projects to import water from somewhere to meet the increased demand caused by population growth. As Leopold said, "Violence (to the land) varies with human population density; a dense population requires a more violent conversion" (see chapter 1).

In the case of chemical herbicides and pesticides applied to the soil, the kinds and quantities produced in ever-increasing amounts exceed the ability of the Environmental Protection Agency to keep abreast of practices. The problems caused by the avalanche of new products and product combinations have resulted in a vast increase in regulatory legislation and a huge bureaucracy faced with an almost superhuman task. That the chemical intermediates and products are basically lethal to many forms of life was dramatically demonstrated on December 3, 1984, in Bhopal, India, when a pesticide intermediate, methyl isocyanate, leaked from a storage tank and killed at least 2,000 residents in the vicinity and injured about 200,000. The justification for the use of toxic chemicals is always a twofold argument—that increased crop yields show a favorable cost/benefit ratio in economic terms,

and that increased yields are necessary to feed a hungry and expanding world population.

The Environmental Fund is on record as believing "that every major problem facing the United States as a nation and humanity as a whole becomes more difficult to solve as population increases."[32] Their supporters would have to be classified in the present context as idealistic survivalists, pursuing the twin goals of a healthy ecosystem and a stabilized healthy population with a balance between births and deaths. Their position, supported by many Catholics as well as by non-Catholics, would appear to be on a collision course with the repeated admonitions of Pope John Paul II against artificial contraception and sterilization which, the pontiff said, are "always seriously illicit."[33] In the opinion of many, the Pope would appear to be advocating a course irrevocably committed to irresponsible and, indeed, miserable survival, in terms of net results.[34] Only by continued dialogue between religious leaders and dedicated idealistic survivalists, and between medical ethicists and ecological bioethicists, can some kind of agreement on priorities be reached.

Another example of seemingly irresponsible behavior with respect to future generations and of the effect of economic pressure on priorities is the case of the tobacco industry. The American Cancer Society has for some years pointed to the connection between cigarette smoking and lung cancer. Recently they have publicized dangers to the offspring of mothers who smoke during pregnancy. Cigarette smoking has been credited with causing 30 percent of the total cancer incidence in America. Now the National Advisory Council on Drug Abuse has in effect said that it is irresponsible to promote the sale of cigarettes by advertising in newspapers, magazines, and billboards, and they have proposed a total ban on such advertising.[35] Cigarette advertising on television broadcasts was banned fourteen years ago. Lloyd Johnston, chairman of the council's subcommittee on prevention, said that cigarettes are the most widely advertised product in America, with the industry spending some

$1.5 billion a year on advertising. The Federal Trade Commission has estimated that half of all billboards in America advertise cigarettes. Now the economic losses to the industry and to the advertising media will have to be weighed against the fact that smoking is estimated to kill about 350,000 Americans each year, according to the council.

But of all the forms of irresponsible survival with respect to future generations, ignorance, superstition, and illiteracy are the greatest barriers to a hopeful future for our descendants. It has always been said that our children are the hope of the future; but unless they can read and develop skills and an ethical understanding of the natural world, they cannot develop into or select leaders who can plan for tomorrow's world. Leopold said, "Perhaps the most serious obstacle impeding the evolution of a land ethic is the fact that our educational and economic system is headed away from, rather than toward, an intense consciousness of land."

Acceptable Survival

Aldo Leopold was concerned with the concept of "carrying-capacity" of the physical environment for the plants, animals, and humans that occupied a given space. We can judge that he was thinking about survival when he wrote in "The Land Ethic" that "North America has a better chance for permanence than Europe, if she can contrive to limit her density." *Contriving* to limit density may suggest limiting human fertility or total immigration; he did not comment on these matters. But with respect to acceptable survival, it is in *Song of the Gavilan* (*Almanac*, 149–54) that we find his critique of technology and his own idea of the good life:

> One of the facts hewn to by science
> is that every river needs more people,
> and all people need more inventions,
> and hence more science; the good life

depends on the indefinite extension of this chain of logic. That the good life on any river may likewise depend on the perception of its music, and the preservation of some music to perceive, is a form of doubt not yet entertained by science. (154)

And it is in the foreword to the *Almanac* that we find the comment

> But wherever the truth may lie, this much is crystal-clear: our bigger-and-better society is now like a hypochondriac, so obsessed with its own economic health as to have lost the capacity to remain healthy. ... Nothing could be more salutary at this stage than a little healthy contempt for a plethora of material blessings. (ix)

In more recent times Lester R. Brown, president and director of The Worldwatch Institute, Washington, D.C., has done the most to urge thought and action to preserve what we can of the natural world in the interests of acceptable survival, or, in his terms, a "sustainable society." In a series of books and brochures from the institute we find a wealth of well-documented material, all of which is relevant to the concept of acceptable survival, including *Losing Ground: Environmental Stress and World Food Prospects* by Erik P. Eckholm.[36] In a powerful effort entitled *Building a Sustainable Society* (1981),[37] Brown describes "The Shape of a Sustainable Society"—which to me is a first attempt to describe acceptable survival—as well as "The Means of Transition," "The Institutional Challenge," and "Changing Values and Shifting Priorities." Summing up the present situation, he said, "We have not inherited the earth from our fathers, we are borrowing it from our children" (359). It is interesting to note that although he seems unfamiliar with Aldo Leopold, he speaks like a true disciple when he comments, "A world that now has over four billion human inhabitants desperately needs a land ethic, a new reverence for land, and a better understanding of the need to use carefully a resource that is too often taken for granted" (352).

1. Norman J. Berrill, *Man's Emerging Mind* (New York: Dodd, Mead and Co., 1955).
2. Alan Gregg, "A Medical Aspect of the Population Problem," *Science* 121 (1955): 681–82.
3. Leopold, *Sand County Almanac*, 1987 ed., 216. The page references herein are from the 1987 edition (see chapter 1, n. 1).
4. Garrett Hardin, "The Tragedy of the Commons," *Science* 162 (1968): 1243–48. This essay has been reprinted in countless subsequent publications.
5. Garrett Hardin, *Exploring New Ethics for Survival* (New York: The Viking Press, 1972; reprint ed., Baltimore: Penguin Books, 1973).
6. Eugene P. Odum and H. T. Odum, *Fundamentals of Ecology*, 3d ed. (Philadelphia: Saunders, 1971), 10.
7. Eugene P. Odum, "Environmental Ethic and Attitude Revolution," in *Philosophy and Environmental Crisis*, ed. Wm. T. Blackstone (Athens: University of Georgia Press, 1974), 14. In this article Odum quoted from Leopold's "Land Ethic."
8. Eugene P. Odum, "The Emergence of Ecology as a New Integrative Discipline,"
9. Alex B. Novikoff, "The Concept of Integrative Levels and Biology," *Science* 101 (1945): 209–15.
10. Richard Falk, *This Endangered Planet: Prospects and Proposals for Human Survival* (New York: Vintage Books, Random House, 1971), 187.
11. V. R. Potter et al., "Purpose and Function of the University," *Science* 167 (1970): 1590–93.
12. V. R. Potter, *Bioethics, Bridge to the Future* (Englewood Cliffs, N.J.: Prentice-Hall, Inc., 1971), 1–3.
13. J. E. Trosko, "Scientific Views of Human Nature: Implications for the Ethics of Technological Intervention," in *The Culture*
14. *of Biomedicine*, vol. 1, *Studies in Science and Culture*, ed. D. H. Brock (Cranbury, N.J.: Association of University Presses, Inc.), 70–97.
14. Charles Darwin, *The Origin of Species*, 6th ed. (London: John Murray, 1872), 428.
15. W. Alvarez et al., "The End of the Cretaceous: Sharp Boundary or Gradual Transition," *Science* 223 (1984): 1183–85. See also W. Alvarez et al., "Impact Theory of Mass Extinctions and the Invertebrate Fossil Record," *Science* 223 (1984): 1135–41.
16. R. R. Turco et al., "Nuclear Winter: Global Consequences of Multiple Nuclear Explosions," *Science* 222 (1983): 1283–92. See also P. R. Ehrlich et al., "Long-Term Biological Consequences of Nuclear War," *Science* 222 (1983): 1293–1300.
17. Jonathan Schell, *The Fate of the Earth* (New York: Knopf, 1982), 21, 130, 184.
18. Lewis Mumford, *Values for Survival* (New York: Harcourt, Brace, 1946).
19. Vogt, *Road to Survival*. The author later published *People: Challenge to Survival* (New York: W. Sloane Associates, 1960).
20. Barry Commoner, *Science and Survival* (New York: Viking Press, 1966).
21. *The Progressive, The Crisis of Survival* (Glenview, Ill.: Scott, Foresman, 1970).
22. Garrett Hardin, *Exploring New Ethics for Survival*, (NY Viking Press, 1972), 75.
23. Joseph W. Meeker, *The Comedy of Survival* (New York: Charles Scribners Sons, 1972).
24. Daniel Callahan, *The Tyranny of Survival* (New York: Macmillan, 1973).
25. Leonard Williams, *Challenge to Survival* (New York: Harper Colophon Books, Harper and Row, 1977).
26. V. R. Potter, "Bioethics and the Human Prospect," in *Studies in Science and Culture*, vol. 1, *The Culture of Biomedicine*, ed. D. H. Brock (Cranbury, N.J.: Association of University Presses, Inc., 1984), 124–37.
27. John Yellen, "Bushmen," *Science* 85, May 1985, 40–48. Dr. Yellen is director of the

anthropology program at the National Science Foundation.

28. Lloyd Timberlake and Anders Wijkman, *Natural Disasters: Acts of God or Acts of Man* (Washington, D.C.: Earthscan, 1984).

29. "Natural Disasters Said Man-Made," *Wisconsin State Journal*, 15 November 1984.

30. *Wisconsin State Journal*, 17 October 1984. Dr. Jonas Salk was quoted.

31. The Environmental Fund, "Water Availability and Population Growth," TEF Data, No. 16, October 1984. The report was based on data from the U.S. Geological Survey, *National Water Summary* (1983), 26–27; and Bureau of the Census, *Estimates of the Population of the States*, July 1, 1981 to 1983, 2.

32. Stated on most literature from The Environmental Fund, e.g., TEF Data No. 16, October 1984, cited in n. 31.

33. AP, *New York Times; Wisconsin State Journal*, 27 January 1985. Dispatch from Caracas, Venezuela, 27 January 1985.

34. Lester Brown, *Building a Sustainable Society* (New York: W. W. Norton, 1981), 330. Brown commented, "As for population issues, few religious organizations have been at the forefront of social activism and some—among them the Catholic Church and the more fundamentalist Muslim sects—can only be counted as deterrents to progress."

35. National Advisory Council on Drug Abuse, reported in *Wisconsin State Journal*, 27 January 1985.

36. Erik P. Eckholm, *Losing Ground: Environmental Stress and World Food Prospects* (New York: W. W. Norton, 1976).

37. Brown, *Building a Sustainable Society*. This book is by far the most authoritative and best documented with respect to the many issues involved in population, resources, and human survival in the long term.

3. The Epistemological Shift

The Tuskegee experiment, along with other controversial research, such as hepatitis studies carried out between 1963 and 1966 on mentally handicapped children at the Willowbrook State School in New York City, impulsed the evaluation of biomedical progress and the need to morally regulate experimentation with human subjects.

Alerted by those events and aware that a change was needed in the way of conducting scientific research, the Congress of the United States established in 1974 the National Commission for the Protection of Human Subjects of Biomedical and Behavioral Research. The National Commission's main purposes were: i) to discuss and reflect about the limits of techno scientific research, ii) to evaluate the balance between the risks and benefits of the human research, iii) to provide guidelines for an equitable selection of human subjects participating in such experiments, and iv) to think about the nature, scope and meaning of informed consent in scientific research.

Thus, the National Commission's general goal was to create a theoretical framework to deliberate on complex problems inherent to scientific experimentation. That framework is widely known as the Belmont Report, which was published in the *Federal Register* on April 18, 1979. In that document we can find the following reflection:

> Scientific research has produced substantial social benefits. It has also posed some troubling ethical questions. Public attention was drawn to these questions by reported abuses of human subjects in biomedical experiments, especially during the Second World War. During the Nuremberg War Crime Trials, the Nuremberg Code was drafted as a set of standards for judging physicians and scientist who had conducted biomedical experiments on concentration camp prisoners. This code became the prototype of many later codes intended to assure that research involving human subjects would be carried out in an ethical manner.[1]

---

1   National Commission for the Protection of Human Subjects of Biomedical and Behavioral Research, *Belmont Report. Ethical Principles and Guidelines for the Protection of Human Subjects of Research*, US Government Printing Office, Reprint from the collection of the University of Michigan Library, 2009, Appendix Volume I, 78-0012.

In this regard, the Belmont Report identified as its primary purposes:

> Identify the basic ethical principles that should underlie the conduct of biomedical and behavioral research involving human subjects and to develop guidelines, which should be followed to assure that such research is conducted in accordance with those principles.[2]

The Belmont Report gathered and summarized all the results of the National Commission's work by defining three principles to inform specific guidelines for research with human subjects.

The idea was, first, to eliminate excessive paternalism from scientific practice which traditionally did not take into account human subjects' autonomy to carry out scientific research. Thus, the Belmont Report meant, at least in theory, the attempt to rethink how scientists could conduct research more ethically.

Secondly, the Belmont Report attempted to restore the respect for human dignity by trying to maximize benefits for subjects of experimentation, and reduce the risks that could cause them harm or injury.

And third, the Belmont Report showed the need for justice at different stages of research: 1. Fair methods and clear procedures to choose subjects of experimentation, 2. Fair distribution of efforts to safeguard the dignity, health and life of those involved in treatment and research, and 3. Avoidance of any type of discrimination in research whatever the origin, race or status of people.

Therefore, the Belmont Report can be understood as the first formulation of theoretical guidelines to configure a structure of deliberation for bioethics. Those principles had a rapid and growing acceptance by extending their scope into the field of medicine in which they started regulating important aspects of

physician-patient relationship. Also, the Belmont Report's principles were general criteria to assist deliberation on particularly complex cases, guide decision-making process, and objectify reasoning on moral controversies. Finally, those principles should be a sufficiently solid theoretical framework to generate more specific rules and determine plausible procedures to be applied at a practical level. In this fashion, the Belmont Report emphasized the importance of clearly distinguishing between nature of research, its limits, scope and possible implications for human lives.

The report was structured in three sections in which various aspects of their implementation were discussed: A. Boundaries between Practice and Research; B. Basic Ethical Principles; and C. Applications. I will briefly explain each one of them.

A. Boundaries between Practice and Research

In this section, the report stressed the need to distinguish between biomedical behavioral research and therapeutic treatment. The fundamental objective of this distinction was to determine which activities and procedures should be thoroughly reviewed to improve the standards of protection for subjects of experimentation. Moreover, this part emphasized the distinction between practice and research by stressing that practice was an external intervention that sought for subjects' welfare by providing proper diagnosis and timely treatment. Instead, research was an activity whose main purposes were to test a hypothesis, reach conclusions and develop a general knowledge on biomedical issues. These three purposes should be reached by 1) taking into account respect for dignity, integrity and well-being of human subjects, and 2) having a high degree of scientific conviction and certainty regarding therapy's safety and effectiveness.

---

2 Ibid., Appendix Volume I, 78-0012.

B. Basic Ethical Principles

The expression "Basic Ethical Principles" referred to the main moral milestones of our Western cultural tradition. At this point, the National Commission's specific aim was to identify the most universally accepted principles of our ethical tradition and determine which ones best suited moral demands of research on human subjects. According to the above mentioned, the National Commission proposed the following principles:

1. *Respect for Persons*: This principle recognized persons as free agents and, at the same time, as worthy of protection in the event that their autonomy was diminished or absent. It implied, on the one hand, an individual right which was related to the ability that most persons have to make decisions and, on the other, it pointed out the duty to respect that autonomy. Also, this principle involved the explicit recognition of individual freedom and the capacity of self-determination inherent in every human being. When this ability was notoriously reduced, patients had the right to a surrogate decision.
2. *Beneficence*: According to the report this principle should be understood beyond traditional kindness, benevolence or charity. Rather, it pointed out the moral obligation to guarantee and promote individuals' welfare at every stage of research and avoid harming them under any circumstance. In this sense, the document stated "two general rules as complementary expressions of beneficent actions: (1) do no harm and (2) maximize possible benefits and minimize possible harms."
3. *Justice*: This principle emphasized the duty to equitably distribute benefits of research to avoid risks for the most vulnerable groups and it also sought to ensure objectivity and fairness in the allocation of burdens. It was conceived, therefore, as a principle of distributive justice which raised important questions, such as who should determine what "to be equal" means or what criterion should be set to determine what a "fair treatment" is. In this regard, the report recognized five criteria of distribution: (1) to each person an equal share, (2) to each person according to individual need, (3) to each person according to individual effort, (4) to each person according to societal contribution, and (5) to each person according to merit. However, those criteria were mutually exclusive and the report did not provide enough deliberative elements to determine which one of them should take preeminence over others and why.

C. Applications

In this section, the report identified three fundamental requirements to implement each one of the principles:

1. *Informed Consent* (required for the application of the principle of Respect for Persons): It considered three elements as conditions of possibility for its fulfillment
   Information: The person must be fully and opportunely informed about possible risks associated with experimentation or treatment.
   Comprehension: The procedure should ensure that subjects of experimentation reasonably understand the nature and scope of biomedical interventions. By considering that intelligence, rationality, maturity and language skills are different among persons, this procedure must be administrated regarding individual capacities.
   Voluntariness: Consent is valid if it is informed as well as voluntary. This means that persons must express their agreement for biomedical experimentation free from external coercion. Hence, this procedure pointed out the need to distinguish between justifiable persuasion and undue influences. However and despite its specifications, informed consent

is a controversial issue that raises important questions still unresolved. Is informed consent main purpose to actively involve human subjects and patients in biomedical decisions? If informed consent implies to recognize and promote individual autonomy, should persons make the final decision by themselves? Are experimentation subjects and patients co-responsible for detrimental consequences of biomedical procedures? Is informed consent purpose to protect scientists and physicians from legal punishment when experimentation outcomes are harmful for individuals? If a person does not consent, should scientists or physicians respect his/her decision regardless eventual negative consequences?

2. *Assessment of Risks and Benefits* (required for the application of the principle of beneficence): It implied that both risks and benefits of experimentation must be balanced through a systematic evaluation of each. Hence, this procedure should help the researcher to determine whether the prospective study was properly designed or not. Also, it should be, on the one hand, a method to clarify if risks were justified and, on the other, a criterion for persons to decide their eventual participation in biomedical experimentation.

3. *Selection of Subjects* (required for the application of the principle of justice): It implied fair procedures in the selection of research subjects. This selection would have two levels on which the principle of justice should be applied: individual and social. Individual justice implied the fairness of researchers, namely, "they should not offer potentially beneficial research only to some patients" or select only "undesirable" subjects for risky experimentation. Social justice meant that there should be a distinction and order of preference in the selection of classes of subjects who ought, or ought not to participate in any kind of research based on their ability and conditions to bear burdens (e.g., adults before children).

Undoubtedly, the Belmont Report was a key guideline in the development of bioethical deliberation and in the improvement of public policies about experimentation with human subjects. Also, its scope has been extended beyond its initial meaning into medical and health care contexts. Thus, that short but influential document can be considered as a valuable set of "basic ethical principles" to scrutinize moral controversies in the biomedical field and, as such, it deserved to be revisited even in this so synoptic way.

Readings

National Commission for the Protection of Human Subjects of Biomedical and Behavioral Research, "The Belmont Report," in Childress, James F., et al, *Belmont Revisited: Ethical Principles for Research with Human Subjects*, USA, Georgetown University Press, 2005: 253–265.

Beauchamp, Tom L., "The Origins and Evolution of the Belmont Report," in Childress, James F., et al, *Belmont Revisited: Ethical Principles for Research with Human Subjects*, USA, Georgetown University Press, 2005: 12–25.

Study Questions

1. Explain the main purposes of the National Commission.
2. Explain the main purposes of the Belmont Report.
3. What are the theoretical and procedural scopes of the Belmont Report's principles?
4. Why is it important to distinguish between biomedical behavioral research and therapeutic treatment?
5. Explain briefly every Belmont Report's principle and its applications?

The Belmont Report

National Commission for the Protection of Human Subjects of
Biomedical and Behavioral Research

Office of the Secretary

Ethical Principles and Guidelines for the
Protection of Human Subjects of Research

The National Commission for the Protection
of Human Subjects of Biomedical and
Behavioral Research

April 18, 1979

AGENCY: Department of Health, Education, and
Welfare.

ACTION: Notice of Report for Public
Comment.

SUMMARY: On July 12, 1974, the National
Research Act (Pub. L. 93-348) was signed into
law, there-by creating the National Commission
for the Protection of Human Subjects of
Biomedical and Behavioral Research. One of the
charges to the Commission was to identify the
basic ethical principles that should underlie the
conduct of biomedical and behavioral research
involving human subjects and to develop guidelines which should be followed to assure that
such research is conducted in accordance with
those principles. In carrying out the above, the
Commission was directed to consider: (i) the
boundaries between biomedical and behavioral
research and the accepted and routine practice

of medicine, (ii) the role of assessment of risk-
benefit criteria in the determination of the
appropriateness of research involving human
subjects, (iii) appropriate guidelines for the
selection of human subjects for participation in
such research and (iv) the nature and definition
of informed consent in various research settings.

The Belmont Report attempts to summarize
the basic ethical principles identified by the
Commission in the course of its deliberations.
It is the outgrowth of an intensive four-day period of discussions that were held in February
1976 at the Smithsonian Institution's Belmont
Conference Center supplemented by the
monthly deliberations of the Commission that
were held over a period of nearly four years. It
is a statement of basic ethical principles and
guidelines that should assist in resolving the
ethical problems that surround the conduct of
research with human subjects. By publishing
the Report in the *Federal Register*, and providing
reprints upon request, the Secretary intends that
it may be made readily available to scientists,
members of Institutional Review Boards, and
Federal employees. The two-volume Appendix,
containing the lengthy reports of experts and
specialists who assisted the Commission in
fulfilling this part of its charge, is available as

DHEW Publication No. (OS) 78-0013 and No. (OS) 78-0014, for sale by the Superintendent of Documents, U.S. Government Printing Office, Washington, D.C. 20402.

Unlike most other reports of the Commission, the Belmont Report does not make specific recommendations for administrative action by the Secretary of Health, Education, and Welfare. Rather, the Commission recommended that the Belmont Report be adopted in its entirety, as a statement of the Department's policy. The Department requests public comment on this recommendation.

National Commission for the Protection of Human Subjects of Biomedical and Behavioral Research

Members of the Commission

Kenneth John Ryan, M.D., Chairman, Chief of Staff, Boston Hospital for Women.

Joseph V. Brady, Ph.D., Professor of Behavioral Biology, Johns Hopkins University.

Robert E. Cooke, M.D., President, Medical College of Pennsylvania.

Dorothy I. Height, President, National Council of Negro Women, Inc.

Albert R. Jonsen, Ph.D., Associate Professor of Bioethics, University of California at San Francisco.

Patricia King, J.D., Associate Professor of Law, Georgetown University Law Center.

Karen Lebacqz, Ph.D., Associate Professor of Christian Ethics, Pacific School of Religion.

***David W. Louisell, J.D., Professor of Law, University of California at Berkeley.

Donald W. Seldin, M.D., Professor and Chairman, Department of Internal Medicine, University of Texas at Dallas.

***Eliot Stellar, Ph.D.,

Provost of the University and Professor of Physiological Psychology, University of Pennsylvania.

***Robert H. Turtle, LL.B., Attorney, VomBaur, Coburn, Simmons & Turtle, Washington, D.C.

*** Deceased.

Table of Contents

Ethical Principles & Guidelines for Research Involving Human Subjects

Scientific research has produced substantial social benefits. It has also posed some troubling ethical questions. Public attention was drawn to these questions by reported abuses of human subjects in biomedical experiments, especially during the Second World War. During the Nuremberg War Crime Trials, the Nuremberg code was drafted as a set of standards for judging physicians and scientists who had conducted biomedical experiments on concentration camp prisoners. This code became the prototype of many later codes[1] intended to assure that research involving human subjects would be carried out in an ethical manner.

The codes consist of rules, some general, others specific, that guide the investigators or the reviewers of research in their work. Such rules often are inadequate to cover complex situations; at times they come into conflict, and they are frequently difficult to interpret or apply. Broader ethical principles will provide a basis on which specific rules may be formulated, criticized and interpreted.

Three principles, or general prescriptive judgments, that are relevant to research involving human subjects are identified in this statement. Other principles may also be relevant. These three are comprehensive, however, and are stated at a level of generalization that should assist scientists, subjects, reviewers and interested citizens to understand the ethical issues inherent in research involving human subjects. These principles cannot always be applied so as to resolve beyond dispute particular ethical problems. The objective is to provide an analytical framework that will guide the resolution of ethical problems arising from research involving human subjects.

This statement consists of a distinction between research and practice, a discussion of the three basic ethical principles, and remarks about the application of these principles.

Part A: Boundaries between Practice & Research

A. Boundaries between Practice and Research

It is important to distinguish between biomedical and behavioral research, on the one hand, and the practice of accepted therapy on the other, in order to know what activities ought to undergo review for the protection of human subjects of research. The distinction between research and practice is blurred partly because both often occur together (as in research designed to evaluate a therapy) and partly because notable departures from standard practice are often called "experimental" when the terms "experimental" and "research" are not carefully defined.

For the most part, the term "practice" refers to interventions that are designed solely to enhance the well-being of an individual patient or client and that have a reasonable expectation of success. The purpose of medical or behavioral practice is to provide diagnosis, preventive treatment or therapy to particular individuals.[2] By contrast, the term "research" designates an activity designed to test an hypothesis, permit conclusions to be drawn, and thereby to develop or contribute to generalizable knowledge (expressed, for example, in theories, principles, and statements of relationships). Research is usually described in a formal protocol that sets forth an objective and a set of procedures designed to reach that objective.

When a clinician departs in a significant way from standard or accepted practice, the innovation does not, in and of itself, constitute research. The fact that a procedure is "experimental," in the sense of new, untested or different, does not automatically place it in the category of research. Radically new procedures of this description should, however, be made the object of formal research at an early stage in order to determine whether they are safe and effective. Thus, it is the responsibility of medical practice committees, for example, to insist that a major innovation be incorporated into a formal research project.[3]

Research and practice may be carried on together when research is designed to evaluate the safety and efficacy of a therapy. This need not cause any confusion regarding whether or not the activity requires review; the general rule is that if there is any element of research in an activity, that activity should undergo review for the protection of human subjects.

Part B: Basic Ethical Principles

B. Basic Ethical Principles

The expression "basic ethical principles" refers to those general judgments that serve as a basic justification for the many particular ethical prescriptions and evaluations of human actions. Three basic principles, among those generally accepted in our cultural tradition, are particularly relevant to the ethics of research involving human subjects: the principles of respect of persons, beneficence and justice.

1. Respect for Persons

Respect for persons incorporates at least two ethical convictions: first, that individuals should be treated as autonomous agents, and second, that persons with diminished autonomy are entitled to protection. The principle of respect for persons thus divides into two separate moral requirements: the requirement to acknowledge autonomy and the requirement to protect those with diminished autonomy.

An autonomous person is an individual capable of deliberation about personal goals and of acting under the direction of such deliberation. To respect autonomy is to give weight to autonomous persons' considered opinions and choices while refraining from obstructing their actions unless they are clearly detrimental to others. To show lack of respect for an autonomous agent is to repudiate that person's considered judgments, to deny an individual the freedom to act on those considered judgments, or to withhold information necessary to make a considered judgment, when there are no compelling reasons to do so.

However, not every human being is capable of self-determination. The capacity for self-determination matures during an individual's life, and some individuals lose this capacity wholly or in part because of illness, mental disability, or circumstances that severely restrict liberty. Respect for the immature and the incapacitated may require protecting them as they mature or while they are incapacitated.

Some persons are in need of extensive protection, even to the point of excluding them from activities which may harm them; other persons require little protection beyond making sure they undertake activities freely and with awareness of possible adverse consequence. The extent of protection afforded should depend upon the risk of harm and the likelihood of benefit. The judgment that any individual lacks autonomy should be periodically reevaluated and will vary in different situations.

In most cases of research involving human subjects, respect for persons demands that subjects enter into the research voluntarily and with adequate information. In some situations, however, application of the principle is not obvious. The involvement of prisoners as subjects of research provides an instructive example. On the one hand, it would seem that the principle of respect for persons requires that prisoners not be deprived of the opportunity to volunteer for research. On the other hand, under prison conditions they may be subtly coerced or unduly influenced to engage in research activities for which they would not otherwise volunteer. Respect for persons would then dictate that prisoners be protected. Whether to allow prisoners to "volunteer" or to "protect" them presents a dilemma. Respecting persons, in most hard cases, is often a matter of balancing competing claims urged by the principle of respect itself.

2. Beneficence

Persons are treated in an ethical manner not only by respecting their decisions and protecting them from harm, but also by making efforts to secure their well-being. Such treatment falls under the principle of beneficence. The term "beneficence" is often understood to cover acts of kindness or charity that go beyond strict obligation. In this document, beneficence is understood in a stronger sense, as an obligation. Two general rules have been formulated as complementary expressions of beneficent actions in this sense: (1) do not harm and (2) maximize possible benefits and minimize possible harms.

The Hippocratic maxim "do no harm" has long been a fundamental principle of medical ethics. Claude Bernard extended it to the realm of research, saying that one should not injure one person regardless of the benefits that might come to others. However, even avoiding harm requires learning what is harmful; and, in the process of obtaining this information, persons may be exposed to risk of harm. Further, the Hippocratic Oath requires physicians to benefit their patients "according to their best judgment." Learning what will in fact benefit may require exposing persons to risk. The problem posed by these imperatives is to decide when it is justifiable to seek certain benefits despite the risks involved, and when the benefits should be foregone because of the risks.

The obligations of beneficence affect both individual investigators and society at large, because they extend both to particular research projects and to the entire enterprise of research. In the case of particular projects, investigators and members of their institutions are obliged to give forethought to the maximization of benefits and the reduction of risk that might occur from the research investigation. In the case of scientific research in general, members of the larger society are obliged to recognize the longer term benefits and risks that may result from the improvement of knowledge and from the development of novel medical, psychotherapeutic, and social procedures.

The principle of beneficence often occupies a well-defined justifying role in many areas of research involving human subjects. An example is found in research involving children. Effective ways of treating childhood diseases and fostering healthy development are benefits that serve to justify research involving children—even when individual research subjects are not direct beneficiaries. Research also makes it possible to avoid the harm that may result from the application of previously accepted routine practices that on closer investigation turn out to be dangerous. But the role of the principle of beneficence is not always so unambiguous. A difficult ethical problem remains, for example, about research that presents more than minimal risk without immediate prospect of direct benefit to the children involved. Some have argued that such research is inadmissible, while others have pointed out that this limit would rule out much research promising great benefit to children in the future. Here again, as with all hard cases, the different claims covered by the principle of beneficence may come into conflict and force difficult choices.

3. Justice

Who ought to receive the benefits of research and bear its burdens? This is a question of justice, in the sense of "fairness in distribution" or "what is deserved." An injustice occurs when some benefit to which a person is entitled is denied without good reason or when some burden is imposed unduly. Another way of conceiving the principle of justice is that equals ought to be treated equally. However, this statement requires explication. Who is equal and who is unequal? What considerations justify departure from equal distribution? Almost all commentators allow that distinctions based on experience, age, deprivation, competence, merit and position do sometimes constitute criteria justifying differential treatment for certain purposes. It is necessary, then, to explain in what respects people should be treated equally. There are several widely accepted formulations of just ways to distribute burdens and benefits. Each formulation mentions some relevant property on the basis of which burdens and benefits should be distributed. These formulations are **(1)** to each person an equal share, **(2)** to each person according to individual need, **(3)** to each person according to individual effort, **(4)** to each person according to societal contribution, and **(5)** to each person according to merit.

Questions of justice have long been associated with social practices such as punishment, taxation and political representation. Until recently these questions have not generally been associated with scientific research. However, they are foreshadowed even in the earliest reflections on the ethics of research involving human subjects. For example, during the 19th and early 20th centuries the burdens of serving as research subjects fell largely upon poor ward patients, while the benefits of improved medical care flowed primarily to private patients. Subsequently, the exploitation of unwilling prisoners as research subjects in Nazi concentration camps was condemned as a particularly flagrant injustice. In this country, in the 1940s, the Tuskegee syphilis study used disadvantaged, rural black men to study the untreated course of a disease that is by no means confined to that population. These subjects were deprived of demonstrably effective treatment in order not to interrupt the project, long after such treatment became generally available.

Against this historical background, it can be seen how conceptions of justice are relevant to research involving human subjects. For example, the selection of research subjects needs to be scrutinized in order to determine whether some classes (e.g., welfare patients, particular racial and ethnic minorities, or persons confined to institutions) are being systematically selected simply because of their easy availability, their compromised position, or their manipulability, rather than for reasons directly related to the problem being studied. Finally, whenever research supported by public funds leads to the development of therapeutic devices and procedures, justice demands both that these not provide advantages only to those who can afford them and that such research should not unduly involve persons from groups unlikely to be among the beneficiaries of subsequent applications of the research.

C. Applications

Applications of the general principles to the conduct of research leads to consideration of the following requirements: informed consent, risk/benefit assessment, and the selection of subjects of research.

1. Informed Consent

Respect for persons requires that subjects, to the degree that they are capable, be given the opportunity to choose what shall or shall not happen to them. This opportunity is provided when adequate standards for informed consent are satisfied.

While the importance of informed consent is unquestioned, controversy prevails over the nature and possibility of an informed consent. Nonetheless, there is widespread agreement that the consent process can be analyzed as containing three elements: information, comprehension and voluntariness.

Information. Most codes of research establish specific items for disclosure intended to assure that subjects are given sufficient information. These items generally include: the research procedure, their purposes, risks and anticipated benefits, alternative procedures (where therapy is involved), and a statement offering the subject the opportunity to ask questions and to withdraw at any time from the research. Additional items have been proposed, including how subjects are selected, the person responsible for the research, etc.

However, a simple listing of items does not answer the question of what the standard should be for judging how much and what sort of information should be provided. One standard frequently invoked in medical practice, namely the information commonly provided by practitioners in the field or in the locale, is inadequate since research takes place precisely when a common understanding does not exist. Another standard, currently popular in malpractice law, requires the practitioner to reveal the information that reasonable persons would wish to know in order to make a decision regarding their care. This, too, seems insufficient since the research subject, being in essence a volunteer, may wish to know considerably more about risks gratuitously undertaken than do patients who deliver themselves into the hand of a clinician for needed care. It may be that a standard of "the reasonable volunteer" should be proposed: the extent and nature of information should be such that persons, knowing that the procedure is neither necessary for their care nor perhaps fully understood, can decide whether they wish to participate in the furthering of knowledge. Even when some direct benefit to them is anticipated, the subjects should understand clearly the range of risk and the voluntary nature of participation.

A special problem of consent arises where informing subjects of some pertinent aspect of the research is likely to impair the validity of the research. In many cases, it is sufficient to indicate to subjects that they are being invited to participate in research of which some features will not be revealed until the research is concluded. In all cases of research involving incomplete disclosure, such research is justified only if it is clear that (1) incomplete disclosure is truly necessary to accomplish the goals of the research, (2) there are no undisclosed risks to subjects that are more than minimal, and (3) there is an adequate plan for debriefing subjects, when appropriate, and for dissemination of research results to them. Information about risks should never be withheld for the purpose of eliciting the cooperation of subjects, and truthful answers should always be given to direct questions about the research. Care should be taken to distinguish cases in which disclosure would destroy or invalidate the research from cases in which disclosure would simply inconvenience the investigator.

Comprehension. The manner and context in which information is conveyed is as important as the information itself. For example, presenting information in a disorganized and rapid fashion, allowing too little time for consideration or curtailing opportunities for questioning, all may adversely affect a subject's ability to make an informed choice.

Because the subject's ability to understand is a function of intelligence, rationality, maturity and language, it is necessary to adapt the presentation of the information to the subject's capacities.

Investigators are responsible for ascertaining that the subject has comprehended the information. While there is always an obligation to ascertain that the information about risk to subjects is complete and adequately comprehended, when the risks are more serious, that obligation increases. On occasion, it may be suitable to give some oral or written tests of comprehension.

Special provision may need to be made when comprehension is severely limited — for example, by conditions of immaturity or mental disability. Each class of subjects that one might consider as incompetent (e.g., infants and young children, mentally disable patients, the terminally ill and the comatose) should be considered on its own terms. Even for these persons, however, respect requires giving them the opportunity to choose, to the extent they are able, whether or not to participate in research. The objections of these subjects to involvement should be honored, unless the research entails providing them a therapy unavailable elsewhere. Respect for persons also requires seeking the permission of other parties in order to protect the subjects from harm. Such persons are thus respected both by acknowledging their own wishes and by the use of third parties to protect them from harm.

The third parties chosen should be those who are most likely to understand the incompetent subject's situation and to act in that person's best interest. The person authorized to act on behalf of the subject should be given an opportunity to observe the research as it proceeds in order to be able to withdraw the subject from the research, if such action appears in the subject's best interest.

Voluntariness. An agreement to participate in research constitutes a valid consent only if voluntarily given. This element of informed consent requires conditions free of coercion and undue influence. Coercion occurs when an overt threat of harm is intentionally presented by one person to another in order to obtain compliance. Undue influence, by contrast, occurs through an offer of an excessive, unwarranted, inappropriate or improper reward or other overture in order to obtain compliance. Also, inducements that would ordinarily be acceptable may become undue influences if the subject is especially vulnerable.

Unjustifiable pressures usually occur when persons in positions of authority or commanding influence—especially where possible sanctions are involved—urge a course of action for a subject. A continuum of such influencing factors exists, however, and it is impossible to state precisely where justifiable persuasion ends and undue influence begins. But undue influence would include actions such as manipulating a person's choice through the controlling influence of a close relative and threatening to withdraw health services to which an individual would otherwise be entitled.

2. Assessment of Risks and Benefits

The assessment of risks and benefits requires a careful arrayal of relevant data, including, in some cases, alternative ways of obtaining the benefits sought in the research. Thus, the assessment presents both an opportunity and a responsibility to gather systematic and comprehensive information about proposed research. For the investigator, it is a means to examine whether the proposed research is properly designed. For a review committee, it is a method for determining whether the risks that will be presented to subjects are justified. For prospective subjects, the assessment will assist the determination whether or not to participate.

The Nature and Scope of Risks and Benefits. The requirement that research be justified on the basis of a favorable risk/benefit assessment bears a close relation to the principle of beneficence, just as the moral requirement that informed consent be obtained is derived primarily from the principle of respect for persons. The term "risk" refers to a possibility that harm may occur. However, when expressions such as "small risk" or "high risk" are used, they usually refer (often ambiguously) to both the chance (probability) of experiencing a harm and the severity (magnitude) of the envisioned harm.

The term "benefit" is used in the research context to refer to something of positive value related to health or welfare. Unlike "risk," "benefit" is not a term that expresses probabilities. Risk is properly contrasted to probability of benefits, and benefits are properly contrasted with harms rather than risks of harm. Accordingly, so-called risk/benefit assessments are concerned with the probabilities and magnitudes of possible harm and anticipated benefits. Many kinds of possible harms and benefits need to be taken into account. There are, for example, risks of psychological harm, physical harm, legal harm, social harm and economic harm and the corresponding benefits. While the most likely types of harms to research subjects are those of psychological or physical pain or injury, other possible kinds should not be overlooked.

Risks and benefits of research may affect the individual subjects, the families of the individual subjects, and society at large (or special groups of subjects in society). Previous codes and Federal regulations have required that risks to subjects be outweighed by the sum of both the anticipated benefit to the subject, if any, and the anticipated benefit to society in the form of knowledge to be gained from the research. In balancing these different elements, the risks and benefits affecting the immediate research subject will normally carry special weight. On the other hand, interests other than those of the subject may on some occasions be sufficient by themselves to justify the risks involved in the research, so long as the subject's rights have been protected. Beneficence thus requires that we protect against risk of harm to subjects and also that we be concerned about the loss of the substantial benefits that might be gained from research.

The Systematic Assessment of Risks and Benefits. It is commonly said that benefits and risks must be "balanced" and shown to be "in a favorable ratio." The metaphorical character of these terms draws attention to the difficulty of making precise judgments. Only on rare occasions will quantitative techniques be available for the scrutiny of research protocols. However, the idea of systematic, nonarbitrary analysis of risks and benefits should be emulated insofar as possible. This ideal requires those making decisions about the justifiability of research to be thorough in the accumulation and assessment of information about all aspects of the research, and to consider alternatives systematically. This procedure renders the assessment of research more rigorous and precise, while making communication between review board members and investigators less subject to misinterpretation, misinformation and conflicting judgments. Thus, there should first be a determination of the validity of the presuppositions of the research; then the nature, probability and magnitude of risk should be distinguished with as much clarity as possible. The method of ascertaining risks should be explicit, especially where there is no alternative to the use of such vague categories as small or slight risk. It should also be determined whether an investigator's estimates of the probability of harm or benefits are reasonable, as judged by known facts or other available studies.

Finally, assessment of the justifiability of research should reflect at least the following considerations: **(i)** Brutal or inhumane treatment of human subjects is never morally justified. **(ii)** Risks should be reduced to those necessary to achieve the research objective. It should be determined whether it is in fact necessary to use human subjects at all. Risk can perhaps never be entirely eliminated, but it can often be reduced by careful attention to alternative procedures. **(iii)** When research involves significant risk of serious impairment, review committees should be extraordinarily insistent on the justification of the risk (looking usually to the likelihood of benefit to the subject — or, in some rare cases, to the manifest voluntariness of the participation). **(iv)** When vulnerable populations are involved in research, the appropriateness of involving them should itself be demonstrated. A number of variables go into such judgments, including the nature and degree of risk, the condition of the particular population involved, and the nature and level of the anticipated benefits. **(v)** Relevant risks and benefits must be thoroughly arrayed in documents and procedures used in the informed consent process.

3. Selection of Subjects

Just as the principle of respect for persons finds expression in the requirements for consent, and the principle of beneficence in risk/benefit assessment, the principle of justice gives rise to moral requirements that there be fair procedures and outcomes in the selection of research subjects.

Justice is relevant to the selection of subjects of research at two levels: the social and the individual. Individual justice in the selection of subjects would require that researchers exhibit fairness: thus, they should not offer potentially beneficial research only to some patients who are in their favor or select only "undesirable" persons for risky research. Social justice requires that distinction be drawn between classes of subjects that ought, and ought not, to participate in any particular kind of research, based on the ability of members of that class to bear burdens and on the appropriateness of placing further burdens on already burdened persons. Thus, it can be considered a matter of social justice that there is an order of preference in the selection of classes of subjects (e.g., adults before children) and that some classes of potential subjects (e.g., the institutionalized mentally infirm or prisoners) may be involved as research subjects, if at all, only on certain conditions.

Injustice may appear in the selection of subjects, even if individual subjects are selected fairly by investigators and treated fairly in the course of research. Thus injustice arises from social, racial, sexual and cultural biases institutionalized in society. Thus, even if individual researchers are treating their research subjects fairly, and even if IRBs are taking care to assure that subjects are selected fairly within a particular institution, unjust social patterns may nevertheless appear in the overall distribution of the burdens and benefits of research. Although individual institutions or investigators may not be able to resolve a problem that is pervasive in their social setting, they can consider distributive justice in selecting research subjects.

Some populations, especially institutionalized ones, are already burdened in many ways by their infirmities and environments. When research is proposed that involves risks and does not include a therapeutic component, other less burdened classes of persons should be called upon first to accept these risks of research, except where the research is directly related to the specific conditions of the class involved. Also, even though public funds for research may often flow in the same directions as public funds for health care, it seems unfair that populations dependent on public health care constitute a pool of preferred research subjects if more advantaged populations are likely to be the recipients of the benefits.

One special instance of injustice results from the involvement of vulnerable subjects. Certain groups, such as racial minorities, the economically disadvantaged, the very sick, and the institutionalized, may continually be sought as research subjects, owing to their ready availability in settings where research is conducted. Given their dependent status and their frequently compromised capacity for free consent, they should be protected against the danger of being involved in research solely for administrative convenience, or because they are easy to manipulate as a result of their illness or socioeconomic condition.

Notes

1. Since 1945, various codes for the proper and responsible conduct of human experimentation in medical research have been adopted by different organizations. The best known of these codes are the Nuremberg Code of 1947, the Helsinki Declaration of 1964 (revised in 1975), and the 1971 Guidelines (codified into Federal Regulations in 1974) issued by the U.S. Department of Health, Education, and Welfare. Codes for the conduct of social and behavioral research have also been adopted, the best known being that of the American Psychological Association, published in 1973.

2. Although practice usually involves interventions designed solely to enhance the well-being of a particular individual, interventions are sometimes applied to one individual for the enhancement of the well-being of another (e.g., blood donation, skin grafts, organ transplants), or an intervention may have the dual purpose of enhancing the well-being of a particular individual, and, at the same time, providing some benefit to others (e.g., vaccination, which protects both the person who is vaccinated and society generally). The fact that some forms of practice have elements other than immediate benefit to the individual receiving an intervention, however, should not confuse the general distinction between research and practice. Even when a procedure applied in practice may benefit some other person, it remains an intervention designed to enhance the well-being of a particular individual or groups of individuals; thus, it is practice and need not be reviewed as research.

3. Because the problems related to social experimentation may differ substantially from those of biomedical and behavioral research, the Commission specifically declines to make any policy determination regarding such research at this time. Rather, the Commission believes that the problem ought to be addressed by one of its successor bodies.

The Origins and Evolution of the Belmont Report

Tom L. Beauchamp

When, on December 22, 1976, I agreed to join the staff of the National Commission for the Protection of Human Subjects of Biomedical and Behavioral Research, my first and only major assignment was to write "The Belmont Paper," as it was then called. At the time, I had already drafted substantial parts of *Principles of Biomedical Ethics* with Jim Childress.[1] Subsequent to my appointment, the two manuscripts were drafted simultaneously, often side by side, the one inevitably influencing the other.

I here explain how the "Belmont Paper" evolved into the *Belmont Report*.[2] I will also correct some common but mistaken speculation about the emergence of frameworks of principles in research ethics and of the connections between *Belmont* and *Principles*.

The Beginnings of *Belmont*

The idea for the "Belmont Paper" originally grew from a vision of shared moral principles governing research that emerged during a breakout session at a four-day retreat held February 13–16, 1976, at the Smithsonian Institution's Belmont Conference Center in Maryland.[3] Earlier in this volume Albert Jonsen reports on the contributions of Stephen Toulmin, Karen Lebacqz, Joe Brady, and others. This meeting predates my work on the *Belmont Report*, and I leave it to Jonsen and others in attendance to relate these events.

A few months after this conference at Belmont, I received two phone calls, the first from Toulmin, staff philosopher at the National Commission, and the second from Michael Yesley, staff director. They asked me to write a paper for the National Commission on the nature and scope of the notion of justice. Yesley told me that the commissioners sought help in understanding theories of justice and their application to moral problems of human subject research. I wrote this paper and assumed that my work for the National Commission was concluded.[4]

However, shortly after I submitted the paper, Toulmin returned to fulltime teaching at the University of Chicago, and Yesley inquired whether I was available to replace him on the staff. This appointment met some resistance. Two commissioners who later became my close friends—namely, Brady and Donald Seldin

—were less than enthusiastic about my appointment. Nonetheless, Yesley prevailed, likely with the help of Chairperson Kenneth Ryan and my colleague Patricia King, and I joined the National Commission staff.

On my first morning in the office, Yesley told me that he was assigning me the task of writing the "Belmont Paper."[5] I asked Yesley what the task was. He pointed out that the National Commission had been charged by Congress to investigate the ethics of research and to *explore basic ethical principles.*[6] Members of the staff were at work on various topics in research ethics, he reported, but no one was working on basic principles. He said that an opening round of discussions of the principles had been held at the Belmont retreat. The National Commission had delineated a rough schema of three basic ethical principles: respect for persons, beneficence, and justice. I asked Yesley what these moral notions meant to the commissioners, to which he responded that he had no well-formed idea and that it was my job to figure out what the commissioners meant—or, more likely, to figure out what they should have meant.

So, I found myself with the job of giving shape and substance to something called the "Belmont Paper," though at that point I had never heard of Belmont or the paper. It struck me as an odd title for a publication. Moreover, this document had never been mentioned during my interview for the job or at any other time until Yesley gave me the assignment. My immediate sense was that I was the new kid on the block and had been given the dregs of National Commission work. I had thought, when I decided to join the National Commission staff, that I would be working on the ethics of psychosurgery and research involving children—heated and perplexing controversies at the time. I was chagrined to learn that I was to write something on which no one else was working and that had its origins in a retreat that I had not attended. Moreover, the mandate to do the work had its roots in a federal law that I had not until that morning seen.

Yesley proceeded to explain that no one had yet worked seriously on the sections of the report on *principles* because no one knew what to do with it. This moment of honesty was not heartening, but I was not discouraged either, because Childress and I were at that time well into the writing of our book on the role of basic principles in biomedical ethics. It intrigued me that we had worked relatively little on research ethics, which was the sole focus of the National Commission. I saw in my early conversations with Yesley that these two projects — *Principles* and *Belmont* — had many points of intersecting interest and could be mutually beneficial.

Yesley also gave me some hope by saying that a crude draft of the "Belmont Paper" already existed, though a twinkle in his eye warned me not to expect too much. That same morning I read the "Belmont draft."[7] Scarce could a new recruit have been more dismayed. So little was said about the principles that to call it a "draft" of principles is like calling a dictionary entry a scholarly treatise. Some sections were useful, especially a few pages that had been written largely by Robert Levine on the subject of "The Boundaries Between Biomedical and Behavioral Research and Accepted and Routine Practice" (later revised under the subtitle "Boundaries Between Practice and Research" and made the first section of the *Belmont Report)*, but this draft of *Belmont* had almost nothing to say about the principles that were slated to be its heart.

In the next few weeks virtually everything in this draft pertaining to principles would be thrown away either because it contained too little on principles or because it had too much on peripheral issues. At the time, these peripheral issues constituted almost the entire document (with the exception of the section written by Levine, which was not peripheral, but also not on principles). The major topics addressed were the National Commission's mandate, appropriate review mechanisms, compensation for injury, national and international regulations and codes, research design, and other items that did not belong in the "Belmont Paper."

These topics, being peripheral, were therefore eliminated. Except for Levine's section on boundaries, everything in this draft landed on the cutting-room floor.[8]

Once the Belmont "draft" was left with nothing in the section on principles, Yesley suggested that I might find the needed content from the massive compendium on research titled *Experimentation with Human Beings*, edited by Jay Katz with the assistance of Alexander Capron and Eleanor Swift Glass.[9] Drawn from sociology, psychology, medicine, and law, this book was at the time the most thorough collection of materials on research ethics and law. Yesley informed me that I should endeavor to learn all the information presented in this book, but after days of poring over this rich resource, I found that it offered virtually nothing on *principles* suitable for an analytical discussion of research ethics. The various codes and statements by professional associations found in this book had occasional connections with my task and with the National Commission's objectives, but only distant ones.[10]

The Historical Origins of the Principles of the *Belmont* Report

Fortunately, Childress and I had gathered a useful collection of materials on principles and theories, largely in the writings of philosophers. I had been influenced by the writings of W. D. Ross and William Frankena. My training led me to turn to these and other philosophical treatments, which had already proved helpful in my work on *Principles*.

However, it would be misleading to suggest that the principles featured in the *Belmont Report* derived from the writings of philosophers. Their grounding is ultimately in what I would eventually call (following Alan Donagan) "the common morality." The *Belmont Report* makes reference to "our cultural tradition" as the basis of its principles, and it is clear that these principles derive from the common morality rather than a particular philosophical work or tradition. However, what *Belmont* means by our "tradition" is unclear, and I believe the import of the *Belmont* principles cannot be tied to a particular tradition, but rather to a conviction that there is a universally valid point of view. I believe, and I think that the commissioners believed, that these principles are norms shared by all morally decent persons.

The commissioners almost certainly believed that these principles are already embedded in public morality and are presupposed in the formulation of public and institutional policies. The principles do not deviate from what every morally sensitive person knows to be right, based on their own moral training and experience. That is, every morally sensitive person believes that a moral way of life requires that we respect persons and take into account their well-being in our actions. *Belmont's* principles are so woven into the fabric of morality in morally sensitive cultures that no responsible research investigator could conduct research without reference to them.[11]

The Relationship Between the *Belmont* Principles and the Principles in *Principles of Biomedical Ethics*

Many have supposed that the *Belmont Report* provided the starting point and the abstract framework for *Principles of Biomedical Ethics*.[12] They have wrongly assumed that *Belmont* preceded and grounded *Principles*.[13] The two works were written simultaneously, the one inevitably influencing the other.[14] There was reciprocity in the drafting, and influence ran bilaterally. I was often simultaneously drafting material on the same principle or topic both for the National Commission and for my colleague

Childress, while he was at the same time writing material for me to inspect. I would routinely write parts of the *Belmont Report* during the day at the National Commission headquarters on Westbard Avenue in Bethesda, then go to my office at Georgetown in the evening and draft parts of chapters for Childress to review. Despite their entirely independent origins, these projects grew up and matured together.

Once I grasped the moral vision of the National Commission initiated at Belmont, I could see that Childress and I had major substantive disagreements with the National Commission. The names of the principles articulated in the *Belmont Report* bear notable similarities to some of the names Childress and I were using and continued to use, but the two schemas of principles are far from constituting a uniform name, number, or conception. Indeed, the two frameworks are not consistent.

I thought at the time, and still do, that the National Commission was confused in the way it delineated the principle of respect for persons. It seemed to blend two independent principles: a principle of respect for autonomy and a principle of protecting and avoiding the causation of harm to incompetent persons. Furthermore, Childress and I both thought that we should stick to our thesis that the principle of beneficence must be distinguished from the principle of nonmaleficence, though the National Commission failed to make any such distinction. This matter was connected to another problem that later bothered me, namely, that the National Commission had an all too utilitarian vision of beneficence—one with inadequate internal controls in its moral framework to protect subjects against abuse when there was the promise of major benefit for other sick or disabled persons.

The differences between the philosophy in *Principles* and the National Commission's views in *Belmont* have occasionally been the subject of published commentary.[15] Some commentators correctly see that we developed substantially different moral visions and that neither approach

was erected on the foundations of the other. By early 1977, I had come to the view that the National Commission, especially in the person of its chair, Kenneth Ryan, was sufficiently rigid in its vision of the principles that there was no way to substantially alter the National Commission's conception, although I thought that all three principles were either defective or underanalyzed. From this point forward, I attempted to analyze principles for the National Commission exclusively as I thought the commissioners would find acceptable. *Principles of Biomedical Ethics* became the only work that reflected my own deepest philosophical convictions about principles.

The Drafting and Redrafting of *Belmont*

While Yesley gave me free rein in the drafting and redrafting of *Belmont*, the drafts were always subject to revisions and improvements made by the commissioners and staff members.[16] All members of the staff did their best to formulate ideas that were responsive to changes suggested by the commissioners. Commissioner Seldin encouraged me with as much vigor as he could muster (which was—and remains today—considerable) to make my drafts as philosophical as possible. Seldin wanted some Mill here, some Kant there, and the signature of philosophical argument sprinkled throughout the document. I tried this style, but other commissioners wanted a streamlined document and minimalist statement relatively free of the trappings of philosophy. Seldin, Yesley, and I ultimately relented,[17] and bolder philosophical defenses of the principles were gradually stripped from the body of *Belmont*.

Public deliberations in National Commission meetings were a staple source of ideas, but a few commissioners spoke privately to me or to Yesley about desired changes, and a few commissioners proposed changes to Assistant Staff

Director Barbara Mishkin, who passed them on to me. Most of these suggestions were accepted, and a serious attempt was made to implement them. In this respect, the writing of this document was a joint product of commissioner-staff interactions. However, most of the revisions made by the commissioners (other than through their comments in public deliberations) concerned small matters, and the commissioners were rarely involved in making written changes.

One meeting on *Belmont* involving a few members of the staff and a few commissioners occurred in September 1977 in the belvedere—rooftop study—of Jonsen's home in San Francisco. The small group in attendance attempted to revise the "Belmont Paper" for presentation at the next meetings during which the commissioners were scheduled to debate it. As Jonsen reports in *The Birth of Bioethics* and in the present volume, the purpose of this meeting was to revisit previous drafts and deliberations of the commissioners.[18]

The history of drafting and redrafting that I have outlined may suggest that the document grew in size over time, but the reverse is true. The document grew quickly in the early drafting and then was contracted over time. I wrote much more for the National Commission about respect for persons, beneficence, and justice than eventually found its way into the *Belmont Report*. When various materials I had written were eliminated from *Belmont*, I would scoop up the reject piles and fashion them for *Principles of Biomedical Ethics*. Several late-written chunks of this book on research ethics were fashioned from the more philosophical, but abjured parts of what I wrote for the National Commission that never found its way into the final draft of *Belmont*.

Explicit and Implicit Ideas about an Applied Research Ethics

Michael Yesley deserves credit for one key organizing conception in this report. He and I were in almost daily discussion about the "Belmont Paper." We spent many hours discussing the best way to develop the principles, to express what the commissioners wanted to say, and even how to sneak in certain lines of thought that the commissioners might not notice. One late afternoon we were discussing the overall enterprise. We discussed each principle, whether the principles were truly independent, and how the principles related to the topics in research ethics under consideration by the National Commission. Yesley said, as a way of summarizing our reflections, "What these principles come to is really quite simple for our purposes: Respect for persons applies to informed consent, beneficence applies to risk-benefit assessment, and justice applies to the selection of subjects." Yesley had articulated the following abstract schema:

Principle of	Applies to	Guidelines for
Respect for Persons		Informed Consent
Beneficence		Risk-Benefit Assessment
Justice		Selection of Subjects

This schema may seem trifling; certainly it was already nascent in preexisting drafts of the report and in the National Commission's deliberations. But no one at the time had articulated the schema in precisely this way, and Yesley's summary was immensely helpful in peering through countless hours of discussion to see the underlying structure and commitment at work in the principles destined to be the backbone of *Belmont*. Yesley had captured what would soon become the major portion of the table of contents of the *Belmont Report*, as well as the rationale of its organization. I then attempted to draft the document so that the basic principles could be "applied" to develop guidelines in specific areas and could also serve as justification for guidelines.

In light of this schema, a general strategy emerged for handling problems of research ethics, namely, that each principle made moral demands in a specific domain of responsibility for research. For example, the principle of respect for persons demands informed and voluntary consent. Under this conception, the *purpose* of consent provisions is not protection from risk, as many earlier federal policies seemed to imply, but the protection of autonomy and personal dignity, including the personal dignity of incompetent persons incapable of acting autonomously, for whose involvement a duly authorized third party must consent.

I wrote the sections on principles in the *Belmont Report* based on this model of each principle applying to a zone of moral concern. In this drafting, the focus of the document shifted to include not only abstract principles and their analysis but also a moral view that is considerably more concrete and meaningful for those engaged in the practice of research. Explication of the values being advanced was heavily influenced by the context of biomedicine (and rather less influenced by contexts of the social and behavioral sciences). *Belmont*, in this way, moved toward an applied, professional morality of research ethics.

Although *Belmont* takes this modest step in the direction of an applied research ethics, there was never any ambition or attempt to make this document specific and practical. This objective was to be accomplished by the other volumes the National Commission issued. *Belmont* was meant to be, and should be remembered as, a moral framework for research ethics. Commissioners and staff were always aware that this framework is too indeterminate *by itself* to decide practice or policy or to resolve moral conflicts. The process of making the general principles in *Belmont* sufficiently concrete is a

progressive process of reducing the indeterminateness and abstractness of the general principles to give them increased action-guiding capacity.[19] *Belmont* looks to educational institutions, professional associations, government agencies, and the like to provide the particulars of research ethics.

Principlism, Casuistry, or Both?

The final editing of the *Belmont Report* was done by three people in a small classroom at NIH.[20] Al Jonsen, Stephen Toulmin, and I were given this assignment by the National Commission. Some who have followed the later writings of Jonsen and Toulmin on casuistry may be surprised to learn that throughout the National Commission's deliberations, as well as in this final drafting, Jonsen and Toulmin contributed to the clarification of the *principles* in the report. There was never an objection by either that a strategy of using principles should be other than central to the National Commission's statement of its ethical framework. Jonsen repeats his support for these principles in the present volume.

However, Jonsen also says in this volume, "The commissioners believed as principlists; they worked as casuists." He is suggesting that the National Commission's deliberations constituted a casuistry of reasoning about historical and contemporary cases,[21] despite the commissioners' commitment to and frequent reference to *Belmont* principles. Jonsen and Toulmin once explicated this understanding of the National Commission's work as follows:

> The one thing [*individual* commissioners] could not agree on was *why* they agreed. ... Instead of securely established universal principles, ... giving them intellectual grounding for particular judgments about specific

kinds of cases, it was the other way around.

> The *locus of certitude* in the Commissioners' discussions ... lay in a shared perception of what was specifically at stake in particular kinds of human situations. ... That could never have been derived from the supposed theoretical certainty of the principles to which individual Commissioners appealed in their personal accounts.[22]

This interpretation gives insight into the National Commission, but it needs careful qualification to avoid misunderstanding. Casuistical reasoning more so than moral theory or universal abstraction often did function to forge agreement during National Commission deliberations. The commissioners appealed to particular cases and families of cases, and consensus was reached through agreement on cases and generalization from cases when agreement on an underlying theoretical rationale would have been impossible.[23] Commissioners would never have been able to agree on a single ethical theory, nor did they even attempt to buttress the *Belmont* principles with a theory. Jonsen and Toulmin's treatment of the National Commission is, in this regard, entirely reasonable, and a similar line of argument can be taken to explicate the methods of reasoning at work in other bioethics commissions.[24]

Nonetheless, this methodological appraisal is consistent with a firm commitment to moral principles; the commissioners, including Jonsen, were emphatic in their support of and appeals to the general moral principles delineated in the *Belmont Report*.[25] The transcripts of the National Commission's deliberations show a constant movement from principle to case, and from case to principle. Principles supported argument about how to handle a case, and precedent cases supported the importance of commitment to principles. Cases or examples favorable to one point of view were brought forward, and counterexamples then advanced. Principles

were invoked to justify the choice and use of both examples and counterexamples. On many occasions an argument was offered that a case judgment was irrelevant or immoral in light of the commitments of a principle.[26] The National Commission's deliberations and conclusions are best understood in terms of reasoning in which principles are interpreted and specified by the force of examples and counterexamples that emerge from experience with cases.

It is doubtful that Jonsen ever intended to deny this understanding of principles and their roles, despite the widely held view that casuistry dispenses with principles. Jonsen has said that "casuistic analysis does not deny the relevance of principle and theory,"[27] and, in an insightful statement in his later work, he has written that

> when maxims such as "Do no harm," or "Informed consent is obligatory," are invoked, they represent, as it were, cut-down versions of the major principles relevant to the topic, such as beneficence and autonomy, cut down to fit the nature of the topic and the kinds of circumstances that pertain to it.[28]

Jonsen goes on to point out that casuistry is "complementary to principles" and that "casuistry is not an alternative to principles: No sound casuistry can dispense with principles."[29]

Casuists and those who support frameworks of principles like those in *Belmont* and *Principles* should be able to agree that when they reflect on cases and policies, they rarely have in hand *either* principles that were formulated without reference to experience with cases *or* paradigm cases lacking a prior commitment to general norms. Only a false dilemma makes us choose between the National Commission as principlist or casuist. It was both.

Notes

This chapter was written for a conference on the *Belmont Report* held in Charlottesville, Virginia. It draws in part on my chapter in *The Story of Bioethics*, published by Georgetown University Press, 2003.

1. A contract for the book was issued by the Oxford University Press on August 19, 1976. The manuscript was completed in late 1977; galleys arrived in October 1978, bearing the 1979 copyright date.

2. See also *Appendices I and II* to the *Belmont Report*. The *Belmont Report* was completed in late 1977 and published on September 30, 1978. *The Belmont Report: Ethical Guidelines for the Protection of Human Subjects of Research* (Washington, DC: DHEW Publication OS 78-0012). It first appeared in the *Federal Register* on April 18, 1979.

   The National Commission for the Protection of Human Subjects of Biomedical and Behavioral Research was established July 12, 1974, under the National Research Act, Public Law 93-348, Title II. The first meeting was held December 3–4, 1974. The 43rd and final meeting was on September 8, 1978.

3. See the archives of the National Commission, 15th meeting, February 13–16,1976, vol. 15 A—a volume prepared for the Belmont meeting. This meeting book contains a "staffsummary" on the subject of "ethical principles" as well as expert papers prepared by Kurt Baier, Alasdair MacIntyre, James Childress, H. Tristram Engelhardt, Alvan Feinstein, and LeRoy Walters. The papers by Engelhardt and Walters most closely approximate the moral considerations ultimately treated in the "Belmont Paper," but neither quite matches the National Commission's three principles. Walters, however, comes very close to a formulation of the concerns in practical ethics to which the National Commission *applies* its principles.

All meeting books are housed in the archives of the Kennedy Institute of Ethics Library, storage facility, Georgetown University.

4. The paper was published as "Distributive Justice and Morally Relevant Differences" in *Appendix I to the Belmont Report*, pp. 6.1–6.20. This paper was distributed at the 22nd meeting of the National Commission, held in September 1976, seven months after the retreat at the Belmont Conference House.

5. My first day was the Saturday meeting of the National Commission on January 8, 1977. Yesley and I met the following Monday.

6. The National Research Act, P.L. 93-348, July 12, 1974. Congress charged the National Commission with recommending regulations to the Department of Health, Education, and Welfare (DHEW) to protect the rights of research subjects and developing ethical principles to govern the conduct of research. In this respect, the *Belmont Report* was at the core of the tasks the National Commission had been assigned by Congress. DHEWs conversion of its grants administration *policies* governing the conduct of research involving human subjects into formal *regulations* applicable to the entire department was relevant to the creation of the National Commission. In the U.S. Senate, Senator Edward Kennedy, with Jacob Javits's support, was calling for a permanent, *regulatory* commission independent of the National Institutes of Health (NIH) to protect the welfare and rights of human subjects. Paul Rogers in the House supported NIH in advocating that the commission be *advisory* only. Kennedy agreed to yield to Rogers if DHEW published satisfactory regulations. This compromise was accepted. Regulations were published on May 30, 1974; then, on July 12, 1974, P.L. 93-348 was modified to authorize the National Commission as an advisory body. Charles McCarthy helped me understand this history. For a useful framing of the more general regulatory history, see Joseph V. Brady

and Albert R. Jonsen (two commissioners), "The Evolution of Regulatory Influences on Research with Human Subjects," in *Human Subjects Research*, ed. Robert Greenwald, Mary Kay Ryan, and James E. Mulvihill, 3–18 (New York: Plenum Press, 1982).

7. This draft had a history beginning with the 16th meeting (March 12–14, 1976), which contained a draft dated March 1, 1976, and titled "Identification of Basic Ethical Principles." This document summarized the relevant historical background and set forth the three "underlying ethical principles" that came to form the National Commission's framework. Each principle was discussed in a single paragraph. This document was slightly recast in a draft of June 3, 1976 (prepared for the 19th meeting, June 11–13, 1976), in which the discussion of principles was shortened to little more than one page devoted to all three principles. Surprisingly, in the summary statement (p. 9), "respect for persons" is presented as the principle of "autonomy." No further draft is presented to the National Commission until ten months later, at the 29th meeting (April 8–9, 1977). I began work on the document in January 1977.

Transcripts of the National Commission's meetings are also available in the archives of the Kennedy Institute of Ethics at Georgetown University. See National Commission for the Protection of Human Subjects of Biomedical and Behavioral Research. Archived Materials 1974–78, General Category: "Transcript of the Meeting Proceedings" (for discussion of the "Belmont Paper" at the following meetings: February 11–13, 1977; July 8–9, 1977; April 14–15, 1978; and June 9–10, 1978).

8. Cf. the radical differences between the draft available at the 19th meeting (June 11–13, 1976) and the draft at the 29th meeting (April 8–9, 1977). The drafts show that the critical period that gave shape to the *Belmont* principles was the period between January and April 1977. Less dramatic

improvements were made between April 1977 and eventual publication more than a year later.

9. Jay Katz, with the assistance of Alexander Capron and Eleanor Glass, eds., *Experimentation with Human Beings* (New York: Russell Sage Foundation, 1972).

10. The first and only footnote in the *Belmont Report* is a reference to this background reading. Typical materials that I examined during this period include *United States v. Karl Brandt, Trials of War Criminals Before the Nuremberg Military Tribunals Under Control Council Law No. 10*, 1948–49, Military Tribunal I (Washington, DC: U.S. Government Printing Office, 1948–1949), vols, 1 and 2, reproduced in part in Katz, *Experimentation with Human Beings*, 292–306; American Medical Association, House of Delegates, Judicial Council, "Supplementary Report of the Judicial Council," *Journal of the American Medical Association* 132 (1946): 90; World Health Organization, 18th World Medical Assembly, Helsinki, Finland, "Declaration of Helsinki: Recommendations Guiding Medical Doctors in Biomedical Research Involving Human Subjects," *New England Journal of Medicine* 271 (1964): 473, reprinted in Katz, *Experimentation with Human Beings*, 312–13. Less helpful than I had hoped was Henry Beecher, "Some Guiding Principles for Clinical Investigation," *Journal of the American Medical Association* 195 (1966): 1135–36. For behavioral research, I started with Stuart E. Golann, "Ethical Standards for Psychology: Development and Revisions, 1938–1968," *Annals of the New York Academy of Sciences* 169 (1970): 398–405, and American Psychological Association, Inc., *Ethical Principles in the Conduct of Research with Human Participants* (Washington, DC: APA, 1973).

11. For a clearer presentation of this viewpoint in a later document by a government-initiated commission, see several chapters in Advisory Committee on Human Radiation

Experiments (ACHRE), *Final Report of the Advisory Committee on Human Radiation Experiments* (New York: Oxford University Press, 1996).

12. See, e.g., Eric Meslin et al., "Principlism and the Ethical Appraisal of Clinical Trials," *Bioethics* 9 (1995): 399–403; Bernard Gert, Charles M. Culver, and K. Danner Clouser, *Bioethics: A Return to Fundamentals* (New York: Oxford University Press, 1997), 72–74; and Jonathan D. Moreno, *Deciding Together: Bioethics and Consensus* (New York: Oxford University Press, 1995), 76–78. Meslin et al. say that "Beauchamp and Childress's *Principles of Biomedical Ethics* ... is the most rigorous presentation of the principles initially described in the *Belmont Report*" (p. 403). Gert et al. see *Principles* as having "emerged from the work of the National Commission" (p. 73). Moreno presumes that Beauchamp and Childress "brought the three *[Belmont]* principles into bioethical analysis more generally." The thesis that the idea of an abstract framework of principles for bioethics originated with the National Commission has been sufficiently prevalent that authors and lecturers have occasionally cited the principles as Childress and I have named and articulated them, and then felt comfortable in attributing these same principles to the National Commission.

13. The draft of *Belmont* that appeared in typescript for the National Commission meeting of December 2, 1977 (37th meeting) shows several similarities to various passages in the first edition of *Principles of Biomedical Ethics*. Childress and I had completed our manuscript by this date, but *Belmont* would be taken through five more drafts presented to the commissioners, the last being presented at the final (43rd) meeting (September 8, 1978).

14. Prior to my involvement with the National Commission, and prior to the Belmont retreat, Childress and I had lectured and written about principles of biomedical ethics. In

early 1976, coincidentally at about the same time of the Belmont retreat, Childress and I wrote a programmatic idea for the book (based on our lectures), which we submitted to the Oxford University Press. We had already developed a general conception of what later came to be called by some commentators "mid-level principles."

For more on the nature, history, and defensibility of a commitment to such mid-level principles in bioethics, see Gert, Culver, and Clouser, *Bioethics: A Return to Fundamentals*, 72ff; Beauchamp and David DeGrazia, "Principlism," in *Bioethics: A Philosophical Overview*, vol. 1 of *Handbook of the Philosophy of Medicine*, ed. George Khusfh (Dordrecht, Neth.: Kluwer, 2002); James Childress, "Ethical Theories, Principles, and Casuistry in Bioethics: An Interpretation and Defense of Principlism," in *Religious Methods and Resources in Bioethics*, ed. Paul F. Camenisch, 181–201 (Boston: Kluwer, 1994); Tom Beauchamp, "Principles and Other Emerging Paradigms for Bioethics," *Indiana Law Journal* 69 (1994): 1–17; Beauchamp, "The Four Principles Approach to Medical Ethics," in *Principles of Health Care Ethics*, ed. R. Gillon, 3–12 (London: John Wiley & Sons, 1994); Beauchamp, "The Role of Principles in Practical Ethics," in *Philosophical Perspectives on Bioethics*, ed. L. W. Sumner and J. Boyle (Toronto: University of Toronto Press, 1996); and Earl Winkler, "Moral Philosophy and Bioethics: Contextualism versus the Paradigm Theory," in *Philosophical Perspectives on Bioethics*, ed. L. W. Sumner and J. Boyle (Toronto: University of Toronto Press, 1996).

15. Particularly insightful is Ernest Marshall, "Does the Moral Philosophy of the *Belmont Report* Rest on a Mistake?" *IRB: A Review of Human Subjects Research* 8 (1986): 5–6. See also John Fletcher, "Abortion Politics, Science, and Research Ethics: Take Down the Wall of Separation," *Journal of Contemporary Health Law and Policy* 8 (1992):

95–121, esp. sect. 4, "Resources in Research Ethics: Adequacy of the *Belmont Report.*"

16. Albert Jonsen, a commissioner, reports in *The Birth of Bioethics* (New York: Oxford University Press, 1998) that I was "working with [Stephen] Toulmin on subsequent drafts" of the *Belmont Report* in 1977. Although I sat next to Stephen in National Commission meetings and conversed with him about many subjects during meetings of the National Commission throughout 1977, we never jointly drafted, worked on, or discussed *Belmont* until it was in near final form and already approved by the commissioners. Stephen had been assigned to a project on recombinant DNA and did not participate in *Belmont* drafts after I came to the National Commission.

17. Yesley was my constant critic, more so than anyone else. Seldin was my constant counsel, forever exhorting me to make the document more philosophically credible. Patricia King taught me more about the National Commission and its commissioners than anyone else. It was she who helped me understand why a really philosophical document was not the most desirable result.

18. Jonsen reports in *The Birth of Bioethics* (p. 103) that "the date is uncertain" of this meeting at his home, but the date is the afternoon of September 21 through September 23, 1977 (including travel period). Jonsen correctly remarks that one purpose of this meeting was to revisit "the February 1977 deliberations" of the commissioners, but he incorrectly reports that the meeting was called "to revise the June 1976 draft." Except for a section on boundaries written by Robert Levine, the June 1976 draft had been so heavily recast that *Belmont* was by September a completely different document. Seven months of continual redrafting of *Belmont* had occurred (from February to September 1977) prior to the meeting at his home. The National Commission did not discuss the draft reports at its meetings during those

seven months (the last discussion having occurred in February). However, "staff drafts" of the "Belmont Paper" were distributed at two meetings during this period, namely, the 29th meeting (April 8–9, 1977) and the 30th meeting (May 13–14, 1977). All drafts are now housed in the archives of the Kennedy Institute of Ethics Library.

19. See Henry S. Richardson, "Specifying Norms as a Way to Resolve Concrete Ethical Problems," *Philosophy and Public Affairs* 19 (1990): 279–310; Richardson, "Specifying, Balancing, and Interpreting Bioethical Principles," *Journal of Medicine and Philosophy* 25 (2000): 285–307, a version of which appears in this volume; Tom Beauchamp and James Childress, *Principles of Biomedical Ethics*, 5th ed. (New York: Oxford University Press, 2001), 15–19; David DeGrazia, "Moving Forward in Bioethical Theory: Theories, Cases, and Specified Principlism," *Journal of Medicine and Philosophy* 17 (1992): 511–39; DeGrazia and Beauchamp, "Philosophical Foundations and Philosophical Methods," in *Methods in Medical Ethics*, ed. Jeremy Sugarman and Daniel P. Sulmasy (Washington, DC: Georgetown University Press, 2001), esp. 31–46.

20. I have diary notes that our editing meetings occurred May 31-June 1, 1978, just prior to the National Commission's 42nd and penultimate meeting, on June 9–10, 1978. Thus, the wording at the 42nd meeting was the final wording unless a commissioner raised an objection at that meeting or the next.

21. As used here, *casuistry* implies that some forms of moral reasoning and judgment neither appeal to nor rely upon principles and rules, but rather involve appeals to the grounding of moral judgment in narratives, paradigm cases, analogies, models, classification schemes, and even immediate intuition and discerning insight. Each change in the circumstances changes the case. The casuistic method begins with cases

whose moral features and conclusions have already been decided and then compares the salient features in the paradigm cases with the features of cases that require a decision. See Albert Jonsen and Stephen Toulmin, *Abuse of Casuistry* (Berkeley: University of California Press, 1988), 11–19, 251–54, 296–99; Jonsen, "Casuistry as Methodology in Clinical Ethics," *Theoretical Medicine* 12 (1991): 299–302; John Arras, "Principles and Particularity: The Role of Cases in Bioethics," *Indiana Law Journal* 69 (1994): 983–1014. See also Toulmin, "The Tyranny of Principles," *Hastings Center Report* 11 (1981): 31–39.

22. Jonsen and Toulmin, *Abuse of Casuistry*, 16–19.

23. A few years ago, I reviewed all the National Commission transcripts pertaining to *Belmont*, primarily to study the National Commission's method of treating issues in research ethics. I found that Jonsen and Toulmin had occasionally mentioned casuistry, but they clearly understood the National Commission's casuistry as consistent with its invocation of moral principles. For additional discussion, see Stephen Toulmin, "The National Commission on Human Experimentation: Procedures and Outcomes," in *Scientific Controversies: Case Studies in the Resolution and Closure of Disputes in Science and Technology*, ed. H. T. Engelhardt Jr. and A. Caplan, 599–613 (New York: Cambridge University Press, 1987),

and Jonsen, "Casuistry as Methodology in Clinical Ethics."

24. See, e.g., Alexander Capron, "Looking Back at the President's Commission," *Hastings Center Report* 13, no. 5 (1983): 8–9.

25. See Jonsen's own summation to this effect in "Casuistry," in *Methods of Bioethics*, ed. Sugarman and Sulmasy, pp. 112–13, and his Introduction to a reprinting of the *Belmont Report* in *Source Book in Bioethics*, ed. Albert Jonsen, Robert M. Veatch, and LeRoy Walters, 22 (Washington, DC: Georgetown University Press, 1998).

26. See, e.g., National Commission for the Protection of Human Subjects of Biomedical and Behavioral Research, "Transcript of the Meeting Proceedings" for the following meetings: February 11–13, 1977, 11–155; July 8–9, 1977, 104–17; April 14–15, 1978, 155–62; and June 9–10, 1978, 113–19.

27. Albert Jonsen, "Case Analysis in Clinical Ethics," *The Journal of Clinical Ethics* 1 (1990): 65.

28. Albert Jonsen, "Casuistry: An Alternative or Complement to Principles?" *Kennedy Institute of Ethics Journal* 5 (1995): 237–51.

29. Jonsen, "Casuistry: An Alternative or Complement to Principles?" 244–49. See also Jonsen, "The Weight and Weighing of Ethical Principles," in *The Ethics of Research Involving Human Subjects: Facing the 21st Century*, ed. Harold Y. Vanderpool, 59–82 (Frederick, MD: University Publishing Group, 1996).

4. Philosophical Foundations of Bioethics

Diverse milestones in the history of Western ethics have inspired the bioethical principles. Beauchamp and Childress have recognized great proximity to recent authors, such as Ross and Frankena, and it is possible to verify that classical thinkers, such as Aristotle, Hume Kant and Mill, also influenced their principles' configuration. Also, I have considered other contemporary authors whose ideas are strongly related to the current understanding of bioethics.

Aristotle

Several key Aristotelian concepts, such as justice, good and virtue are either explicitly or tacitly present in Beauchamp and Childress' principles definition and epistemological scope. However, Aristotle's influence is especially notorious regarding the teleological aspects of bioethical principles.

Aristotle defined moral action as certain human activity directed towards the full realization of what we potentially are. What we potentially are points out an end "given by nature" which can only be reached through a tenacious and constant moral behavior. That end (happiness) is human life's most perfect good and means the farther reward for our efforts.

Aristotle affirmed that "the virtue of man also will be the state of character which makes a man good and which makes him do his own work well". Therefore, virtue is not a mere passion or faculty. Virtue is a way of being, an expression of character since it reveals the internal and natural tendency towards good.

In more specific terms, Aristotle defined virtue as a middle term between two vices: excess and deficiency. Also, virtue is "the mean relative to us, this being determined by a rational principle, and by that principle by which the man of practical wisdom would determine it". He who possesses the virtue of practical wisdom (*phronesis*) also would have the ability to act well and correctly. In other words, that person would have the capacity to know what to do to resolve complex situations and how to deliberate on and objectively resolve moral dilemmas.

This particular kind of virtue is not only acquired through practice but by intellectual learning. The ability of deliberation needs time and preparation to be developed; it does not bloom spontaneously. Hence, only that individual who is wise in practice and knows how to deliberate and make decisions, will be able to recognize the middle way to think and act with prudence and wisdom since only "the man who is capable of deliberating has practical wisdom."

In conclusion, diverse Aristotelian concepts such as, excellence, perfection, practical wisdom (prudence), justice, fairness and virtue, have been important benchmarks for Beauchamp and Childress' principles. In specific terms, Aristotelian virtue allows proper and objective deliberation as well as the application of plausible and reasonable procedures to resolve private and public conflicts.

Finally, Aristotelian ethics provides another important element for bioethics. Since the emergence of Modern science, ethics had been confined to a subjective realm whereas positivism maintained the monopoly of rationality and objectivity. However, the effort of enlightened philosophers to give a scientific character to ethics was in vain. That failure did nothing but confirm the validity of several aspects of Aristotelian ethics since this proposes a different idea of practical rationality beyond that formal understanding of Enlightenment.

By following Aristotle, Beauchamp and Childress stressed a central point for bioethical deliberation: a practical ethics that considers the procedural dimension of morality seems to be the only plausible way to think about, deepen and resolve complex moral controversies originated by current biotechnological power.

David Hume

Hume's ethics is based on the assumption that human beings have a natural interest in sustaining and preserving society. In *An Inquiry Concerning the Principles of Morals,* Hume characterized morality as an inter-subjective phenomenon determined by natural inclinations. Passions, which are motivated by feelings of pleasure and displeasure, define our goals, and the only purpose of reason is to specify means to achieve ends already pointed out by our feelings. In this sense, feelings are criteria of morality and imply a mechanistic conception of human behavior: we pursue pleasure and avoid pain.

Pleasure implies permanent states of happiness, and pain involves misery in a similar degree of intensity. By virtue of experience, human beings associate the concept of good to happiness and evil to misery. In this way, the mechanistic tendency to pleasures becomes a criterion to determine the morality of actions.

By following Aristotle, Hume thought that pleasures must not necessarily be separated from virtue. In fact, the virtuous or moral action is that which produces pleasure (happiness) and the vicious or immoral one is that which causes displeasure (misery). Apparently, this reasoning introduces a relative concept of morality since feelings can differ between individuals. However, Hume resolved the problem by affirming that human beings share the same nature and, hence, they will pursue the same pleasures and will finally coincide on moral judgments.

Regarding levels of morality, Hume considered that social virtues take precedence over private ones. Social virtues can sustain and promote common life as well as to enable social cohesion. In this sense, social virtues reveal themselves as useful for society and therefore for every individual. Thereby, any society will tend to approve that which implies more utility and disapprove that which causes more pain and discomfort. Virtue does not mean to act according to right reason but according to feelings which leads us to choose some ends over others.

Acting according to virtue also means to act according to the principle of greatest utility for us and for all. Therefore, acting according to the principle of utility implies to consider justice and benevolence as superior principles of morality. Both of them are social virtues and their observance permit to achieve social cohesion and peaceful coexistence. Justice points out the intrinsic equality between individuals who share the same natural inclinations. Benevolence implies the capacity to feel the same and see others like oneself.

Beuchamp and Childress have borrowed from Hume some important epistemological elements to determine the meaning and scope of the principles of beneficence and justice. Also, these authors stress, like Hume, the need to link the abstract concept of virtue with good practices; namely, reinforce it with eminent skills and qualities that exalt its concrete dimension. A classical Hume's paragraph can help us to ratify the above mentioned:

> It may be esteemed, perhaps, a superfluous task to prove, that the benevolent or softer affections are estimable, and wherever they appear, engage the approbation and good-will of mankind. The epithets sociable, good-natured, humane, merciful, grateful, friendly, generous, beneficent, or their equivalents, are known in all languages, and universally express the highest merit, which human nature is capable of attaining. Where these amiable qualities are attended with birth and power and eminent abilities, and display themselves in the good government or useful instruction of mankind, they seem even to raise the possessors of them above the rank of human nature, and make them approach in some measure to the divine.[1]

Hume's thought speaks by itself.

John Stuart Mill

The main exponent of Modern utilitarianism is John Stuart Mill. Strongly influenced at first by Bentham's ideas, his philosophy's starting point was to rethink the liberal British empiricist tradition begun by Locke. In his book *A System of Logic, Ratiocinative and Inductive* (1843), Mill argued that empiricism, a philosophy based on experience, optimizes the structure of society whereas moral cohesion, which is necessary and useful in the civil space, arises from an utilitarian understanding of morality.

His main contribution to utilitarian theory, which leads us away from a purely quantitative position, is his distinction between high and low pleasures. They correspond to different declinations of human passions, which do not necessarily lead to happiness, and may be determined by pseudo moral criteria or concupiscent inclinations. Thus, Mill faced with the following objection to Bentham's conception. If the majority of people were accustomed to lower pleasures and considered them desirable, would they necessarily be happy? Maybe not, as society would not be able to sustain itself if the conduct of its citizens was only inspired in the pursuit of passionate happiness:

> It is better to be a human being dissatisfied than a pig satisfied; better to be Socrates dissatisfied than a fool satisfied. And if the fool, or the pig, are of a different opinion, it is because they only know their own side of the question. The other party to the comparison knows both sides.[2]

Therefore Mill moved away from Bentham's conception because he introduced the concept of quality of pleasure as a criterion of moral rightness, against the set of arithmetic principles that Bentham proposed. How can we

---

1 Hume, David, *An Enquiry Concerning the Principles of Morals*, USA, Wilder Publications, 2008, p. 9.

2 Mill, John Stuart, *Utilitarianism*, New York, The Liberal Arts Press, 1948, p. 14.

know the superiority of one type of pleasure over another? The answer is simple: we need to experience both of them; namely, bodily and spiritual pleasures. Only in this way we will be 1) A competent moral agency, equally related to both ends and, 2) Capable to distinguish between the lowest and highest pleasures. Mill rejected the identification of utilitarianism with a "doctrine of swine." Therefore, it would be an error to think that pleasures do not differ between them either in degree or kind.

Beyond the concept of utility that underlies Beauchamp and Childress' principlism, the Millean distinction between quality and quantity of pleasures is essential to understand that it is unreasonable to carry out any action just because it is evaluated as useful. In fact, a serious and timely consideration of this distinction would have prevented many deaths and suffering that have been caused by an indiscriminate use of technology from 1940 onwards.

However, the hedonistic principle of *sacrifice of minorities*, present in the utilitarian theory, seems inconsistent with the moral standards of any civilized society. Is it morally plausible to achieve the greatest happiness of the greatest number by indefinitely postponing the welfare of those who do not belong to that majority? Is it possible to configure any ethics by demanding minorities to renounce their identity, tradition and legitimate aspirations because they are not the majority? These questions, still unanswered, underlie principlism as well.

Immanuel Kant

Unlike Aristotle, Kant considered that all metaphysics of morals should transcend the sphere in which good is identified with being. Thus, morality should be understood in terms of "right" or "wrong" as concepts associated to the observance or not observance of law of reason. From that premise, Kant established a

new foundation for ethics, characterized by an *a priori*, universal and necessary conception of rationality: *a priori* because experience is not required to sanction morality of actions; universal since reason is shared by all humans beings; and necessary because the condition of possibility of moral action is an apodictic or categorical mandate of reason that points out an unconditional and objective obligation without any empirical limitation.

According to Kant, the big error of ethics has been to analyze human behavior through principles of contingent nature. As human will implies the capacity to determine action through the representation of certain laws called imperatives, most of imperatives through which rational beings conduct their lives are hypothetical, that is, assertoric. This means that humans often act only if their actions imply favorable consequences for them. Thereby, Kant thought that a rational foundation for ethics could not be obtained from those kind of imperatives since their subjectivity and relativistic nature only leads to an eclectic set of diverse and contradictory moral foundations.

Kantian ethical imperative should represent in itself a universal rational law and a rational criterion of morality, free from contingent and emotive elements. It is, in sum, a categorical imperative or unconditional mandate.

Kant stated the first formulation of the categorical imperative as follows: "Act only according to that maxim whereby you can at the same time will that it should become a universal law."[3] This formulation implies a rational law in itself as well as a criterion to distinguish moral actions from those, which are not. In this sense, any maxim able to be universalized will imply a moral action. The adequacy between our particular principles (maxims) and the categorical imperative (rational law), implies the objective, universal and necessary morality of

---

3   Kant, Immanuel, *Grounding for the Metaphysics of Morals,* 3rd ed., Hackett. pp. 30: Translate by James W. Ellington. Also see: *Fondements de la métaphysique des moeurs,* Paris, Librairie Delagrave, 1939; Translate by Victor Delbos.

actions. Therefore, moral actions must be able to be thought without self-contradiction, that is, without inconsistency between the rational creature and the rational law.

The ability to adjust maxims to the rational law belongs to a good will, that is, a will able to follow the categorical mandate of reason. This ability of self-legislation points out moral duty as a pure expression of human liberty. In moral terms, freedom means unconditional will, that is, a will able of self-legislation, and able to impose itself its own rules and obey them by virtue of the duty involved in that act and by mere respect for the rational law. Thus, freedom, as autonomy of will, is the only source of moral action and the unique condition of possibility of all ethics.

Although Kantian concept of autonomy differs from Beauchamp and Childress' (which does not necessarily imply unconditional actions), the fact of being morally unconditioned (autonomous) has an absolute, universal, rational and objective moral value. In other words, autonomy is inherent to morality and acquires practical relevance in bioethics when opinions and decisions of persons are considered for deliberation and decision-making processes.

Hans Jonas

Jonas distinguishes two stages in the history of technology: Premodern technology, related to "traditional" ethics or "ethics given so far," and Modern technology, which must be addressed by his principle of responsibility.[4]

As the search for progress, strongly linked with technological advances, provokes science to discover with a syncopated rhythm without any kind of contemplations either for mankind or nature, Jonas' ethics seeks to avoid total disaster and emphasizes the obligation

to foresee, with a high degree of accuracy, true consequences of technological action.

Nature is unable to reverse by itself damage and devastation caused by relentless technological colonization. Also, the scope of current human action seems to be beyond any possibility of calculation:

All this has decisively changed. Modern technology has introduced actions of such novel scale, objects and consequences that the framework of former ethics can no longer contain them. The *Antigone* chorus on the *demotes*, the wondrous power, of man would have to read differently now; and its admonition to the individual to honor the laws of the land would no longer be enough. The goods, too, whose venerable right could check the headlong rush of human action, are long gone. To be sure, the old prescriptions of the "neighbor" ethics—of justice, charity, honesty and so on—still hold in their intimate immediacy for the nearest, day-by-day sphere of human interaction. But this sphere is overshadowed by a growing realm of collective action where doer, deed, and effect are no longer the same as they were in the proximate sphere, and which by the enormity of its power forces upon ethics a new dimension of responsibility never dreamed of before.[5]

Technology has accompanied human beings since their appearance. The use of tools has allowed the satisfaction of human needs. At the same time, *Homo Faber* has preceded *Homo Sapiens* on the evolutionary chain. The capacity to make has preceded the ability to foresee. Subsequently, *Homo Sapiens* has reaffirmed

4 See, Jonas, Hans, *Das Prinzip Veranwortung: Versuchi einer Ethic für die Tecnologische Zivilisation*, Francfort am Main, Insel Verlag, 1988, p. 17 and following.

5 Jonas, Hans, *The Imperative of Responsibility. In Search of an Ethics for the Technological Age*, The University of Chicago Press, 1985, p. 6.

himself as an individual capable of making science as well as able to calculate and prevent the consequences of his actions. However, the ability to foresee is not equivalent with the capacity to make. Scientists are only able to presuppose possible consequences of technological action. Technology is no longer a controllable and finite instrument. Nowadays, it has turned into an unstoppable impulse for discovering which surpasses itself. Thereby, technology, beyond its questionable moral neutrality, is becoming a dangerous and multifactorial conjunction of subjective ends determined by economic and political factors.

This development generates, according to Jonas, an independent dynamic that overpowers human will through a sort of technological challenge that requires the implementation of all that which in theory is seen as possible. This basically means that we are losing control of technology and hence, we are losing freedom. Technological progress has been consolidated in the current world and it is able to act even against human will. The source of this dynamic movement points out a close relationship between scientific progress and technological development. Science requires for its development increasingly sophisticated instruments and thus it transforms technology into a kind of giant laboratory that must make all necessary elements to continue to discover.

As a result of that circular dynamic, nature has become vulnerable to human action. Therefore, there has existed a gap between technology and traditional ethical reflection since this has not considered any kind of responsibilities towards environment. The unusual power that contemporary subject displays shows the urgency to find grounds for universally valid moral rules. However, the difficulty of finding these foundations would come, according to Jonas, from the chasm that contemporary philosophy opened between reality, axiologically neutral, and human beings who are considered as the only source of moral value. The formulation of new basis for an ethics of responsibility that reduces

that gap between being (nature) and consciousness (humans) is necessary.

Jonas proposes to extend the moral scope of human responsibility in accordance with the expansion of human action's scope. Thereby, and in close harmony with bioethics' goals, Jonas suggests a new foundation for contemporary morality; a new imperative that orders the preservation of an authentic human life and the respect for the genetic identity of our specie. That new imperative says in its first formulation: "Act so that the effects of your action are compatible with the permanence of genuine human life".[6] Unlike Kant, who appealed to the encapsulated correlation between act and subject, the new imperative implies a wider tuning between consequences of acts and human beings' survival.

Thus, while premodern technological actions require only traditional ethics rules, Jonas intends to respond to the current conditions of existence in which human action has been modified by technoscientific by proposing a more reaching imperative that demands new moral standards to configure "a real future as an opened place to our responsibility".

Therefore, Kantian moral reasoning is complemented by the new imperative since this adds a perspective of future which categorical imperative lacks of. Thereby, Jonas' imperative overcomes the enlightened subjectivity of Kantian imperative because it implies a concrete and objective future as the horizon of human responsibility. In fact, Jonas considers real and concrete consequences of human action and a futuristic factor in responsibility as a moral foundation of universal value. His idea of the future, unlike an Utopian conception, is conceived more as a threat than a harbinger of a promised dawn.

According to Jonas, genuine human life involves two basic elements: first, the preservation of environment and biodiversity, and second, the conservation of human genetic identity.

---

6 Ibid.,p. 32–33.

Anthropocentrism rooted in "traditional" ethics does not include a concern for the preservation of nature. However, Jonas thinks that nature has its own moral rights as an end in itself which new imperative simply takes as an axiom. At the same time, the threat to modify and alter human beings' genetic codes with all its moral controversies was never considered by previous ethical reflection.

Jonas' thought involves the assumption that freedom, creative skills, and evaluative abilities have been present in nature even before mankind's emergence. Thus, human beings must be preserved because they are the repository of a magnificent natural heritage that is committed to existence. Jonas thinks that we must answer for mankind and future world in terms of a commitment to an infinite and universal plan of creation. This onto-theological argument (controversial in itself) also points out a fundamental duty of Jonas' ethics: to care of being, that is, to conserve, respect and ensure human life and environment for the benefit of future generations.

Apel and Habermas

Karl-Otto Apel and Jürgen Habermas' dialogical ethics emphasizes the concept of co-responsibility as a starting point for the post metaphysical transformation of Kantian philosophy. In the *Critique of Pure Reason*, Kant asks what would be the conditions of possibility to a valid knowledge. To answer that question he introduces the separation between a *noumenal* world (the thing in itself) that is unknowable, and a *phenomenal* world that is presented to consciousness. Apel and Habermas do not need to draw on this distinction because in their ethics the starting point of reflection migrates from individual consciousness to language that can, in principle, be shared by all.

All those who are endowed with communicative competence, that is, able to understand, agree and interpret are valid interlocutors.

Therefore, the central question of dialogical ethics, unlike Kant, is: Is an intersubjective agreement about the truth and the meaning of statements possible? The answer is yes. However, all interlocutors will share the responsibility for their actions and their consequences in society. The mere use of language and the presence of conventional rules, show the interlocutor his belonging to a community. The Kantian "I think" that refers to a philosophy of consciousness based on the Cartesian *Cogito Ergo Sum* becomes in Apel and Habermas a "We argue."

At this point, the question about the relation between dialogical ethics and the historical responsibility this discipline for its own application arises. In this regard, in "Über Moralität und Sittlichkeit" Habermas proposes the formulation of the principle of universalization (U):

> (U) A [moral norm] is valid just in case the foreseeable consequences and side-effects of its general observance for the interests and value-orientations of *each individual* could be *jointly* accepted by *all* concerned without coercion (i.e., in a sufficiently reasonable discourse).

This principle replaces Kant's categorical imperative and implies, only in a partial and fragmentary way, a discursive and post metaphysical transformation of Kant's philosophy. At first, (U) would be able to respond to common responsibility's demands as well as to the global impact of current collective activities. From this requirement, dialogical ethics orders speakers to participate in real discourses. Then, through that communicative process, the specific rules that will be valid for all those who have participated on equal terms in their formulation, are defined by consensus.

However, (U) is not sufficient to ensure that consensus. According to Apel, this principle should and could be applied to the regulation of conflicts, which in practice is impossible without addressing necessary exceptions in its application. This philosopher proposes a principle of complementary reciprocity (C), which commands public collaboration for progressive installation of (U) conditions of possibility conditions. Therefore, (C) is a formal principle that works as a regulative idea of teleological actions by revealing the true claim of universality of dialogical ethics. If (C) is not recognized, we should assume that doctrines as Human Rights could be only applied in the Western world (where, at least in theory, there are more conditions for its implementation). Therefore, the recognition of this principle implies an acceptance of a responsibility, which requires speakers to assist in its implementation in speaking communities.

Habermas and Apel's ethics attempts to break down the subject-object paradigm of modernity that has drawn a big gap between individuals (the subject) and world (the object). There exist a close relationship between our destiny as social beings and the preservation of public space, understood as an eminently argumentative place. This idea does not only represents a condition of possibility for bioethics but, above all, indicates that every person is a being-in-the-world, whose welfare is unthinkable without considering the good of other human and extra-human entities.

Engelhardt

In an effort to elucidate the basic bioethical problems of pluralistic and secular societies, Engelhardt identifies the basic principles that govern the possibility of communication and collaboration between morally-strange secular communities, that is, communities with different moral viewpoints, values and principles. These problems have an immense importance since, according to Engelhardt, they are the conflict at the roots of bioethics.[7]

He introduces the principles of permission and beneficence, which are at the base of all ethical relationships between morally strange communities, by introducing them presented as "the source, beginnings, commencements or origins of particular areas of the moral life." Even though they are not "fundamental", at least they are useful in moral deliberation and the solution of ethical issues. Thereby, Engelhardt assumes *a priori* that human beings reject force as being a solution for ethical differences.

The principle of permission states the limits in the interaction between different morally strange individuals and communities. Only through authorization (willful agreement of parts involved) can one act involving others due to the impossibility of stating a binding rational universal morality in a secular society. Since differences in values and viewpoints are inescapable, only through valid permit we can act affecting others, the moral strangers. This principle also states the authority to decide whether a particular moral action is good or bad. However, it neither entails a general binding understanding of morality nor intends to establish one. Since general agreements of what is right and wrong cannot be meeting, either "through rational arguments or common beliefs," the authority to decide and sanction what is wrong or right is left to what is agreed between parts in the particular case. Now, if actions are done against authorized acts, one *can* expect licit (but not mandatory) retaliation by force from the offended. These sanctions for immorality are justified because we commit to a "peaceable society" as soon as we start talking about moral communication across moral communities. Thus, violating the principle of permission justify "circumscription of the autonomy of the offender" as a punitive answer to his acts. One should also expect the consequence of being set aside of that moral community due to that misbehavior

On the other hand, the principle of beneficence is related to the goal of morality, namely, to *do* the good and *avoid* the bad. Humans, as

---

7 Engelhardt, H. Tristam, *The Foundations of Bioethics*, Second Edition, Oxford University Press, 1996.

social animals, always participate in communities with diverse moral contents and when doing so, if one desires to be morally right one must act in a beneficent way and "do to others their good." Thus, this principle "reflects the circumstance that moral concerns encompass the pursuit of goods and the avoidance of harms." Beneficence has an important role in unveiling a characteristic of human nature, as we tend to state our goals in social terms, involving others, and it is there that differences express. Beneficence is the bone and flesh of morality, "because without a commitment to beneficence the moral life has no content," and it "grounds what can be termed the morality of welfare and social sympathies."

Sanctions for immoral actions at the level of the principle of beneficence can only be intellectual; if one has failed to act beneficently according to one moral community "one has at most cut oneself off from the beneficent community."

Engelhadrt then forwards a question concerning malevolence, understood as an action against beneficence. What happens to those that *act malevolently*? If such is the case, acting against the good of a community or individual, but with permission, should not be answered with force, since permission is the basis for secular morality. Now, if the case is that the action is done without permission and against the good of an individual or community, the offender must surely be answered with force since he/she is not legitimized to act in such way.

Due to the nature of these principles, Engelhardt states that permission is "conceptually prior to beneficence." One can imagine a situation in which one would actually violate the principle of permission without even knowing what concept of beneficence is present in that particular community, "one can act in non-beneficient ways without being in conflict with the minimal notion of morality."

Regarding to another principle of bioethics that has been put forward by authors such as Beauchamp and Childress, called principle of justice, claims on it are also seen by Engelhardt

as being "at root a concern with beneficence," since those judgments of justice presuppose a particular content- rich viewpoint. Bioethical matters such as health care resource allocation and physician-patient relationships are taken into consideration by this appeals to justice (*"what ought to be done"*) and are part of the global moral issues.

In relation to the socio-political implications of these principles, Engelhardt thinks that we need to secure basis for a neutral democracy that commits itself "to not being committed to a particular vision of the good." Democracies should focus on allowing individuals and communities the fulfillment of personal values and ends, as long as these respect the minimum right of other individuals and communities of not being acted upon without authorization and allowing them too the pursuit of their own "good."

Until now, the rules of traditional ethics have sought to regulate human relationships. It is now, however, that we should keep in mind the valuative, ideological, religious and philosophical discrepancies that can be seen in globalization. This axiological diversity involves generating procedures to ensure tolerance and respect for our differences, in addition to forming a basis for recognizing, on behalf of moral strangeness, a certain minimum of morality that would allow protecting the equality of human beings in the exercise of their rights and fulfillment of their duties. At this point, evidently bioethics has a relevant responsibility.

Readings

Aristotle, *Nicomachean Ethics*, in McKeon, Richard, *The Basic Works of Aristotle*, New York, The Modern Library, 2001: **952-964; 1022–1029.**

Kant, Immanuel, *Groundwork of the Metaphysics of Morals,* Radford VA, A & D Publishing, 2008: **12–20; 31-39; 45–53.**

Mill, John Stuart, *Utilitarianism*, New York, Dover Publications Inc., 2007: **5-17; 35–41.**

Jonas, Hans, *The Imperative of Responsibility. In Search of an Ethics for the Technological Age*, USA, The University of Chicago Press, 1984: **1–24.**

Study Questions

1. Why virtue is important in bioethical deliberation?
2. Why the Aristotelian concept of prudence (practical wisdom) and the Kantian concept of dignity may be useful in bioethical deliberation.
3. Identify other Aristotelian concepts that can be workable in bioethics? Justify your answer.
4. How could we apply the Hume's concept of experience on moral deliberation?
5. Why can the concept of utility be considered as a criterion to resolve moral quandaries?
6. What are the connections between Jonas' ethics of responsibility and bioethics?
7. What are the relationships between Apel and Habermas' dialogical ethics and bioethics?
8. Explain briefly the bioethical principles that Engelhardt considers more suitable with the current conditions of existence.

Nicomachean Ethics

Aristotle

Book II

1 Virtue, then, being of two kinds, intellectual and moral, intellectual virtue in the main owes both its birth and its growth to teaching (for which reason it requires experience and time), while moral virtue comes about as a result of habit, whence also its name *ethike* is one that is formed by a slight variation from the word *ethos* (habit). From this it is also plain that none of the moral virtues arises in us by nature; for nothing that exists by nature can form a habit contrary to its nature. For instance the stone which by nature moves downwards cannot be habituated to move upwards, not even if one tries to train it by throwing it up ten thousand times; nor can fire be habituated to move downwards, nor can anything else that by nature behaves in one way be trained to behave in another. Neither by nature, then, nor contrary to nature do the virtues arise in us; rather we are adapted by nature to receive them, and are made perfect by habit.

Again, of all the things that come to us by nature we first acquire the potentiality and later exhibit the activity (this is plain in the case of the senses; for it was not by often seeing or often hearing that we got these senses, but on the contrary we had them before we used them, and did not come to have them by using them);

but the virtues we get by first exercising them, as also happens in the case of the arts as well. For the things we have to learn before we can do them, we learn by doing them, e. g. men become builders by building and lyre-players by playing the lyre; so too we become just by doing just acts, temperate by doing temperate acts, brave by doing brave acts.

This is confirmed by what happens in states; for legislators make the citizens good by forming habits in them, and this is the wish of every legislator, and those who do not effect it miss their mark, and it is in this that a good constitution differs from a bad one.

Again, it is from the same causes and by the same means that every virtue is both produced and destroyed, and similarly every art; for it is from playing the lyre that both good and bad lyre-players are produced. And the corresponding statement is true of builders and of all the rest; men will be good or bad builders as a result of building well or badly. For if this were not so, there would have been no need of a teacher, but all men would have been born good or bad at their craft. This, then, is the case with the virtues also; by doing the acts that we do in our transactions with other men we become just or unjust, and by doing the acts that we do in the presence of danger, and being habituated to

1103^b

feel fear or confidence, we become brave or cowardly. The same is true of appetites and feelings of anger; some men become temperate and good-tempered, others self-indulgent and irascible, by behaving in one way or the other in the appropriate circumstances. Thus, in one word, states of character arise out of like activities. This is why the activities we exhibit must be of a certain kind; it is because the states of character correspond to the differences between these. It makes no small difference, then, whether we form habits of one kind or of another from our very youth; it makes a very great difference, or rather *all* the difference.

2   Since, then, the present inquiry does not aim at theoretical knowledge like the others (for we are inquiring not in order to know what virtue is, but in order to become good, since otherwise our inquiry would have been of no use), we must examine the nature of actions, namely how we ought to do them; for these determine also the nature of the states of character that are produced, as we have said.[1] Now, that we must act according to the right rule is a common principle and must be assumed—it will be discussed later,[2] i.e. both what the right rule is, and how it is related to the other virtues. But this must be agreed upon beforehand, that the whole account of matters of conduct must be given in outline and not precisely, as we said at the very beginning[3] that the accounts we demand must be in accordance with the subject-matter; matters concerned with conduct and questions of what is good for us have no fixity, any more than matters of health. The general account being of this nature, the account of particular cases is yet more lacking in exactness; for they do not fall under any art or precept but the agents themselves must in each case consider what is appropriate to the occasion, as happens also in the art of medicine or of navigation.

But though our present account is of this nature we must give what help we can. First, then, let us consider this, that it is the nature of such things to be destroyed by defect and excess, as we see in the case of strength and of health (for to gain light on things imperceptible we must use the evidence of sensible things); both excessive and defective exercise destroys the strength, and similarly drink or food which is above or below a certain amount destroys the health, while that which is proportionate both produces and increases and preserves it. So too is it, then, in the case of temperance and courage and the other virtues. For the man who flies from and fears everything and does not stand his ground against anything becomes a coward, and the man who fears nothing at all but goes to meet every danger becomes rash; and similarly the man who indulges in every pleasure and abstains from none becomes self-indulgent, while the man who shuns every pleasure, as boors do, becomes in a way insensible; temperance and courage, then, are destroyed by excess and defect, and preserved by the mean.

But not only are the sources and causes of their origination and growth the same as those of their destruction, but also the sphere of their actualization will be the same; for this is also true of the things which are more evident to sense, e.g. of strength; it is produced by taking much food and undergoing much exertion, and it is the strong man that will be most able to do these things. So too is it with the virtues; by abstaining from pleasures we become temperate, and it is when we have become so that we are most able to abstain from them; and similarly too in the case of courage; for by being habituated to despise things that are terrible and to stand our ground against them we become brave, and it is when we have become so that we shall be most able to stand our ground against them.

3   We must take as a sign of states of character the pleasure or pain that ensues on acts; for the

---

[1] a 31–b 25.   [2] vi. 13.   [3] 1094b 11–27.

man who abstains from bodily pleasures and delights in this very fact is temperate, while the man who is annoyed at- it is self-indulgent, and he who stands his ground against things that are terrible and delights in this or at least is not pained is brave, while the man who is pained is a coward. For moral excellence is concerned with pleasures and pains; it is on account of the plea-
10 sure that we do bad things, and on account of the pain that we abstain from noble ones. Hence we ought to have been brought up in a particular way from our very youth, as Plato says,[4] so as both to delight in and to be pained by the things that we ought; for this is the right education.

Again, if the virtues are concerned with ac-
tions and passions, and every passion and every action is accompanied by pleasure and pain, for
15 this reason also virtue will be concerned with pleasures and pains. This is indicated also by the fact that punishment is inflicted by these means; for it is a kind of cure, and it is the nature of cures to be effected by contraries.

Again, as we said but lately,[5] every state of soul has a nature relative to and concerned with
20 the kind of things by which it tends to be made worse or better; but it is by reason of pleasures and pains that men become bad, by pursuing and avoiding these—either the pleasures and pains they ought not or when they ought not or as they ought not, or by going wrong in one of the other similar ways that may be distin-
25 guished. Hence men[6] even define the virtues as certain states of impassivity and rest; not well, however, because they speak absolutely, and do not say 'as one ought' and 'as one ought not' and 'when one ought or ought not', and the other things that may be added. We assume, then, that this kind of excellence tends to do what is best with regard to pleasures and pains, and vice does the contrary.

The following facts also may show us that
30 virtue and vice are concerned with these same things. There being three objects of choice and

three of avoidance, the noble, the advantageous, the pleasant, and their contraries, the base, the injurious, the painful, about all of these the good man tends to go right and the bad man to go wrong, and especially about pleasure; for this is common to the animals, and also it accompanies all objects of choice; for even the noble and 35 the advantageous appear pleasant.

Again, it has grown up with us all from our 1105ª infancy; this is why it is difficult to rub off this passion, engrained as it is in our life. And we measure even our actions, some of us more and 5 others less, by the rule of pleasure and pain. For this reason, then, our whole inquiry must be about these; for to feel delight and pain rightly or wrongly has no small effect on our actions.

Again, it is harder to fight with pleasure than with anger, to use Heraclitus' phrase, but both art and virtue are always concerned with what is harder; for even the good is better when it is 10 harder. Therefore for this reason also the whole concern both of virtue and of political science is with pleasures and pains; for the man who uses these well will be good, he who uses them badly bad.

That virtue, then, is concerned with plea-
sures and pains, and that by the acts from which it arises it is both increased and, if they are done differently, destroyed, and that the acts from 15 which it arose are those in which it actualizes itself—let this be taken as said.

4   The question might be asked, what we mean by saying[7] that we must become just by doing just acts, and temperate by doing temperate acts; for if men do just and temperate acts, they are already just and temperate, exactly as, if 20 they do what is in accordance with the laws of grammar and of music, they are grammarians and musicians.

Or is this not true even of the arts? It is possible to do something that is in accordance with the laws of grammar, either by chance or

---

[4] *Laws*, 653 A ff., *Rep.* 401 E–402 A.
[6] Probably Speusippus is referred to.

[5] ª 27–ᵇ 3.
[7] 1103ª 31–ᵇ 25, 1104ª 27–ᵇ 3.

at the suggestion of another. A man will be a grammarian, then, only when he has both done something grammatical and done it grammatically; and this means doing it in accordance with the grammatical knowledge in himself.

Again, the case of the arts and that of the virtues are not similar; for the products of the arts have their goodness in themselves, so that it is enough that they should have a certain character, but if the acts that are in accordance with the virtues have themselves a certain character it does not follow that they are done justly or temperately. The agent also must be in a certain condition when he does them; in the first place he must have knowledge, secondly he must choose the acts, and choose them for their own sakes, and thirdly his action must proceed from a firm and unchangeable character. These are not reckoned in as conditions of the possession of the arts, except the bare knowledge; but as a condition of the possession of the virtues knowledge has little or no weight, while the other conditions count not for a little but for everything, i.e. the very conditions which result from often doing just and temperate acts.

Actions, then, are called just and temperate when they are such as the just or the temperate man would do; but it is not the man who does these that is just and temperate, but the man who also does them *as* just and temperate men do them. It is well said, then, that it is by doing just acts that the just man is produced, and by doing temperate acts the temperate man; without doing these no one would have even a prospect of becoming good.

But most people do not do these, but take refuge in theory and think they are being philosophers and will become good in this way, behaving somewhat like patients who listen attentively to their doctors, but do none of the things they are ordered to do. As the latter will not be made well in body by such a course of treatment, the former will not be made well in soul by such a course of philosophy.

5 Next we must consider what virtue is. Since things that are found in the soul are of three kinds—passions, faculties, states of character, virtue must be one of these. By passions I mean appetite, anger, fear, confidence, envy, joy, friendly feeling, hatred, longing, emulation, pity, and in general the feelings that are accompanied by pleasure or pain; by faculties the things in virtue of which we are said to be capable of feeling these, e. g. of becoming angry or being pained or feeling pity; by states of character the things in virtue of which we stand well or badly with reference to the passions, e. g. with reference to anger we stand badly if we feel it violently or too weakly, and well if we feel it moderately; and similarly with reference to the other passions.

Now neither the virtues nor the vices are *passions*, because we are not called good or bad on the ground of our passions, but are so called on the ground of our virtues and our vices, and because we are neither praised nor blamed for our passions (for the man who feels fear or anger is not praised, nor is the man who simply feels anger blamed, but the man who feels it in a certain way), but for our virtues and our vices we *are* praised or blamed.

Again, we feel anger and fear without choice, but the virtues are modes of choice or involve choice. Further, in respect of the passions we are said to be moved, but in respect of the virtues and the vices we are said not to be moved but to be disposed in a particular way.

For these reasons also they are not *faculties*; for we are neither called good nor bad, nor praised nor blamed, for the simple capacity of feeling the passions; again, we have the faculties by nature, but we are not made good or bad by nature; we have spoken of this before.[8]

If, then, the virtues are neither passions nor faculties, all that remains is that they should be *states of character*.

Thus we have stated what virtue is in respect of its genus.

---

[8] 1103ᵃ 18–ᵇ 2.

6   We must, however, not only describe virtue
15 as a state of character, but also say what sort of
state it is. We may remark, then, that every virtue
or excellence both brings into good condition
the thing of which it is the excellence and makes
the work of that thing be done well; e. g. the
excellence of the eye makes both the eye and its
work good; for it is by the excellence of the eye
20 that we see well. Similarly the excellence of the
horse rakes a horse both good in itself and good
at running and at carrying its rider and at await-
ing the attack of the enemy. Therefore, if this is
true in every case, the virtue of man also will be
the state of character which makes a man good
and which makes him do his own work well.

How this is to happen we have stated already,[9]
25 but it will be made plain also by the following
consideration of the specific nature of virtue. In
everything that is continuous and divisible it is
possible to take more, less, or an equal amount,
and that either in terms of the thing itself or
relatively to us; and the equal is an intermediate
between excess and defect. By the intermediate
30 in the object I mean that which is equidistant
from each of the extremes, which is one and the
same for all men; by the intermediate relatively
to us that which is neither too much nor too little—and this is not one, nor the same for all. For
instance, if ten is many and two is few, six is the
intermediate, taken in terms of the object; for
it exceeds and is exceeded by an equal amount;
35 this is intermediate according to arithmetical
proportion. But the intermediate relatively to us
1106ᵇ is not to be taken so; if ten pounds are too much
for a particular person to eat and two too little,
it does not follow that the trainer will order six
pounds; for this also is perhaps too much for
the person who is to take it, or too little—too
5 little for Milo,[10] too much for the beginner in
athletic exercises. The same is true of running
and wrestling. Thus a master of any art avoids
excess and defect, but seeks the intermediate
and chooses this—the intermediate not in the
object but relatively to us.

If it is thus, then, that every art does its work
well—by looking to the intermediate and judging its works by this standard (so that we often
say of good works of art that it is not possible 10
either to take away or to add anything, implying that excess and defect destroy the goodness of works of art, while the mean preserves
it; and good artists, as we say, look to this in
their work), and if, further, virtue is more exact
and better than any art, as nature also is, then
virtue must have the quality of aiming at the 15
intermediate. I mean moral virtue; for it is
this that is concerned with passions and actions, and in these there is excess, defect, and
the intermediate. For instance, both fear and
confidence and appetite and anger and pity and
in general pleasure and pain may be felt both
too much and too little, and in both cases not
well; but to feel them at the right times, with 20
reference to the right objects, towards the right
people, with the right motive, and in the right
way, is what is both intermediate and best, and
this is characteristic of virtue. Similarly with
regard to actions also there is excess, defect,
and the intermediate. Now virtue is concerned
with passions and actions, in which excess is 25
a form of failure, and so is defect, while the
intermediate is praised and is a form of success;
and being praised and being successful are both
characteristics of virtue. Therefore virtue is a
kind of mean, since, as we have seen, it aims at
what is intermediate.

Again, it is possible to fail in many ways (for
evil belongs to the class of the unlimited, as the
Pythagoreans conjectured, and good to that of
the limited), while to succeed is possible only in 30
one way (for which reason also one is easy and
the other difficult—to miss the mark easy, to hit
it difficult); for these reasons also, then, excess
and defect are characteristic of vice, and the
mean of virtue;

For men are good in but one way, but   35
bad in many.

---

[9] 1104ª 11–27.

[10] A famous wrestler.

1107ª Virtue, then, is a state of character concerned with choice, lying in 'a mean, i. e. the mean relative to us, this being determined by a rational principle, and by that principle by which the man of practical wisdom would determine it. Now it is a mean between two vices, that which depends on excess and that which depends on defect; and again it is a mean because the vices respectively fall short of or exceed what is right in both passions and actions, while virtue both finds and chooses that which is intermediate. Hence in respect of its substance and the definition which states its essence virtue is a mean, with regard to what is best and right an extreme.

But not every action nor every passion admits of a mean; for some have names that already imply badness, e. g. spite, shamelessness, envy, and in the case of actions adultery, theft, murder; for all of these and suchlike things imply by their names that they are themselves bad, and not the excesses or deficiencies of them. It is not possible, then, ever to be right with regard to them; one must always be wrong. Nor does goodness or badness with regard to such things depend on committing adultery with the right woman, at the right time, and in the right way, but simply to do any of them is to go wrong. It would be equally absurd, then, to expect that in unjust, cowardly, and voluptuous action there should be a mean, an excess, and a deficiency; for at that rate there would be a mean of excess and of deficiency, an excess of excess, and a deficiency of deficiency. But as there is no excess and deficiency of temperance and courage because what is intermediate is in a sense an extreme, so too of the actions we have mentioned there is no mean nor any excess and deficiency, but however they are done they are wrong; for in general there is neither a mean of excess and deficiency, nor excess and deficiency of a mean.

7 We must, however, not only make this general statement, but also apply it to the individual facts. For among statements about conduct those which are general apply more widely, but those which are particular are more genuine, since conduct has to do with individual cases, and our statements must harmonize with the facts in these cases. We may take these cases from our table. With regard to feelings of fear and confidence courage is the mean; of the 1107ᵇ people who exceed, he who exceeds in fearlessness has no name (many of the states have no name), while the man who exceeds in confidence is rash, and he who exceeds in fear and falls short in confidence is a coward. With regard to pleasures and pains—not all of them, and not so much with regard to the pains—the mean is temperance, the excess self-indulgence. Persons deficient with regard to the pleasures are not often found; hence such persons also have received no name. But let us call them 'insensible'.

With regard to giving and taking of money the mean is liberality, the excess and the defect prodigality and meanness. In these actions people exceed and fall short in contrary ways; the prodigal exceeds in spending and falls short in taking, while the mean man exceeds in taking and falls short in spending. (At present we are giving a mere outline or summary, and are satisfied with this; later these states will be more exactly determined.[11]) With regard to money there are also other dispositions—a mean, magnificence (for the magnificent man differs from the liberal man; the former deals with large sums, the latter with small ones), an excess, tastelessness and vulgarity, and a deficiency, niggardliness; these differ from the states opposed to liberality, and the mode of their difference will be stated later.[12]

With regard to honour and dishonour the mean is proper pride, the excess is known as a sort of 'empty vanity', and the deficiency is undue humility; and as we said[13] liberality was related to magnificence, differing from it by dealing with small sums, so there is a state similarly related to proper pride, being concerned with small honours while that is concerned with great.

---

[11] iv. 1. [12] 1122ª 20–9, ᵇ 10–18. [13] II. 17–19.

For it is possible to desire honour as one ought, and more than one ought, and less, and the man who exceeds in his desires is called ambitious, the man who falls short unambitious, while the intermediate person has no name. The dispositions also are nameless, except that that of the ambitious man is called ambition. Hence the people who are at the extremes lay claim to the middle place; and we ourselves sometimes call the intermediate person ambitious and 1108ᵃ sometimes unambitious, and sometimes praise the ambitious man and sometimes the unambitious. The reason of our doing this will be stated in what follows;[14] but now let us speak of the remaining states according to the method which has been indicated.

With regard to anger also there is an excess, 5 a deficiency, and a mean. Although they can scarcely be said to have names, yet since we call the intermediate person good-tempered let us call the mean good temper; of the persons at the extremes let the one who exceeds be called irascible, and his vice irascibility, and the man who falls short an inirascible sort of person, and the deficiency inirascibility.

There are also three other means, which have 10 a certain likeness to one another, but differ from one another: for they are all concerned with intercourse in words and actions, but differ in that one is concerned with truth in this sphere, the other two with pleasantness; and of this one kind is exhibited in giving amusement, the other in all the circumstances of life. We must therefore speak of these too, that we 15 may the better see that in all things the mean is praiseworthy, and the extremes neither praiseworthy nor right, but worthy of blame. Now most of these states also have no names, but we must try, as in the other cases, to invent names ourselves so that we may be clear and easy to 20 follow. With regard to truth, then, the intermediate is a truthful sort of person and the mean

may be called truthfulness, while the pretence which exaggerates is boastfulness and the person characterized by it a boaster, and that which 25 understates is mock modesty and the person characterized by it mock-modest. With regard to pleasantness in the giving of amusement the intermediate person is ready-witted and the disposition ready wit, the excess is buffoonery and the person characterized by it a buffoon, while the man who falls short is a sort of boor and his state is boorishness. With regard to the remaining kind of pleasantness, that which is exhibited in life in general, the man who is pleasant in the right way is friendly and the mean is friendliness, while the man who exceeds is an obsequious person if he has no end in view, a flatterer if he is aiming at his own advantage, and the man who falls short and is unpleasant in all circumstances is a quarrelsome and surly sort of person.

There are also means in the passions and 30 concerned with the passions; since shame is not a virtue, and yet praise is extended to the modest man. For even in these matters one man is said to be intermediate, and another to exceed, as for instance the bashful man who is ashamed of everything; while he who falls short or is not ashamed of anything at all is shameless, and the intermediate person is modest. Righteous 35 indignation is a mean between envy and spite, 1108ᵇ and these states are concerned with the pain and pleasures that are felt at the fortunes of our neighbours; the man who is characterized by righteous indignation is pained at undeserved good fortune, the envious man, going beyond 5 him, is pained at all good fortune, and the spiteful man falls so far short of being pained that he even rejoices. But these states there will be an opportunity of describing elsewhere;[15] with regard to justice, since it has not one simple meaning, we shall, after describing the other states, distinguish its two kinds and say how

---

[14] ᵇ 11–26, 1125ᵇ 14–18.

[15] The reference may be to the whole treatment of the moral virtues in iii. 6–iv. 9, or to the discussion of shame in iv. 9 and an intended corresponding discussion of righteous indignation, or to the discussion of these two states in *Rhet.* ii. 6, 9, 10.

10 each of them is a mean;[16] and similarly we shall treat also of the rational virtues.[17]

8   There are three kinds of disposition, then, two of them vices, involving excess and deficiency respectively, and one a virtue, viz. the mean, and all are in a sense opposed to all; for the extreme states are contrary both to the intermediate state 15 and to each other, and the intermediate to the extremes; as the equal is greater relatively to the less, less relatively to the greater, so the middle states are excessive relatively to the deficiencies, deficient relatively to the excesses, both in passions and in actions. For the brave man appears rash relatively 20 to the coward, and cowardly relatively to the rash man; and similarly the temperate man appears self-indulgent relatively to the insensible man, insensible relatively to the self-indulgent, and the liberal man prodigal relatively to the mean man, mean relatively to the prodigal. Hence also the people at the extremes push the intermediate man each over to the other, and the brave man is 25 called rash by the coward, cowardly by the rash man, and correspondingly in the other cases.

These states being thus opposed to one another, the greatest contrariety is that of the extremes to each other, rather than to the intermediate; for these are further from each other than from the intermediate, as the great is further from the 30 small and the small from the great than both are from the equal. Again, to the intermediate some extremes show a certain likeness, as that of rashness to courage and that of prodigality to liberality; but the extremes show the greatest unlikeness to each other; now contraries are defined as the things that are furthest from each 35 other, so that things that are further apart are more contrary.

1109ª   To the mean in some cases the deficiency, in some the excess is more opposed; e.g. it is not rashness, which is an excess, but cowardice, which is a deficiency, that is more opposed to courage, and not insensibility, which is a deficiency, but self-indulgence, which is an excess, that is more 5 opposed to temperance. This happens from two reasons, one being drawn from the thing itself; for because one extreme is nearer and liker to the intermediate, we oppose not this but rather its contrary to the intermediate. E.g., since rashness is thought liker and nearer to courage, and cowardice more unlike, we oppose rather the 10 latter to courage; for things that are further from the intermediate are thought more contrary to it. This, then, is one cause, drawn from the thing itself; another is drawn from ourselves; for the things to which we ourselves more naturally tend seem more contrary to the intermediate. For instance, we ourselves tend more naturally to 15 pleasures, and hence are more easily carried away towards self-indulgence than towards propriety. We describe as contrary to the mean, then, rather the directions in which we more often go to great lengths; and therefore self-indulgence, which is an excess, is the more contrary to temperance.

9   That moral virtue is a mean, then, and in 20 what sense it is so, and that it is a mean between two vices, the one involving excess, the other deficiency, and that it is such because its character is to aim at what is intermediate in passions and in actions, has been sufficiently stated. Hence also it is no easy task to be good. For in everything it 25 is no easy task to find the middle, e.g. to find the middle of a circle is not for every one but for him who knows; so, too, any one can get angry—that is easy—or give or spend money; but to do this to the right person, to the right extent, at the right time, with the right motive, and in the right way, *that* is not for every one, nor is it easy; wherefore goodness is both rare and laudable and noble.

Hence he who aims at the intermediate must 30 first depart from what is the more contrary to it, as Calypso advises—

Hold the ship out beyond that surf and spray.[18]

---

[16] 1129ª 26–ᵇ 1, 1130ª 14–ᵇ 5, 1131ᵇ 9–15, 1132ª 24–30, 1133ᵇ 30–1134ª 1.   [17] Bk. vi.

[18] *Od.* xii. 219 f. (Mackail's trans.). But it was Circe who gave the advice (xii. 108), and the actual quotation is from Odysseus' orders to his steersman.

For of the extremes one is more erroneous, one less so; therefore, since to hit the mean is hard in the extreme, we must as a second best, as people 35 say, take the least of the evils; and this will be done best in the way we describe.

1109ᵇ   But we must consider the things towards which we ourselves also are easily carried away; for some of us tend to one thing, some to another; and this will be recognizable from the 5 pleasure and the pain we feel. We must drag ourselves away to the contrary extreme; for we shall get into the intermediate state by drawing well away from error, as people do in straightening sticks that are bent.

Now in everything the pleasant or pleasure is most to be guarded against; for we do not judge it impartially. We ought, then, to feel towards pleasure as the elders of the people felt towards Helen, and in all circumstances repeat their say-10 ing;¹⁹ for if we dismiss pleasure thus we are less likely to go astray. It is by doing this, then, (to sum the matter up) that we shall best be able to hit the mean.

But this is no doubt difficult, and especially 15 in individual cases; for it is not easy to determine both how and with whom and on what provocation and how long one should be angry; for we too sometimes praise those who fall short and call them good-tempered, but sometimes we praise those who get angry and call them manly. The man, however, who deviates little from goodness is not blamed, whether he do so in the direction of the more or of the less, but only the man who deviates more widely; for *he* 20 does not fail to be noticed. But up to what point and to what extent a man must deviate before he becomes blameworthy it is not easy to determine by reasoning, any more than anything else that is perceived by the senses; such things depend on particular facts, and the decision rests with perception. So much, then, is plain, that the 25 intermediate state is in all things to be praised, but that we must incline sometimes towards the

excess, sometimes towards the deficiency; for so shall we most easily hit the mean and what is right.

Book VI

1   Since we have previously said that one ought to choose that which is intermediate, not the excess nor the defect,¹ and that the intermediate is determined by the dictates of the right rule,² let us discuss the nature of these dictates. In all the 20 states of character we have mentioned,³ as in all other matters, there is a mark to which the man who has the rule looks, and heightens or relaxes his activity accordingly, and there is a standard which determines the mean states which we say are intermediate between excess and defect, being in accordance with the right rule. But such 15 a statement, though true, is by no means clear; for not only here but in all other pursuits which are objects of knowledge it is indeed true to say that we must not exert ourselves nor relax our efforts too much nor too little, but to an intermediate extent and as the right rule dictates; but if a man had only this knowledge he would be none the wiser—e.g. we should not know what 30 sort of medicines to apply to our body if some one were to say 'all those which the medical art prescribes, and which agree with the practice of one who possesses the art.' Hence it is necessary with regard to the states of the soul also not only that this true statement should be made, but also that it should be determined what is the right rule and what is the standard that fixes it.

We divided the virtues of the soul and said 35 that some are virtues of character and others of intellect.⁴ Now we have discussed in detail the moral virtues;³ with regard to the others let 1139ᵃ us express our view as follows, beginning with some remarks about the soul. We said before⁵

¹⁹ *Il.* iii. 156–60.
² 1107ᵃ 1, Cf. 1103ᵇ 31, 1114ᵇ 29.
²⁴ Cf. 1134ᵇ 15–17.
³ In iii. 6–v. 11.
¹ 1104ᵃ 11–27, 1106ᵃ 26–1107ᵃ 27.
⁴ 1103ᵃ 3–7.

that there are two parts of the soul—that which grasps a rule or rational principle, and the irrational; let us now draw a similar distinction within the part which grasps a rational principle. And let it be assumed that there are two parts which grasp a rational principle—one by which we contemplate the kind of things whose originative causes are invariable, and one by which we contemplate variable things; for where objects differ in kind the part of the soul answering to each of the two is different in kind, since it is in virtue of a certain likeness and kinship with their objects that they have the knowledge they have. Let one of these parts be called the scientific and the other the calculative; for to deliberate and to calculate are the same thing, but no one deliberates about the invariable. Therefore the calculative is one part of the faculty which grasps a rational principle. We must, then, learn what is the best state of each of these two parts; for this is the virtue of each.

2   The virtue of a thing is relative to its proper work. Now there are three things in the soul which control action and truth—sensation, reason, desire.

Of these sensation originates no action; this is plain from the fact that the lower animals have sensation but no share in action.

What affirmation and negation are in thinking, pursuit and avoidance are in desire; so that since moral virtue is a state of character concerned with choice, and choice is deliberate desire, therefore both the reasoning must be true and the desire right, if the choice is to be good, and the latter must pursue just what the former asserts. Now this kind of intellect and of truth is practical; of the intellect which is contemplative, not practical nor productive, the good and the bad state are truth and falsity respectively (for this is the work of everything intellectual); while of the part which is practical and intellectual the good state is truth in agreement with right desire.

The origin of action—its efficient, not its final cause—is choice, and that of choice is desire and reasoning with a view to an end. This is why choice cannot exist either without reason and intellect or without a moral state; for good action and its opposite cannot exist without a combination of intellect and character. Intellect itself, however, moves nothing, but only the intellect which aims at an end and is practical; for this rules the productive intellect as well, since every one who makes makes for an end, and that which is made is not an end in the unqualified sense (but only an end in a particular relation, and the end of a particular operation)—only that which is *done* is that; for good action is an end, and desire aims at this. Hence choice is either desiderative reason or ratiocinative desire, and such an origin of action is a man. (It is to be noted that nothing that is past is an object of choice, e. g. no one chooses to have sacked Troy; for no one *deliberates* about the past, but about what is future and capable of being otherwise, while what is past is not capable of not having taken place; hence Agathon is right in saying

For this alone is lacking even to God,   10
To make undone things that have
    once been done.)

The work of both the intellectual parts, then, is truth. Therefore the states that are most strictly those in respect of which each of these parts will reach truth are the virtues of the two parts.

3   Let us begin, then, from the beginning, and discuss these states once more. Let it be assumed that the states by virtue of which the soul possesses truth by way of affirmation or denial are five in number, i. e. art, scientific knowledge, practical wisdom, philosophic wisdom, intuitive reason; we do not include judgement and opinion because in these we may be mistaken.

Now what *scientific knowledge* is, if we are to speak exactly and not follow mere similarities,

---

5 1102ᵃ 26–8.

is plain from what follows. We all suppose that
20 what we know is not even capable of being otherwise; of things capable of being otherwise we do not know, when they have passed outside our observation, whether they exist or not. Therefore the object of scientific knowledge is of necessity. Therefore it is eternal; for things that are of necessity in the unqualified sense are all eternal; and things that are eternal are ungenerated and imperishable. Again, every sci-
25 ence is thought to be capable of being taught, and its object of being learned. And all teaching starts from what is already known, as we maintain in the *Analytics*[6] also; for it proceeds sometimes through induction and sometimes by
30 syllogism. Now induction is the starting-point which knowledge even of the universal presupposes, while syllogism proceeds *from* universals. There are therefore starting-points from which syllogism proceeds, which are not reached by syllogism; it is therefore by induction that they are acquired. Scientific knowledge is, then, a state of capacity to demonstrate, and has the other limiting characteristics which we specify in the *Analytics*;[7] for it is when a man believes in a certain way and the starting-points are known to him that he has scientific knowledge, since if they are not better known to him than the conclusion, he will have his knowledge only incidentally.
35 Let this, then, be taken as our account of scientific knowledge.

4 In the variable are included both things made and things done; making and acting are different (for their nature we treat even the discussions outside our school as reliable); so that the reasoned state of capacity to act is
5 different from the reasoned state of capacity to make. Hence too they are not included one in the other; for neither is acting making nor is making acting. Now since architecture is an art and is essentially a reasoned state of capacity to make, and there is neither any art that is not

such a state nor any such state that is not an art, *art* is identical with a state of capacity to make, 10 involving a true course of reasoning. All art is concerned with coming into being, i.e. with contriving and considering how something may come into being which is capable of either being or not being, and whose origin is in the maker and not in the thing made; for art is concerned neither with things that are, or come into being, by necessity, nor with things that do so in accordance with nature (since these have their origin in themselves). Making and acting being 15 different, art must be a matter of making, not of acting. And in a sense chance and art are concerned with the same objects; as Agathon says, 'art loves chance and chance loves art'. Art, then, as has been said,[8] is a state concerned with mak- 20 ing, involving a true course of reasoning, and lack of art on the contrary is a state concerned with making, involving a false course of reasoning; both are concerned with the variable.

5 Regarding *practical wisdom* we shall get at the truth by considering who are the persons we 25 credit with it. Now it is thought to be the mark of a man of practical wisdom to be able to deliberate well about what is good and expedient for himself, not in some particular respect, e. g. about what sorts of thing conduce to health or to strength, but about what sorts of thing conduce to the good life in general. This is shown by the fact that we credit men with practical wisdom in some particular respect when they have calculated well with a view to some good end which is one of those that are not the object 30 of any art. It follows that in the general sense also the man who is capable of deliberating has practical wisdom. Now no one deliberates about things that are invariable, nor about things that it is impossible for him to do. Therefore, since scientific knowledge involves demonstration, but there is no demonstration of things whose first principles are variable (for all such things 35 might actually be otherwise), and since it is

---

[6] *An. Post.* 71[a] 1.   [7] Ib. [b] 9–23.   [8] I. 9.

impossible to deliberate about things that are of necessity, practical wisdom cannot be scien-

1140ᵇ tific knowledge nor art; not science because that which can be done is capable of being otherwise, not art because action and making are different kinds of thing. The remaining alternative, then,

5 is that it is a true and reasoned state of capacity to act with regard to the things that are good or bad for man. For while making has an end other than itself, action cannot; for good action itself is its end. It is for this reason that we think Pericles and men like him have practical wis- dom, viz. because they can see what is good for

10 themselves and what is good for men in general; we consider that those can do this who are good at managing households or states. (This is why we call temperance (*sophrosyne*) by this name; we imply that it preserves one's practical wisdom (*sodsousa ten phronesin*). Now what it preserves is a judgement of the kind we have described. For it is not any and every judgement that pleasant and painful objects destroy and pervert, e. g. the judgement that the triangle has or has not

15 its angles equal to two right angles, but only judgements about what is to be done. For the originating causes of the things that are done consist in the end at which they are aimed; but the man who has been ruined by pleasure or pain forthwith fails to see any such originating cause—to see that for the sake of this or because of this he ought to choose and do whatever he chooses and does; for vice is destructive of the originating cause of action.)

20 Practical wisdom, then, must be a reasoned and true state of capacity to act with regard to human goods. But further, while there is such a thing as excellence in art, there is no such thing as excellence in practical wisdom; and in art he who errs willingly is preferable, but in practi- cal wisdom, as in the virtues, he is the reverse. Plainly, then, practical wisdom is a virtue and

25 not an art. There being two parts of the soul that can follow a course of reasoning, it must be the virtue of one of the two, i.e. of that part which forms opinions; for opinion is about the variable and so is practical wisdom. But yet it is

not only a reasoned state; this is shown by the fact that a state of that sort may be forgotten but practical wisdom cannot. 30

6 Scientific knowledge is judgement about things that are universal and necessary, and the conclusions of demonstration, and all scientific knowledge, follow from first principles (for sci- entific knowledge involves apprehension of a ra- tional ground). This being so, the first principle from which what is scientifically known follows cannot be an object of scientific knowledge, of art, or of practical wisdom; for that which can 35 be scientifically known can be demonstrated, and art and practical wisdom deal with things that are variable. Nor are these first principles 1141ᵃ the objects of philosophic wisdom, for it is a mark of the philosopher to have *demonstration* about some things. If, then, the states of mind by which we have truth and are never deceived about things invariable or even variable are scientific knowledge, practical wisdom, philo- sophic wisdom, and intuitive reason, and it 5 cannot be any of the three (i.e. practical wisdom, scientific knowledge, or philosophic wisdom), the remaining alternative is that it is *intuitive reason* that grasps the first principles.

7 *Wisdom* (1) in the arts we ascribe to their most finished exponents, e. g. to Phidias as a sculptor and to Polyclitus as a maker of portrait- 10 statues, and here we mean nothing by wisdom except excellence in art; but (2) we think that some people are wise in general, not in some particular field or in any other limited respect, as Homer says in the *Margites*,

Him did the gods make neither a 15
digger nor yet a ploughman Nor wise
in anything else.

Therefore wisdom must plainly be the most finished of the forms of knowledge. It follows that the wise man must not only know what follows from the first principles, but must also possess truth about the first principles.

Therefore wisdom must be intuitive reason combined with scientific knowledge—scientific knowledge of the highest objects which has received as it were its proper completion.

20   Of the highest objects, we say; for it would be strange to think that the art of politics, or practical wisdom, is the best knowledge, since man is not the best thing in the world. Now if what is healthy or good is different for men and for fishes, but what is white or straight is always the

25   same, any one would say that what is wise is the same but what is practically wise is different; for it is to that which observes well the various matters concerning itself that one ascribes practical wisdom, and it is to this that one will entrust such matters. This is why we say that some even of the lower animals have practical wisdom, viz. those which are found to have a power of foresight with regard to their own life. It is evident also that philosophic wisdom and the art of politics cannot be the same; for if the state of mind concerned with a man's own interests

30   is to be called philosophic wisdom, there will be many philosophic wisdoms; there will not be one concerned with the good of all animals (any more than there is one art of medicine for all existing things), but a different philosophic wisdom about the good of each species.

But if the argument be that man is the best

1141ᵇ of the animals, this makes no difference; for there are other things much more divine in their nature even than man, e.g., most conspicuously, the bodies of which the heavens are framed. From what has been said it is plain, then, that philosophic wisdom is scientific knowledge, combined with intuitive reason, of the things that are highest by nature. This is why we say Anaxagoras, Thales, and men like them have

5   philosophic but not practical wisdom, when we see them ignorant of what is to their own advantage, and why we say that they know things that are remarkable, admirable, difficult, and divine, but useless; viz. because it is not human goods that they seek.

Practical wisdom on the other hand is concerned with things human and things about which it is possible to deliberate; for we say this is above all the work of the man of practical wisdom, to deliberate well, but no one deliberates about things invariable, nor about things which have not an end, and that a good that can be brought about by action. The man who is without qualification good at deliberating is the man who is capable of aiming in accordance with calculation at the best for man of things attainable by action. Nor is practical wisdom concerned with universals only—it must also   15 recognize the particulars; for it is practical, and practice is concerned with particulars. This is why some who do not know, and especially those who have experience, are more practical than others who know; for if a man knew that light meats are digestible and wholesome, but did not know which sorts of meat are light, he   20 would not produce health, but the man who knows that chicken is wholesome is more likely to produce health.

Now practical wisdom is concerned with action; therefore one should have both forms of it, or the latter in preference to the former. But of practical as of philosophic wisdom there must be a controlling kind.

8   Political wisdom and practical wisdom are the same state of mind, but their essence is not the same. Of the wisdom concerned with the city, the practical wisdom which plays a controlling part is legislative wisdom, while that which is related to this as particulars to their universal   25 is known by the general name 'political wisdom'; this has to do with action and deliberation, for a decree is a thing to be carried out in the form of an individual act. This is why the exponents of this art are alone said to 'take part in politics'; for these alone 'do things' as manual labourers 'do things'.

Practical wisdom also is identified especially with that form of it which is concerned with a man himself—with the individual; and this is known by the general name 'practical wisdom';   30 of the other kinds one is called household management, another legislation, the third politics, and of the latter one part is called deliberative and the other judicial. Now knowing what is good for oneself will be one kind of knowledge, 1142ᵃ but it is very different from the other kinds; and the man who knows and concerns himself with his own interests is thought to have practical wisdom, while politicians are thought to be busybodies; hence the words of Euripides,

> But how could I be wise, who might at ease,
> Numbered among the army's multitude,
> Have had an equal share? ...
> 5 For those who aim too high and do too much. ...

Those who think thus seek their own good, and consider that one ought to do so. From this opinion, then, has come the view that such men have practical wisdom; yet perhaps one's own good cannot exist without household man-10 agement, nor without a form of government. Further, how one should order one's own affairs is not clear and needs inquiry.

What has been said is confirmed by the fact that while young men become geometricians and mathematicians and wise in matters like these, it is thought that a young man of practical wisdom cannot be found. The cause is that such wisdom is concerned not only with universals but with particulars, which become 15 familiar from experience, but a young man has no experience, for it is length of time that gives experience; indeed one might ask this question too, why a boy may become a mathematician, but not a philosopher or a physicist. Is it because the objects of mathematics exist by abstraction, while the first principles of these other subjects come from experience, and because young men have no conviction about the latter but merely use the proper language, while the essence of mathematical objects is plain enough to them?

20 Further, error in deliberation may be either about the universal or about the particular;

we may fail to know either that all water that weighs heavy is bad, or that this particular water weighs heavy.

That practical wisdom is not scientific knowledge is evident; for it is, as has been said,"⁹ concerned with the ultimate particular fact, since the thing to be done is of this nature. It is 25 opposed, then, to intuitive reason; for intuitive reason is of the limiting premises, for which no reason can be given, while practical wisdom is concerned with the ultimate particular, which is the object not of scientific knowledge but of perception—not the perception of qualities peculiar to one sense but a perception akin to that by which we perceive that the particular figure before us is a triangle; for in that direction as well as in that of the major premiss there will be a limit. But this is rather perception than practical wisdom, though it is another kind of 30 perception than that of the qualities peculiar to each sense.

9 There is a difference between inquiry and deliberation; for deliberation is inquiry into a particular kind of thing. We must grasp the nature of excellence in deliberation as well—whether it is a form of scientific knowledge, or opinion, or skill in conjecture, or some other kind of thing. *Scientific knowledge* it is not; for men do not inquire about the things they know about, but 1142ᵇ good deliberation is a kind of deliberation, and he who deliberates inquires and calculates. Nor is it *skill in conjecture*; for this both involves no reasoning and is something that is quick in its operation, while men deliberate a long time, and they say that one should carry out quickly the conclusions of one's deliberation, but should 5 deliberate slowly. Again, *readiness of mind* is different from excellence in deliberation; it is a sort of skill in conjecture. Nor again is excellence in deliberation *opinion* of any sort. But since the man who deliberates badly makes a mistake, while he who deliberates well does so correctly, excellence in deliberation is clearly a kind of correctness,

---

9 1141ᵇ 14–22.

but neither of knowledge nor of opinion; for there is no such thing as correctness of knowledge (since there is no such thing as error of knowledge), and correctness of opinion is truth; and at the same time everything that is an object of opinion is already determined. But again excellence in deliberation involves reasoning. The remaining alternative, then, is that it is *correctness of thinking*; for this is not yet assertion, since, while even opinion is not inquiry but has reached the stage of assertion, the man who is deliberating, whether he does so well or ill, is searching for something and calculating.

But excellence in deliberation is a certain correctness of deliberation; hence we must first inquire what deliberation is and what it is about. And, there being more than one kind of correctness, plainly excellence in deliberation is not any and every kind; for (1) the incontinent man and the bad man, if he is clever, will reach as a result of his calculation what he sets before himself, so that he will have deliberated correctly, but he will have got for himself a great evil. Now to have deliberated well is thought to be a good thing; for it is this kind of correctness of deliberation that is excellence in deliberation, viz. that which tends to attain what is good. But (2) it is possible to attain even good by a false syllogism, and to attain what one ought to do but not by the right means, the middle term being false; so that this too is not yet excellence in deliberation—this state in virtue of which one attains what one ought but not by the right means. Again (3) it is possible to attain it by long deliberation while another man attains it quickly. Therefore in the former case we have not yet got excellence in deliberation, which is rightness with regard to the expedient—rightness in respect both of the end, the manner, and the time. (4) Further it is possible to have deliberated well either in the unqualified sense or with reference to a particular end. Excellence in deliberation in the unqualified sense, then, is that which succeeds with reference to what is the end in the unqualified sense, and excellence in deliberation in a particular sense is that

which succeeds relatively to a particular end. If, then, it is characteristic of men of practical wisdom to have deliberated well, excellence in deliberation will be correctness with regard to what conduces to the end of which practical wisdom is the true apprehension.

10 Understanding, also, and goodness of understanding, in virtue of which men are said to be men of understanding or of good understanding, are neither entirely the same as opinion or scientific knowledge (for at that rate all men would have been men of understanding), nor are they one of the particular sciences, such as medicine, the science of things connected with health, or geometry, the science of spatial magnitudes. For understanding is neither about things that are always and are unchangeable, nor about any and every one of the things that come into being, but about things which may become subjects of questioning and deliberation. Hence it is about the same objects as practical wisdom; but understanding and practical wisdom are not the same. For practical wisdom issues commands, since its end is what ought to be done or not to be done; but understanding only judges. (Understanding is identical with goodness of understanding, men of understanding with men of good understanding.) Now understanding is neither the having nor the acquiring of practical wisdom; but as learning is called understanding when it means the exercise of the faculty of knowledge, so 'understanding' is applicable to the exercise of the faculty of opinion for the purpose of judging of what some one else says about matters with which practical wisdom is concerned—and of judging soundly; for 'well' and 'soundly' are the same thing. And from this has come the use of the name 'understanding' in virtue of which men are said to be 'of good understanding', viz. from the application of the word to the grasping of scientific truth; for we often call such grasping understanding.

11 What is called judgement, in virtue of which men are said to 'be sympathetic judges' 20

1143ᵃ

5

10

15

and to 'have judgement', is the right discrimination of the equitable. This is shown by the fact that we say the equitable man is above all others a man of sympathetic judgement, and identify equity with sympathetic judgement about certain facts. And sympathetic judgement is judgement which discriminates what is equitable and does so correctly; and correct judgement is that which judges what is true.

25 Now all the states we have considered converge, as might be expected, to the same point; for when we speak of judgement and understanding and practical wisdom and intuitive reason we credit the same people with possessing judgement and having reached years of reason and with having practical wisdom and understanding. For all these faculties deal with ultimates, i.e. with particulars; and being a man of understanding and of good or sympathetic
30 judgement consists in being able to judge about the things with which practical wisdom is concerned; for the equities are common to all good men in relation to other men. Now all things which have to be done are included among particulars or ultimates; for not only must the man of practical wisdom know particular facts, but understanding and judgement are' also concerned with things to be done, and these
35 are ultimates. And intuitive reason is concerned with the ultimates in both directions; for both the first terms and the last are objects of intui-
1143ᵇ tive reason and not of argument, and the intuitive reason which is presupposed by demonstrations grasps the unchangeable and first terms, while the intuitive reason involved in practical reasonings grasps the last and variable fact, i. e. the minor premiss. For these variable facts are the starting-points for the apprehension of the
5 end, since the universals are reached from the particulars; of these therefore we must have perception, and this perception is intuitive reason.

This is why these states are thought to be natural endowments—why, while no one is thought to be a philosopher by nature, people are thought to have by nature judgement, understanding, and intuitive reason. This is shown

by the fact that we think our powers correspond to our time of life, and that a particular age brings with it intuitive reason and judgement; this implies that nature is the cause. [Hence intuitive reason is both beginning and end; for 10 demonstrations are from these and about these.] Therefore we ought to attend to the undemonstrated sayings and opinions of experienced and older people or of people of practical wisdom not less than to demonstrations; for because experience has given them an eye they see aright.

We have stated, then, what practical and philosophic wisdom are, and with what each of them is concerned, and we have said that each is 15 the virtue of a different part of the soul.

12 Difficulties might be raised as to the utility of these qualities of mind. For (1) philosophic wisdom will contemplate none of the things that will make a man happy (for it is not concerned with any coming into being), and 20 though practical wisdom has *this* merit, for what purpose do we need it? Practical wisdom is the quality of mind concerned with things just and noble and good for man, but these are the things which it is the mark of a *good* man to do, and we are none the more able to act for *knowing* them if the virtues are states of *character*, just as we 25 are none the better able to act for knowing the things that are healthy and sound, in the sense not of producing but of issuing from the state of health; for we are none the more able to act for having the art of medicine or of gymnastics. But (2) if we are to say that a man should have practical wisdom not for the sake of knowing moral truths but for the sake of becoming good, practical wisdom will be of no use to those who 30 *are* good; but again it is of no use to those who have *not* virtue; for it will make no difference whether they have practical wisdom themselves or obey others who have it, and it would be enough for us to do what we do in the case of health; though we wish to become healthy, yet we do not learn the art of medicine. (3) Besides this, it would be thought· strange if practical wisdom, being inferior to philosophic wisdom,

is to be put in authority over it, as seems to be implied by the fact that the art which produces anything rules and issues commands about that thing.

35   These, then, are the questions we must discuss; so far we have only stated the difficulties.

1144ᵃ   (1) Now first let us say that in themselves these states must be worthy of choice because they are the virtues of the two parts of the soul respectively, even if neither of them produce anything.

(2) Secondly, they do produce something, not as the art of medicine produces health, however, but as health produces health;[10] so does philosophic wisdom produce happiness; for, 5 being a part of virtue entire, by being possessed and by actualizing itself it makes a man happy.

(3) Again, the work of man is achieved only in accordance with practical wisdom as well as with moral virtue; for virtue makes us aim at the right mark, and practical wisdom makes us take the right means. (Of the fourth part of the soul—the nutritive[11]—there is no such virtue; for 10 there is nothing which it is in its power to do or not to do.)

(4) With regard to our being none the more able to do because of our practical wisdom what is noble and just, let us begin a little further back; starting with the following principle. As we say that some people who do just acts are not necessarily just, i.e. those who do the acts 15 ordained by the laws either unwillingly or owing to ignorance or for some other reason and not for the sake of the acts themselves (though, to be sure, they do what they should and all the things that the good man ought), so is it, it seems, that in order to be good one must be in a certain state when one does the several acts, 20 i. e. one must do them as a result of choice and for the sake of the acts themselves. Now virtue makes the choice right, but the question of the things which should naturally be done to carry out our choice belongs not to virtue but to

another faculty. We must devote our attention to these matters and give a clearer statement about them. There is a faculty which is called 25 cleverness; and this is such as to be able to do the things that tend towards the mark we have set before ourselves, and to hit it. Now if the mark be noble, the cleverness is laudable, but if the mark be bad, the cleverness is mere smartness; hence we call even men of practical wisdom clever or smart. Practical wisdom is not the faculty, but it does not exist without this faculty. And this eye of the soul acquires its formed state not 30 without the aid of virtue, as has been said[12] and is plain; for the syllogisms which deal with acts to be done are things which involve a starting-point, viz. 'since the end, i.e. what is best, is of such and such a nature', whatever it may be (let it for the sake of argument be what we please); and this is not evident except to the good man; for wickedness perverts us and causes us to be 35 deceived about the starting-points of action. Therefore it is evident that it is impossible to be practically wise without being good.

13   We must therefore consider virtue also 1144ᵇ once more; for virtue too is similarly related; as practical wisdom is to cleverness—not the same, but like it—so is natural virtue to virtue in the strict sense. For all men think that each type of character belongs to its possessors in some sense by nature; for from the very moment of 5 birth we are just or fitted for self-control or brave or have the other moral qualities; but yet we seek something else as that which is good in the strict sense—we seek for the presence of such qualities in another way. For both children and brutes have the natural dispositions to these qualities, but without reason these are evidently hurtful. Only we seem to see this much, that, 10 while one may be led astray by them, as a strong body which moves without sight may stumble badly because of its lack of sight, still, if a man once acquires reason, that makes a difference in

---

[10] i. e. as health, as an inner state, produces the activities which we know as constituting health.
[11] The other three being the scientific, the calculative, and the desiderative.
[12] ll. 6–26.

action; and his state, while still like what it was, will then be virtue in the strict sense. Therefore, as in the part of us which forms opinions there 15 are two types, cleverness and practical wisdom, so too in the moral part there are two types, natural virtue and virtue in the strict sense, and of these the latter involves practical wisdom. This is why some say that all the virtues are forms of practical wisdom, and why Socrates in one respect was on the right track while in another he went astray; in thinking that all the virtues were forms of practical wisdom he was wrong, but in saying they implied practical 20 wisdom he was right. This is confirmed by the fact that even now all men, when they define virtue, after naming the state of character and its objects add 'that (state) which is in accordance with the right rule'; now the right rule is that which is in accordance with practical wisdom. All men, then, seem somehow to divine that this kind of state is virtue, viz. that which is in 25 accordance with practical wisdom. But we must go a little further. For it is not merely the state in accordance with the right rule, but the state that implies the *presence* of the right rule, that is virtue; and practical wisdom is a right rule about such matters. Socrates, then, thought the virtues were rules or rational principles (for he thought they were, all of them, forms of scientific knowledge), while we think they *involve* a rational principle.

It is clear, then, from what has been said, that 30 it is not possible to be good in the strict sense without practical wisdom, nor practically wise without moral virtue. But in this way we may also refute the dialectical argument whereby it might be contended that the virtues exist in separation from each other; the same man, it might be said, is not best equipped by nature for all the virtues, so that he will have already acquired 35 one when he has not yet acquired another. This is possible in respect of the natural virtues, but 1145ᵃ not in respect of those in respect of which a man is called without qualification good; for with the presence of the one quality, practical wisdom, will be given all the virtues. And it is plain that, even if it were of no practical value, we should have needed it because it is the virtue of the part of us in question; plain too that the choice will not be right without practical wisdom any more than without virtue; for the one determines the 5 end and the other makes us do the things that lead to the end.

But again it is not *supreme* over philosophic wisdom, i.e. over the superior part of us, any more than the art of medicine is over health; for it does not use it but provides for its coming into being; it issues orders, then, for its sake, but 10 not to it. Further, to maintain its supremacy would be like saying that the art of politics rules the gods because it issues orders about all the affairs of the state.

Groundwork of the Metaphysics of Morals

Immanuel Kant

Transition from the Metaphysic of Morals to the Critique of Pure Practical Reason

The Concept of Freedom is the Key that explains the Autonomy of the Will

The will is a kind of causality belonging to living beings in so far as they are rational, and freedom would be this property of such causality that it can be efficient, independently of foreign causes determining it; just as physical necessity is the property that the causality of all irrational beings has of being determined to activity by the influence of foreign causes.

The preceding definition of freedom is negative and therefore unfruitful for the discovery of its essence, but it leads to a positive conception which is so much the more full and fruitful.

Since the conception of causality involves that of laws, according to which, by something that we call cause, something else, namely the effect, must be produced; hence, although freedom is not a property of the will depending on physical laws, yet it is not for that reason lawless; on the contrary it must be a causality acting according to immutable laws, but of a peculiar kind; otherwise a free will would be an absurdity. Physical necessity is a heteronomy of the efficient causes, for every effect is possible only according to this law, that something else determines the efficient cause to exert its causality. What else then can freedom of the will be but autonomy, that is, the property of the will to be a law to itself? But the proposition: "The will is in every action a law to itself," only expresses the principle: "To act on no other maxim than that which can also have as an object itself as a universal law." Now this is precisely the formula of the categorical imperative and is the principle of morality, so that a free will and a will subject to moral laws are one and the same.

On the hypothesis, then, of freedom of the will, morality together with its principle follows from it by mere analysis of the conception. However, the latter is a synthetic proposition; viz., an absolutely good will is that whose maxim can always include itself regarded as a universal law; for this property of its maxim can never be discovered by analysing the conception of an absolutely good will. Now such synthetic propositions are only possible in this way: that the two cognitions are connected together by their union with a third in which they are both to be found. The positive concept of freedom furnishes this third cognition, which cannot, as with physical causes, be the nature of the sensible world (in the concept of which we find conjoined the concept of something in relation as cause to something else as effect). We cannot now at once show what this third is to which freedom points us and of which we have an idea a priori, nor can we make intelligible how the concept of freedom is shown to be legitimate from principles of pure practical reason and with it the possibility of a categorical imperative; but some further preparation is required.

Freedom Must Be Presupposed as a Property of the Will of All Rational Beings

It is not enough to predicate freedom of our own will, from Whatever reason, if we have not sufficient grounds for predicating the same of all rational beings. For as morality serves as a law for us only because we are rational beings, it must also hold for all rational beings; and as it must be deduced simply from the property of freedom, it must be shown that freedom also is a property of all rational beings. It is not enough, then, to prove it from certain, supposed experiences of human nature (which indeed is quite impossible, and it can only be shown a priori), but we must show that it belongs to the activity of all rational beings endowed with a will. Now I say every being that cannot act except under the idea of freedom is just for that reason in a practical point of view really free, that is to say, all laws which are inseparably connected with freedom have the same force for him as if his will had been shown to be free in itself by a proof theoretically conclusive. [I adopt this method of assuming freedom merely as an idea which rational beings suppose in their actions, in order to avoid the necessity of proving it in its theoretical aspect also. The former is sufficient for my purpose; for even though the speculative proof should not be made out, yet a being that cannot

act except with the idea of freedom is bound by the same laws that would oblige a being who was actually free. Thus we can escape here from the onus which presses on the theory.] Now I affirm that we must attribute to every rational being which has a will that it has also the idea of freedom and acts entirely under this idea. For in such a being we conceive a reason that is practical, that is, has causality in reference to its objects. Now we cannot possibly conceive a reason consciously receiving a bias from any other quarter with respect to its judgements, for then the subject would ascribe the determination of its judgement not to its own reason, but to an impulse. It must regard itself as the author of its principles independent of foreign influences. Consequently as practical reason or as the will of a rational being it must regard itself as free, that is to say, the will of such a being cannot be a will of its own except under the idea of freedom. This idea must therefore in a practical point of view be ascribed to every rational being.

Of the Interest Attaching to the Ideas of Morality

We have finally reduced the definite conception of morality to the idea of freedom. This latter, however, we could not prove to be actually a property of ourselves or of human nature; only we saw that it must be presupposed if we would conceive a being as rational and conscious of its causality in respect of its actions, i.e., as endowed with a will; and so we find that on just the same grounds we must ascribe to every being endowed with reason and will this attribute of determining itself to action under the idea of its freedom.

Now it resulted also from the presupposition of these ideas that we became aware of a law that the subjective principles of action, i.e., maxims, must always be so assumed that they can also hold as objective, that is, universal principles, and so serve as universal laws of our own dictation. But why then should I subject myself to this principle and that simply as a rational being, thus also subjecting to it all other being endowed with reason? I will allow that no interest urges me to this, for that would not give a categorical imperative, but I must take an interest in it and discern how this comes to pass; for this properly an "I ought" is properly an "I would," valid for every rational being, provided only that reason determined his actions without any hindrance. But for beings that are in addition affected as we are by springs of a different kind, namely, sensibility, and in whose case that is not always done which reason alone would do, for these that necessity is expressed only as an "ought," and the subjective necessity is different from the objective.

It seems then as if the moral law, that is, the principle of autonomy of the will, were properly speaking only presupposed in the idea of freedom, and as if we could not prove its reality and objective necessity independently. In that case we should still have gained something considerable by at least determining the true principle more exactly than had previously been done; but as regards its validity and the practical necessity of subjecting oneself to it, we should not have advanced a step. For if we were asked why the universal validity of our maxim as a law must be the condition restricting our actions, and on what we ground the worth which we assign to this manner of acting—a worth so great that there cannot be any higher interest; and if we were asked further how it happens that it is by this alone a man believes he feels his own personal worth, in comparison with which that of an agreeable or disagreeable condition is to be regarded as nothing, to these questions we could give no satisfactory answer.

We find indeed sometimes that we can take an interest in a personal quality which does not involve any interest of external condition, provided this quality makes us capable of participating in the condition in case reason were to effect the allotment; that is to say, the mere being worthy of happiness can interest of itself

even without the motive of participating in this happiness. This judgement, however, is in fact only the effect of the importance of the moral law which we before presupposed (when by the idea of freedom we detach ourselves from every empirical interest); but that we ought to detach ourselves from these interests, i.e., to consider ourselves as free in action and yet as subject to certain laws, so as to find a worth simply in our own person which can compensate us for the loss of everything that gives worth to our condition; this we are not yet able to discern in this way, nor do we see how it is possible so to act—in other words, whence the moral law derives its obligation.

It must be freely admitted that there is a sort of circle here from which it seems impossible to escape. In the order of efficient causes we assume ourselves free, in order that in the order of ends we may conceive ourselves as subject to moral laws: and we afterwards conceive ourselves as subject to these laws, because we have attributed to ourselves freedom of will: for freedom and self-legislation of will are both autonomy and, therefore, are reciprocal conceptions, and for this very reason one must not be used to explain the other or give the reason of it, but at most only logical purposes to reduce apparently different notions of the same object to one single concept (as we reduce different fractions of the same value to the lowest terms).

One resource remains to us, namely, to inquire whether we do not occupy different points of view when by means of freedom we think ourselves as causes efficient a priori, and when we form our conception of ourselves from our actions as effects which we see before our eyes.

It is a remark which needs no subtle reflection to make, but which we may assume that even the commonest understanding can make, although it be after its fashion by an obscure discernment of judgement which it calls feeling, that all the "ideas" that come to us involuntarily (as those of the senses) do not enable us to know objects otherwise than as they affect us; so that what they may be in themselves remains unknown to us, and consequently that as regards "ideas" of this kind even with the closest attention and clearness that the understanding can apply to them, we can by them only attain to the knowledge of appearances, never to that of things in themselves. As soon as this distinction has once been made (perhaps merely in consequence of the difference observed between the ideas given us from without, and in which we are passive, and those that we produce simply from ourselves, and in which we show our own activity), then it follows of itself that we must admit and assume behind the appearance something else that is not an appearance, namely, the things in themselves; although we must admit that as they can never be known to us except as they affect us, we can come no nearer to them, nor can we ever know what they are in themselves. This must furnish a distinction, however crude, between a world of sense and the world of understanding, of which the former may be different according to the difference of the sensuous impressions in various observers, while the second which is its basis always remains the same, Even as to himself, a man cannot pretend to know what he is in himself from the knowledge he has by internal sensation. For as he does not as it were create himself, and does not come by the conception of himself a priori but empirically, it naturally follows that he can obtain his knowledge even of himself only by the inner sense and, consequently, only through the appearances of his nature and the way in which his consciousness is affected. At the same time beyond these characteristics of his own subject, made up of mere appearances, he must necessarily suppose something else as their basis, namely, his ego, whatever its characteristics in itself may be. Thus in respect to mere perception and receptivity of sensations he must reckon himself as belonging to the world of sense; but in respect of whatever there may be of pure activity in him (that which reaches consciousness immediately and not through affecting the senses), he must reckon himself as belonging to the intellectual world, of which, however, he has no further knowledge. To such

a conclusion the reflecting man must come with respect to all the things which can be presented to him: it is probably to be met with even in persons of the commonest understanding, who, as is well known, are very much inclined to suppose behind the objects of the senses something else invisible and acting of itself. They spoil it, however, by presently sensualizing this invisible again; that is to say, wanting to make it an object of intuition, so that they do not become a whit the wiser.

Now man really finds in himself a faculty by which he distinguishes himself from everything else, even from himself as affected by objects, and that is reason. This being pure spontaneity is even elevated above the understanding. For although the latter is a spontaneity and does not, like sense, merely contain intuitions that arise when we are affected by things (and are therefore passive), yet it cannot produce from its activity any other conceptions than those which merely serve to bring the intuitions of sense under rules and, thereby, to unite them in one consciousness, and without this use of the sensibility it could not think at all; whereas, on the contrary, reason shows so pure a spontaneity in the case of what I call ideas [ideal conceptions] that it thereby far transcends everything that the sensibility can give it, and exhibits its most important function in distinguishing the world of sense from that of understanding, and thereby prescribing the limits of the understanding itself.

For this reason a rational being must regard himself qua intelligence (not from the side of his lower faculties) as belonging not to the world of sense, but to that of understanding; hence he has two points of view from which he can regard himself, and recognise laws of the exercise of his faculties, and consequently of all his actions: first, so far as he belongs to the world of sense, he finds himself subject to laws of nature (heteronomy); secondly, as belonging to the intelligible world, under laws which being independent of nature have their foundation not in experience but in reason alone.

As a rational being, and consequently belonging to the intelligible world, man can never conceive the causality of his own will otherwise than on condition of the idea of freedom, for independence of the determinate causes of the sensible world (an independence which reason must always ascribe to itself) is freedom. Now the idea of freedom is inseparably connected with the conception of autonomy, and this again with the universal principle of morality which is ideally the foundation of all actions of rational beings, just as the law of nature is of all phenomena.

Now the suspicion is removed which we raised above, that there was a latent circle involved in our reasoning from freedom to autonomy, and from this to the moral law, viz.: that we laid down the idea of freedom because of the moral law only that we might afterwards in turn infer the latter from freedom, and that consequently we could assign no reason at all for this law, but could only [present] it as a petitio principii which well disposed minds would gladly concede to us, but which we could never put forward as a provable proposition. For now we see that, when we conceive ourselves as free, we transfer ourselves into the world of understanding as members of it and recognise the autonomy of the will with its consequence, morality; whereas, if we conceive ourselves as under obligation, we consider ourselves as belonging to the world of sense and at the same time to the world of understanding.

How Is a Categorical Imperative Possible?

Every rational being reckons himself qua intelligence as belonging to the world of understanding, and it is simply as an efficient cause belonging to that world that he calls his causality a will. On the other side he is also conscious of himself as a part of the world of sense in which his actions, which are mere appearances [phenomena] of that causality, are displayed; we cannot, however, discern how they are possible from this causality which we do not know; but instead of that, these actions as belonging to the sensible world must be viewed as determined by other phenomena, namely, desires and inclinations. If therefore I were only a member of the world of understanding, then all my actions would perfectly conform to the principle of autonomy of the pure will; if I were only a part of the world of sense, they would necessarily be assumed to conform wholly to the natural law of desires and inclinations, in other words, to the heteronomy of nature. (The former would rest on morality as the supreme principle, the latter on happiness.) Since, however, the world of understanding contains the foundation of the world of sense, and consequently of its laws also, and accordingly gives the law to my will (which belongs wholly to the world of understanding) directly, and must be conceived as doing so, it follows that, although on the one side I must regard myself as a being belonging to the world of sense, yet on the other side I must recognize myself as subject as an intelligence to the law of the world of understanding, i.e., to reason, which contains this law in the idea of freedom, and therefore as subject to the autonomy of the will: consequently I must regard the laws of the world of understanding as imperatives for me and the actions which conform to them as duties.

And thus what makes categorical imperatives possible is this, that the idea of freedom makes me a member of an intelligible world, in consequence of which, if I were nothing else, all my actions would always conform to the autonomy of the will; but as I at the same time intuite myself as a member of the world of sense, they ought so to conform, and this categorical "ought" implies a synthetic a priori proposition, inasmuch as besides my will as affected by sensible desires there is added further the idea of the same will but as belonging to the world of the understanding, pure and practical of itself, which contains the supreme condition according to reason of the former will; precisely as to the intuitions of sense there are added concepts of the understanding which of themselves signify nothing but regular form in general and in this way synthetic a priori propositions become possible, on which all knowledge of physical nature rests.

The practical use of common human reason confirms this reasoning. There is no one, not even the most consummate villain, provided only that he is otherwise accustomed to the use of reason, who, when we set before him examples of honesty of purpose, of steadfastness in following good maxims, of sympathy and general benevolence (even combined with great sacrifices of advantages and comfort), does not wish that he might also possess these qualities. Only on account of his inclinations and impulses he cannot attain this in himself, but at the same time he wishes to be free from such inclinations which are burdensome to himself. He proves by this that he transfers himself in thought with a will free from the impulses of the sensibility into an order of things wholly different from that of his desires in the field of the sensibility; since he cannot expect to obtain by that wish any gratification of his desires, nor any position which would satisfy any of his actual or supposable inclinations (for this would destroy the preeminence of the very idea which wrests that wish from him): he can only expect a greater intrinsic worth of his own person. This better person, however, he imagines himself to be when be transfers himself to the point of view of a member of the world of the understanding, to which he is involuntarily forced by the idea of freedom, i.e., of independence on determining causes of the world of sense; and from this point of view he is conscious of a good will, which by his own confession constitutes the law for the bad will that he possesses as a member of the world of sense—a law whose authority he recognizes while transgressing it. What he morally "ought" is then what he necessarily "would," as a member of the world of the understanding, and is conceived by him as an "ought" only inasmuch as he likewise considers himself as a member of the world of sense.

Of the Extreme Limits of all Practical Philosophy.

All men attribute to themselves freedom of will. Hence come all judgements upon actions as being such as ought to have been done, although they have not been done. However, this freedom is not a conception of experience, nor can it be so, since it still remains, even though experience shows the contrary of what on supposition of freedom are conceived as its necessary consequences. On the other side it is equally necessary that everything that takes place should be fixedly determined according to laws of nature. This necessity of nature is likewise not an empirical conception, just for this reason, that it involves the motion of necessity and consequently of a priori cognition. But this conception of a system of nature is confirmed by experience; and it must even be inevitably presupposed if experience itself is to be possible, that is, a connected knowledge of the objects of sense resting on general laws. Therefore freedom is only an idea of reason, and its objective reality in itself is doubtful; while nature is a concept of the understanding which proves, and must necessarily prove, its reality in examples of experience.

There arises from this a dialectic of reason, since the freedom attributed to the will appears to contradict the necessity of nature, and placed between these two ways reason for speculative purposes finds the road of physical necessity much more beaten and more appropriate than that of freedom; yet for practical purposes the narrow footpath of freedom is the only one on which it is possible to make use of reason in our conduct; hence it is just as impossible for the subtlest philosophy as for the commonest reason of men to argue away freedom. Philosophy must then assume that no real contradiction will be found between freedom and physical necessity of the same human actions, for it cannot give up the conception of nature any more than that of freedom.

Nevertheless, even though we should never be able to comprehend how freedom is possible, we must at least remove this apparent contradiction in a convincing manner. For if the thought of freedom contradicts either itself or nature, which is equally necessary, it must in competition with physical necessity be entirely given up.

It would, however, be impossible to escape this contradiction if the thinking subject, which seems to itself free, conceived itself in the same sense or in the very same relation when it calls itself free as when in respect of the same action it assumes itself to be subject to the law of nature. Hence it is an indispensable problem of speculative philosophy to show that its illusion respecting the contradiction rests on this, that we think of man in a different sense and relation when we call him free and when we regard him as subject to the laws of nature as being part and parcel of nature. It must therefore show that not only can both these very well co-exist, but that both must be thought as necessarily united in the same subject, since otherwise no reason could be given why we should burden reason with an idea which, though it may possibly without contradiction be reconciled with another that is sufficiently established, yet entangles us in a perplexity which sorely embarrasses reason in its theoretic employment. This duty, however; belongs only to speculative philosophy. The philosopher then has no option whether he will remove the apparent contradiction or leave it untouched; for in the latter case the theory respecting this would be bonum vacans, into the possession of which the fatalist would have a right to enter and chase all morality out of its supposed domain as occupying it without title.

We cannot however as yet say that we are touching the bounds of practical philosophy. For the settlement of that controversy does not belong to it; it only demands from speculative reason that it should put an end to the discord in which it entangles itself in theoretical questions, so that practical reason may have rest and security from external attacks which might make the ground debatable on which it desires to build.

The claims to freedom of will made even by common reason are founded on the consciousness and the admitted supposition that reason is independent of merely subjectively determined causes which together constitute what belongs to sensation only and which consequently come under the general designation of sensibility. Man considering himself in this way as an intelligence places himself thereby in a different order of things and in a relation to determining grounds of a wholly different kind when on the one hand he thinks of himself as an intelligence endowed with a will, and consequently with causality, and when on the other he perceives himself as a phenomenon in the world of sense (as he really is also), and affirms that his causality is subject to external determination according to laws of nature. Now he soon becomes aware that both can hold good, nay, must hold good at the same time. For there is not the smallest contradiction in saying that a thing in appearance (belonging to the world of sense) is subject to certain laws, of which the very same as a thing or being in itself is independent, and that he must conceive and think of himself in this twofold way, rests as to the first on the consciousness of himself as an object affected through the senses, and as to the second on the consciousness of himself as an intelligence, i.e., as independent on sensible impressions in the employment of his reason (in other words as belonging to the world of understanding).

Hence it comes to pass that man claims the possession of a will which takes no account of anything that comes under the head of desires and inclinations and, on the contrary, conceives actions as possible to him, nay, even as necessary which can only be done by disregarding all desires and sensible inclinations. The causality of such actions lies in him as an intelligence and in the laws of effects and actions [which depend] on the principles of an intelligible world, of which indeed he knows nothing more than that in it pure reason alone independent of sensibility gives the law; moreover since it is only in that world, as an intelligence, that he is his proper self (being as man only the appearance of himself), those laws apply to him directly and categorically, so that the incitements of inclinations and appetites (in other words the whole nature of the world of sense) cannot impair the laws of his volition as an intelligence. Nay, he does not even hold himself responsible for the former or ascribe them to his proper self, i.e., his will: he only ascribes to his will any indulgence which he might yield them if he allowed them to influence his maxims to the prejudice of the rational laws of the will.

When practical reason thinks itself into a world of understanding, it does not thereby transcend its own limits, as it would if it tried to enter it by intuition or sensation. The former is only a negative thought in respect of the world of sense, which does not give any laws to reason in determining the will and is positive only in this single point that this freedom as a negative characteristic is at the same time conjoined with a (positive) faculty and even with a causality of reason, which we designate a will, namely a faculty of so acting that the principle of the actions shall conform to the essential character of a rational motive, i.e., the condition that the maxim have universal validity as a law. But were it to borrow an object of will, that is, a motive, from the world of understanding, then it would overstep its bounds and pretend to be acquainted with something of which it knows nothing. The conception of a world of the understanding is then only a point of view which reason finds itself compelled to take outside the appearances in order to conceive itself as practical, which would not be possible if the influences of the sensibility had a determining power on man, but which is necessary unless he is to be denied the consciousness of himself as an intelligence and, consequently, as a rational cause, energizing by reason, that is, operating freely. This thought certainly involves the idea of an order and a system of laws different from that of the mechanism of nature which belongs to the sensible world; and it makes the conception of an intelligible world necessary (that is to say, the whole system of

rational beings as things in themselves). But it does not in the least authorize us to think of it further than as to its formal condition only, that is, the universality of the maxims of the will as laws, and consequently the autonomy of the latter, which alone is consistent with its freedom; whereas, on the contrary, all laws that refer to a definite object give heteronomy, which only belongs to laws of nature and can only apply to the sensible world.

But reason would overstep all its bounds if it undertook to explain how pure reason can be practical, which would be exactly the same problem as to explain how freedom is possible.

For we can explain nothing but that which we can reduce to laws, the object of which can be given in some possible experience. But freedom is a mere idea, the objective reality of which can in no wise be shown according to laws of nature, and consequently not in any possible experience; and for this reason it can never be comprehended or understood, because we cannot support it by any sort of example or analogy. It holds good only as a necessary hypothesis of reason in a being that believes itself conscious of a will, that is, of a faculty distinct from mere desire (namely, a faculty of determining itself to action as an intelligence, in other words, by laws of reason independently on natural instincts). Now where determination according to laws of nature ceases, there all explanation ceases also, and nothing remains but defence, i.e., the removal of the objections of those who pretend to have seen deeper into the nature of things, and thereupon boldly declare freedom impossible. We can only point out to them that the supposed contradiction that they have discovered in it arises only from this, that in order to be able to apply the law of nature to human actions, they must necessarily consider man as an appearance: then when we demand of them that they should also think of him qua intelligence as a thing in itself, they still persist in considering him in this respect also as an appearance. In this view it would no doubt be a contradiction to suppose the causality of the same subject (that is, his will) to be withdrawn from all the natural laws of the sensible world. But this contradiction disappears, if they would only bethink themselves and admit, as is reasonable, that behind the appearances there must also lie at their root (although hidden) the things in themselves, and that we cannot expect the laws of these to be the same as those that govern their appearances.

The subjective impossibility of explaining the freedom of the will is identical with the impossibility of discovering and explaining an interest [Interest is that by which reason becomes practical, i.e., a cause determining the will. Hence we say of rational beings only that they take an interest in a thing; irrational beings only feel sensual appetites. Reason takes a direct interest in action then only when the universal validity of its maxims is alone sufficient to determine the will. Such an interest alone is pure. But if it can determine the will only by means of another object of desire or on the suggestion of a particular feeling of the subject, then reason takes only an indirect interest in the action, and, as reason by itself without experience cannot discover either objects of the will or a special feeling actuating it, this latter interest would only be empirical and not a pure rational interest. The logical interest of reason (namely, to extend its insight) is never direct, but presupposes purposes for which reason is employed.] which man can take in the moral law. Nevertheless he does actually take an interest in it, the basis of which in us we call the moral feeling, which some have falsely assigned as the standard of our moral judgement, whereas it must rather be viewed as the subjective effect that the law exercises on the will, the objective principle of which is furnished by reason alone.

In order indeed that a rational being who is also affected through the senses should will what reason alone directs such beings that they ought to will, it is no doubt requisite that reason should have a power to infuse a feeling of pleasure or satisfaction in the fulfilment of duty, that is to say, that it should have a causality by which it determines the sensibility according to

its own principles. But it is quite impossible to discern, i.e., to make it intelligible a priori, how a mere thought, which itself contains nothing sensible, can itself produce a sensation of pleasure or pain; for this is a particular kind of causality of which as of every other causality we can determine nothing whatever a priori; we must only consult experience about it. But as this cannot supply us with any relation of cause and effect except between two objects of experience, whereas in this case, although indeed the effect produced lies within experience, yet the cause is supposed to be pure reason acting through mere ideas which offer no object to experience, it follows that for us men it is quite impossible to explain how and why the universality of the maxim as a law, that is, morality, interests. This only is certain, that it is not because it interests us that it has validity for us (for that would be heteronomy and dependence of practical reason on sensibility, namely, on a feeling as its principle, in which case it could never give moral laws), but that it interests us because it is valid for us as men, inasmuch as it had its source in our will as intelligences, in other words, in our proper self, and what belongs to mere appearance is necessarily subordinated by reason to the nature of the thing in itself.

The question then, "How a categorical imperative is possible," can be answered to this extent, that we can assign the only hypothesis on which it is possible, namely, the idea of freedom; and we can also discern the necessity of this hypothesis, and this is sufficient for the practical exercise of reason, that is, for the conviction of the validity of this imperative, and hence of the moral law; but how this hypothesis itself is possible can never be discerned by any human reason. On the hypothesis, however, that the will of an intelligence is free, its autonomy, as the essential formal condition of its determination, is a necessary consequence. Moreover, this freedom of will is not merely quite possible as a hypothesis (not involving any contradiction to the principle of physical necessity in the connexion of the phenomena of the sensible world) as speculative philosophy can show: but further, a rational being who is conscious of causality through reason, that is to say, of a will (distinct from desires), must of necessity make it practically, that is, in idea, the condition of all his voluntary actions. But to explain how pure reason can be of itself practical without the aid of any spring of action that could be derived from any other source, i.e., how the mere principle of the universal validity of all its maxims as laws (which would certainly be the form of a pure practical reason) can of itself supply a spring, without any matter (object) of the will in which one could antecedently take any interest; and how it can produce an interest which would be called purely moral; or in other words, how pure reason can be practical- to explain this is beyond the power of human reason, and all the labour and pains of seeking an explanation of it are lost.

It is just the same as if I sought to find out how freedom itself is possible as the causality of a will. For then I quit the ground of philosophical explanation, and I have no other to go upon. I might indeed revel in the world of intelligences which still remains to me, but although I have an idea of it which is well founded, yet I have not the least knowledge of it, nor an I ever attain to such knowledge with all the efforts of my natural faculty of reason. It signifies only a something that remains over when I have eliminated everything belonging to the world of sense from the actuating principles of my will, serving merely to keep in bounds the principle of motives taken from the field of sensibility; fixing its limits and showing that it does not contain all in all within itself, but that there is more beyond it; but this something more I know no further. Of pure reason which frames this ideal, there remains after the abstraction of all matter, i.e., knowledge of objects, nothing but the form, namely, the practical law of the universality of the maxims, and in conformity with this conception of reason in reference to a pure world of understanding as a possible efficient cause, that is a cause determining the will. There must here be a total absence of springs; unless this idea of

an intelligible world is itself the spring, or that in which reason primarily takes an interest; but to make this intelligible is precisely the problem that we cannot solve.

Here now is the extreme limit of all moral inquiry, and it is of great importance to determine it even on this account, in order that reason may not on the one band, to the prejudice of morals, seek about in the world of sense for the supreme motive and an interest comprehensible but empirical; and on the other hand, that it may not impotently flap its wings without being able to move in the (for it) empty space of transcendent concepts which we call the intelligible world, and so lose itself amidst chimeras. For the rest, the idea of a pure world of understanding as a system of all intelligences, and to which we ourselves as rational beings belong (although we are likewise on the other side members of the sensible world), this remains always a useful and legitimate idea for the purposes of rational belief, although all knowledge stops at its threshold, useful, namely, to produce in us a lively interest in the moral law by means of the noble ideal of a universal kingdom of ends in themselves (rational beings), to which we can belong as members then only when we carefully conduct ourselves according to the maxims of freedom as if they were laws of nature.

Concluding Remark

The speculative employment of reason with respect to nature leads to the absolute necessity of some supreme cause of the world: the practical employment of reason with a view to freedom leads also to absolute necessity, but only of the laws of the actions of a rational being as such. Now it is an essential principle of reason, however employed, to push its knowledge to a consciousness of its necessity (without which it would not be rational knowledge). It is, however, an equally essential restriction of the same reason that it can neither discern the necessity of what is or what happens, nor of what ought to happen, unless a condition is supposed on which it is or happens or ought to happen. In this way, however, by the constant inquiry for the condition, the satisfaction of reason is only further and further postponed. Hence it unceasingly seeks the unconditionally necessary and finds itself forced to assume it, although without any means of making it comprehensible to itself, happy enough if only it can discover a conception which agrees with this assumption. It is therefore no fault in our deduction of the supreme principle of morality, but an objection that should be made to human reason in general, that it cannot enable us to conceive the absolute necessity of an unconditional practical law (such as the categorical imperative must be). It cannot be blamed for refusing to explain this necessity by a condition, that is to say, by means of some interest assumed as a basis, since the law would then cease to be a supreme law of reason. And thus while we do not comprehend the practical unconditional necessity of the moral imperative, we yet comprehend its incomprehensibility, and this is all that can be fairly demanded of a philosophy which strives to carry its principles up to the very limit of human reason.

Utilitarianism

John Stuart Mill

What Utilitarianism Is

A PASSING REMARK is all that needs be given to the ignorant blunder of supposing that those who stand up for utility as the test of right and wrong use the term in that restricted and merely colloquial sense in which utility is opposed to pleasure. An apology is due to the philosophical opponents of utilitarianism for even the momentary appearance of confounding them with anyone capable of so absurd a misconception; which is the more extraordinary, inasmuch as the contrary accusation, of referring everything to pleasure, and that, too, in its grossest form, is another of the common charges against utilitarianism: and, as has been pointedly remarked by an able writer, the same sort of persons, and often the very same persons, denounce the theory "as impracticably dry when the word 'utility' precedes the word 'pleasure,' and as too practically voluptuous when the word 'pleasure' precedes the word 'utility.'" Those who know anything about the matter are aware that every writer, from Epicurus to Bentham, who maintained the theory of utility meant by it, not something to be contradistinguished from pleasure, but pleasure itself, together with exemption from pain; and instead of opposing the useful to the agreeable or the ornamental, have always declared that the useful means these, among other things. Yet the common herd, including the herd of writers, not only in newspapers and periodicals, but in books of weight and pretension, are perpetually falling into this shallow mistake. Having caught up the word "utilitarian," while knowing nothing whatever about it but its sound, they habitually express by it the rejection or the neglect of pleasure in some of its forms: of beauty, of ornament, or of amusement. Nor is the term thus ignorantly misapplied solely in disparagement, but occasionally in compliment, as though it implied superiority to frivolity and the mere pleasures of the moment. And this perverted use is the only one in which the word is popularly known, and the one from which the new generation are acquiring their sole notion of its meaning. Those who introduced the word, but who had for many years discontinued it as a distinctive appellation, may well feel themselves called upon to resume it if by doing so they can hope to contribute anything toward rescuing it from this utter degradation.[1]

The creed which accepts as the foundation of morals "utility" or the "greatest happiness principle" holds that actions are right in proportion as they tend to promote happiness; wrong as they tend to produce the reverse of happiness. By happiness is intended pleasure and the absence of pain; by unhappiness, pain and the privation of pleasure. To give a clear view of the moral standard set up by the theory, much more requires to be said; in particular, what things it includes in the ideas of pain and pleasure, and to what extent this is left an open question. But these supplementary explanations do not affect the theory of life on which this theory of morality is grounded—namely, that pleasure and freedom from pain are the only things desirable as ends; and that all desirable things (which are as numerous in the utilitarian as in any other scheme) are desirable either for pleasure inherent in themselves or as means to the promotion of pleasure and the prevention of pain.

Now such a theory of life excites in many minds, and among them in some of the most estimable in feeling and purpose, inveterate dislike. To suppose that life has (as they express it) no higher end than pleasure—no better and nobler object of desire and pursuit—they designate as utterly mean and groveling, as a doctrine worthy only of swine, to whom the followers of Epicurus were, at a very early period, contemptuously likened; and modern holders of the doctrine are occasionally made the subject of equally polite comparisons by its German, French, and English assailants.

------

1   The author of this essay has reason for believing himself to be the first person who brought the word "utilitarian" into use. He did not invent it, but adopted it from a passing expression in Mr. Galt's *Annals of the Parish*. After using it as a designation for several years, he and others abandoned it from a growing dislike to anything resembling a badge or watchword of sectarian distinction. But as a name for one single opinion, not a set of opinions—to denote the recognition of utility as a standard, not any particular way of applying it—the term supplies a want in the language, and offers, in many cases, a convenient mode of avoiding tiresome circumlocution.

When thus attacked, the Epicureans have always answered that it is not they, but their accusers, who represent human nature in a degrading light, since the accusation supposes human beings to be capable of no pleasures except those of which swine are capable. If this supposition were true, the charge could not be gainsaid, but would then be no longer an imputation; for if the sources of pleasure were precisely the same to human beings and to swine, the rule of life which is good enough for the one would be good enough for the other. The comparison of the Epicurean life to that of beasts is felt as degrading, precisely because a beast's pleasures do not satisfy a human being's conceptions of happiness. Human beings have faculties more elevated than the animal appetites and, when once made conscious of them, do not regard anything as happiness which does not include their gratification. I do not, indeed, consider the Epicureans to have been by any means faultless in drawing out their scheme of consequences from the utilitarian principle. To do this in any sufficient manner, many Stoic, as well as Christian, elements require to be included. But there is no known Epicurean theory of life which does not assign to the pleasures of the intellect, of the feelings and imagination, and of the moral sentiments a much higher value as pleasures than to those of mere sensation. It must be admitted, however, that utilitarian writers in general have placed the superiority of mental over bodily pleasures chiefly in the greater permanency, safety, uncostliness, etc., of the former—that is, in their circumstantial advantages rather than in their intrinsic nature. And on all these points utilitarians have fully proved their case; but they might have taken the other and, as it may be called, higher ground with entire consistency. It is quite compatible with the principle of utility to recognize the fact that some kinds of pleasure are more desirable and more valuable than others. It would be absurd that, while in estimating all other things quality is considered as well as quantity, the estimation of pleasure should be supposed to depend on quantity alone.

If I am asked what I mean by difference of quality in pleasures, or what makes one pleasure more valuable than another, merely as a pleasure, except its being greater in amount, there is but one possible answer. Of two pleasures, if there be one to which all or almost all who have experience of both give a decided preference, irrespective of any feeling of moral obligation to prefer it, that is the more desirable pleasure. If one of the two is, by those who are competently acquainted with both, placed so far above the other that they prefer it, even though knowing it to be attended with a greater amount of discontent, and would not resign it for any quantity of the other pleasure which their nature is capable of, we are justified in ascribing to the preferred enjoyment a superiority in quality so far outweighing quantity as to render it, in comparison, of small account.

Now it is an unquestionable fact that those who are equally acquainted with and equally capable of appreciating and enjoying both do give a most marked preference to the manner of existence which employs their higher faculties. Few human creatures would consent to be changed into any of the lower animals for a promise of the fullest allowance of a beast's pleasures; no intelligent human being would consent to be a fool, no instructed person would be an ignoramus, no person of feeling and conscience would be selfish and base, even though they should be persuaded that the fool, the dunce, or the rascal is better satisfied with his lot than they are with theirs. They would not resign what they possess more than he for the most complete satisfaction of all the desires which they have in common with him. If they ever fancy they would, it is only in cases of unhappiness so extreme that to escape from it they would exchange their lot for almost any other, however undesirable in their own eyes. A being of higher faculties requires more to make him happy, is capable probably of more acute suffering, and certainly accessible to it at more points, than one of an inferior type; but in spite of these liabilities, he can never really wish to sink into what he feels to be a lower grade of existence. We may give what explanation we please of this unwillingness; we may attribute it to pride, a name which is given indiscriminately to some of the most and to some of the least estimable feelings of which mankind are capable; we may refer it to the love of liberty and personal independence, an appeal to which was with the Stoics one of the most effective means for the inculcation of it; to the love of power or to the love of excitement, both of which do really enter into and contribute to it; but its most appropriate appellation is a sense of dignity, which all human beings possess in one form or other, and in some, though by no means in exact, proportion to their higher faculties, and which is so essential a part of the happiness of those in whom it is strong that nothing which conflicts with it could be otherwise than momentarily an object of desire to them. Whoever supposes that this preference takes place at a sacrifice of happiness—that the superior being, in anything like equal circumstances, is not happier than the inferior—confounds the two very different ideas of happiness and content. It is indisputable that the being whose capacities of enjoyment are low has the greatest chance of having them fully satisfied; and a highly endowed being will always feel that any happiness which he can look for, as the world is constituted, is imperfect. But he can learn to bear its imperfections, if they are at all bearable; and they will not make him envy the being who is indeed unconscious of the imperfections, but only because he feels not at all the good which those imperfections qualify. It is better to be a human being dissatisfied than a pig satisfied; better to be Socrates dissatisfied than a fool satisfied. And if the fool, or the pig, are of a different opinion, it is because they only know their own side of the question. The other party to the comparison knows both sides.

It may be objected that many who are capable of the higher pleasures occasionally, under the influence of temptation, postpone them to the lower. But this is quite compatible with a full appreciation of the intrinsic superiority of the higher. Men often, from infirmity of character, make their election for the nearer good, though they know it to be the less valuable; and this no less when the choice is between two bodily pleasures than when it is between bodily and mental. They pursue sensual indulgences to the injury of health, though perfectly aware that health is the greater good. It may be further objected that many who begin with youthful enthusiasm for everything noble, as they advance in years, sink into indolence and selfishness. But I do not believe that those who undergo this very common change voluntarily choose the lower description of pleasures in preference to the higher. I believe that, before they devote themselves exclusively to the one, they have already become incapable of the other. Capacity for the nobler feelings is in most natures a very tender plant, easily killed, not only by hostile influences, but by mere want of sustenance; and in the majority of young persons it speedily dies away if the occupations to which their position in life has devoted them, and the society into which it has thrown them, are not favorable to keeping that higher capacity in exercise. Men lose their high aspirations as they lose their intellectual tastes, because they have not time or opportunity for indulging them; and they addict themselves to inferior pleasures, not because they deliberately prefer them, but because they are either the only ones to which they have access or the only ones which they are any longer capable of enjoying. It may be questioned whether anyone who has remained equally susceptible to both classes of pleasures ever knowingly and calmly preferred the lower, though many, in all ages, have broken down in an ineffectual attempt to combine both.

From this verdict of the only competent judges, I apprehend there can be no appeal. On a question which is the best worth having of two pleasures, or which of two modes of existence is the most grateful to the feelings, apart from its moral attributes and from its consequences, the judgment of those who are qualified by knowledge of both, or, if they differ, that of the majority among them, must be admitted as final. And

there needs be the less hesitation to accept this judgment respecting the quality of pleasures, since there is no other tribunal to be referred to even on the question of quantity. What means are there of determining which is the acutest of two pains, or the intensest of two pleasurable sensations, except the general suffrage of those who are familiar with both? Neither pains nor pleasures are homogeneous, and pain is always heterogeneous with pleasure. What is there to decide whether a particular pleasure is worth purchasing at the cost of a particular pain, except the feelings and judgment of the experienced? When, therefore, those feelings and judgment declare the pleasures derived from the higher faculties to be preferable *in kind*, apart from the question of intensity, to those of which the animal nature, disjoined from the higher faculties, is susceptible, they are entitled on this subject to the same regard.

I have dwelt on this point as being a necessary part of a perfectly just conception of utility or happiness considered as the directive rule of human conduct. But it is by no means an indispensable condition to the acceptance of the utilitarian standard; for that standard is not the agent's own greatest happiness, but the greatest amount of happiness altogether; and if it may possibly be doubted whether a noble character is always the happier for its nobleness, there can be no doubt that it makes other people happier, and that the world in general is immensely a gainer by it. Utilitarianism, therefore, could only attain its end by the general cultivation of nobleness of character, even if each individual were only benefited by the nobleness of others, and his own, so far as happiness is concerned, were a sheer deduction from the benefit. But the bare enunciation of such an absurdity as this last renders refutation superfluous.

According to the greatest happiness principle, as above explained, the ultimate end, with reference to and for the sake of which all other things are desirable—whether we are considering our own good or that of other people—is an existence exempt as far as possible from pain, and as rich as possible in enjoyments, both in point of quantity and quality; the test of quality and the rule for measuring it against quantity being the preference felt by those who, in their opportunities of experience, to which must be added their habits of self-consciousness and self-observation, are best furnished with the means of comparison. This, being according to the utilitarian opinion the end of human action, is necessarily also the standard of morality, which may accordingly be defined "the rules and precepts for human conduct," by the observance of which an existence such as has been described might be, to the greatest extent possible, secured to all mankind; and not to them only, but, so far as the nature of things admits, to the whole sentient creation.

Against this doctrine, however, arises another class of objectors who say that happiness, in any form, cannot be the rational purpose of human life and action; because, in the first place, it is unattainable; and they contemptuously ask, What right hast thou to be happy?—a question which Mr. Carlyle clinches by the addition, What right, a short time ago, hadst thou even *to be?* Next they say that men can do *without* happiness; that all noble human beings have felt this, and could not have become noble but by learning the lesson of *Entsagen*, or renunciation; which lesson, thoroughly learned and submitted to, they affirm to be the beginning and necessary condition of all virtue.

The first of these objections would go to the root of the matter were it well founded; for if no happiness is to be had at all by human beings, the attainment of it cannot be the end of morality or of any rational conduct. Though, even in that case, something might still be said for the utilitarian theory, since utility includes not solely the pursuit of happiness, but the prevention or mitigation of unhappiness; and if the former aim be chimerical, there will be all the greater scope and more imperative need for the latter, so long at least as mankind think fit to live and do not take refuge in the simultaneous act of suicide recommended under

certain conditions by Novalis.[2] When, however, it is thus positively asserted to be impossible that human life should be happy, the assertion, if not something like a verbal quibble, is at least an exaggeration. If by happiness be meant a continuity of highly pleasurable excitement, it is evident enough that this is impossible. A state of exalted pleasure lasts only moments or in some cases, and with some intermissions, hours or days, and is the occasional brilliant flash of enjoyment, not its permanent and steady flame. Of this the philosophers who have taught that happiness is the end of life were as fully aware as those who taunt them. The happiness which they meant was not a life of rapture, but moments of such, in an existence made up of few and transitory pains, many and various pleasures, with a decided predominance of the active over the passive, and having as the foundation of the whole not to expect more from life than it is capable of bestowing. A life thus composed, to those who have been fortunate enough to obtain it, has always appeared worthy of the name of happiness. And such an existence is even now the lot of many during some considerable portion of their lives. The present wretched education and wretched social arrangements are the only real hindrance to its being attainable by almost all.

The objectors perhaps may doubt whether human beings, if taught to consider happiness as the end of life, would be satisfied with such a moderate share of it. But great numbers of mankind have been satisfied with much less. The main constituents of a satisfied life appear to be two, either of which by itself is often found sufficient for the purpose: tranquillity and excitement. With much tranquillity, many find that they can be content with very little pleasure; with much excitement, many can reconcile themselves to a considerable quantity of pain. There is assuredly no inherent impossibility of enabling even the mass of mankind to

2 [Pseudonym of Friedrich Leopold Freiherr von Hardenberg (1772-1801), German poet and leader of early German Romanticism.]

unite both, since the two are so far from being incompatible that they are in natural alliance, the prolongation of either being a preparation for, and exciting a wish for, the other. It is only those in whom indolence amounts to a vice that do not desire excitement after an interval of repose; it is only those in whom the need of excitement is a disease that feel the tranquillity which follows excitement dull and insipid, instead of pleasurable in direct proportion to the excitement which preceded it. When people who are tolerably fortunate in their outward lot do not find in life sufficient enjoyment to make it valuable to them, the cause generally is caring for nobody but themselves. To those who have neither public nor private affections, the excitements of life are much curtailed, and in any case dwindle in value as the time approaches when all selfish interests must be terminated by death; while those who leave after them objects of personal affection, and especially those who have also cultivated a fellow-feeling with the collective interests of mankind, retain as lively an interest in life on the eve of death as in the vigor of youth and health. Next to selfishness, the principal cause which makes life unsatisfactory is want of mental cultivation. A cultivated mind—I do not mean that of a philosopher, but any mind to which the fountains of knowledge have been opened, and which has been taught, in any tolerable degree, to exercise its faculties—finds sources of inexhaustible interest in all that surrounds it: in the objects of nature, the achievements of art, the imaginations of poetry, the incidents of history, the ways of mankind, past and present, and their prospects in the future. It is possible, indeed, to become indifferent to all this, and that too without having exhausted a thousandth part of it, but only when one has had from the beginning no moral or human interest in these things and has sought in them only the gratification of curiosity.

Now there is absolutely no reason in the nature of things why an amount of mental culture sufficient to give an intelligent interest in these objects of contemplation should not be the inheritance of everyone born in a civilized country. As little is there an inherent necessity that any human being should be a selfish egotist, devoid of every feeling or care but those which center in his own miserable individuality. Something far superior to this is sufficiently common even now, to give ample earnest of what the human species may be made. Genuine private affections and a sincere interest in the public good are possible, though in unequal degrees, to every rightly brought up human being. In a world in which there is so much to interest, so much to enjoy, and so much also to correct and improve, everyone who has this moderate amount of moral and intellectual requisites is capable of an existence which may be called enviable; and unless such a person, through bad laws or subjection to the will of others, is denied the liberty to use the sources of happiness within his reach, he will not fail to find this enviable existence, if he escape the positive evils of life, the great sources of physical and mental suffering—such as indigence, disease, and the unkindness, worthlessness, or premature loss of objects of affection. The main stress of the problem lies, therefore, in the contest with these calamities from which it is a rare good fortune entirely to escape; which, as things now are, cannot be obviated, and often cannot be in any material degree mitigated. Yet no one whose opinion deserves a moment's consideration can doubt that most of the great positive evils of the world are in themselves removable, and will, if human affairs continue to improve, be in the end reduced within narrow limits. Poverty, in any sense implying suffering, may be completely extinguished by the wisdom of society combined with the good sense and providence of individuals. Even that most intractable of enemies, disease, may be indefinitely reduced in dimensions by good physical and moral education and proper control of noxious influences, while the progress of science holds out a promise for the future of still more direct conquests over this detestable foe. And every advance in that direction relieves us from some, not only of the chances which cut short our own lives, but, what concerns us still more, which deprive us of those in whom our happiness is wrapt up. As for vicissitudes of fortune and other disappointments connected with worldly circumstances, these are principally the effect either of gross imprudence, of ill-regulated desires, or of bad or imperfect social institutions. All the grand sources, in short, of human suffering are in a great degree, many of them almost entirely, conquerable by human care and effort; and though their removal is grievously slow—though a long succession of generations will perish in the breach before the conquest is completed, and this world becomes all that, if will and knowledge were not wanting, it might easily be made—yet every mind sufficiently intelligent and generous to bear a part, however small and inconspicuous, in the endeavor will draw a noble enjoyment from the contest itself, which he would not for any bribe in the form of selfish indulgence consent to be without.

And this leads to the true estimation of what is said by the objectors concerning the possibility and the obligation of learning to do without happiness. Unquestionably it is possible to do without happiness; it is done involuntarily by nineteen-twentieths of mankind, even in those parts of our present world which are least deep in barbarism; and it often has to be done voluntarily by the hero or the martyr, for the sake of something which he prizes more than his individual happiness. But this something, what is it, unless the happiness of others or some of the requisites of happiness? It is noble to be capable of resigning entirely one's own portion of happiness, or chances of it; but, after all, this self-sacrifice must be for some end; it is not its own end; and if we are told that its end is not happiness but virtue, which is better than happiness, I ask, would the sacrifice be made if the hero or martyr did not believe that it would earn for others immunity from similar sacrifices? Would it be made if he thought that his renunciation of happiness for himself would produce

no fruit for any of his fellow creatures, but to make their lot like his and place them also in the condition of persons who have renounced happiness? All honor to those who can abnegate for themselves the personal enjoyment of life when by such renunciation they contribute worthily to increase the amount of happiness in the world; but he who does it or professes to do it for any other purpose is no more deserving of admiration than the ascetic mounted on his pillar. He may be an inspiriting proof of what men *can* do, but assuredly not an example of what they *should*.

Though it is only in a very imperfect state of the world's arrangements that anyone can best serve the happiness of others by the absolute sacrifice of his own, yet, so long as the world is in that imperfect state, I fully acknowledge that the readiness to make such a sacrifice is the highest virtue which can be found in man. I will add that in this condition of the world, paradoxical as the assertion may be, the conscious ability to do without happiness gives the best prospect of realizing such happiness as is attainable. For nothing except that consciousness can raise a person above the chances of life by making him feel that, let fate and fortune do their worst, they have not power to subdue him; which, once felt, frees him from excess of anxiety concerning the evils of life and enables him, like many a Stoic in the worst times of the Roman Empire, to cultivate in tranquillity the sources of satisfaction accessible to him, without concerning himself about the uncertainty of their duration any more than about their inevitable end.

Meanwhile, let utilitarians never cease to claim the morality of self-devotion as a possession which belongs by as good a right to them as either to the Stoic or to the Transcendentalist. The utilitarian morality does recognize in human beings the power of sacrificing their own greatest good for the good of others. It only refuses to admit that the sacrifice is itself a good. A sacrifice which does not increase or tend to increase the sum total of happiness, it considers as wasted. The only self-renunciation which it applauds is devotion to the happiness, or to some of the means of happiness, of others, either of mankind collectively or of individuals within the limits imposed by the collective interests of mankind.

I must again repeat what the assailants of utilitarianism seldom have the justice to acknowledge, that the happiness which forms the utilitarian standard of what is right in conduct is not the agent's own happiness but that of all concerned. As between his own happiness and that of others, utilitarianism requires him to be as strictly impartial as a disinterested and benevolent spectator. In the golden rule of Jesus of Nazareth, we read the complete spirit of the ethics of utility. "To do as you would be done by," and "to love your neighbor as yourself," constitute the ideal perfection of utilitarian morality. As the means of making the nearest approach to this ideal, utility would enjoin, first, that laws and social arrangements should place the happiness or (as, speaking practically, it may be called) the interest of every individual as nearly as possible in harmony with the interest of the whole; and, secondly, that education and opinion, which have so vast a power over human character, should so use that power as to establish in the mind of every individual an indissoluble association between his own happiness and the good of the whole, especially between his own happiness and the practice of such modes of conduct, negative and positive, as regard for the universal happiness prescribes; so that not only he may be unable to conceive the possibility of happiness to himself, consistently with conduct opposed to the general good, but also that a direct impulse to promote the general good may be in every individual one of the habitual motives of action, and the sentiments connected therewith may fill a large and prominent place in every human being's sentient existence. If the impugners of the utilitarian morality represented it to their own minds in this its true character, I know not what recommendation possessed by any other morality they could possibly affirm to be wanting to it; what

more beautiful or more exalted developments of human nature any other ethical system can be supposed to foster, or what springs of action, not accessible to the utilitarian, such systems rely on for giving effect to their mandates.

The objectors to utilitarianism cannot always be charged with representing it in a discreditable light. On the contrary, those among them who entertain anything like a just idea of its disinterested character sometimes find fault with its standard as being too high for humanity. They say it is exacting too much to require that people shall always act from the inducement of promoting the general interests of society. But this is to mistake the very meaning of a standard of morals and confound the rule of action with the motive of it. It is the business of ethics to tell us what are our duties, or by what test we may know them; but no system of ethics requires that the sole motive of all we do shall be a feeling of duty; on the contrary, ninety-nine hundredths of all our actions are done from other motives, and rightly so done if the rule of duty does not condemn them. It is the more unjust to utilitarianism that this particular misapprehension should be made a ground of objection to it, inasmuch as utilitarian moralists have gone beyond almost all others in affirming that the motive has nothing to do with the morality of the action, though much with the worth of the agent. He who saves a fellow creature from drowning does what is morally right, whether his motive be duty or the hope of being paid for his trouble; he who betrays the friend that trusts him is guilty of a crime, even if his object be to serve another friend to whom he is under greater obligations.[3] But to speak only of actions done

---

3   An opponent, whose intellectual and moral fairness it is a pleasure to acknowledge (the Rev. J. Llewellyn Davies), has objected to this passage, saying, "Surely the rightness or wrongness of saving a man from drowning does depend very much upon the motive with which it is done. Suppose that a tyrant, when his enemy jumped into the sea to escape from him, saved him from drowning simply in order that he might inflict upon him more exquisite tortures, would it tend to clearness to speak of that rescue as 'a morally right action'? Or suppose again, according

from the motive of duty, and in direct obedience to principle: it is a misapprehension of the utilitarian mode of thought to conceive it as implying that people should fix their minds upon so wide a generality as the world, or society at large. The great majority of good actions are intended not for the benefit of the world, but for that of individuals, of which the good of the world is made up; and the thoughts of the most virtuous man need not on these occasions travel beyond the particular persons concerned, except so far as is necessary to assure himself that in benefiting them he is not violating the rights, that is, the legitimate and authorized expectations, of anyone else. The multiplication of happiness is, according to the utilitarian ethics, the object of virtue: the occasions on which any person (except one in a thousand) has it in his power to do this on an extended scale—in other words, to be a public benefactor—are but exceptional; and on these occasions alone is he called on to consider public utility; in every other case, private utility, the interest or happiness of some few persons, is all he has to attend to. Those alone the influence of whose actions extends to society in general need concern themselves habitually about so large an object. In the case of abstinences indeed—of things which people forbear to do from moral considerations, though the consequences in the particular case might be beneficial—it would be unworthy of an intelligent agent not to be consciously aware that the action is of a class which, if practiced generally, would be generally injurious, and that this is the ground of the obligation to abstain from it. The amount of regard for the public interest implied in this recognition is no greater than is demanded by every system of morals, for they all enjoin to abstain from whatever is manifestly pernicious to society.

The same considerations dispose of another reproach against the doctrine of utility, founded on a still grosser misconception of the purpose of a standard of morality and of the very meaning of the words "right" and "wrong." It is often affirmed that utilitarianism renders men cold and unsympathizing; that it chills their moral feelings toward individuals; that it makes them regard only the dry and hard consideration of the consequences of actions, not taking into their moral estimate the qualities from which those actions emanate. If the assertion means that they do not allow their judgment respecting the rightness or wrongness of an action to be influenced by their opinion of the qualities of the person who does it, this is a complaint not against utilitarianism, but against any standard of morality at all; for certainly no known ethical standard decides an action to be good or bad because it is done by a good or a bad man, still less because done by an amiable, a brave, or a benevolent man, or the contrary. These considerations are relevant, not to the estimation of actions, but of persons; and there is nothing in the utilitarian theory inconsistent with the fact that there are other things which interest us in persons besides the rightness and wrongness

---

to one of the stock illustrations of ethical inquiries, that a man betrayed a trust received from a friend, because the discharge of it would fatally injure that friend himself or someone belonging to him, would utilitarianism compel one to call the betrayal 'a crime' as much as if it had been done from the meanest motive?"

I submit that he who saves another from drowning in order to kill him by torture afterwards does not differ only in motive from him who does the same thing from duty or benevolence; the act itself is different. The rescue of the man is, in the case supposed, only the necessary first step of an act far more atrocious than leaving him to drown would have been. Had Mr. Davies said, "The rightness or wrongness of saving a man from drowning does depend very much"— not upon the motive, but—"upon the *intention*," no utilitarian would have differed from him. Mr. Davies, by an oversight too common not to be quite venial, has in this case confounded the very different ideas of Motive and Intention. There is no point which utilitarian thinkers (and Bentham pre-eminently) have taken more pains to illustrate than this. The morality of the action depends entirely upon the intention—that is, upon what the agent *wills to do*. But the motive, that is, the feeling which makes him will so to do, if it makes no difference in the act, makes none in the morality: though it makes a great difference in our moral estimation of the agent, especially if it indicates a good or a bad habitual *disposition*—a bent of character from which useful, or from which hurtful actions are likely to arise.

[The foregoing note appeared in the second (1864) edition of *Utilitarianism* but was dropped in succeeding ones.]

of their actions. The Stoics, indeed, with the paradoxical misuse of language which was part of their system, and by which they strove to raise themselves above all concern about anything but virtue, were fond of saying that he who has that has everything; that he, and only he, is rich, is beautiful, is a king. But no claim of this description is made for the virtuous man by the utilitarian doctrine. Utilitarians are quite aware that there are other desirable possessions and qualities besides virtue, and are perfectly willing to allow to all of them their full worth. They are also aware that a right action does not necessarily indicate a virtuous character, and that actions which are blamable often proceed from qualities entitled to praise. When this is apparent in any particular case, it modifies their estimation, not certainly of the act, but of the agent. I grant that they are, notwithstanding, of opinion that in the long run the best proof of a good character is good actions; and resolutely refuse to consider any mental disposition as good of which the predominant tendency is to produce bad conduct. This makes them unpopular with many people, but it is an unpopularity which they must share with everyone who regards the distinction between right and wrong in a serious light; and the reproach is not one which a conscientious utilitarian need be anxious to repel.

If no more be meant by the objection than that many utilitarians look on the morality of actions, as measured by the utilitarian standards, with too exclusive a regard, and do not lay sufficient stress upon the other beauties of character which go toward making a human being lovable or admirable, this may be admitted. Utilitarians who have cultivated their moral feelings, but not their sympathies, nor their artistic perceptions, do fall into this mistake; and so do all other moralists under the same conditions. What can be said in excuse for other moralists is equally available for them, namely, that, if there is to be any error, it is better that it should be on that side. As a matter of fact, we may affirm that among utilitarians, as among adherents of other systems, there is every imaginable degree

of rigidity and of laxity in the application of their standard; some are even puritanically rigorous, while others are as indulgent as can possibly be desired by sinner or by sentimentalist. But on the whole, a doctrine which brings prominently forward the interest that mankind have in the repression and prevention of conduct which violates the moral law is likely to be inferior to no other in turning the sanctions of opinion against such violations. It is true, the question "What does violate the moral law?" is one on which those who recognize different standards of morality are likely now and then to differ. But difference of opinion on moral questions was not first introduced into the world by utilitarianism, while that doctrine does supply, if not always an easy, at all events a tangible and intelligible, mode of deciding such differences.

It may not be superfluous to notice a few more of the common misapprehensions of utilitarian ethics, even those which are so obvious and gross that it might appear impossible for any person of candor and intelligence to fall into them; since persons, even of considerable mental endowment, often give themselves so little trouble to understand the bearings of any opinion against which they entertain a prejudice, and men are in general so little conscious of this voluntary ignorance as a defect that the vulgarest misunderstandings of ethical doctrines are continually met with in the deliberate writings of persons of the greatest pretensions both to high principle and to philosophy. We not uncommonly hear the doctrine of utility inveighed against as a *godless* doctrine. If it be necessary to say anything at all against so mere an assumption, we may say that the question depends upon what idea we have formed of the moral character of the Deity. If it be a true belief that God desires, above all things, the happiness of his creatures, and that this was his purpose in their creation, utility is not only not a godless doctrine, but more profoundly religious than any other. If it be meant that utilitarianism does not recognize the revealed will of God as the supreme law of morals, I answer that a utilitarian who believes in the perfect goodness and wisdom of *God* necessarily believes that whatever God has thought fit to reveal on the subject of morals must fulfill the requirements of utility in a supreme degree. But others besides utilitarians have been of opinion that the Christian revelation was intended, and is fitted, to inform the hearts and minds of mankind with a spirit which should enable them to find for themselves what is right, and incline them to do it when found, rather than to tell them, except in a very general way, what it is; and that we need a doctrine of ethics, carefully followed out, to *interpret* to us the will of God. Whether this opinion is correct or not, it is superfluous here to discuss; since whatever aid religion, either natural or revealed, can afford to ethical investigation is as open to the utilitarian moralist as to any other. He can use it as the testimony of God to the usefulness or hurtfulness of any given course of action by as good a right as others can use it for the indication of a transcendental law having no connection with usefulness or with happiness.

Again, utility is often summarily stigmatized as an immoral doctrine by giving it the name of "expediency," and taking advantage of the popular use of that term to contrast it with principle. But the expedient, in the sense in which it is opposed to the right, generally means that which is expedient for the particular interest of the agent himself; as when a minister sacrifices the interests of his country to keep himself in place. When it means anything better than this, it means that which is expedient for some immediate object, some temporary purpose, but which violates a rule whose observance is expedient in a much higher degree. The expedient, in this sense, instead of being the same thing with the useful, is a branch of the hurtful. Thus it would often be expedient, for the purpose of getting over some momentary embarrassment, or attaining some object immediately useful to ourselves or others, to tell a lie. But inasmuch as the cultivation in ourselves of a sensitive feeling on the subject of veracity is one of the most useful, and the enfeeblement of that feeling one of the most hurtful, things to which our conduct can be instrumental; and inasmuch as any, even unintentional, deviation from truth does that much toward weakening the trustworthiness of human assertion, which is not only the principal support of all present social well-being, but the insufficiency of which does more than any one thing that can be named to keep back civilization, virtue, everything on which human happiness on the largest scale depends—we feel that the violation, for a present advantage, of a rule of such transcendent expediency is not expedient, and that he who, for the sake of convenience to himself or to some other individual, does what depends on him to deprive mankind of the good, and inflict upon them the evil, involved in the greater or less reliance which they can place in each other's word, acts the part of one of their worst enemies. Yet that even this rule, sacred as it is, admits of possible exceptions is acknowledged by all moralists; the chief of which is when the withholding of some fact (as of information from a malefactor, or of bad news from a person dangerously ill) would save an individual (especially an individual other than oneself) from great and unmerited evil, and when the withholding can only be effected by denial. But in order that the exception may not extend itself beyond the need, and may have the least possible effect in weakening reliance on veracity, it ought to be recognized and, if possible, its limits defined; and, if the principle of utility is good for anything, it must be good for weighing these conflicting utilities against one another and marking out the region within which one or the other preponderates.

Again, defenders of utility often find themselves called upon to reply to such objections as this—that there is not time, previous to action, for calculating and weighing the effects of any line of conduct on the general happiness. This is exactly as if anyone were to say that it is impossible to guide our conduct by Christianity because there is not time, on every occasion on which anything has to be done, to read through the Old and New Testaments. The answer to the objection is that there has been ample time, namely, the whole past duration of the human species. During all that time mankind have been learning by experience the tendencies of actions; on which experience all the prudence as well as all the morality of life are dependent. People talk as if the commencement of this course of experience had hitherto been put off, and as if, at the moment when some man feels tempted to meddle with the property or life of another, he had to begin considering for the first time whether murder and theft are injurious to human happiness. Even then I do not think that he would find the question very puzzling; but, at all events, the matter is now done to his hand. It is truly a whimsical supposition that, if mankind were agreed in considering utility to be the test of morality, they would remain without any agreement as to what *is* useful, and would take no measures for having their notions on the subject taught to the young and enforced by law and opinion. There is no difficulty in proving any ethical standard whatever to work ill if we suppose universal idiocy to be conjoined with it; but on any hypothesis short of that, mankind must by this time have acquired positive beliefs as to the effects of some actions on their happiness; and the beliefs which have thus come down are the rules of morality for the multitude, and for the philosopher until he has succeeded in finding better. That philosophers might easily do this, even now, on many subjects; that the received code of ethics is by no means of divine right; and that mankind have still much to learn as to the effects of actions on the general happiness, I admit or rather earnestly maintain. The corollaries from the principle of utility, like the precepts of every practical art, admit of indefinite improvement, and, in a progressive state of the human mind, their improvement is perpetually going on. But to consider the rules of morality as improvable is one thing; to pass over the intermediate generalization entirely and endeavor to test each individual action directly by the first principle is another. It is a strange notion that the acknowledgment of a first principle is inconsistent with the admission of secondary

ones. To inform a traveler respecting the place of his ultimate destination is not to forbid the use of landmarks and direction-posts on the way. The proposition that happiness is the end and aim of morality does not mean that no road ought to be laid down to that goal, or that persons going thither should not be advised to take one direction rather than another. Men really ought to leave off talking a kind of nonsense on this subject, which they would neither talk nor listen to on other matters of practical concernment. Nobody argues that the art of navigation is not founded on astronomy because sailors cannot wait to calculate the Nautical Almanac. Being rational creatures, they go to sea with it ready calculated; and all rational creatures go out upon the sea of life with their minds made up on the common questions of right and wrong, as well as on many of the far more difficult questions of wise and foolish. And this, as long as foresight is a human quality, it is to be presumed they will continue to do. Whatever we adopt as the fundamental principle of morality, we require subordinate principles to apply it by; the impossibility of doing without them, being common to all systems, can afford no argument against any one in particular; but gravely to argue as if no such secondary principles could be had, and as if mankind had remained till now, and always must remain, without drawing any general conclusions from the experience of human life is as high a pitch, I think, as absurdity has ever reached in philosophical controversy.

The remainder of the stock arguments against utilitarianism mostly consist in laying to its charge the common infirmities of human nature, and the general difficulties which embarrass conscientious persons in shaping their course through life. We are told that a utilitarian will be apt to make his own particular case an exception to moral rules, and, when under temptation, will see a utility in the breach of a rule, greater than he will see in its observance. But is utility the only creed which is able to furnish us with excuses for evil-doing and means of cheating our own conscience? They are afforded in abundance by all doctrines which recognize as a fact in morals the existence of conflicting considerations, which all doctrines do that have been believed by sane persons. It is not the fault of any creed, but of the complicated nature of human affairs, that rules of conduct cannot be so framed as to require no exceptions, and that hardly any kind of action can safely be laid down as either always obligatory or always condemnable. There is no ethical creed which does not temper the rigidity of its laws by giving a certain latitude, under the moral responsibility of the agent, for accommodation to peculiarities of circumstances; and under every creed, at the opening thus made, self-deception and dishonest casuistry get in. There exists no moral system under which there do not arise unequivocal cases of conflicting obligation. These are the real difficulties, the knotty points both in the theory of ethics and in the conscientious guidance of personal conduct. They are overcome practically, with greater or with less success, according to the intellect and virtue of the individual; but it can hardly be pretended that anyone will be the less qualified for dealing with them, from possessing an ultimate standard to which conflicting rights and duties can be referred. If utility is the ultimate source of moral obligations, utility may be invoked to decide between them when their demands are incompatible. Though the application of the standard may be difficult, it is better than none at all; while in other systems, the moral laws all claiming independent authority, there is no common umpire entitled to interfere between them; their claims to precedence one over another rest on little better than sophistry, and, unless determined, as they generally are, by the unacknowledged influence of consideration of utility, afford a free scope for the action of personal desires and partialities. We must remember that only in these cases of conflict between secondary principles is it requisite that first principles should be appealed to. There is no case of moral obligation in which some secondary principle is not involved; and if only one, there can seldom be any real doubt which one it is, in the mind of any person by whom the principle itself is recognized.

The Imperative of Responsibility: In Search of an Ethics for the Technological Age

Hans Jonas

1 The Altered Nature of Human Action

All previous ethics—whether in the form of issuing direct enjoinders to do and not to do certain things, or in the form of defining principles for such enjoinders, or in the form of establishing the ground of obligation for obeying such principles—had these interconnected tacit premises in common: that the human condition, determined by the nature of man and the nature of things, was given once for all; that the human good on that basis was readily determinable; and that the range of human action and therefore responsibility was narrowly circumscribed. It will be the burden of the present argument to show that these premises no longer hold, and to reflect on the meaning of this fact for our moral condition. More specifically, it will be my contention that with certain developments of our powers the *nature of human action* has changed, and, since ethics is concerned with action, it should follow that the changed nature of human action calls for a change in ethics as well: this not merely in the sense that new objects of action have added to the case material on which received rules of conduct are to be applied, but in the more radical sense that the qualitatively novel nature of certain of our actions has opened up a whole new dimension of ethical relevance for which there is no precedent in the standards and canons of traditional ethics.

The novel powers I have in mind are, of course, those of modern *technology*. My first point, accordingly, is to ask how this technology affects the nature of our acting, in what ways it makes acting under its dominion *different* from what it has been through the ages. Since throughout those ages man was never without technology, the question involves the human difference of *modern* from previous technology.

I. The Example of Antiquity

Let us start with an ancient voice on man's powers and deeds which in an archetypal sense itself strikes, as it were, a technological note—the famous Chorus from Sophocles' *Antigone*.

Many the wonders but nothing more
wondrous than man. This thing crosses the
sea in the winter's storm, making his path
through the roaring waves. And she, the
greatest of gods, the Earth—deathless she

is, and unwearied—he wears her away as the ploughs go up and down from year to year and his mules turn up the soil.

The tribes of the lighthearted birds he ensnares, and the races of all the wild beasts and the salty brood of the sea, with the twisted mesh of his nets, he leads captive, this clever man. He controls with craft the beasts of the open air, who roam the hills. The horse with his shaggy mane he holds and harnesses, yoked about the neck, and the strong bull of the mountain.

Speech and thought like the wind and the feelings that make the town, he has taught himself, and shelter against the cold, refuge from rain. Ever resourceful is he. He faces no future helpless. Only against death shall he call for aid in vain. But from baffling maladies has he contrived escape.

Clever beyond all dreams the inventive craft that he has which may drive him one time or another to well or ill. When he honors the laws of the land and the gods' sworn right high indeed is his city; but stateless the man who dares to do what is shameful.

[Lines 335–370]

1. Man and Nature

This awestruck homage to man's powers tells of his violent and violating irruption into the cosmic order, the self-assertive invasion of nature's various domains by his restless cleverness; but also of his building—through the self-taught powers of speech and thought and social sentiment—the home for his very humanity, the artifact of the city. The raping of nature and the civilizing of man go hand in hand. Both are in defiance of the elements, the one by venturing into them and overpowering their creatures, the other by securing an enclave against them in the shelter of the city and its laws. Man is the maker of his life *qua* human, bending circumstances to

his will and needs, and except against death he is never helpless.

Yet there is a subdued and even anxious quality about this appraisal of the marvel that is man, and nobody can mistake it for immodest bragging. Unspoken, but self-evident for those times, is the pervading knowledge behind it all that, for all his boundless resourcefulness, man is still small by the measure of the elements: precisely this makes his sallies into them so daring and allows those elements to tolerate his forwardness. Making free with the denizens of land and sea and air, he yet leaves the encompassing nature of those elements unchanged, and their generative powers undiminished. He cannot harm them by carving out his little kingdom from theirs. They last, while his schemes have their short-lived way. Much as he harries Earth, the greatest of gods, year after year with his plough—she is ageless and unwearied; her enduring patience he must and can trust, and to her cycle he must conform. And just as ageless is the sea. With all his netting of the salty brood, the spawning ocean is inexhaustible. Nor is it hurt by the plying of ships, nor sullied by what is jettisoned into its deeps. And no matter how many illnesses he contrives to cure, mortality does not bow to his cunning.

All this holds because before our time man's inroads into nature, as seen by himself, were essentially superficial and powerless to upset its appointed balance. (Hindsight reveals that they were not always so harmless in reality.) Nor is there a hint, in the *Antigone* chorus or anywhere else, that this is only a beginning and that greater things of artifice and power are yet to come—that man is embarked on an endless course of conquest. He had gone thus far in reducing necessity, had learned by his wits to wrest that much from it for the humanity of his life, and reflecting upon this, he was overcome by awe at his own boldness.

2. The Man-Made Island of the "City"

The room he has thus made was filled by the city of men—meant to enclose, and not to expand—and thereby a new balance was struck within the larger balance of the whole. All the good or ill to which man's inventive craft may drive him one time or another is inside the human enclave and does not touch the nature of things.

The immunity of the whole, untroubled in its depth by the importunities of man, that is, the essential immutability of Nature as the cosmic order, was indeed the backdrop to all of mortal man's enterprises, including his intrusions into that order itself. Man's life was played out between the abiding and the changing: the abiding was Nature, the changing his own works. The greatest of these works was the city, and on it he could confer some measure of abiding by the laws he made for it and undertook to honor. But no long-range certainty pertained to this contrived continuity. As a vulnerable artifact, the cultural construct can grow slack or go astray. Not even within its artificial space, with all the freedom it gives to man's determination of self, can the arbitrary ever supersede the basic terms of his being. The very inconstancy of human fortunes assures the constancy of the human condition. Chance and luck and folly, the great equalizers in human affairs, act like an entropy of sorts and make all definite designs in the long run revert to the perennial norm. Cities rise and fall, rules come and go, families prosper and decline; no change is there to stay, and in the end, with all the temporary deflections balancing each other out, the state of man is as it always was. So here, too, in his very own artifact, the social world, man's control is small and his abiding nature prevails.

Still, this citadel of his own making, clearly set off from the rest of things and entrusted to him, was the whole and sole domain of man's responsible action. Nature was not an object of human responsibility—she taking care of herself and, with some coaxing and worrying, also of man: not ethics, only cleverness applied to her. But in the city, the social work of art, where men deal with men, cleverness must be wedded to morality, for this is the soul of its being. It is in this intrahuman frame, then, that all traditional ethics dwells, and it matches the size of action delimited by this frame.

II. Characteristics of Previous Ethics

Let us extract from the above those characteristics of human action which are relevant for a comparison with the state of things today.

1. All dealing with the nonhuman world, that is, the whole realm of *techne* (with the exception of medicine), was ethically neutral—in respect both of the object and the subject of such action: in respect of the object, because it impinged but little on the self-sustaining nature of things and thus raised no question of permanent injury to the integrity of its object, the natural order as a whole; and in respect of the agent subject it was ethically neutral because *techne* as an activity conceived itself as a determinate tribute to necessity and not as an indefinite, self-validating advance to mankind's major goal, claiming in its pursuit man's ultimate effort and concern. The real vocation of man lay elsewhere. In brief, action on nonhuman things did not constitute a sphere of authentic ethical significance.

2. Ethical significance belonged to the direct dealing of man with man, including the dealing with himself: all traditional ethics is *anthropocentric*.

3. For action in this domain, the entity "man" and his basic condition was considered constant in essence and not itself an object of reshaping *techne*.

4. The good and evil about which action had to care lay close to the act, either in the praxis itself or in its immediate reach, and were not matters for remote planning. This proximity of ends pertained to time as well as space. The effective range of action was small, the time span of foresight, goal-setting, and accountability was

short, control of circumstances limited. Proper conduct had its immediate criteria and almost immediate consummation. The long run of consequences beyond was left to chance, fate, or providence. Ethics accordingly was of the here and now, of occasions as they arise between men, of the recurrent, typical situations of private and public life. The good man was the one who met these contingencies with virtue and wisdom, cultivating these powers in himself, and for the rest resigning himself to the unknown.

All enjoinders and maxims of traditional ethics, materially different as they may be, show this confinement to the immediate setting of the action. "Love thy neighbor as thyself"; "Do unto others as you would wish them to do unto you"; "Instruct your child in the way of truth"; "Strive for excellence by developing and actualizing the best potentialities of your being *qua* man"; "Subordinate your individual good to the common good"; "Never treat your fellow man as a means only but always also as an end in himself"—and so on. Note that in all these maxims the agent and the "other" of his action are sharers of a common present. It is those who are alive now and in some relationship with me who have a claim on my conduct as it affects them by deed or omission. The ethical universe is composed of contemporaries, and its horizon to the future is confined by the foreseeable span of their lives. Similarly confined is its horizon of place, within which the agent and the other meet as neighbor, friend, or foe, as superior and subordinate, weaker and stronger, and in all the other roles in which humans interact with one another. To this proximate range of action all morality was geared.

It follows that the *knowledge* that is required—besides the moral will—to assure the morality of action fitted these limited terms: it was not the knowledge of the scientist or the expert, but knowledge of a kind readily available to all men of good will. Kant went so far as to say that "human reason can, in matters of morality, be easily brought to a high degree of accuracy and completeness even in the most ordinary intelligence";[1] that "there is no need of science or philosophy for knowing what man has to do in order to be honest and good, and indeed to be wise and virtuous. ... [Ordinary intelligence] can have as good hope of hitting the mark as any philosopher can promise himself";[2] and again: "I need no elaborate acuteness to find out what I have to do so that my willing be morally good. Inexperienced regarding the course of the world, unable to anticipate all the contingencies that happen in it," I can yet know how to act in accordance with the moral law.[3]

Not every thinker in ethics, it is true, went so far in discounting the cognitive side of moral action. But even when it received much greater emphasis, as in Aristotle, where the discernment of the situation and what is fitting for it makes considerable demands on experience and judgment, such knowledge has nothing to do with the science of things. It implies, of course, a general conception of the human good as such, a conception predicated on the presumed invariables of man's nature and condition, which may or may not find expression in a theory of its own. But its translation into practice requires a knowledge of the here and now, and this is entirely nontheoretical. This "knowledge" proper to virtue (of the "where, when, to whom, and how") stays with the immediate issue, in whose defined context the action as the agent's own takes its course and within which it terminates. The good or bad of the action is wholly decided within that short-term context. Its authorship is unquestioned, and its moral quality shines forth from it, visible to its witnesses. No one was held responsible for the unintended later effects of his well-intentioned, well-considered, and well-performed act. The short arm of human power did not call for a long arm of predictive knowledge; the shortness of the one is as little culpable as that of the other. Precisely because the human good, known in its generality, is the same for all time, its realization or violation takes place at each time, and its complete locus is always the present.

III. New Dimensions of Responsibility

All this has decisively changed. Modern technology has introduced actions of such novel scale, objects, and consequences that the framework of former ethics can no longer contain them. The *Antigone* chorus on the *deinotes*, the wondrous power, of man would have to read differently now; and its admonition to the individual to honor the laws of the land would no longer be enough. The gods, too, whose venerable right could check the headlong rush of human action, are long gone. To be sure, the old prescriptions of the "neighbor" ethics—of justice, charity, honesty, and so on—still hold in their intimate immediacy for the nearest, day-by-day sphere of human interaction. But this sphere is overshadowed by a growing realm of collective action where doer, deed, and effect are no longer the same as they were in the proximate sphere, and which by the enormity of its powers forces upon ethics a new dimension of responsibility never dreamed of before.

1. The Vulnerability of Nature

Take, for instance, as the first major change in the inherited picture, the critical vulnerability of nature to man's technological intervention—unsuspected before it began to show itself in damage already done. This discovery, whose shock led to the concept and nascent science of ecology, alters the very concept of ourselves as a causal agency in the larger scheme of things. It brings to light, through the effects, that the nature of human action has *de facto* changed, and that an object of an entirely new order—no less than the whole biosphere of the planet—has been added to what we must be responsible for because of our power over it. And of what surpassing importance an object, dwarfing all previous objects of active man! Nature as a human responsibility is surely a *novum* to be pondered in ethical theory. What kind of obligation is operative in it? Is it more than a utilitarian concern? Is it just prudence that bids us not to kill the goose that lays the golden eggs, or saw off the branch on which we sit? But the "we" who sit here and who may fall into the abyss—who is it? And what is *my* interest in its sitting or falling?

Insofar as it is the fate of *man*, as affected by the condition of nature, which makes our concern about the preservation of nature a *moral* concern, such concern admittedly still retains the anthropocentric focus of all classical ethics. Even so, the difference is great. The containment of nearness and contemporaneity is gone, swept away by the spatial spread and time span of the cause-effect trains which technological practice sets afoot, even when undertaken for proximate ends. Their irreversibility conjoined to their aggregate magnitude injects another novel factor into the moral equation. Add to this their cumulative character: their effects keep adding themselves to one another, with the result that the situation for later subjects and their choices of action will be progressively different from that of the initial agent and ever more the fated product of what was done before. All traditional ethics reckoned only with noncumulative behavior.[4] The basic situation between persons, where virtue must prove and vice expose itself, remains always the same, and every deed begins afresh from this basis. The recurring occasions which pose their appropriate alternatives for human conduct—courage or cowardice, moderation or excess, truth or mendacity, and so on—each time reinstate the primordial conditions from which action takes off. These were never superseded, and thus moral actions were largely "typical," that is, conforming to precedent. In contrast with this, the cumulative self-propagation of the technological change of the world constantly overtakes the conditions of its contributing acts and moves through none but unprecedented situations, for which the lessons of experience are powerless. And not even content with changing its beginning to the point of unrecognizability, the cumulation as such may consume the basis of the whole series, the very condition of itself.

All this would have to be cointended in the will of the single action if this is to be a morally responsible one.

2. The New Role of Knowledge in Morality

Knowledge, under these circumstances, becomes a prime duty beyond anything claimed for it heretofore, and the knowledge must be commensurate with the causal scale of our action. The fact that it cannot really be thus commensurate, that is, that the predictive knowledge falls behind the technical knowledge that nourishes our power to act, itself assumes ethical importance. The gap between the ability to foretell and the power to act creates a novel moral problem. With the latter so superior to the former, recognition of ignorance becomes the obverse of the duty to know and thus part of the ethics that must govern the evermore necessary self-policing of our outsized might. No previous ethics had to consider the global condition of human life and the far-off future, even existence, of the race. These now being an issue demands, in brief, a new conception of duties and rights, for which previous ethics and metaphysics provide not even the principles, let alone a ready doctrine.

3. Has Nature "Rights" Also?

And what if the new kind of human action would mean that more than the interest of man alone is to be considered—that our duty extends farther, and the anthropocentric confinement of former ethics no longer holds? It is at least not senseless anymore to ask whether the condition of extrahuman nature, the biosphere as a whole and in its parts, now subject to our power, has become a human trust and has something of a moral claim on us not only for our ulterior sake but for its own and in its own right. If this were the case it would require quite some rethinking in basic principles of ethics. It would mean to seek not only the human good but also the good of things extrahuman, that is, to extend

the recognition of "ends in themselves" beyond the sphere of man and make the human good include the care for them. No previous ethics (outside of religion) has prepared us for such a role of stewardship—and the dominant, scientific view of *Nature* has prepared us even less. Indeed, that view emphatically denies us all conceptual means to think of Nature as something to be honored, having reduced it to the indifference of necessity and accident, and divested it of any dignity of ends. But still, a silent plea for sparing its integrity seems to issue from the threatened plenitude of the living world. Should we heed this plea, should we recognize its claim as morally binding because sanctioned by the nature of things, or dismiss it as a mere sentiment on our part, which we may indulge as far as we wish and can afford to do? If the former, it would (if taken seriously in its theoretical implications) push the necessary rethinking beyond the doctrine of action, that is, ethics, into the doctrine of being, that is, metaphysics, in which all ethics must ultimately be grounded. On this speculative subject I will say no more here than that we should keep ourselves open to the thought that natural science may not tell the whole story about Nature.

IV. Technology as the "Calling" of Mankind

1. Homo Faber over Homo Sapiens

Returning to strictly intrahuman considerations, there is another ethical aspect to the growth of *techne* as a pursuit beyond the pragmatically limited terms of former times. Then, so we found, *techne* was a measured tribute to necessity, not the road to mankind's chosen goal—a means with a finite measure of adequacy to well-defined proximate ends. Now, *techne* in the form of modern technology has turned into an infinite forward-thrust of the race, its most significant enterprise, in whose permanent, self-transcending advance to ever greater things the vocation of man tends to be seen, and whose success of maximal control over things and himself appears as the consummation of his destiny. Thus the triumph of *homo faber* over his external object means also his triumph in the internal constitution of *homo sapiens*, of whom he used to be a subsidiary part. In other words, technology, apart from its objective works, assumes ethical significance by the central place it now occupies in human purpose. Its cumulative creation, the expanding artificial environment, continuously reinforces the particular powers in man that created it, by compelling their unceasing inventive employment in its management and further advance, and by rewarding them with additional success—which only adds to the relentless claim. This positive feedback of functional necessity and reward—in whose dynamics pride of achievement must not be forgotten—assures the growing ascendancy of one side of man's nature over all the others, and inevitably at their expense. If nothing succeeds like success, nothing also entraps like success. Outshining in prestige and starving in resources whatever else belongs to the fullness of man, the expansion of his power is accompanied by a contraction of his self-conception and being. In the image he entertains of himself—the programmatic idea which determines his actual being as much as it reflects it—man now is evermore the maker of what he has made and the doer of what he can do, and most of all the preparer of what he will be able to do next. But who is "he"? Not you or I: it is the aggregate, not the individual doer or deed that matters here; and the indefinite future, rather than the contemporary context of the action, constitutes the relevant horizon of responsibility. This requires imperatives of a new sort. If the realm of making has invaded the space of essential action, then morality must invade the realm of making, from which it has formerly stayed aloof, and must do so in the form of public policy. Public policy has never had to deal before with issues of such inclusiveness and such lengths of anticipation. In fact, the changed nature of human action changes the very nature of politics.

2. The Universal City as a Second Nature

For the boundary between "city" and "nature" has been obliterated: the city of men, once an enclave in the nonhuman world, spreads over the whole of terrestrial nature and usurps its place. The difference between the artificial and the natural has vanished, the natural is swallowed up in the sphere of the artificial, and at the same time the total artifact (the works of man that have become "the world" and as such envelop their makers) generates a "nature" of its own, that is, a necessity with which human freedom has to cope in an entirely new sense.

Once it could be said *Fiat justitia, pereat mundus*, "Let justice be done, and may the world perish"—where "world," of course, meant the renewable enclave in the imperishable whole. Not even rhetorically can the like be said anymore when the perishing of the whole through the doings of man—be they just or unjust—has become a real possibility. Issues never legislated come into the purview of the laws which the total city must give itself so that there will be a world for the generations of man to come.

3. Man's Presence in the World as an Imperative

That there *ought* to be through all future time such a world fit for human habitation, and that it ought in all future time to be inhabited by a mankind worthy of the human name, will be readily affirmed as a general axiom or a persuasive desirability of speculative imagination (as persuasive and as undemonstrable as the proposition that there being a world at all is "better" than there being none): but as a *moral* proposition, namely, a practical *obligation* toward the posterity of a distant future, and a principle of decision in present action, it is quite different from the imperatives of the previous ethics of contemporaneity; and it has entered the moral scene only with our novel powers and range of prescience.

The *presence of man in the world* had been a first and unquestionable given, from which all idea of obligation in human conduct started out.

Now it has itself become an *object* of obligation: the obligation namely to ensure the very premise of all obligation, that is, the *foothold* for a moral universe in the physical world—the existence of mere *candidates* for a moral order. This entails, among other things, the duty to preserve this physical world in such a state that the conditions for that presence remain intact; which in turn means protecting the world's vulnerability from what could imperil those very conditions. The difference this makes for ethics may be illustrated in one example.

V. Old and New Imperatives

1. Kant's categorical imperative said: "Act so that you *can* will that the maxim of your action be made the principle of a universal law." The "can" here invoked is that of reason and its consistency with itself: *Given* the existence of a community of human agents (acting rational beings), the action must be such that it can without self-contradiction be imagined as a general practice of that community. Mark that the basic reflection of morals here is not itself a moral but a logical one: The "I *can* will" or "I *cannot* will" expresses logical compatibility or incompatibility, not moral approbation or revulsion. But there is no self-contradiction in the thought that humanity would once come to an end, therefore also none in the thought that the happiness of present and proximate generations would be bought with the unhappiness or even nonexistence of later ones—as little as, after all, in the inverse thought that the existence or happiness of later generations would be bought with the unhappiness or even partial extinction of present ones. The sacrifice of the future for the present is *logically* no more open to attack than the sacrifice of the present for the future. The difference is only that in the one case the series goes on, and in the other it does not (or: its future ending is contemplated). But that it *ought to go on*, regardless of the distribution of happiness or unhappiness,

even with a persistent preponderance of unhappiness over happiness, nay, of immorality over morality[5]—this cannot be derived from the rule of self-consistency *within* the series, long or short as it happens to be: it is a commandment of a very different kind, lying outside and "prior" to the series as a whole, and its ultimate grounding can only be metaphysical.

2. An imperative responding to the new type of human action and addressed to the new type of agency that operates it might run thus: "Act so that the effects of your action are compatible with the permanence of genuine human life"; or expressed negatively: "Act so that the effects of your action are not destructive of the future possibility of such life"; or simply: "Do not compromise the conditions for an indefinite continuation of humanity on earth"; or, again turned positive: "In your present choices, include the future wholeness of Man among the objects of your will."

3. It is immediately obvious that no rational contradiction is involved in the violation of this kind of imperative. I can will the present good with sacrifice of the future good. Just as I can will my own end, I can will that of humanity. Without falling into contradiction with myself, I can prefer a short fireworks display of the most extreme "self-fulfillment," for myself or for the world, to the boredom of an endless continuation in mediocrity.

However, the new imperative says precisely that we may risk our own life—but not that of humanity; and that Achilles indeed had the right to choose for himself a short life of glorious deeds over a long life of inglorious security (with the tacit premise that a posterity would be there to know and tell of his deeds), but that we do not have the right to choose, or even risk, nonexistence for future generations on account of a better life for the present one. Why we do not have this right, why on the contrary we have an obligation toward that which does not yet exist and never need exist at all—an obligation not only toward its fortunes in case it happens to exist, but toward its coming to exist in the first place, to which as nonexistent "it" surely has no claim: to underpin this proposition theoretically is by no means easy and without religion perhaps impossible. At present, our imperative simply posits it without proof, as an axiom.

4. It is also evident that the new imperative addresses itself to public policy rather than private conduct, which is not in the causal dimension to which that imperative applies. Kant's categorical imperative was addressed to the individual, and its criterion was instantaneous. It enjoined each of us to consider what would happen *if* the *maxim* of my present action were made, or at this moment already were, the principle of a universal legislation; the self-consistency or inconsistency of such a *hypothetical* universalization is made the test for my *private* choice. But it was no part of the reasoning that there is any probability of my private choice in fact becoming universal law, or that it might contribute to its becoming that. Indeed, *real* consequences are not considered at all, and the principle is one not of objective responsibility but of the subjective quality of my self-determination. The new imperative invokes a different consistency: not that of the act with itself, but that of its eventual *effects* with the continuance of human agency in times to come. And the "universalization" it contemplates is by no means hypothetical—that is, a purely logical transference from the individual "me" to an imaginary, causally unrelated "all" ("*if* everybody acted like that"); on the contrary, the actions subject to the new imperative—actions of the collective whole—have their universal reference in their actual scope of efficacy: they "totalize" themselves in the progress of their momentum and thus are bound to terminate in shaping the universal dispensation of things. This adds a *time* horizon to the moral calculus which is entirely absent from the instantaneous logical operation of the Kantian imperative: whereas the latter extrapolates into an ever-present order of abstract compatibility, our imperative extrapolates into a predictable real *future* as the open-ended dimension of our responsibility.

VI. Earlier Forms of "Future-oriented Ethics"

Now it may be objected that with Kant we have chosen an extreme example of the ethics of subjective intention (*Gesinnungsethik*), and that our assertion of the present-oriented character of all former ethics, as holding among contemporaries, is contradicted by several ethical forms of the past. The following three examples come to mind: the conduct of earthly life (to the point of sacrificing its entire happiness) with a view to the eternal salvation of the soul; the long-range concern of the legislator and statesman for the future common weal; and the politics of utopia, with its readiness to use those living now as a mere means to a goal that lies in a future after their time, or to exterminate them as obstacles in its way—of which revolutionary Marxism is the prime example.

1. The Ethics of Fulfillment in the Life Hereafter

Of these three cases the first and third share the trait of placing the future above the present as the possible locus of absolute value, thus demoting the present to a mere preparation for the future. An important difference is that in the religious case the acting down here is not credited with bringing on the future bliss by its own causality (as revolutionary action is supposed to do), but is merely supposed to *qualify* the agent for it, namely, in the eyes of God, to whom faith must entrust its realization. That qualification, however, consists in a life pleasing to God, of which in general it may be assumed that it is the best, most worthwhile life in itself anyway, thus worthy to be chosen for its own sake and not merely for that of eventual future bliss. Indeed, when chosen mainly from that reward motive, the life in question would lose in worth and therewith even in its qualifying strength. That is to say, the latter is the greater, the less intended it is. When we then ask what human qualities are held to procure the qualification, that is, to constitute a life pleasing to God, we must look at the life prescriptions of the particular creeds—and these we may often find to be just those prescriptions of justice, charity, purity of heart, etc., which would, or could, be prescribed by an innerworldly ethic of the classical sort as well. Thus in the "moderate" version of the belief in the soul's salvation (of which, if I am not mistaken, Judaism is an example) we still deal, after all, with an ethics of contemporaneity and immediacy, notwithstanding the transcendent goal; and what ethics it might concretely be in this or that historical case—that is not deducible from the transcendent goal as such (of whose content no idea can be formed anyway), but is told by the way in which the "life pleasing to God," said to be the precondition for it, was in each instance given material content.

It may happen, however, that the content is such—and this is the case in the "extreme" forms of the soul salvation doctrine—that its practice, that is, the fulfillment of the "precondition," can in no way be regarded as of value in itself but is merely the stake in a wager, with whose loss, that is, the failure to attain the eternal reward, all would be lost. For in this case of the dreadful metaphysical bet as elaborated by Pascal, the stake is one's entire earthly existence with all its possibilities of enjoyment and fulfillment, whose very renunciation is made the price of eternal salvation. In this category belong all those forms of radical mortification of the flesh, of life-denying asceticism, whose practitioners would have cheated themselves out of everything if their expectations were disappointed. This otherworldly wager differs from the calculus of ordinary, this-worldly hedonism, with its considered risks of sometime-renunciations and deferments, merely by the totality of its *quid pro quo* and the surpassing nature of the chance for which the stakes are risked. But just this surpassing expectation moves the whole undertaking out of the realm of ethics. Between the finite and the infinite, the temporal and the eternal, there is no commensurability and thus no meaningful comparison; that is, there is neither a qualitative nor a quantitative sense in

which one is *preferable* to the other. Concerning the *value* of the goal, whose informed appraisal ought to form an essential element of *ethical* decision, there is nothing but the empty assertion that it is the ultimate value. Also lacking is the *causal* relation—which at least *ethical* thinking requires—between the action and its (hoped-for) result; that "result," so we saw, is conceived not as being effected by present renunciation but merely as promised from elsewhere in compensation for it.

If one inquires *why* the this-worldly renunciation is considered so meritorious that it may dare to expect this kind of indemnification or reward, one answer might be that the flesh is sinful, desire is evil, and the world is impure. In this case (as in the somewhat different case where individuation as such is regarded as bad) asceticism does represent, after all, a genuine instrumentality of action and a path to internal goal-achievement through one's own performance: the path, namely, from impurity to purity, from sinfulness to sanctity, from bondage to freedom, from selfhood to self-transcendence. Insofar as it is such a "path," asceticism is already in itself the *best* sort of life by the metaphysical criteria assumed. But in this case we are dealing again with an ethic of the here and now: a form—albeit a supremely egotistic and individualistic form—of the ethic of self-perfection, whose inward exertions may indeed attain to those peak moments of spiritual illumination, which are a present foretaste of the future reward: a mystical experience of the Absolute.

In sum, we can say that, insofar as this whole complex of otherworldly striving falls within ethics at all (as do, for instance, the aforementioned "moderate" forms in which a life good in itself forms the condition for eternal reward), it too fits our thesis concerning the orientation of all previous ethics to the present.

2. The Statesman's Responsibility for the Future

What about the examples of *innerworldly* future-oriented ethics, which alone do really belong to rational ethics in that they reckon with a known cause-effect pattern? We mentioned in the second place the long-range care of the legislator and statesman for the future good of the commonwealth. Greek political theory is on the whole silent about the *time* aspect which interests us here; but this silence itself is revealing. Something can be gathered from the praise of great lawgivers like Solon and Lycurgus or from the censure of a statesman like Pericles. The praise of the lawgiver includes, it is true, the durability of his creation, but not his planning ahead of something that is to come about only in aftertimes and not attainable already to his contemporaries. His endeavor is to create a viable political structure, and the test of viability is in the enduring of his creation—a changeless enduring if possible. The best state, so it was thought, is also the best for the future, precisely because the stable equilibrium of its present ensures its future as such; and it will then, of course, be the best state *in* that future as well, since the criteria of a good order (of which durability is one) do not change. They do not change because human nature does not change, which with its imperfections is included in the conception which the wise lawgiver must have of a viable political order. This conception thus aims not at the ideally perfect state but rather at the realistically best, that is, the best possible state—and this is now just as possible, and just as imperiled, as it will always be. But this very peril, which threatens all order with the disorder of the human passions, makes necessary, in addition to the singular, founding wisdom of the lawgiver, the continuous, governing wisdom of the statesman. The reproach of Socrates against the politics of Pericles, be it noted, is not that, in the end after his death, his grandiose schemes came to nought, but rather that with such grandiose schemes (including their initial successes) he had already in his own time turned the Athenians' heads and corrupted their civic virtues. Athens' current misfortune thus was blamed not on the eventual failure of those policies but on the blemish at their roots,

which even "success" in their own terms would not have made better in retrospect. What would have been good at that time would be that still today and would most probably have survived into the present.

The foresight of the statesman thus consists in the wisdom and moderation he devotes to the *present*. This present is not here for the sake of a future different from (and superior to) it in type, but rather proves itself—luck permitting—in a future still like itself, and so must be as justified already in itself as its succession is hoped to be. Duration, in short, results as a concomitant of what is good now and at all times. Certainly, political action has a wider time span of effect and responsibility than private action, but its ethics, according to the premodern view, is still none other than the present-oriented one, applied to a life form of longer duration.

3. The Modern Utopia

a) This changes only with what, in my third example, I called the politics of utopia, which is a thoroughly modern phenomenon and presupposes a previously unknown, dynamic eschatology of history. The religious eschatologies of earlier times do not yet represent this case, although they prepare for it. Messianism, for example, does not ordain a messianic politics, but leaves the coming of the Messiah to divine dispensation. Human behavior is implicated in it only in the sense that it can make itself worthy of the event through fulfilling those very norms to which it is subject even without such a prospect. Here we find to hold on the collective scale what we previously found to hold on the personal scale with regard to otherworldly hopes: the here and now is certainly overarched by them, but is not entrusted with their active realization. It serves them the better, the more faithful it remains to its own God-given law, whose fulfillment lies entirely within itself.

b) Here, too, there did occur the extreme form, where the "urgers of the end" took matters into their own hands and with one last thrust of earthly action tried to bring about the messianic kingdom or millennium, for which they considered the time ripe. In fact, some of the chiliastic movements, especially at the beginning of the modern era, lead into the neighborhood of utopian politics, particularly when they are not content with merely having made a start and clearing the path, but when they make a positive beginning with the Kingdom of God, of whose *contents* they have a definite conception. Insofar as ideas of social equality and justice play a role in this conception, the characteristic motivation of modern utopian ethics is already there: but not yet the yawning gulf, stretching across generations, between now and later, means and end, action and goal, which marks the modern, secularized eschatology, that is, modern political utopianism. It is still an ethic of the self-vindicating present, not of the retroactively vindicating future: the true man is already there, and even, in the "community of the saints," the kingdom of God from the moment they realize it in their own midst, as ordained and held to be possible in the dawning fulness of time. The assault, however, against the establishments of the world that still oppose its spreading, is made in the expectation of a Jericho-like miracle, not as a mediated process of historical causation. The last step to the innerworldly utopian ethic of history is yet to be taken.

c) Only with the advent of modern *progress*, both as a fact and as an idea, did the possibility emerge of conceiving everything past as a stepping-stone to the present and of everything present as a stepping-stone to the future. When this notion (which in itself, as unlimited, distinguishes no stage as final and leaves to each the immediacy of its own present) is wed with a secularized eschatology which assigns to the absolute, defined in terms of this world, a finite place in time, and when to this is added a conception of a teleological dynamism which leads to the final state of affairs—then we have the conceptual prerequisites for a utopian politics. "To found the kingdom of heaven already upon earth" (Heinrich Heine) presupposes some idea of what such an earthly kingdom of heaven would look like (or so one would think—but on this point the theory displays a remarkable blank). In any case, even lacking such an idea, the resolute secular eschatology entails a conception of human events that radically demotes to provisional status all that goes before, stripping it of its independent validity and at best making it the vehicle for reaching the promised state of things that is yet to come—a means to the future end which alone is worthy in itself.

Here in fact is a break with the past, and what we have said concerning the present-oriented character of all previous ethics and their common premise of the persistence of human nature is no longer true of the teaching which represents this break most clearly, the Marxist philosophy of history and its corresponding ethic of action. Action takes place for the sake of a future which neither the agent nor the victim nor their contemporaries will live to enjoy. The obligations upon the now issue from that goal, not from the good and ill of the contemporary world; and the norms of action are just as provisional, indeed just as "inauthentic," as the conditions which it will transmute into the higher state. The ethic of revolutionary eschatology considers itself an ethic of transition, while the consummate, true ethic (essentially still unknown) will only come into its own after the harsh interim morality (which can last a long time) has created the conditions for it and thereby abrogated itself.

Thus there already exists, in Marxism, a future-oriented ethic, with a distance of vision, a time span of affirmed responsibility, a scope of object (= all of future humanity), and a depth of concern (the whole future nature of man)— and, as we might already add, with a sense for the powers of technology—which in all these respects stands comparison with the ethic for which we want to plead here. All the more important it is to determine the relation between these two ethical positions which, as answers to the unprecedented modern situation and especially to its technology, have so much in common over against premodern ethics and yet are so different from one another. This must wait until we have heard more about the problems and tasks which the ethic here envisaged has to deal with, and which are posed by the colossal progress of technology. For technology's power over human destiny has overtaken even that of communism, which no less than capitalism thought merely to make use of it. We say this much in advance: while both positions concern themselves with the utopian possibilities of this technology, the ethic we are looking for is *not* eschatological and, in a sense yet to be specified, is anti-utopian.

VII. Man as an Object of Technology

Our comparison dealt with the historical forms of the ethics of contemporaneity and immediacy, for which the Kantian case served only as an example. What stands in question is not their validity within their own frame of reference but their sufficiency for those new dimensions of human action which transcend that frame. Our thesis is that the new kinds and dimensions of action require a commensurate ethic of foresight and responsibility which is as novel as the eventualities which it must meet. We have seen that these are the eventualities that arise out of the works of *homo faber* in the era of technology. But among those novel works we have not mentioned yet the potentially most ominous class. We have considered *techne* only as applied to the nonhuman realm. But man himself has been added to the objects of technology. *Homo faber* is turning upon himself and gets ready to make over the maker of all the rest. This consummation of his power, which may well portend the overpowering of man, this final imposition of art on nature, calls upon the utter resources of ethical thought, which never before has been faced with elective alternatives to what were considered the definite terms of the human condition.

1. Extension of Life Span

Take, for instance, the most basic of these "givens," man's *mortality*. Who ever before had to make up his mind on its desirable and *eligible* measure? There was nothing to choose about the upper limit, the "threescore years and ten, or by reason of strength fourscore." Its inexorable rule was the subject of lament, submission, or vain (not to say foolish) wish-dreams about possible exceptions—strangely enough, almost never of affirmation. The intellectual imagination of a George Bernard Shaw and a Jonathan Swift speculated on the privilege of not having to die, or the curse of not being able to die. (Swift with the latter was the more perspicacious of the two.) Myth and legend toyed with such themes against the acknowledged background of the unalterable, which made the earnest man rather pray "teach us to number our days that we may get a heart of wisdom" (Psalm 90). Nothing of this was in the realm of doing and effective decision. The question was only how to relate to the stubborn fact.

But lately the dark cloud of inevitability seems to lift. A practical hope is held out by certain advances in cell biology to prolong, perhaps indefinitely extend, the span of life by counteracting biochemical processes of aging. Death no longer appears as a necessity belonging to the nature of life, but as an avoidable, at least in principle tractable and long-delayable, organic malfunction. A perennial yearning of mortal man seems to come nearer fulfillment. And for the first time we have in earnest to ask the questions "How desirable is this? How desirable for the individual, and how for the species?" These questions involve the very meaning of our finitude, the attitude toward death, and the general biological significance of the balance of death and procreation. Even prior to such ultimate questions are the more pragmatic ones of who should be eligible for the boon: Persons of particular quality and merit? Of social eminence? Those who can pay for it? Everybody? The last would seem the only just course. But it would have to be paid for at the opposite end, at the source.

For clearly, on a population-wide scale, the price of extended age must be a proportional slowing of replacement, that is, a diminished access of new life. The result would be a decreasing proportion of youth in an increasingly aged population. How good or bad would that be for the general condition of man? Would the species gain or lose? And how *right* would it be to preempt the place of youth? Having to die is bound up with having been born: mortality is but the other side of the perennial spring of "natality" (to use Hannah Arendt's term). This had always been ordained; now its meaning has to be pondered in the sphere of decision.

To take the extreme (not that it will ever be obtained): if we abolish death, we must abolish procreation as well, for the latter is life's answer to the former, and so we would have a world of old age with no youth, and of known individuals with no surprises of such that had never been before. But this perhaps is precisely the wisdom in the harsh dispensation of our mortality: that it grants us the eternally renewed promise of the freshness, immediacy, and eagerness of youth, together with the supply of otherness as such. There is no substitute for this in the greater accumulation of prolonged experience: it can never recapture the unique privilege of seeing the world for the first time and with new eyes; never relive the wonder which, according to Plato, is the beginning of philosophy; never the curiosity of the child, which rarely enough lives on as thirst for knowledge in the adult, until it wanes there too. This ever renewed beginning, which is only to be had at the price of ever repeated ending, may well be mankind's hope, its safeguard against lapsing into boredom and routine, its chance of retaining the spontaneity of life. Also, the role of the *memento mori* in the individual's life must be considered, and what its attenuation to indefiniteness may do to it. Perhaps a nonnegotiable limit to our expected time is necessary for each of us as the incentive to number our days and make them count.

So it could be that what by intent is a philanthropic gift of science to man, the partial granting of his oldest wish—to escape the curse of mortality—turns out to be to the detriment of man. I am not indulging in prediction and, in spite of my noticeable bias, not even in valuation. My point is that already the promised gift raises questions that had never to be asked before in terms of practical choice, and that no principle of former ethics, which took the human constants for granted, is competent to deal with them. And yet they must be dealt with ethically and by principle and not merely by the pressure of interests.

2. Behavior Control

It is similar with all the other, quasi-utopian possibilities which progress in the biomedical sciences has partly already placed at our disposal and partly holds in prospect for eventual translation into technological know-how. Of these, *behavior control* is much nearer to practical readiness than the still hypothetical prospect I have just been discussing, and the ethical questions it raises are less profound but have a more direct bearing on the moral conception of man. Here again, the new kind of intervention exceeds the old ethical categories. They have not equipped us to rule, for example, on mental control by chemical means or by direct electrical action on the brain via implanted electrodes—undertaken, let us assume, for defensible and even laudable ends. The mixture of beneficial and dangerous potentials is obvious, but the lines are not easy to draw. Relief of mental patients from distressing and disabling symptoms seems unequivocally beneficial. But from the relief of the *patient*, a goal entirely in the tradition of the medical art, there is an easy passage to the relief of *society* from the inconvenience of difficult individual behavior among its members: that is, the passage from medical to social application; and this opens up an indefinite field with grave potentials. The troublesome problems of rule and unruliness in modern mass society make the extension of such control methods to nonmedical categories extremely tempting for social management. Numerous questions of human rights and dignity arise. The difficult question of preempting versus enabling care insists on concrete answers. Shall we induce learning attitudes in schoolchildren by the mass administration of drugs, circumventing the appeal to autonomous motivation? Shall we overcome aggression by electronic pacification of brain areas? Shall we generate sensations of happiness or pleasure or at least contentment through independent stimulation (or tranquilizing) of the appropriate centers—independent, that is, of the objects of happiness, pleasure, or content and their attainment in personal living and achieving? Candidacies could be multiplied. Business firms might become interested in some of these techniques for performance increase among their employees.

Regardless of the question of compulsion or consent, and regardless also of the question of undesirable side-effects, each time we thus bypass the human way of dealing with human problems, short-circuiting it by an impersonal mechanism, we have taken away something from the dignity of personal selfhood and advanced a further step on the road from responsible subjects to programmed behavior systems. Social functionalism, important as it is, is only one side of the question. Decisive is the question of what kind of individuals the society is composed of—to make its existence valuable as a whole. Somewhere along the line of increasing social manageability at the price of individual autonomy, the question of the worthwhileness of the whole human enterprise must pose itself. Answering it involves the image of man we entertain. We must think it anew in light of the things we can do with it or to it now and could never do before.

3. Genetic Manipulation

This holds even more with respect to the last object of a technology applied on man himself—the *genetic* control of future men. This is too wide a subject for the cursory treatment of these

prefatory remarks, and it will have its own chapter in a later "applied part" to succeed this volume. Here I merely point to this most ambitious dream of *homo faber*, summed up in the phrase that man will take his own evolution in hand, with the aim of not just preserving the integrity of the species but of modifying it by improvements of his own design. Whether we have the right to do it, whether we are qualified for that creative role, is the most serious question that can be posed to man finding himself suddenly in possession of such fateful powers. Who will be the image-makers, by what standards, and on the basis of what knowledge? Also, the question of the moral right to experiment on future human beings must be asked. These and similar questions, which demand an answer before we embark on a journey into the unknown, show most vividly how far our powers to act are pushing us beyond the terms of all former ethics.

VIII. The "Utopian" Dynamics of Technical Progress and the Excessive Magnitude of Responsibility

The ethically relevant common feature in all the examples adduced is what I like to call the inherently "utopian" drift of our actions under the conditions of modern technology, whether it works on nonhuman or on human nature, and whether the "utopia" at the end of the road be planned or unplanned. By the kind and size of its snowballing effects, technological power propels us into goals of a type that was formerly the preserve of Utopias. To put it differently, technological power has turned what used and ought to be tentative, perhaps enlightening plays of speculative reason into competing blueprints for projects, and in choosing between them we have to choose between extremes of remote effects. The one thing we can really know of them is their extremism as such—that they concern the total condition of nature on our globe and the very kind of creatures that shall, or shall not, populate it. In consequence of the inevitably "utopian" scale of modern technology, the salutary gap between everyday and ultimate issues, between occasions for common prudence and occasions for illuminated wisdom, is steadily closing. Living now constantly in the shadow of unwanted, built-in, automatic utopianism, we are constantly confronted with issues whose positive choice requires supreme wisdom—an impossible situation for man in general, because he does not possess that wisdom, and in particular for contemporary man, because he denies the very existence of its object, namely, objective value and truth. We need wisdom most when we believe in it least.

If the new nature of our acting then calls for a new ethics of long-range responsibility, coextensive with the range of our power, it calls in the name of that very responsibility also for a new kind of humility—a humility owed, not like former humility to the smallness of our power, but to the excessive magnitude of it, which is the excess of our power to act over our power to foresee and our power to evaluate and to judge. In the face of the quasi-eschatological potentials of our technological processes, ignorance of the ultimate implications becomes itself a reason for responsible restraint—as the second best to the possession of wisdom itself.

One other aspect of the required new ethics of responsibility for and to a distant future is worth mentioning: the doubt it casts on the capacity of representative government, operating by its normal principles and procedures, to meet the new demands. For according to those principles and procedures, only *present* interests make themselves heard and felt and enforce their consideration. It is to them that public agencies are accountable, and this is the way in which concretely the respecting of rights comes about (as distinct from their abstract acknowledgment). But the *future* is not represented, it is not a force that can throw its weight into the scales. The nonexistent has no lobby, and the unborn are powerless. Thus accountability to

them has no political reality behind it in present decision-making, and when they can make their complaint, then we, the culprits, will no longer be there.

This raises to an ultimate pitch the old question of the power of the wise, or the force of ideas not allied to self-interest, in the body politic. What force shall represent the future in the present? That is a question for political philosophy, and one on which I dare not voice my woefully uncertain ideas. They would be premature here anyway. For before that question of enforcement can become practical, the new ethics must find its theory, on which do's and don'ts can be based. That is: before the question of what *force*, comes the question of what *insight* or value-knowledge will represent the future in the present.

IX. The Ethical Vacuum

And here is where I come to a standstill, where we all come to a standstill. For the very same movement which put us in possession of the powers that have now to be regulated by norms—the movement of modern knowledge called science—has by a necessary complementarity eroded the foundations from which norms could be derived; it has destroyed the very idea of norm as such. Not, fortunately, the feeling for norm and even for particular norms. But this feeling becomes uncertain of itself when contradicted by alleged knowledge or at least denied all support by it. It always has a difficult time against the loud clamors of greed and fear. Now it must in addition blush before the frown or smirk of superior knowledge which has certified it as unfounded and incapable of foundation. First it was nature that was "neutralized" with respect to value, then man himself. Now we shiver in the nakedness of a nihilism in which near-omnipotence is paired with near-emptiness, greatest capacity with knowing least for what ends to use it.

It is moot whether, without restoring the category of the sacred, the category most thoroughly destroyed by the scientific enlightenment, we can have an ethics able to cope with the extreme powers which we possess today and constantly increase and are almost compelled to wield. Regarding those consequences that are imminent enough still to hit ourselves, fear can do the job—fear which is so often the best substitute for genuine virtue or wisdom. But this means fails us toward the more distant prospects, which here matter the most, especially as the beginnings seem mostly innocent in their smallness. Only awe of the sacred with its unqualified veto is independent of the computations of mundane fear and the solace of uncertainty about distant consequences. However, religion in eclipse cannot relieve ethics of its task; and while of faith it can be said that as a moving force it either is there or is not, of ethics it is true to say that it must be there.

It must be there because men act, and ethics is for the ordering of actions and for regulating the power to act. It must be there all the more, then, the greater the powers of acting that are to be regulated; and as it must fit their size, the ordering principle must also fit their kind. Thus, novel powers to act require novel ethical rules and perhaps even a new ethics.

"Thou shalt not kill" was enunciated because man has the power to kill and often the occasion and even the inclination for it—in short, because killing is actually done. It is only under the *pressure* of real habits of action, and generally of the fact that always action already takes place, without *this* having to be commanded first, that ethics as the ruling of such acting under the standard of the good or the permitted enters the stage. Such a *pressure* emanates from the novel technological powers of man, whose exercise is given with their existence. *If* they really are as novel in kind as here contended, and if by the kind of their potential consequences they really have abolished the moral neutrality which the technical commerce with matter hitherto enjoyed—then their pressure bids us to seek for new prescriptions in ethics which are competent to assume their guidance, but which first of all can hold their own theoretically against that very pressure.

In this chapter we have developed our *premises*, namely, first, that our collective technological practice constitutes a new kind of human action, and this not just because of the novelty of its methods but more so because of the unprecedented nature of some of its objects, because of the sheer magnitude of most of its enterprises, and because of the indefinitely cumulative propagation of its effects. From all three of these traits, our second premise follows: that what we are doing in this manner is, regardless of the particulars of any of its immediate purposes, no longer ethically neutral as a whole. With this exposition of the ethical question, the task of seeking an answer, and first of all a rational principle for it, only begins.

5. Reasoning on Biomedical Issues

In their acclaimed book *Principles of Biomedical Ethics*, Beauchamp and Childress carry out a defense of principlism as a deliberative method to reason on moral controversies arisen in biomedical field. Their four-principles approach (also known as "Georgetown Mantra") derives from what they call common morality and also from professional traditions in health care.

In general terms, principlism implies and recognizes theoretical and practical aspects of moral reasoning. According to the authors, those aspects are traditional and display themselves at two levels: deliberative (theoretical) and procedural (practical). In order to properly address these two levels, and before examining the meanings of morality and professional ethics, Beauchamp and Childress start clarifying what "ethics" means and what kinds of ethics we can distinguish, task that at this point, reveals itself as methodologically necessary.

On the one hand, the authors define the concept of normative ethics which seeks norms for the guidance and evaluation of conducts and practices. As ethical theories attempt to identify and justify those norms, theoretical guidelines are often called "principles." In this fashion, practical or applied ethics is normative and

implies the attempt to interpret general norms to apply them in specific contexts of moral deliberation.

Therefore, in the framework of normative ethics, general norms are broader frameworks to start moral deliberation (they are not concrete). Instead, practical norms are specific and work in particular scenarios.

On the other hand, we have nonnormative ethics which can be divided into two types:

1. *Descriptive ethics* that implies a factual investigation of moral conceptions, beliefs and conducts. In other words, it observes and describes moral values by using a scientific method and it is able to establish sociological, psychological and historical elements of morality. It also investigates how people reason, judge an act but it doesn't take a moral position regarding its object of study.

2. *Metaethics* which carries out an analysis of language, concepts and methods of reasoning in normative ethics as well as studies the meaning of classical terms of moral connotation such as right, obligation, virtue, morality, responsibility, pluralism, equality, among others. Also, metaethics addresses problems such as whether morality is

objective or subjective, relative or universal, and rational or nonrational. In short, metaethics implies a conceptual analysis far from facts.

Beyond this division of ethics into diverse types and to determine the field in which bioethics works, Beauchamp and Childress go further and distinguish between common and particular moralities. They characterize common morality as universal morality. This point is, certainly, controversial. We need to consider that morality refers to norms about right and wrong human conducts. The balance of what is right and wrong is carried out through rules apparently of universal scope and accepted by all people committed to morality. However, those rules are shared and agreed in an incomplete way since our agreement regarding them is tacit rather than explicit. For instance, we can agree that the principle of just distribution of benefit and burdens, as a *prima facie* principle, namely, a self-evident mandate, is necessary to maintain the social cohesion. But it occurs that we do not necessarily share the meaning of social justice or which the best criterion for distribution of benefit and burdens in a society is. However, and by virtue of that tacit consensus, common morality becomes a universal morality although we must understand the term "universal" in a narrowed scope since the precepts of that common morality are only valid inside determined groups such as religions, cultures, communities, societies, traditions and the like. Hence, those precepts bind only the members of those groups. For example, as a non-Muslim person, I am not morally obliged to observe the Koran's mandates. In a plural and pluralistic society I should respect those Koran's precepts and ideas as part of a legitimate moral diversity but nobody can force me to perform Muslim duties.

However, there are moral concepts that go beyond culture and tradition, such as freedom and dignity, among others. Those intercultural or transcultural principles are specified into norms that order to respect the autonomy, rights, views, beliefs and life of others. But, once again, when we agree with others regarding those issues, the agreement is formal and work properly only in general and noncontroversial contexts since we differ with respect to the content of those moral standards. Therefore, when moral controversies become more specific and complex a formal agreement is not sufficient; we certainly need a material one. At that point, we need to dialogue, debate on, reason about and agree the meaning, content, scope and applicability of moral principles. That is the only way those principles are able to point out specific procedures and rules for decision-making.

Despite these considerations, Beauchamp and Childress affirm that common morality is a set of norms shared by all persons committed to morality. It is, in other words and theoretically speaking, applicable to all persons in all places. According to this, Beauchamp and Childress define ten norms of common morality applicable in the bioethical field: 1. Do not kill, 2. Do not cause pain or suffering to others, 3. Prevent harm, 4. Rescue persons in danger, 5. Tell the truth, 6. Nurture the young and dependent, 7. Keep your promises, 8. Do not steal, 9. Do not punish the innocent, 10. Obey the law.

These norms are self-evident to reason and should be accepted by all rational people committed to morality. However, in practical terms, the observance of these norms is not absolute since each one of them is susceptible of being violated with or without moral justification.

In the same way, Beauchamp and Childress identify ten virtues of common morality: 1. Nonmalevolence; 2. Honesty; 3. Integrity; 4. Conscientiousness; 5. Trustworthiness; 6. Fidelity; 7. Gratitude; 8. Truthfulness; 9. Lovingness; and 10. Kindness. These virtues are also self-evident and represent a criterion of universal admiration. I fact, a person who lacks them could be considered immoral or, al least, defective morally speaking.

Therefore, we could characterize the concept of common morality according to the following elements:

1. It is the product of human experience and history.
2. It represents a universally shared product.
3. It is founded on several cultures.
4. It is not relative to specific cultures or individuals. It transcends both.
5. It comprises moral beliefs not formal standards prior to formal beliefs.
6. There is not only one theory of common morality.
7. There may be different epistemological dimensions of common morality.

It is expected that all people committed to morality adhere to common morality' standards. However, not all people care about or identify themselves with moral demands.

Now, although particular moralities share some dimension of common morality (general moral principles) they specifically come from culture, that is, they are traditional. In this fashion, particular moralities demand some types of conducts according to specific moral codes and procedures (standards of practice). Also, they oblige only within a specific cultural or professional framework. Hence, they cannot force people who live outside that framework to observe specific rules or moral standards. For instance, I am not morally forced to observe Koran's principles and mandates since I am not Muslim. In the same way, I am not morally forced to keep a secret of confession because I am not a priest, or I am not morally bounded to perform a surgery with excellence (in the case of an emergency) since I am not a surgeon.

In conclusion, particular moralities are concrete (they have specific rules and procedures to regulate moral behavior), non-universal (their rules are only valid inside a specific context; they are contingent) and content/rich norms (rules and procedures are well defined and specified). Instead, common morality is abstract (it only works with general theoretical guidelines: principles), universal (it should be shared for most of people committed to morality; it does not only work within a determined cultural context), content/thin norms (Principles are vague and have a broad epistemological and methodological scope).

Reading

Beauchamp, Tom L.; Childress, James F., *Principles of Biomedical Ethics*, 7th Edition, Oxford University Press, 2012: **1–13**.

Study Questions

1. Why could bioethics be considered as a normative ethics?
2. What are the main differences between common morality and particular moralities?
3. Where are the principles of bioethics coming from? From a common morality? From a particular one? Justify your answer.
4. Identify and explain the main elements of moral reasoning in bioethics.

Principles of Biomedical Ethics

Tom L. Beauchamp and James F. Childress

1
Moral Norms

Medical ethics enjoyed remarkable continuity from the time of Hippocrates until the middle of the twentieth century, when developments in the biological and health sciences created concerns about the adequacy of traditional moral guidelines.[1] The Hippocratic tradition had neglected ethical problems of truthfulness, privacy, the distribution of health care resources, communal responsibility, the use of research subjects, and the like. To avoid a similar narrowness, we primarily use philosophical reflection on morality that is distanced from the history of professional medical ethics. This philosophical reflection is not a fully adequate basis for professional ethics, but it allows us to examine and, where appropriate, depart from dominant assumptions in approaches to the biomedical sciences and health care.

Normative and Nonnormative Ethics

The term *ethics* needs attention before we turn to the meanings of *morality* and *professional ethics*. *Ethics* is a generic term covering several different ways of examining and understanding the moral life. Some approaches to ethics are normative, others nonnormative.

Normative Ethics

General normative ethics attempts to answer the question, "Which general moral norms for the guidance and evaluation of conduct should we accept, and why?" Ethical theories attempt to identify and justify these norms, which are often called principles. In Chapter 9 we examine several theories and offer criteria for assessing them.

Many practical questions would remain unanswered even if a fully satisfactory general ethical theory were available. *Practical ethics* (used here as synonymous with *applied ethics*, and by contrast to *theoretical ethics*) is the attempt to interpret general norms for the purpose of addressing particular problems and contexts. The term *practical* refers to the use of norms in the course of deliberating about moral problems, practices, and policies in professions, institutions, and government. Often no straightforward movement from norms—in the form of theories, principles, or precedents—to particular judgments is available. General norms are usually only starting points for the development of concrete norms of conduct.

Nonnormative Ethics

There are two types of nonnormative ethics. The first type is *descriptive ethics*, which is the factual investigation of moral beliefs and conduct. It uses scientific techniques to study how people reason and act. For example, anthropologists, sociologists, psychologists, and historians determine which moral norms and attitudes are expressed in professional practice, in professional codes, in institutional mission statements and rules, and in public policies. They study phenomena such as surrogate decision making, treatment of the dying, and the nature of consent obtained from patients.

The second type is *metaethics*, which involves analysis of the language, concepts, and methods of reasoning in normative ethics. For example, metaethics addresses the meanings of terms such as *right, obligation, virtue, justification, morality,* and *responsibility*. It is also concerned with moral epistemology (the theory of moral knowledge), the logic and patterns of moral reasoning and justification, and the possibility and nature of moral truth. Whether morality is objective or subjective, relative or nonrelative, and rational or nonrational are all important topics in metaethics.

Descriptive ethics and metaethics are nonnormative because their objective is to establish what factually or conceptually *is* the case, not what ethically *ought to be* the case or what is ethically *valuable*. Often in this book we rely on reports in descriptive ethics, for example, when discussing the nature of professional codes of ethics. However, our underlying interest is usually in whether the prescriptions found in such codes are *justifiable*, which is a normative issue.[2]

The Common Morality as Universal Morality

In its most familiar sense, *morality* refers to norms about right and wrong human conduct that are so widely shared that they form a stable (although incomplete) social agreement. As a social institution, morality encompasses many standards of conduct, including moral principles, rules, rights, and virtues. We learn about morality as we grow up, and we also learn to distinguish the universal morality that holds for everyone from norms that bind only members of special groups, such as physicians, nurses, or public health officials. All persons living a moral life grasp the core dimensions of morality. They know not to lie, not to steal others' property, to keep promises, to respect the rights of others, not to kill or cause harm to innocent persons, and the like. All persons committed to morality do not doubt the relevance and importance of these rules. They know that violating these norms is unethical and will likely generate feelings of remorse and provoke the moral censure of others. Because we are already convinced about these matters, the literature of ethics does not usually debate the merit or acceptability of these basic moral commitments. However, debates do occur about their precise meaning, scope, weight, and strength, often in relation to hard cases.

The Nature of the Common Morality

The common morality is the set of norms shared by all persons committed to morality. The common morality is not merely *a* morality, in contrast to other moralities.[3] The common morality is applicable to all persons in all places, and we rightly judge all human conduct by its standards. The following are norms that are examples (though not a complete list) of *standards of action* (rules of obligation) found in the common morality: (1) Do not kill, (2) Do not cause pain or suffering to others, (3) Prevent evil or harm from occurring, (4) Rescue persons in danger, (5) Tell the truth, (6) Nurture the young and dependent, (7) Keep your promises, (8) Do not steal, (9) Do not punish the innocent, and (10) Obey the law.

The common morality contains, in addition, standards other than rules of obligation. Here are ten examples (again, not a complete list) of *moral character traits*, or virtues, recognized in the common morality: (1) nonmalevolence, (2) honesty, (3) integrity, (4) conscientiousness, (5) trustworthiness, (6) fidelity, (7) gratitude, (8) truthfulness, (9) lovingness, and (10) kindness. These virtues are universally admired traits of character.[4] A person is deficient in moral character if he or she lacks such traits. Negative traits that are the opposite of these virtues are *vices* (malevolence, dishonesty, lack of integrity, cruelty, etc.). They are universally recognized as substantial moral defects. In this chapter we say no more about character and the virtues and vices, reserving this area of investigation for Chapter 2.

It should not be thought that our account of universal morality (in the remainder of this chapter and in Chapter 10) conceives of the common morality as ahistorical or as a priori, whereas other parts of morality are historical products relative to cultures.[5] We do not embrace an ahistorical conception, but can we demonstrate that there is a nonrelativist, or universalist, way of avoiding ahistoricism? This is an important and complicated problem in moral theory that we cannot engage in depth here. We offer only four simple clarifications of our position: First, we hold that the common morality is a product of human experience and history and is a universally shared product. The origin of the norms of the common morality is no different in principle from the origin of the norms of a particular morality in that both are learned and transmitted in communities. The primary difference is that the common morality is found in all cultures,[6] whereas particular moralities are found only in one or more cultures forming a subset of all cultures. Second, we accept moral pluralism (some would say relativism) in *particular* moralities (see pp. 5–8), but we reject a historical moral pluralism (or relativism) in the *common* morality. The common morality is not relative to cultures or individuals, because it transcends both. Third, the common morality comprises moral beliefs (what all morally committed persons believe), not standards prior to moral belief. Fourth, explications of the common morality—in books such as this one—are historical products, and every *theory* of the common morality has a history of development by the authors of the theory. (See, further, Chapter 10, pp. 387-88, 391.)

Theses about the Common Morality

The appeals that we make to the common morality might be understood as normative, nonnormative, or both. If the appeals are *normative*, the claim is that the common morality has normative force: It establishes moral standards for everyone, and failing to abide by these standards is unethical. If the appeals are *nonnormative*, the claim is that we can empirically study whether the common morality is present in all cultures. We accept both the normative force of the common morality and the possibility of studying it empirically.

Some critics of our account in this book assert that scant anthropological or historical evidence supports the empirical hypothesis that a universal common morality exists.[7] In light of this criticism, we need to consider how good the evidence is both for and against the existence of a universal common morality. This is a nuanced problem. In principle, scientific research could either confirm or falsify the hypothesis of a universal morality. However, as with all empirical research, it is essential to be clear about the hypothesis being tested. Our hypothesis is simply that all persons *committed to morality* adhere to the standards that we are calling the common morality. It would, of course, be absurd to assert that all persons do, in fact, accept the norms of the common morality. Clearly many amoral, immoral, or selectively moral persons do not care about or identify with moral demands.

We explore this hypothesis in Chapter 10 rather than here in Chapter 1 (see pp. 387–88). For now we say only that when we claim that the normative judgments found in many parts of this book are derived from the common morality, we do not mean that our *theory* of the common morality gets this morality just right or that it extends the common morality in just the right ways. There may be dimensions of the common morality that we do not correctly capture or depict. Moreover, to say that we attempt to *build* on the common morality in this book by extending it into new areas is not to say that we can validly claim its authority at every level of our account.

Particular Moralities as Nonuniversal

The Nature of Particular Moralities

We shift now from *universal morality* (the common morality) to *particular moralities*. Many moral norms are not shared by all cultures, groups, and individuals. Whereas the common morality contains general moral norms that are abstract, universal, and content-thin, particular moralities present concrete, nonuniversal, and content-rich norms. (More precisely, particular moralities accept norms at all levels of generality, whereas common morality is comprised only of abstract, universal, and content-thin norms. Particular moralities are distinguished by their particular norms, but share the common morality with all other particular moralities.) These specific moralities include the many responsibilities, aspirations, ideals, sympathies, attitudes, and sensitivities found in diverse cultural traditions, religious traditions, professional practice standards, institutional expectations, and the like. In some cases explication of the values in these moralities requires a special knowledge and may involve refinement by experts or scholars—as, for example, in the body of Jewish religious, legal, and moral norms in the Talmudic tradition. There may also be well-structured moral systems to adjudicate conflicts and provide methods for judgments in borderline cases—as, for example, within the norms and methods in Roman Catholic casuistry.

Professional moralities, which include moral codes and standards of practice, are one form of particular morality. These moralities often legitimately vary from other moralities in the way in which they handle conflicts of interest, protocol review, advance directives, and other subjects. (See the next section, "Professional and Public Moralities.") *Moral ideals* such as charitable goals and aspirations that exceed obligations provide a second instructive example of particular moralities. Moral ideals such as charitable beneficence, by definition, are not required of all persons; indeed they are not *required* of any person.[8] Actions performed from these ideals are morally praiseworthy, but persons who fail to fulfill their ideals cannot be blamed or criticized by others. Moral ideals can be universally praised even though they are not universally required. It is reasonable to presume that all morally committed persons share an admiration of and endorsement of *some* moral ideals, and in this respect those ideals can be said to be shared moral beliefs in the common morality. However, they are not universally shared as *demands* of the moral life. When they become requirements of conduct (e.g., in a monastic tradition), such beliefs are part of a particular morality, not part of universal morality. These ideals and their supererogatory nature are discussed in Chapter 2.

Morality, then, consists of more than principles and rules of the common morality. Morality includes nonbinding moral ideals that individuals and groups accept and act on, communal norms that bind only members of specific moral communities, extraordinary virtues, and the like.

Persons who accept a particular morality often suppose that they speak with an authoritative moral voice for all persons. They operate under the false belief that they have the force of the common morality (that is, universal morality) behind them. The particular moral viewpoints that these persons hold may be morally acceptable and even praiseworthy, but they do not bind other persons or communities. For example, persons who believe intensely that scarce medical resources, such as transplantable organs, should be distributed only by lottery rather than by medical need may have very good moral reasons for their views, but they cannot claim the support of the common morality for those views.

Professional and Public Moralities

Just as the common morality is accepted by all morally committed persons, most professions have, at least implicitly, a professional morality with standards of conduct that are generally acknowledged by those in the profession who are serious about their moral responsibilities. In medicine, professional morality specifies general moral norms for the institutions and practices of medicine. Special roles and relationships in medicine require rules that other professions may not need. For example, as we argue in Chapters 4 and 8, rules of informed consent and medical confidentiality are rooted in the more general moral requirements of respecting the autonomy of persons and protecting them from harm. These rules may not be serviceable or appropriate outside of medicine and research.

Members of professions often *informally* adhere to widely accepted moral guidelines—such as rules prohibiting discrimination against colleagues on the basis of gender, race, religion, or national origin. In recent years *formal* codifications of and instruction in professional morality have increased through codes of medical and nursing ethics, codes of research ethics, and the reports and recommendations of public commissions. Before we assess these developments, the nature of professions needs brief discussion.

According to Talcott Parsons, a profession is "a cluster of occupational roles, that is, roles in which the incumbents perform certain functions valued in the society in general, and, by these activities, typically earn a living at a fulltime job."[9] Under this definition, circus performers, exterminators, and garbage collectors are professionals; prostitutes probably are not (because their function is not "valued in the society in general"), despite prostitution's reputation as "the world's oldest profession." Today, it is not surprising to find all such activities characterized as professions, inasmuch as the word *profession* has come, in common use, to mean almost any occupation by which a person earns a living. The once honorific sense of *profession* is now better reflected in the term *learned profession*, which assumes an extensive education in the arts, sciences, technologies, and the like.

Professionals in the relevant sense are usually distinguished by their specialized knowledge and training as well as by their commitment to provide important services to patients, clients, or consumers. Professions maintain self-regulating organizations that control entry into occupational roles by formally certifying that candidates have acquired the necessary knowledge and skills. In learned professions, such as medicine, nursing, and public health, the professional's background knowledge is partly acquired through closely supervised training, and the professional is committed to providing a service to others.

Health care professions specify and enforce obligations for their members, thereby seeking to ensure that persons who enter into relationships with these professionals will find them competent and trustworthy. The obligations that professions attempt to enforce are determined by an accepted role. These obligations comprise the "ethics" of the profession, although there may also be role-specific ideals such as self-effacement that are not obligatory. Problems of professional ethics usually arise either from conflicts over appropriate professional standards or conflicts between professional commitments and the commitments professionals have to activities outside the profession. Because the traditional rules of professional morality are often vague, some professions codify their standards in detailed statements aimed at reducing the vagueness.

Codes often specify rules of etiquette in addition to rules of ethics. For example, one historically significant version of the code of the American Medical Association (AMA) instructed physicians not to criticize fellow physicians who have previously been in charge of a case."[10] Such professional codes tend to foster and reinforce member identification with the prevailing values of the profession. These codes are beneficial when they effectively incorporate defensible moral norms, but some professional codes oversimplify moral requirements, make them indefensibly rigid, or make excessive and unwarranted claims about their completeness and authoritativeness. As a consequence, professionals may mistakenly suppose that they are satisfying all relevant moral requirements by strictly following the rules of the code, just as many people believe that they fully discharge their moral obligations when they meet all relevant legal requirements.

We can and should ask whether the codes specific to areas of science, medicine, and health care are coherent, defensible, and comprehensive within their domain. Historically, few codes have had much to say about the implications of several moral principles and rules such as veracity, respect for autonomy, and justice that have been the subjects of intense discussion in contemporary biomedical ethics. From ancient medicine to the present, physicians have often generated codes for themselves without subjecting them to the scrutiny or acceptance of patients and the public. These codes have rarely appealed to more general ethical standards or to a source of moral authority beyond the traditions and judgments of physicians. The articulation of professional norms in these circumstances has often appeared to protect the profession's interests more than to offer a broad and impartial moral viewpoint or to address issues of importance to patients and society.[11]

Psychiatrist Jay Katz once poignantly expressed his reservations about such codes of medical ethics. Initially inspired by his outrage over the fate of Holocaust victims, Katz became convinced that only a persistent improvement in professional ethics and an educational effort that reaches beyond traditional codes could provide meaningful guidance for research involving human subjects:

> As I became increasingly involved in the world of law, I learned much that was new to me from my colleagues and students about such complex issues as the right to self-determination and privacy and the extent of the authority of governmental, professional, and other institutions to intrude into private life. ... These issues ... had rarely been discussed in my medical education. Instead it had been all too uncritically assumed that they could be resolved by fidelity to such undefined principles as *primum non nocere* ["First, do no harm"] or to visionary codes of ethics.[12]

Public Regulation of Professional Conduct

Additional moral direction for health professionals and scientists comes through the public policy process, which includes regulations and guidelines promulgated by governmental bodies. The term *public policy* is used here to refer to a set of nonnative, enforceable guidelines accepted by an official public body, such as an agency of government or a legislature, to govern a particular area of conduct. The policies of corporations, hospitals, trade groups, and professional societies sometimes have a deep impact on public policy, but these policies are private, not public—though these bodies are frequently regulated by public policies. A close connection exists between law and public policy: All laws constitute public policies, but not all public policies are, in the conventional sense, laws. In contrast to laws, public policies need not be explicitly formulated or codified. For example, an official who decides not to fund a newly recommended government program with no prior history of funding is formulating a public policy. Decisions not to act, as well as decisions to act, can constitute public policies.

Public policies, such as those that fund health care for the indigent or protect subjects of biomedical research, usually incorporate moral considerations. Moral analysis is part of good policy *formation*, not merely a method for evaluating *existing* policy. Efforts to protect the rights of patients and research subjects provide instructive examples. Over the past thirty-five years the U.S. government has created several national commissions, advisory committees, and councils to formulate guidelines for research involving human subjects, as well as for other areas of biomedical ethics. Morally informed policies have guided decision making about the choice of treatments as well. For example, the U.S. Congress passed the Patient Self-Determination Act (PSDA) as the first federal legislation to ensure that health care institutions inform patients about institutional policies that allow them to accept or refuse medical treatment and about their rights under state law, including a right to formulate advance directives.[13] The relevance of bioethics to public policy is now recognized in most developed countries, several of which have influential national bioethics committees.

Many courts have been active in developing case law that sets standards for science, medicine, and health care. Legal decisions often express communal moral norms and stimulate ethical reflection that over time alters those norms. For example, the line of court decisions in the U.S. starting with the Karen Ann Quinlan case in the mid-1970s has constituted a nascent tradition of moral reflection that has been influenced by, and has influenced, literature in ethics on topics such as whether life-saving medical technologies should be viewed as medical treatments that are subject to the same standards of decision making as other forms of treatment.

Policy formation and criticism involve more complex forms of moral judgment than ethical theories, principles, and rules can handle on their own.[14] Public policy is often formulated in contexts that are marked by profound social disagreements, uncertainties, and differing interpretations of history. No body of abstract moral principles and rules can fix policy in such circumstances, because abstract norms do not contain enough specific information to provide direct and discerning guidance. The implementation of moral principles and rules must take into account factors such as feasibility, efficiency, cultural pluralism, political procedures, pertinent legal requirements, uncertainty about risk, and noncompliance by patients. Principles and rules provide the moral background for policy formation and evaluation, but a policy must also be shaped by empirical data and by information available in fields such as medicine, nursing, public health, economics, law, biotechnology, and psychology.

When using moral norms to formulate or criticize public policies, we cannot move with assurance from a judgment that an *act* is morally right (or wrong) to a judgment that a corresponding *law* or *policy* is morally right (or wrong). The judgment that an act is morally wrong does not necessarily lead to the judgment that the government should prohibit it or refuse to allocate funds to support it. For example, one can argue, without inconsistency, that sterilization and abortion are morally wrong but that the law should not prohibit them, because they are fundamentally matters of personal choice beyond the authority of government (or, alternatively, because many persons would seek dangerous and unsanitary procedures from unlicensed practitioners). Similarly, the judgment that an act is morally acceptable does not imply that the law should permit it. For example, the belief that active euthanasia is morally justified for terminally ill infants who face uncontrollable pain and suffering is consistent with the belief that the government should legally prohibit such active euthanasia because it would not be possible to control abuses if it were legalized.

We are not defending any of these moral judgments. We are maintaining that the connections between moral norms and judgments about policy or law are complicated and that a judgment about the morality of *acts* does not entail a corresponding judgment about *law* and *policy*. Factors such as the symbolic value of law, the costs of a program and its enforcement, and the demands of competing programs often must be considered.

Moral Dilemmas

Reasoning through dilemmas to conclusions and choices is a familiar feature of decision making. Consider a particular case.[15] Some years ago, the judges on the California Supreme Court had to reach a decision about the legal force and limits of medical confidentiality. A man killed a woman after confiding to a therapist his intention to commit the act. The therapist had attempted unsuccessfully to have the man committed but, in accordance with his duty of medical confidentiality to the patient, did not communicate the threat to the woman when the commitment attempt failed.

The majority opinion of the Court held that "When a therapist determines, or pursuant to the standards of his profession should determine, that his patient presents a serious danger of violence to another, he incurs an obligation to use reasonable care to protect the intended victim against such danger." This obligation extends to notifying the police and directly warning the intended victim. The justices in the majority opinion argued that therapists generally ought to observe the rule of medical confidentiality, but that this rule must yield in this case to the "public interest in safety from violent assault." Although these justices recognized that rules of professional ethics have substantial public value, they held that matters of greater importance, such as protecting others against violent assault, can override these rules.

In a minority opinion, one judge disagreed and argued that doctors violate patients' rights if they fail to observe standard rules of confidentiality. If it were common practice to break these rules, he reasoned, the fiduciary nature of the relationship between physicians and patients would erode. The mentally ill would refrain from seeking aid or divulging critical information because of the loss of trust that is essential for effective treatment. As a result, violent assaults would increase.

This case presents straightforward moral and legal dilemmas in which both judges cite relevant reasons to support their conflicting judgments. Moral dilemmas are circumstances in which moral obligations demand or appear to demand that a person adopt each of two (or more) alternative but incompatible actions, such that the person cannot perform all the required actions. These dilemmas occur in at least two forms.[16] (1) Some evidence or argument indicates that an act is morally permissible and some evidence or argument indicates that it is morally wrong, but the evidence or strength of argument on both sides is inconclusive. Abortion, for example, is sometimes said to be a terrible dilemma for women who see the evidence in this way. (2) An agent believes that, on moral grounds, he or she is obligated to perform two or more mutually exclusive actions. In a moral dilemma of this form, one or more moral norms obligate an agent to do x and one or more moral norms obligate the agent to do y. but the agent cannot do both in the circumstance. The reasons behind alternatives x and y are weighty and neither set of reasons is overriding. If one acts on either set of reasons, one's actions will be morally acceptable in some respects and morally unacceptable in others. Some have viewed the intentional cessation of life-prolonging therapies in the case of patients in a persistent vegetative state, such as Karen Ann Quinlan, Nancy Cruzan, and Terri Schiavo, as dilemmatic in this second way.

Conflicting moral principles and rules may create difficult dilemmas, as popular literature, novels, and films often illustrate. For example, an impoverished person who steals to save a family from starvation or a person who lies to protect a confidential family document confronts such a dilemma. The only way to comply with one obligation in such situations is to contravene another obligation. No matter which course is chosen, some obligation must be overridden or compromised. It is misleading to say that we are obligated to perform both actions in these dilemmatic circumstances. We should discharge the obligation that, in the circumstances, we judge to override or to compromise what we would have been firmly obligated to perform were it not for the conflict.

Conflicts between moral requirements and self-interest sometimes create a *practical* dilemma, but not, strictly speaking, a *moral* dilemma. If moral reasons compete with non-moral reasons, questions about priority can still arise even though no moral dilemma is present. Examples appear in the work of anthropologist William R. Bascom, who collected hundreds of "African dilemma tales" transmitted for decades and sometimes centuries in African tribal societies. One traditional dilemma posed by the Hausa tribe of Nigeria is called *cure for impotence:*

> A friend gave a man a magical armlet that cured his impotence. Later he [the man with the armlet] saw his mother, who had been lost in a slave raid, in a gang of prisoners. He begged his friend to use his magic to release her. The friend agreed on one condition—that the armlet be returned. What shall his choice be?[17]

Hard choice? Perhaps, but presumably not a hard *moral* choice. The obligation to the mother is moral in character, whereas retaining the armlet is a matter of self-interest. We are assuming that no moral obligation exists to a sexual partner; in some circumstances, such an obligation would produce a moral dilemma. In any event, it is not clear that a moral reason in conflict with a personal reason entails that the moral reason is overriding. If a physician, in a situation of scarcity of available drugs, must choose between saving his own life or that of a patient, the moral obligation to take care of the patient may not be overriding.

Some moral philosophers and theologians have argued that although many practical dilemmas involving moral reasons exist, no irresolvable moral dilemmas exist. They do not deny that agents experience moral perplexity, conflict, and disagreement in difficult cases, but they insist that the purpose of a moral theory is to provide a principled procedure for resolving all deep conflicts. Some major figures in the history of ethics have defended this conclusion, because they accept one supreme moral value as overriding all other conflicting values (moral and nonmoral) and because they regard it as incoherent to allow contradictory obligations in a properly structured moral theory. The only *ought*, they maintain, is the *ought* generated by the supreme value.[18] We examine such theories (e.g., utilitarian and Kantian theories) in Chapter 9.

In contrast to the account of moral obligation found in these theories, we maintain throughout this book that various moral principles can and do conflict in the moral life. These conflicts sometimes produce irresolvable moral dilemmas. When forced to a choice, we may "resolve" the situation by choosing one option over another, but we still may believe that neither option is morally preferable to the competing option. A physician with a limited supply of medicine may have to choose to save the life of one patient rather than another and still find her moral dilemma irresolvable. Explicit acknowledgment of such dilemmas helps deflate unwarranted expectations of moral principles and theories. Although we often find ways of reasoning about what we should do, we may not be able to reach a reasoned resolution in many instances. In some cases, the dilemma may only become more difficult and remain unresolved even after the most careful reflection.

A Framework of Moral Norms

The common morality contains moral norms that are basic for biomedical ethics. These norms are treated individually in four chapters in Part 2 of this book (Chapters 4–7). Most classical ethical theories include these principles in some form,[19] and traditional medical codes presuppose at least some of them.

Basic Principles

The set of moral principles defended in this book functions as an analytical framework intended to express general norms of the common morality that are a suitable starting point for biomedical ethics. These principles should function as general guidelines for the formulation of the more specific rules. In Chapters 4 through 7 we defend four clusters of moral principles: (1) *respect for autonomy* (a norm of respecting and supporting autonomous decisions), (2) *nonmaleficence* (a norm of avoiding the causation of harm), (3) *beneficence* (a group of norms pertaining to relieving, lessening, or preventing harm and providing benefits and balancing benefits against risks and costs), and

(4) *justice* (a group of norms for fairly distributing benefits, risks, and costs).

Nonmaleficence and beneficence have played a central historical role in medical ethics. By contrast, respect for autonomy and justice were neglected in traditional medical ethics and have risen to prominence only recently. As an example, consider the work of British physician Thomas Percival. In 1803, he published *Medical Ethics*, the first comprehensive account of medical ethics in the long history of the subject. This book served as the prototype for the AMA's first code of ethics in 1847. Percival argued (using somewhat different language) that nonmaleficence and beneficence fix the physician's primary obligations and triumph over the patient's preferences and decision-making rights in circumstances of serious conflict.[20] Percival failed to appreciate the depth of the importance of principles of respect for autonomy and distributive justice for physician conduct (despite their presence in the common morality, which he arguably did recognize as relevant for medical practice). However, in fairness to him, these considerations are now prominent in discussions of biomedical ethics in a way they were not when he wrote at the turn of the nineteenth century.

That four clusters of moral "principles" or "general norms" are central to biomedical ethics is a conclusion the authors of this work have reached by examining *considered moral judgments* and the way *moral beliefs cohere*, two notions we discuss in Chapter 10. The selection of these four principles, rather than some other cluster of principles, does not receive an argued defense in Chapters 1 through 3. However, in Chapters 4 through 7, we do defend the vital role of each principle in biomedical ethics.

Rules

Our framework encompasses several types of moral norms, including principles, rules, obligations, and rights. We treat principles as the most general and comprehensive norms, but we draw only a loose distinction between rules and principles. Both are general norms of obligation. The difference is that rules are more specific in content and more restricted in scope than principles. Principles do not function as precise guides to action that direct us in each circumstance in the way that more detailed rules and judgments do. Finally, principles and rules usually establish rights as well as obligations, as we explain in Chapter 9.

We defend several types of rules that specify principles: substantive rules, authority rules, and procedural rules.

Substantive rules. Rules of truth telling, confidentiality, privacy, forgoing treatment, informed consent, and rationing health care provide more specific guides to action than do abstract principles. An example of a rule that sharpens the requirements of the principle of respect for autonomy in certain contexts is, "Follow an incompetent patient's advance directive whenever it is clear and relevant." To indicate how this rule specifies the principle of respect for autonomy, we may state it more fully as, "Respect the autonomy of incompetent patients by following all clear and relevant formulations in their advance directives." This formulation shows how the initial norm of respect for autonomy endures while becoming specified. (See, further, the section "Specifying Principles and Rules" later in this chapter.)

Authority rules. We also defend rules about decisional authority—that is, rules regarding who may and should make decisions and perform actions. For example, *rules of surrogate authority* determine who should serve as surrogate agents when making decisions for incompetent persons, while *rules of professional authority* determine who in professional ranks should make decisions to override or to accept a patient's decisions. Another example appears in *rules of distributional authority* that determine who

should make decisions about allocating scarce medical resources.

Authority rules do not delineate substantive standards or criteria for making decisions. However, authority rules and substantive rules interact. For instance, authority rules are justified, in part, by how well particular authorities can be expected to respect and express substantive rules and principles.

Procedural rules. We also defend rules that establish procedures to be followed in certain circumstances. Procedures for determining eligibility for organ transplantation and procedures for reporting grievances to higher authorities are typical examples. We often resort to procedural rules when we run out of substantive rules and when authority rules are incomplete or inconclusive. For example, if substantive or authority rules are inadequate to determine which patients should receive scarce medical resources, we resort to procedural rules such as queuing and lottery.[21] (See pp. 277–78 in Chapter 7.)

Virtues, Emotions, and Other Moral Considerations

This framework of principles and rules does not mention character and virtues, moral ideals, or moral emotions. Yet they are as important as principles and rules for a comprehensive vision of the moral life. These aspects of the moral life receive attention in Chapters 2, 9, and 10.

Conflicting Moral Norms

Norms as Prima Facie Binding

Principles, rules, obligations, and rights are not wooden standards that disallow compromise.

Although "a person of principle" is sometimes regarded as strict and unyielding, we must specify principles so they can function in particular circumstances, and we must often weigh them against other moral norms. It is no objection to moral norms that, in some circumstances, they can be justifiably overridden by other moral norms with which they conflict. All general moral norms are justifiably overridden in some circumstances. For example, we might justifiably not tell the truth to prevent someone from killing another person; and we might justifiably disclose confidential information about a person to protect the rights of another person. Principles, duties, and rights are not absolute merely because they are universal.

W. D. Ross's distinction between *prima facie* and *actual* obligations informs our analysis. A *prima facie* obligation is one that must be fulfilled unless it conflicts, on a particular occasion, with an equal or stronger obligation. This type of obligation is always binding *unless* a competing moral obligation outweighs it in a particular circumstance. Some acts are at once prima facie wrong and prima facie right, because two or more norms conflict in the circumstances. Agents must then determine what they ought to do by finding an actual or overriding (in contrast to prima facie) obligation. That is, they must locate what Ross called "the greatest balance" of right over wrong. Agents can determine their *actual* obligations in such situations by examining the respective weights of the competing prima facie obligations (the relative weights of all competing prima facie norms). What agents ought to do is, in the end, determined by what they ought to do all things considered.[22]

For example, imagine that a psychiatrist has confidential medical information about a patient who also happens to be an employee in the hospital where the psychiatrist practices. The employee is seeking advancement in a stress-filled position, but the psychiatrist has good reason to believe that this advancement would be devastating for both the employee and the hospital. The psychiatrist has several duties in these circumstances, including those of confidentiality, nonmaleficence, beneficence, and respect for autonomy. Should the psychiatrist break confidence in this circumstance to meet these other duties? Could the psychiatrist make "confidential" disclosures to a hospital administrator and not to the personnel office? Addressing such questions through a process of moral deliberation and justification is required to establish an agent's actual duty in the face of conflicting prima facie duties.

No moral theory or professional code of ethics has successfully presented a system of moral rules free of conflicts and exceptions, but this fact should not generate either skepticism or alarm. Ross's distinction between prima facie and actual obligations conforms closely to our experience as moral agents and provides indispensable categories for biomedical ethics. Almost daily we confront situations that force us to choose among conflicting values in our personal lives. Some choices are moral, and many are nonmoral. For example, a person's financial situation might require that he or she choose between buying books and buying a train ticket to see friends. Not having the books will be an inconvenience and a loss, and not visiting home will leave the friends disappointed. Such a choice is not easy, but we are usually able to think through the alternatives, deliberate, and reach a conclusion. The moral life presents similar problems of choice.

Moral Regret and Residual Obligation

An agent who is able to determine which act is the best act to perform under circumstances of a conflict of obligations may still not discharge all aspects of moral obligation by performing the selected act. Even the morally best action under many circumstances of conflict is regrettable and will leave a moral residue, which is also referred to as a "moral trace."[23] Regret and residue can arise even if the right choice of action is clear and uncontested.

This point is about *continuing obligation*, not merely about *feelings* of regret and residue. Moral residue results because an overridden prima facie obligation does not simply go away when overridden. Often persons have residual obligations because the obligations they were unable to discharge create new obligations. As Ross puts it in the case of breaking a promise, we feel not only "compunction" (here meaning deep regret and a sting of conscience) but realize that "it is our duty to make up somehow to the promisee for the breaking of the promise."[24] We both feel regret and recognize continuing obligation. Although we cannot keep an obligation that we failed to perform, we can make up for it in a variety of ways, depending on the circumstance. For example, we may be able to notify persons in advance that we will not be able to keep a promise; we may be able to apologize in a manner that heals a relationship; we may be able to create a change of circumstance so that the conflict does not occur again; or we may be able to provide adequate compensation.

Regret and a sense of moral residue may exist whether or not residual obligations can be discharged. They are the natural result of the fact that an overruled prima facie obligation does not mean that the obligation winds up counting for nothing.

Specifying Principles and Rules

The four clusters of principles we present in this book do not constitute a general ethical theory and provide only a framework of norms with which we can start in biomedical ethics. Our framework is spare, because prima facie principles do not contain sufficient content to address the nuances of moral problems. However, the principles can be specified to provide more specific guidance. The reason why directives in particular moralities often differ is that abstract starting points in the common morality can be coherently specified in more than one way to create practical guidelines and procedures.

Specification is a process of reducing the indeterminate character of abstract norms and generating more specific, action-guiding content.[25] For example, without further specification, "do no harm" is too bare a starting point for thinking through problems such as whether it is permissible to hasten the death of a terminally ill patient. Specification is not a process of producing or defending general norms such as those in the common morality; it assumes that they are available. Specifying the norms with which one starts (whether those in the common morality or norms previously specified to some extent) is accomplished by narrowing the scope of the norms, not by explaining what the general norms mean. The scope is narrowed, as Henry Richardson puts it, by "spelling out where, when, why, how, by what means, to whom, or by whom the action is to be done or avoided."[26] For example, the norm that we are obligated to "respect the autonomy of persons" cannot, unless specified, handle complicated problems of what to disclose or demand in clinical medicine and research involving human subjects. A definition of "respect for autonomy" (as, say, "allowing competent persons to exercise their liberty rights") might clarify one's meaning in using the norm, but would not narrow the general norm or render it more specific.

Specification, then, does not merely analyze meaning; it adds content. For example, as noted previously, one possible specification of "respect the autonomy of persons" is "respect the autonomy of competent patients by following their advance directives when they become incompetent." This specification will work well in some medical contexts, but it will confront limits in others, necessitating additional specification. Progressive specification can continue indefinitely, but to qualify all along the way as a specification some transparent connection must be maintained to the initial general norm that gives moral authority to the resulting string of specifications.

An example of specification arises when psychiatrists conduct forensic evaluations of patients in a legal context. Psychiatrists cannot always obtain an informed consent and risk violating their obligations to respect autonomy. However, obtaining informed consent is a vital rule of medical ethics. A specification aimed at handling this problem is "Respect the autonomy of persons who are the subjects of forensic evaluations, where consent is not legally required, by disclosing to the evaluee the nature and purpose of the evaluation." We do not claim that this formulation is the best specification, but it is roughly the provision recommended in the "Ethical Guidelines for the Practice of Forensic Psychiatry" of the American Academy of Psychiatry and the Law.[27] This specification attempts to guide forensic psychiatrists in discharging their diverse moral obligations.

A more extended example of specification involves the oft-cited rule "Doctors should put their patients' interests first." In some countries patients can receive the best treatment strategy only if their physicians falsify information on insurance forms or at least thinly spread the truth; yet the rule of patient priority does not imply that a physician should act illegally by lying or distorting the description of a patient's problem on an insurance form. Rules against deception, on the one hand, and for patient priority, on the other, are not categorical demands. When they conflict, they need specification.

A survey of practicing physicians' attitudes toward deception illustrates how some physicians reconcile their dual commitment to patients and to nondeception. Dennis H. Novack and several colleagues used a questionnaire to obtain physicians' responses to four difficult ethical problems that potentially could be resolved by deception. In one scenario, a physician recommends an annual screening mammography for a fifty-two-year-old woman who protests that last year her insurance company would not cover the test and that she had to pay herself, although she could not afford it. A secretary suggests that the patient's insurance company would cover the costs of the mammography if the physician stated the reason as "rule out cancer" rather than "screening mammography," although the latter alone was the true reason. Almost 70% of the physicians responding to this survey indicated that they would state that they were attempting to "rule out cancer," and 85% of this group (85% of the 70%) insisted that their act would not involve "deception."[28]

We can interpret these physicians' decisions as crude attempts to specify the rule that "Doctors should put their patients' interests first." Some doctors seem to think that it should be specified as follows: "Doctors should put their patients' interests first by withholding information from or misleading someone who has no *right* to that information, including an insurance company with unjust policies of coverage, who thereby forfeits his or her right to accurate information." In addition, most physicians in the study apparently did not operate with the definition of deception favored by the researchers, which is "to deceive is to make another believe what is not true, to mislead." Some physicians apparently believed that "deception" occurs when one person *unjustifiably* misleads another, and that it was *justifiable* to mislead the insurance company in these circumstances. It appears that these physicians would not agree on how to specify rules against deception or rules assigning priority to patients' interests.

All moral rules are, in principle, subject to specification. They all will need some additional content, because, as Richardson puts it, "the complexity of the moral phenomena always outruns our ability to capture them in general norms."[29] Many already specified rules will need further specification to handle new circumstances of conflict. Progressive specification often must occur to handle the variety of problems that arise, gradually reducing the conflicts that abstract principles themselves cannot resolve.

These conclusions are connected to our earlier discussion of *particular moralities*. Different persons and groups will offer conflicting specifications, potentially creating multiple particular moralities. In any problematic case, competing specifications are likely to be offered by reasonable and fair-minded parties, all of whom are committed to the common morality. Nothing in the model of specification suggests that we can avoid all circumstances of conflicting judgments.

To say that a problem or conflict is resolved or dissolved by specification is to say that norms have been made sufficiently determinate in content that, when cases fall under them, we know what ought to be done. Obviously some *proposed* specifications will not provide the most adequate or justified resolution. When competing specifications emerge, we should seek to discover which is superior. Proposed specifications should be based on deliberative processes of reasoning. The specification best supported by argument would seem the one that ought to prevail. In Chapter 10, we argue that we also need to link specification to a method of justification that allows for a reflective testing of our moral principles and other relevant moral beliefs to make them as coherent as possible. The goal is to adjust specifications, as needed, to render them coherent with the premises of other justified moral commitments. If proposed specifications are shown to have incoherent results, we must continue to readjust the guides further. (See Chapter 10, pp. 381–87.) In this way, we connect specification as a method with a model of justification that will support some specifications and not others.

Finally, some specified norms are virtually absolute and need no further specification. Examples include prohibitions of cruelty that involve the unnecessary infliction of pain and suffering.[30] More interesting are norms that are intentionally formulated with the goal of including all legitimate exceptions. An example is. "Always obtain oral or written informed consent for medical interventions with competent patients, *except* in emergencies, in forensic examinations, in low-risk situations, or when patients have waived their right to adequate information." This norm needs further interpretation, including an analysis of what constitutes an informed consent, an emergency, a waiver, a forensic examination, and a low risk. However, this rule would be absolute if it were correct that all legitimate exceptions had successfully been incorporated in its formulation.

If such rules exist, they are rare. In light of the range of possibilities for contingent conflicts among rules, even the firmest rules are likely to encounter exceptive cases. If professional medical associations, health care institutions, religious groups, and government bureaus had more often taken this lesson to heart, we would have been spared many stubbornly imperious pronouncements in biomedical ethics.

Weighing and Balancing

The process of weighing and balancing. Principles, rules, professional obligations, and rights often need to be balanced. Is balancing different from specification? Each conception seems to address a separate dimension of moral norms. Balancing is the process of finding reasons to support beliefs about which moral norms should prevail. Balancing is concerned with the relative weights and strengths of different moral norms, whereas specification is concerned primarily with their scope (i.e., range). Accordingly, balancing consists of deliberation and judgment about the relative weights or strengths of norms. At first glance, balancing seems best suited for reaching judgments in particular cases, whereas specification seems especially useful for developing more specific policies from already accepted general norms. But are the two conceptions really different?

The metaphor of larger and smaller weights moving a scale up and down has often been invoked to depict the balancing process, but this metaphor may obscure what happens in balancing. Justified acts of balancing can be supported by good reasons. They need not rest merely on intuition or feeling (although intuitive balancing is one form of balancing). Suppose a physician encounters an emergency case that would require her to extend an already long day, making her unable to keep a promise to take her son to the local library. She then engages in a process of deliberation that leads her to consider how urgently her son needs to get to the library, whether they could go later to the library, whether another physician could handle the emergency case, and so on. If she determines to stay deep into the night with the patient, this obligation will have become overriding because, let us assume, she has found a good and sufficient reason for her action. The reason might be that a life hangs in the balance and she alone may have the knowledge to deal adequately with the circumstances. Canceling her evening with her son, distressing as it may be, could be justified by the significance of her reason for doing what she does.

One way of viewing the process of balancing merges it with specification. David DeGrazia and Henry Richardson have argued that the reasons offered in balancing are simply specifications that incorporate those reasons. In our example, the physician's reasons can be generalized for similar cases: "If a patient's life hangs in the balance and the attending physician alone has the knowledge to deal adequately with the full array of the circumstances, then the physician's conflicting domestic obligations must yield." Even if we do not always state the way we balance considerations in the form of a specification, might not all deliberative judgments conform to this model? If so, then deliberative balancing *is* deliberative specification.

The goal of merging specification and balancing is appealing, but it is too streamlined to handle all situations of balancing. Specification requires that a moral agent extend norms by both narrowing their scope and generalizing to relevantly similar circumstances. Thus, "respect the autonomy of competent patients when they become incompetent by following their advance directives" is a rule suited for all incompetent patients with advance directives. However, it often seems that the responses of caring moral agents, such as physicians and nurses, are specific to the needs of *this* patient or *this* family in *this* circumstance. Numerous considerations must be weighed and balanced and any generalizations that could be formed might not hold even in related cases. For example, cases in which risk of harm and burden are involved for a patient are often circumstances unlikely to be decided by expressing *by rule* how much risk is allowable or how heavy the burden can be to secure a certain stated benefit. After levels of risk and burden are determined, these considerations must be balanced with the likelihood of the success of a procedure (in this specific case), the uncertainties involved, whether an adequately informed consent can be obtained, whether the family has a role to play, and the like. In this way, balancing allows for a due consideration of all norms bearing on a complex, very particular circumstance.

Consider the following discussion with a young woman who has just been told that she is HIV-infected, as recorded by physician Timothy Quill and nurse Penelope Townsend:[31]

PATIENT: Please don't tell me that. Oh my God. Oh my children. Oh Lord have mercy. Oh God, why did He do this to me? ...
DR. QUILL: First thing we have to do is learn as much as we can about it, because right now you are okay.
PATIENT: I don't even have a future. Everything I know is that you gonna die anytime. What is there to do? What if I'm a walking time bomb? People will be scared to even touch me or say anything to me.
DR. QUILL: No, that's not so.
PATIENT: Yes they will, 'cause I feel that way ...
DR. QUILL: There is a future for you ...
PATIENT: Okay, alright. I'm so scared. 1 don't want to die. I don't want to die, Dr.

Quill, not yet. I know I got to die, but I don't want to die.

DR. QUILL: We've got to think about a couple of things.

Quill and Townsend work to calm down and reassure this patient, while engaging sympathetically with the patient's feelings and conveying the presence of knowledgeable medical authorities. Their emotional investment in the patient's feelings is joined with a detached evaluation of the patient. Too much compassion and emotional investment may doom the task at hand; too much detachment will be cold and may destroy the patient's trust. A balance in the sense of a right mixture between engagement and detachment must be found. Quill and Townsend could try to *generalize* from norms of respect and beneficence to a specification regarding how caring physicians and nurses should respond to patients who are desperately upset. However, any such generalization will ring hollow and will not be subtle enough to provide practical guidance for this patient, and certainly not for all desperately upset patients. Each encounter calls for a response not adequately captured by general rules and their specifications. Behavior that in the context of one desperate patient is a caring response will intrude on privacy or irritate the next desperate patient. A physician may, for example, find it appropriate to touch or caress a patient in a circumstance in which such behavior would be entirely inappropriate for another patient. How physicians and nurses balance different moral considerations often involves sympathetic insight, humane responsiveness, and the practical wisdom of evaluating a particular patient's circumstance and needs.[32] Balancing is more complex than the simple case of balancing two principles that are in conflict. Considerations of trust, compassion, objective assessment, caring responsiveness, reassurance, and the like must be balanced. For example, to act compassionately may be to undercut objective assessment. Not all of the norms at work

can reasonably be said to be specifications, nor is there a final specification.

In many clinical contexts it may be impossibly complicated to engage in specification. For example, in cases of balancing harms of treatment against the benefits of treatment for incompetent patients, the cases are often so exceptional that it is perilous to generalize a conclusion that would reach out to other cases. These problems are sometimes complicated by disagreements among family members about what constitutes a benefit, poor decisions and indecision by a marginally competent patient, limitations of time and resources, and the like.

We do not suggest that balancing is a matter of on-the-fly, unreflective intuition without reasons. Instead, we propose a model of moral judgment that focuses on how balancing and judgment occur through practical astuteness, discriminating intelligence, and sympathetic responsiveness that are not reducible to the specification of norms. The capacity to balance many moral considerations is connected to what we discuss in Chapter 2 as capacities of moral character. Capacities such as compassion, attentiveness, discernment, caring, and kindness are integral to the way wise moral agents balance diverse, sometimes competing, moral considerations. These capacities tutor us in "what to notice, how to care, what to be sensitive to, how to get beyond one's own biases and narrowness of vision," and the like.[33]

Practicability supplies another reason why the model of specification needs supplementation by the model of balancing. Progressive specification would eventually mushroom into a body of norms so bulky that the normative system would become unwieldy. A scheme of comprehensive specification would constitute a package of potentially hundreds, thousands, or millions of rules, each suited to a narrow range of conduct. In the ideal of specification, every type of action in a circumstance of the contingent conflict of norms would be covered by a rule, but the formulation of rules for every circumstance of contingent conflict would be a body of rules so cumbersome as to become ineffective. The larger the number of rules and the more complex each rule, the less likely it becomes that the system will be achievable, and practicable were it achievable. Moreover, every rule is subject at any time to challenge if a contingent conflict arises or in the face of a newly detected problem of lack of coherence in the rules.

Conditions that constrain balancing. To allay concerns that the model of balancing is too intuitive or too open-ended and lacking in a commitment to firm principles and rigorous reasoning, we here list six conditions that should help reduce intuition, partiality, and arbitrariness. These conditions must be met to justify infringing one prima facie norm to adhere to another. (To the extent these conditions incorporate norms, the norms are prima facie, not absolute.)

1. Good reasons can be offered to act on the overriding norm rather than on the infringed norm.
2. The moral objective justifying the infringement has a realistic prospect of achievement.
3. No morally preferable alternative actions are available.[34]
4. The lowest level of infringement, commensurate with achieving the primary goal of the action, has been selected.
5. Any negative effects of the infringement have been minimized.
6. All affected parties have been treated impartially.

Although some of these conditions are obvious and noncontroversial, some are often not observed in moral deliberation and would lead to different conclusions were they observed. For example, some proposals to use life-extending technologies, despite the objections of patients or their surrogates, violate condition 2 by endorsing actions in which no realistic prospect exists of achieving the goals of a proposed

intervention. Typically, this occurs when health professionals regard the intervention as legally required, but in some cases the standard invoked is merely a traditional or prevailing one.

More commonly violated is condition 3. Actions are frequently performed without serious consideration of alternative actions that might be performed. As a result, agents fail to identify a morally preferable alternative. For example, in animal care and use committees a common conflict involves the obligation to approve a good scientific protocol and the obligation to protect animals against unnecessary suffering. A protocol is often approved if it proposes a *standard* form of anesthesia. However, standard forms of anesthesia are not always the best way to protect the animal, and further inquiry would be required to determine the best anesthetic for the particular interventions proposed. In our schema of conditions, it is unjustifiable to approve the protocol or to conduct the experiment without this additional inquiry, which affects conditions 4 and 5 as well as 3.

Finally, consider this example: The principle of respect for autonomy and the principle of beneficence (which requires acts intended to prevent harm to others) sometimes conflict in responding to the HIV/AIDS epidemic. Respect for autonomy sets a prima facie barrier to invasions of privacy and the mandatory testing of people at risk of HIV infection, yet their actions may put others at risk under conditions in which society has a prima facie obligation to act to prevent harm to those at risk. To justify overriding respect for autonomy, one must show that mandatory testing that invades the privacy of certain individuals is necessary to prevent harm to others and has a reasonable prospect of preventing such harm. If it meets these conditions, mandatory testing still must pass the least-infringement test (condition 4), and health workers must seek to reduce negative effects, such as the consequences that individuals fear from testing (condition 5). As we will see in Chapter 8, many proposed forms of mandatory testing and invasions of privacy are not justified because other available alternatives would have a higher probability of success without infringing rights of autonomy.[35]

Accordingly, the preceding six conditions are morally demanding, at least in some circumstances. When conjoined with requirements of coherence that we propose in Chapter 10, these conditions should help us achieve a reasonable measure of protection against purely intuitive, subjective, or partial balancing judgments. We could try to introduce further criteria or safeguards, such as "rights override nonrights" and "liberty principles override nonliberty principles," but these rules are certain to fail in circumstances in which rights claims and liberty interests are relatively minor. Honesty about the process of balancing, as well as the process of specification, compels us to return to our earlier discussion of moral dilemmas and perplexity and to acknowledge that in some circumstances we will not be able to determine which moral norm to follow.

Moral Diversity and Moral Disagreement

Conscientious and reasonable moral agents understandably disagree over moral priorities in circumstances of a contingent conflict of norms. Morally conscientious persons may disagree, for example, about whether disclosure of a life-threatening condition to a fragile patient is appropriate, whether religious values about brain death have a place in secular biomedical ethics, whether teenagers should be permitted to refuse life-sustaining treatments, and hundreds of other issues in biomedical ethics. Such disagreement does not indicate moral ignorance or moral defect. We simply lack a single, entirely reliable way to resolve many disagreements, despite methods of specifying and balancing.

Neither morality nor ethical theory has the resources to provide a single solution to every moral problem. Moral disagreement can emerge because of (1) factual disagreements (e.g., about the level of suffering that an action will cause), (2) disagreement resulting from insufficient information or evidence, (3) disagreements about which norms are applicable or relevant in the circumstances, (4) disagreement about the relative weights or rankings of the relevant norms, (5) disagreements about appropriate forms of specification or balancing, (6) the presence of a genuine moral dilemma, and (7) scope disagreements about who should be protected by a moral norm (e.g., whether embryos, fetuses, and sentient animals are protected; see Chapter 3); or (8) conceptual disagreements about a crucial moral notion (such as whether removal of nutrition and hydration at a family's request constitutes *killing*).

Different parties may emphasize different principles or assign different weights to principles even when they agree on which principles are relevant. Such disagreement may persist even among morally committed persons who conform to all the demands that morality makes on them. If evidence is incomplete and different sets of evidence are available to different parties, one individual or group may be justified in reaching a conclusion that another individual or group is justified in rejecting. Even when both parties have incorrect beliefs, each party may be justified in holding its beliefs. We cannot hold persons to a higher practical standard than to make judgments conscientiously in light of the relevant norms and relevant evidence. (See our account of justification in Chapter 10, where we argue that we cannot know whether a moral disagreement is irresolvable until we have examined competing views using an appropriate method of justification.)

Disagreement in the moral life may discourage persons who deal with practical problems, but the phenomenon of moral disagreement provides no basis for skepticism about morality or about moral thinking. It offers a reason for taking morality seriously and using the best tools we have to carry our moral projects as far as we can. We frequently do obtain near-complete agreement in our moral judgments, and we always have available the thin set of four clusters of universal principles mentioned earlier in this chapter.

When moral disagreements arise, a moral agent can—and often should—defend his or her decision without disparaging or reproaching others who reach different decisions. Recognition of *legitimate* diversity (by contrast to moral violations that warrant criticism and perhaps even punishment) is vital when we evaluate the actions of others. One person's conscientious assessment of his or her obligations may differ from another's, even when they confront the same moral problem. Both evaluations may be solidly grounded in the common morality. Similarly, what one institution or government determines it should do may differ from what another institution or government determines it should do. In such cases, we can assess one

position as morally preferable to another only if we can show that the position rests on a more coherent specification or interpretation of the common morality.[36]

Conclusion

In this chapter we have explained and initiated a defense of what is sometimes called the *four-principles approach* to biomedical ethics,[37] now increasingly called *principlism*.[38] The four clusters of principles derive from considered judgments in the common morality and professional traditions in health care, particularly medicine and nursing, although we have been critical of certain aspects of medical codes and traditional medical ethics. Our goal in later chapters is to develop, specify, and balance these principles.

6. Principlism and Morality

Principlism can be defined as an analytical framework of general norms of common morality, which, at the same time, provides specific rules of particular moralities with a scope of common morality. I other words, it is a general framework of prima facie norms which are not specific. These norms—principles of Respect for Autonomy, Nonmaleficence, Beneficence and Justice are self-evident from facts and point out moral values that are morally equivalent in theory. Thus, those principles are not absolute. As moral problems are rich in diversity and specificity as well as have several nuances, principles must be specified to provide more concrete guidance in moral deliberation. Those specifications are able to create practical guidelines and procedures.

What is Specification?

Specification is the process of reducing the indeterminate character of abstract norms and generating more specific action-guide content. For example, if we take the principle of nonmaleficence, which orders "do not harm," we can see that mandate is too broad and does not implicitly content the meaning of harm. In this case, the principle of nonmaleficence is not enough by itself to determine whether or not a physician should withhold a treatment in a terminally ill patient. Certainly, we need to narrow the scope of that norm (do no harm), not necessarily to explain what it means. Therefore, we could specify the norm "do no harm" into the more specific norm "do not cause unnecessary pain." The process of specification can continue, but at least we have defined with more certainty what harm can mean given some circumstances. In this case, we can define "harm" as "unnecessary pain." Thereby, we have narrowed the scope of a general principle and, at the same time, we have added content to it.

The specification of any principle does not only imply to analyze its meaning but very especially add content to it. Thus, to specify a principle we need to define conditions, contexts, means, ends and consequences in order to make its application flexible and more workable in practical terms. This means that principles are not categorical or unconditional demands. There are conditions for their application; some of their conditions are consequences and empirical facts.

Problems of Specification

Different persons and groups offer conflicting specifications, potentially creating multiple particular moralities. Also, some specifications do not provide the most adequate or justified resolution. This means that when competing specifications emerge we should seek to discover which one is superior and more morally plausible, objective and impartial. Therefore, proposed specifications should be based on deliberative processes of reasoning.

Some specified norms are virtually absolute and need no further specification, for instance, prohibitions of cruelty that imply the unnecessary infliction of pain and suffering. However, there are other circumstances in which we need to balance not only principles and rules but also obligations and rights, especially when different moral conceptions address a singular/separate dimension of moral norms.

Balancing

Balancing is the process of finding reasons to support beliefs about which moral norms should prevail. In this way, as specification is concerned with moral norms' scopes, balancing addresses the relative weights and strengths of different moral principles.

As balancing may be intuitive, partial or arbitrary, Beauchamp and Childress provide some criteria for reducing intuition, partiality and arbitrariness in balancing:

1. Good reasons can be offered to act on the overriding norm rather than on the infringed norm.
2. The moral objective justifying the infringement has a realistic prospect of achievement.
3. No morally preferable alternative actions are available.

4. The lowest level of infringement, commensurate with achieving the primary goal of the action, has been selected.
5. Any negative effects of the infringement have been minimized.
6. All affected parties have been treated impartially.

However, morally conscientious persons may disagree about several matters. For example, whether or not disclosure of a life-threatening condition to a fragile patient is appropriate, or whether religious values about brain death have a place in secular bioethics. We call this situation "moral disagreement."

Moral Diversity and Moral Disagreement

Moral disagreement can emerge due to multiple situations:

1. Factual disagreement (the level of suffering that an action can cause).
2. Disagreement resulting from a lack of information or evidence.
3. Disagreement about norms and their applicability.
4. Disagreement about relative rankings of norms.
5. Disagreement about specifications or balancing.
6. The presence of a genuine moral dilemma.
7. Disagreement about who should be protected by moral norm (fetuses, embryos, sentient animals)
8. Conceptual disagreement about a crucial moral notion (whether removal of nutrition or hydration constitutes *killing*).

Despite the above mentioned, the phenomenon of moral disagreement provides no basis for skepticism about morality or moral thinking.

Instead, it offers a reason for taking morality seriously and using the best tools to make the best decision possible. At the same time, it promotes the recognition of moral diversity as *legitimate* diversity and urges us to raise impartial, objective and relevant arguments to address and resolve moral conflicts and dilemmas.

Principlism

Every principle identified and described by Beauchamp and Childress has a procedural dimension represented by rules. Thus, Respect for Autonomy (a principle of self-determination) implies rules such as respect and support autonomous decisions, among others. Nonmaleficence (Do not cause harm), orders in more procedural terms, do not kill others. Beneficence (Do good) points out some rules such as prevent harm or provide benefits to others. Justice (all people are intrinsically equal, no discrimination) implies the rule of distributing benefits, risks and costs fairly.

Among the rules that each principle points out, Beauchamp and Childress distinguish three main types: Substantive Rules, Authority Rules, and Procedural Rules:

- Substantive Rules: Truth telling, confidentiality, privacy, forgoing treatment, Informed Consent, Rationing Health Care.
- Authority Rules: Surrogate authority (incompetent persons), professional authority (make decisions to accept or override a patient's decision), distributional authority (who should decide how to allocate scarce medical resources).
- Procedural Rules: It implies specific procedures to be followed in certain circumstances in which both substantive and authority rules do not work properly. Some kinds of procedural rules are those used to distribute benefits or allocate organs: lottery, need, medical condition, queuing, etc.

Therefore, principlism implies norms of common morality (general principles) as well as norms of particular moralities (specific rules and procedures).

Beauchamp and Childress use the term "principles" in a wide sense, by including most of moral norms. However, they sometimes narrow the scope of principles, that is, they refer to broad and general norms as a source of more concrete rules. I fact, the literal meaning of "principle" is *source* or *origin*, and this meaning was also adopted by Beauchamp and Childress. In other words, when we use principles to carry out moral deliberation, we are starting the process of reasoning in order to address moral conflicts and quandaries. Principles represent the beginning of any deliberation process.

Readings

Gert, Bernard; Culver, Charles M.; Clouser, K. Danner, "Principlism," in *Bioethics: A Return to Fundamentals*, Oxford University Press, 1997: **71–92**.

Callahan, Daniel, "Individual Good and Common Good: A Communitarian Approach to Bioethics," in *The Roots of Bioethics: Health, Progress, Technology, Death*, Oxford University Press, 2012: **50–61**.

Study Questions

1. What is specification and why is important in bioethics?
2. What is balancing?
3. Explain the procedural relationships between principles and rules in bioethics.
4. Identify and explain the main elements of moral disagreement?

Principlism

Bernard Gert, Charles M. Culver, and K. Danner Clouser

Having presented our own account of morality, from the foundations to the practical rules and ideals that guide actions, we devote this chapter to highlighting its distinctive differences. In order for our account of morality to be clearly and accurately perceived, we contrast it with the dominant "theory" that has pervaded biomedical ethics for almost two decades. We want to minimize the chances that aspects of this dominant theory might unwittingly and automatically be read into our own account, so we highlight the significant differences between the two accounts. Inasmuch as part of the rationale for this book is to show the relevance of theory to practice, it is appropriate to bring the matter into sharper focus by examining in detail the dominant theory in use. Readers who have neither interest in nor commitment to another theory of ethics can, without significant loss of understanding, skip this chapter.

In arguing that our theory is more adequate and more useful we follow the time-honored tradition of theory replacement. We point out how our theory (1) overcomes the inadequacies of the dominant theory, (2) accounts for what is good in the dominant theory, and (3) is more readily usable, understandable, and intuitively correct than the dominant theory. Thus, in this chapter, we focus particularly on the inadequacies of the theory in question, and show how the good aspects of it are better accounted for by our theory.

The dominant view in question we have labeled "principlism."[1] It is characterized by its citing of four principles which constitute the core of its account of biomedical ethics: beneficence, autonomy, nonmaleficence, and justice. So entrenched is this "theory," that clinical moral problems are often grouped (for conferences, papers, and books) according to which principle is deemed most relevant and necessary for solving them. It has become fashionable and customary to cite one or another of these principles as the key for resolving a particular biomedical ethical problem. Throughout much of the biomedical ethical literature, authors seem to believe that they have brought theory to bear on the problem before them insofar as they have mentioned one or more of the principles. Thus, not only do the principles presumably lead to acceptable solutions, but they are also treated by many as the ultimate grounds of appeal.

We examine principlism by looking at the undeniably leading account of principlism, namely that of Beauchamp and Childress, as manifested in the editions of their book, *Principles of Biomedical Ethics.*[2] Their account is the very best the position has to offer, and it is their account which has so pervaded the world of biomedical ethics. For many years it has provided the conceptual framework of the Georgetown Intensive Bioethics Course, a one-week summer course which has been attended by thousands from the United States as well as from around the world. Beauchamp and Childress's book is outstanding for its insights into particular problems in bioethics and for its sensitivity to important issues and relevant subtleties. Our criticism focuses only on their theoretical account of morality.

As we emphasized in previous articles on principlism, we are not criticizing Beauchamp and Childress as such. We select them as the very best spokesmen for the principle-based approach to bioethics, but we are concerned about the widespread popularization of principlism throughout the biomedical ethics world, where it is not dealt with as carefully as it is in the hands of Beauchamp and Childress. This concern is more important than ever to emphasize, because principlism is still flourishing, even though Beauchamp and Childress have changed their theoretical account considerably. Their fourth edition (1994) has accommodated so well to the criticisms of principlism that Ezekiel Emanuel entitled his review of the book "The Beginning of the End of Principlism."[3] This turn of events helps to reinforce our claim that it is not particularly Beauchamp and Childress that we are criticizing, but a paradigmatic form of principlism, which has been and still is thriving throughout the bioethical world. We do continue occasionally to cite early editions of *Principles of Biomedical Ethics*, but only because those editions are the ones that have been so influential in shaping the paradigmatic form of principlism which persists in the bioethical world at large. Meanwhile, we remind the readers that the fourth edition is very different, and according to Ezekiel Emanuel may no longer even be principlism. In this edition Beauchamp and Childress appeal, as we ourselves have long done, to a basis in common morality, the claims concerning which, Emanuel says,

"constitute a radical change and herald the end of 'principlism.'"[4]

To understand the historical background of principlism's pervasive influence, it is helpful to review the "Belmont Report," which seems to be the progenitor of the principles.

The Principles in Historical Context

The principles emerged from the work of the National Commission for the Protection of Human Subjects of Biomedical and Behavioral Research, which was created by Congress in 1974. One of the charges to the commission was to identify the basic ethical principles that should underlie the conduct of biomedical and behavioral research involving human subjects, and to develop guidelines which should be followed to ensure that such research is conducted in accordance with those principles.[5]

At that time there was frustration over the many and various rules for research that were spelled out in the extant codes covering research using human subjects. These codes included the Nuremberg Code of 1947, the Helsinki Declaration of 1964 (revised in 1975), and the 1971 Guidelines issued by the (then) United States Department of Health, Education, and Welfare. (The "Guidelines" were codified into U.S. federal regulations in 1974.) The assortment of rules seemed at times inadequate, conflicting, and difficult to apply. It therefore became part of the commission's charge to formulate "broader ethical principles [to] provide a basis on which specific rules may be formulated, criticized and interpreted."[6]

The higher level of generality was achieved by the commission and articulated as three ethical principles: the principle of respect for persons, the principle of beneficence, and the principle of justice. These principles comprised the "Belmont Report," so-named because their articulation was the culmination of intense discussions that took place at the Smithsonian Institution's Belmont Conference Center. In effect, these principles sought to frame in a more general and useful way the moral concerns that underlay the diverse, ambiguous, and (sometimes) conflicting rules comprising the various ethical codes related to research on human subjects.

The work of the commission was significant. It was insightful and helpful; it elegantly captured in a more general way the basic moral concerns haltingly expressed in the miscellaneous codes. The commission also went on to delineate some of the more practical consequences of the principles. From the principle of respect for persons came attention to autonomy (which from their discussion seems more like what is now regarded as "competence") and to informed consent. From the principle of beneficence came the obligation to maximize benefits over risks and not to harm. From the principle of justice came attention to fairness in the distribution of the benefits and burdens of research.

These principles were clearly intended to be generalized guides for protecting humans as subjects in biomedical and behavioral research. Also, they seem less to have been derived from a theory of any sort and more to have been abstractions from ethical rules expressing particular moral concerns. In a summary fashion the principles generalize and encapsulate a variety of moral considerations especially applicable to research using human subjects. Very likely these formulations additionally accomplished a crucial maneuver for the commission. They made possible a consensus in a setting where a more detailed account of morality would probably never have been agreed upon.

From these beginnings the application of the principles has grown and now encompasses biomedical ethics in general. Each principle has changed somewhat as its meaning is elaborated, as subdivision takes place, and as another principle or two is added (varying with each author). For example, for Beauchamp and Childress, the principle of beneficence spawns the principle of

nonmaleficence. Nevertheless, in one form or another, these principles have come to dominate the field of bioethics, which is why we are investigating several of them in detail.

Our overall impression of the principles is that they express something very important, something very basic to common moral intuitions. However, for reasons to be seen, they are inadequate and misleading. Our plan is to show how our more comprehensive theoretical framework can encompass and preserve what is good about the principles, while eliminating their unfortunate features. We see them as historically providing a conceptual ladder that allowed the field to achieve certain insights and goals. But having enabled that achievement, the ladder is best set aside because it has become cumbersome and possibly dangerous.

Critique of Principlism: Our General Approach

Although we have been referring to principlism as a theory, it is not in fact a theory, but rather a collection of "principles," which together are popularly but mistakenly thought to function as a theory in guiding action. Principlism puts forward certain principles which it considers to be the high-level "action guides" most relevant for dealing with issues of biomedical ethics. A variety of principles are claimed by different authors to be "the principles of biomedical ethics," but the best known and most frequently cited principles are those labeled "the principle of autonomy," "the principle of nonmaleficence," "the principle of beneficence," and "the principle of justice." Because these four occur by far most frequently together (and thus are more apt to pose as a theory of biomedical ethics), and because these are the ones espoused by the prime expositors of principlism (Beauchamp and Childress), they are the ones we analyze in order to contrast and compare them with our own theory.

In this chapter we show that principlism is mistaken about the nature of morality and is misleading about the foundations of ethics. We argue that its "principles" are really misnomers, since, when examined carefully, they are not action guides at all. Traditionally, principles really are action guides that summarize and encapsulate a whole theory and thus, in a shorthand manner, assist a moral agent in making a moral decision. Those kinds of principles are to be clearly distinguished from those of principlism. We argue that the principles of principlism primarily function as checklists, naming issues worth remembering when one is considering a biomedical moral issue. "Consider this ... consider that ... remember to look for ..." is what they tell the agent; they do not embody an articulated, established, and unified moral system capable of providing useful guidance.

These principles presumably follow from several different moral theories, though that connection is neither explicitly focused on nor clearly stated by the proponents of principlism. This is a matter of significant concern since there seem to be no underlying connections among the principles. They do not grow out of a common foundation and they have no systematic relationship among themselves. Though each may be an expression of one or another important and traditional concern of morality, there is no priority ranking among them nor even any specified procedure for resolving the conflicts that inevitably arise between principles. This serves to perpetuate what we have called the "anthology syndrome." This, as described in Chapter 1, is a kind of relativism espoused (perhaps unwittingly) by many books (usually anthologies) of bioethics. They parade before the reader a variety of "theories" of ethics (Kantianism, deontology, utilitarianism, other forms of consequentialism) and say, in effect, choose the theory, maxim, principle, or rule that best suits you or the situation. Similarly, though each of the principles of principlism embodies a key concern from one or another theory of morality, no account is given of whether (or how) they are related to each other. We conclude that principlism obscures and confuses moral reasoning by its failure to provide genuine action guides and by its eclectic and unsystematic account of morality.

We begin our analysis with a brief discussion of the principles of nonmaleficence and justice in order to set the context for our argument. Then we discuss in more detail the principles of autonomy and beneficence in order to demonstrate the force of our arguments against principlism. These latter two were chosen not only because they are the principles most often employed in discussion of biomedical ethics, but also because they best illustrate the most problematic aspects of principlism. In particular, we show that principlism manifests the inadequacies of most previous accounts of morality by failing to appreciate the significance of the distinction between moral rules and moral ideals, by misrepresenting the ordinary concept of duty, and by failing to realize that morality is a public system that applies to everyone.

The Principle of Nonmaleficence

This is the one principle for which we have a strong affinity because, as Chapter 2 makes clear, the key insight expressed by the principle of nonmaleficence is also a major orientation of our account of morality. It is the only one of the four principles that does not blur the distinction between moral rules and moral ideals. Indeed, this principle is most reasonably interpreted as merely summarizing some of the moral rules. The moral rules "Don't kill," "Don't cause pain," and "Don't disable" are clearly included in this principle, and probably the rule "Don't deprive of pleasure" is as well. Even the rule "Don't deprive of freedom" can be included in the principle of nonmaleficence, but principlism seems to prefer to include it under the principle of autonomy. However, we see no reason for distinguishing "Do not deprive of freedom" from the other four rules, for all five of these rules proscribe causing what are universally recognized as evils (or harms)—death, pain, disability, loss of freedom, and loss of pleasure.

The principle of nonmaleficence does no more than simply collapse four or five moral rules into one more general rule, "Do not cause harm." That general rule, in the form "Primum non nocere," is often taken as the first principle of medicine. It is primarily a matter of purpose and style whether one prefers to list five distinct moral rules or to have one general principle that includes them all. We prefer the former because it makes more salient the fact that there are different kinds of harms (or evils) and that rational persons can and do rank them differently. (Neglecting the fact that there are different rational rankings is one of the primary causes of unjustified paternalism—see Chapter 10.) Thus, insofar as specifying the different harms that one must avoid causing must be explicitly and carefully done sooner or later, the gain in simplicity of having just one general principle is minimal and transitory at best. Nonetheless, this principle, even as it stands, has no major problems. That fact is not surprising, since it is the only one of the principles that is not an invention of philosophers, but is a longstanding principle of medicine.

The Principle of Justice

Our discussion of justice is equally brief, but not for the same reasons. Not only is this principle not similar to any specific moral rules, it does not even pretend to provide a guide to action. It is doubtful that even the proponents of principlism put much stock in it as an action guide. The "principle of justice" is the prime example of a principle functioning simply as a checklist of moral concerns. It amounts to no more than saying that one should be concerned with matters of distribution; it recommends just or fair distribution without endorsing any particular account of justice or fairness. Thus, as used by principlism, the principle of justice, in effect, is merely a chapter heading under which one might find sophisticated discussions of various theories of justice. After reading such a chapter one might be better informed and more sensitive to the differing theories of justice, but when dealing with an actual problem of distribution, one would be baffled by the injunction to "apply the principle of justice."

The principle of justice shares an additional problem with the two remaining principles: it blurs the distinction between what is morally required (obeying the moral rules) and what is morally encouraged (following the moral ideals). Since the principle of justice cannot be taken seriously as an action guide, this blurring is not as obvious as in the two remaining principles. In this, as in other matters, principlism simply takes over errors of those theories which suggested the four principles in the first place. For example: The most prominent contemporary discussion of justice is by John Rawls. In *A Theory of Justice*, Rawls describes what he calls the duty of justice as follows:

> This duty requires us to support and to comply with just institutions that exist and apply to us. It also constrains us to further just arrangements not yet established, at least when this can be done without too much cost to ourselves.[7]

Rawls includes in what he regards as a single duty (1) the moral rule requiring one to obey (just) laws and (2) the moral ideal encouraging one to help make just laws, without even realizing the significant difference between these two guides to action.[8] As we show later, this failure to distinguish between what is morally required (the moral rules) and what is morally encouraged (the moral ideals) also creates significant confusion in both the principle of autonomy and the principle of beneficence.

The Principle of Autonomy

This principle seems to be the centerpiece of principlism. It is cited more frequently than any of the others and has taken on a life of its own. The concept of autonomy has come to dominate discussions of medical ethics to the point that there is a growing and focused opposition to its predominance. Attention is being drawn to concerns that outweigh autonomy; its primacy over all of the other principles is being questioned. (It is to the credit of Beauchamp and Childress that they make it clear that other considerations sometimes outweigh autonomy.)[9] But these developments are only symptomatic of deeper theoretical problems with autonomy as a principle. As close as Beauchamp and Childress get to stating the principle of autonomy is this:

> Hence, we shall here understand the principle of autonomy as follows: *Autonomous actions and choices should not be constrained by others. ...* It asserts a right of noninterference and correlatively an obligation not to constrain autonomous actions—nothing more but also nothing less." (2d ed., p. 62, their emphasis)

And in the third edition (p. 72, their emphasis):

> This principle can be stated in its negative form as follows: *Autonomous actions are not to be subjected to controlling constraints by others.* This principle provides the justificatory basis for the right to make autonomous decisions. The principle should be treated as a broad, abstract principle independent of restrictive or exceptive clauses such as "We must respect individuals' views and rights so long as their thoughts and actions do not seriously harm other persons." Like all moral principles, this principle has only prima facie standing. It asserts a right of noninterference and correlatively an obligation not to constrain autonomous actions.

As stated here it is surprisingly akin to the principle of nonmaleficence and, as such, we of course have little disagreement with it. In fact, it seems to pick out just one evil, the loss of freedom, and gives it a principle all to itself. Interpreted simply as an alternative formulation of the moral rule "Do not deprive of freedom," we have no objection to this principle, for it is a genuine action guide in that it prohibits constraining others' actions. However, the principle does not say simply that one should not constrain another's actions and choices, but rather it says that one should not constrain another's *autonomous* actions and choices. The principle does not prohibit constraining nonautonomous choices and actions. Consequently, the distinction between autonomous and nonautonomous actions takes on great moral significance. What counts as an autonomous choice or action becomes a matter of fundamental moral concern; thus the addition of "autonomous" causes many problems in applying the principle of autonomy.

Autonomous actions and choices. In practice the basic difficulty with autonomy, dogging it throughout all its uses, is knowing whether the actions and choices one is concerned with are autonomous. Is the choice to give up drinking the autonomous choice or is the autonomous choice to continue drinking? Is the choice to withdraw from expensive life-prolonging treatment to save one's family money and anguish the autonomous choice, or is the autonomous choice the decision to go on living a while longer? Which choice is it that one is being admonished not to constrain?

If there is a conflict between people who differ on which choice of the patient is the autonomous one, each side will appeal to the principle of autonomy for support. One side may favor overruling a patient's refusal because the fact that it is irrational shows that the choice is not autonomous; whereas the other side may favor going along with the patient's explicitly stated refusal on the ground that although it is irrational, the patient is competent and therefore the refusal is an autonomous choice. Both sides can sincerely claim that they are acting on the principle of autonomy by respecting the autonomous choice. This is not merely a normal problem of interpretation, for, as discussed in the previous chapter, we realize that all of the moral rules are subject to some interpretation. However autonomy is such a fundamentally ambiguous and disputed concept that "the principle of autonomy" can be used to support two completely opposing ways of acting, even when there is no disagreement on the observable facts of the case and there are no cultural differences. Such a principle is obviously not a useful guide to action.

There may seem to be times when it is appropriate to question whether a patient has made an autonomous choice, such as when he is delirious, or intoxicated, or under the influence of drugs, and the views he expresses significantly differ from those he expresses when he is in a normal state. However, when the significant departure from previously expressed views is not temporary and not explained by medical reasons, then it is misleading and unhelpful to focus on the question of whether a patient's choices are autonomous. The correct application of the label of "autonomous" to a patient's choices is a matter of longstanding philosophical dispute, and there is no clear ordinary use of the term which is helpful in resolving any of the difficult cases. Thus, following the principle of autonomy may encourage one to act with unjustified paternalism, that is, to overrule the patient's explicit refusal, simply because one views that choice as not being autonomous. Thus the principle of autonomy may lead one

to deprive a person of freedom without an adequate justification for doing so.

A much more adequate method for dealing with such problems is by using the concepts of "rational" and "irrational" as we have presented them in Chapter 2. Only if a person's decision concerning his own health care is seriously irrational is overruling it justified (see Chapter 10). If the decision is rational, overruling it is not justified. Suppose, for example, that a patient has thoughtfully and persistently throughout his life insisted that if he contracts terminal cancer, he wants no treatment at all. But now that he has cancer that is regarded as terminal (and is anxious, stressed, and drugged), he says he wants life-prolonging treatment. Health care professionals would be hard pressed to decide what to do on the basis of whether or not this was an autonomous decision (after all, it was a sudden change of mind, under the influence of drugs and stress). However, the patient's current decision in favor of treatment is clearly not irrational, and hence, on our account, should not be overridden. (We discuss this matter in considerable detail in Chapters 6 and 10.)

Moral rules and moral ideals: A fundamental distinction. At the core of many problems with the principle of autonomy, as with other principles, is its general failure to recognize the significance of the distinction between what is morally encouraged (following the moral ideals) and what is morally required (obeying the moral rules). Many philosophers, including Kant and Mill, have made this distinction, or rather one that seems closely related to it, by distinguishing between duties of perfect obligation and duties of imperfect obligation ("perfect" and "imperfect" duties). However, this indiscriminate use of the term "duty" (a matter we discuss later in connection with beneficence) has resulted in this crucial distinction not being made in the correct way. The first five moral rules, discussed in Chapter 2, are examples of perfect duties. So also are the second five moral rules requiring one not to deceive, not to cheat, not to break promises, not to disobey the law, and not to neglect one's duty (in the normal sense of "duty"). Perfect duties must be impartially obeyed all of the time. One is allowed to violate a perfect duty only when one has an adequate justification for doing so.

On the other hand, the moral ideals are imperfect duties, that is, those duties that are impossible to obey either impartially or all of the time. Working to help the downtrodden is an example. One must pick and choose not only which of the downtrodden to help, but also when and where one will provide this help. Furthermore, one may even choose not to act on that imperfect duty at all, but rather to act on some other imperfect duty such as preventing the deprivation of freedom of someone, somewhere. It seems as if an imperfect duty is a duty that one is not required to act on at all; morality certainly does not require one to work for either Oxfam or for Amnesty International, let alone both. It is not morally required to give to or work for any charity, although morality certainly encourages such behavior. Doing so is following an imperfect duty (moral ideal), not a perfect duty (moral rule).

Because this traditional distinction between perfect and imperfect duties embodies a confusion about the notion of duty, we make the distinction in a different and less misleading fashion. Moral rules prohibit acting in ways that cause, or increase the risk of, others suffering some harm. That is precisely what morality requires. Moral ideals, on the other hand, encourage the prevention and relief of harm, but morality does not require following those ideals (unless a moral rule, such as "Do your duty," requires such prevention or relief, but then the circumstances are specified and limited, as discussed in Chapter 3). The moral rules must be followed all the time, toward everyone, impartially, but that is impossible in the case of the moral ideals. Doing what morality requires (obeying the moral rules) is usually not praiseworthy; rather it is expected, and failing to do it makes one liable to punishment. Doing what morality encourages (following the moral

ideals) is usually praiseworthy and failing to do it is not punishable. The distinction between moral rules and moral ideals is crucial for a proper understanding of the moral system.

The phrases "perfect duties" and "imperfect duties" obscure this crucial distinction between moral rules and moral ideals. The ordinary use of "duty" suggests that punishment is deserved when one fails to do one's duty. After all, it is morally required to obey the moral rules impartially all of the time. For example, whenever one deprives persons of freedom (principlism might call this violating their autonomy), one needs an adequate justification for doing so. But one does not need a justification for failing to help them to increase their freedom (principlism might call this promoting their autonomy), unless one has a duty to do so, for example, because of one's profession. In the absence of such a duty, helping someone to increase her freedom is following a moral ideal. Morality certainly encourages doing that, but morality does not require doing it.

Autonomy as rule and ideal. The principle of autonomy requires respect for autonomy, but it fails to distinguish clearly between "respecting (not violating) autonomy" and "promoting autonomy." Not distinguishing clearly between "respecting autonomy" and "promoting autonomy" inevitably leads to confusion. Compounded by the search for the "genuinely" autonomous actions and choices, the principle of autonomy invites a kind of activism in which an agent promotes those choices and actions of another that the agent regards as the other's autonomous choices and actions, even though that involves depriving that person of freedom. For example, suppose a woman is pregnant with a fetus that tests have shown to be severely defective. The woman, wanting an abortion, consults a counselor, informing the counselor that she has "always been a good Catholic." The counselor, seeking to abide by the principle of autonomy, faces a dilemma. The principle commits him not only to never overriding a client's autonomous decision, but to actively promoting the client's autonomy. But what is the pregnant woman's autonomous self in this case? Her "real self" may be her firm and life-long commitment to Catholicism, in which case the counselor should, in the interests of promoting autonomy, lead her back to those foundations. On the other hand, moving her back to her religious commitments could be seen as an intrusion on her apparently autonomous decision to have the abortion. Thus the dual demands of the principle of autonomy not only lead to confusion, but could be seen as leading to immoral manipulation of a vulnerable patient in order to promote what one decides is (or should be) the patient's autonomous choice.[10]

Thus, principlism's centerpiece "principle of autonomy" embodies a dangerous level of confusion. That confusion is created by unclarity as to what counts as autonomous actions and choices and the additional blurring of a basic moral distinction between moral rules and moral ideals. This unnecessary introduction of the confused and disputed concept of autonomy inevitably results in making it more difficult to think clearly about moral problems. The goal of moral philosophy is to clarify moral thinking, not to introduce new and unnecessary complications.

As an aside, it is worth observing that the principle of autonomy probably caught on so tenaciously in the last three decades for many reasons. One is that Kantian ethics was experiencing a renaissance and that Kant's notion of autonomy was central to his account of morality. A second is that the society became increasingly aware that the medical profession was so markedly paternalistic that patient self-determination was almost nonexistent. A third was that the increase in medical technology resulted in alternative treatments for most maladies. A fourth was the aging of the population and the resulting increase in chronic diseases that could not be cured, only managed, and patients often knew almost as much about managing them as their physicians. A fifth, the combination of the increase in medical technology that could keep extremely sick people alive for a long time,

together with an aging population that often had a rational desire not to be kept alive, even made it rational to refuse life-prolonging treatment. So the emphasis on autonomy became the banner under which forces rallied to gain for patients more control over their own health care. Allowing the patient to decide what, if any, treatment he would receive became the main issue, and thus momentum and conviction, rather than conceptual clarity or theoretical soundness, perpetuated the emphasis on autonomy. Even the fact that the principle of autonomy did not really embody Kant's notion of autonomy did not detract from the overwhelming political appeal of invoking the principle.

An example of how confused the general understanding of autonomy is can be seen by examining Kant's view of autonomy. On Kant's view a person is not acting autonomously if he kills himself or allows himself to die because of intractable pain. To do so is to allow pleasure and pain (which, according to Kant, are not part of the rational self) to determine one's actions. Thus, such suicide or allowing oneself to die is not an autonomous action of the rational self. To act autonomously one must always act in accord with the Categorical Imperative. In *The Grounding of the Metaphysics of Morals*, Kant explicitly states that the Categorical Imperative requires one not to commit suicide because of pain. By way of contrast, note that one of the major arguments in favor of allowing people to die when they are suffering from intractable pain is the principle of autonomy. The seeds of confusion were present in the initial planting of the concept of autonomy. This explains, in part, why we prefer the simple rule "Don't deprive of freedom" to the principle of autonomy for protecting patient self-determination.

The Principle of Beneficence

As used by principlism, this principle suffers shortcomings similar to those of autonomy.

As popularly used in the biomedical ethics literature this principle is cited simply to give "validation" both to preventing or relieving harm and to doing good or conferring benefits. Beauchamp and Childress, though much more cautious in their discussion of the principle of beneficence than many, do not avoid the errors. For them the principle of beneficence "asserts the duty to help others further their important and legitimate interests."[11] As such it is morally required. In the biomedical context, the principle becomes the duty to confer benefits and to actively prevent and remove harms, in addition to balancing the possible goods against the possible harms of an action. Even though Beauchamp and Childress are well aware that many philosophers treat beneficent acts as "morally ideal," they still regard beneficence as morally required. But how can benefiting others always be morally required of everyone? As we have shown, impartiality is an essential feature of moral requirements, but the requirement of beneficence cannot be impartially followed toward everyone all the time.

Thus the principle of beneficence not only succumbs to the same criticisms that we earlier leveled at the principle of autonomy, by ignoring the distinction between moral ideals (preventing harms) and moral rules (avoiding causing harms), but it adds a new one, namely, failing to distinguish between the preventing or relieving of harms and the conferring of benefits (promoting goods). This distinction is especially important for medicine, inasmuch as preventing or relieving harm often justifies violating a moral rule without consent, whereas conferring benefits (or promoting goods) rarely, if ever, does.

Beneficence and the concept of duty. Another major confusion perpetuated by the principle of beneficence concerns the concept of duty. Although it arises from the mistake of turning moral ideals into duties, the problem itself has nothing to do with the rules/ideals distinction. Principlism considers it a duty to follow the principles. This becomes especially clear in the frequent references to "the duty of beneficence." That beneficence is a moral ideal is not the only reason it is incorrect to call it a duty; it is equally incorrect to call "not killing" a duty, even though it is a moral rule. Rather it is incorrect because such usage distorts and obscures the primary meaning of "duty," which specifically refers to the particular duties that come with one's role, occupation, or profession. Though it is correct to say "one ought not to kill" or "one ought to help the downtrodden," it creates significant confusion to regard these "oughts" as duties. For some philosophers "Do your duty" has come to mean no more than "Do what you morally ought to do." But using the term "duty" in this way makes it very difficult to talk about real duties, such as those associated with people's occupations and whose content is determined by the members of those occupations or professions and the society in which they live. For reasons of conceptual soundness and clarity, we use the term "duty" only in its ordinary sense, that is, to refer to what is required by one's role in society, particularly by one's occupation, profession, or relationship as family member. It is not only misleading to talk of the moral ideals as imperfect duties, it is also misleading to talk of the moral rules as perfect duties.

Thus "Do your duty" is a distinct moral rule and on a par with the other moral rules; it is not a metarule telling one to obey the other moral rules. However, morality does put a limit on what counts as a duty: there can be no duty to violate unjustifiably any of the other moral rules. "Do your duty" is justified as a moral rule because of the harm, or significantly increased risk of harm, that is caused by one's failure to do that which others are justifiably counting on being done. One is morally required to do his duty, but it generates confusion to say that one has a duty to do his duty.

In medicine it is especially misleading to use the principle of beneficence as if it creates a general duty for all health care workers. Again, this obscures the role of real duties, that is, the specific duties that come with one's role or profession. Beauchamp and Childress seem to recognize the significant difference between what they call the general duty of beneficence and the specific duties of beneficence. They state: "Even if our general duty of beneficence derives in part from reciprocity and fair play, our specific duties of beneficence often derive from special moral relationships with persons, frequently through institutional roles."[12] A later version (third edition) is even clearer: "Even if the general obligation of beneficence derives largely from reciprocity, specific obligations of beneficence often derive from special moral relationships with persons, frequently through institutional roles and contractual arrangements ..."[13] They are clear that doctors, nurses, and others in the health care field have specific duties to their patients that are determined by their profession and by the practices of their specific institution. However, to lump these varied and detailed professional duties together with the misconceived "general duty of beneficence" and place it all under one principle of beneficence is to substitute a slogan for substance.

Beneficence and "morality as a public system."
Principlism fails to appreciate that morality is a "public system," that is, it must be known and understood by all moral agents, and it cannot be irrational for them to follow it. This failure to recognize that all justified violations of a moral rule must be part of a public system that applies to everyone, that is, that everyone must know that this kind of violation is allowed, is a serious flaw. This failure to appreciate that morality is a public system is most clearly seen in act utilitarianism (see Chapter 2). If act utilitarianism is thought of as a code of conduct requiring everyone always to act so as to produce the best overall consequences, regardless of the consequences of everyone knowing that they are allowed to act in that way, then it is appropriately criticized for not recognizing the public nature of morality, that is, that morality must be a public system that applies to all moral agents.

Rule utilitarianism is, properly speaking, not a consequentialist moral system, for rules as well as consequences seem to be involved in making a moral judgment on a particular act. Nonetheless, even rule utilitarianism does not appreciate the fact that morality is a public system. It claims that those rules which would have the best consequences if generally obeyed, are the moral rules. It does not require that those rules be known by all those who are subject to them. More important, a rule utilitarian has significant problems in dealing with exceptions to the rules. If a rule utilitarian tries to avoid the problem of justified exceptions by incorporating the exceptions into the rule itself, the rule becomes indefinitely long; as such, it cannot be part of a public system, because it cannot be understood by all rational persons. Common morality has rules that are simple and general.

If a rule utilitarian adopts simple and general rules, she must determine how particular violations of a rule are justified. She must decide whether to (1) consider only the consequences of her doing this particular act at this particular time or (2) consider the consequences of everyone knowing that they are allowed to do that act in the same morally relevant circumstances. If a rule utilitarian is contemplating cheating on an exam or deceiving someone and chooses (1), then her decision is often at odds with what morality requires. If she chooses (2) she is no longer a rule utilitarian. Rule utilitarianism must determine justified exceptions by appealing to actual or foreseeable consequences of the particular act. Common morality determines justified exceptions by appealing to the purely hypothetical consequences of *everyone knowing* that they are allowed to break the rule in the same morally relevant circumstances. If they are better than the consequences of *everyone knowing* that they are not allowed to break the rule, the violation is justified. Common morality requires consideration of these hypothetical consequences because such consideration is essential for impartially obeying the moral rules.

Neither act nor rule utilitarianism appreciates that for an act to be morally acceptable it must be one that can be publicly allowed. Thus, no principle derived from utilitarianism, such as the principle of beneficence, can be relied on to produce valid moral conclusions. Not surprisingly, the principle of beneficence, more than the other principles, is most affected by this failure to appreciate that morality is a public system. When the consequences of a particular rule violation, such as cheating, are good, but the consequences of that kind of violation being publicly allowed are bad, principlism has serious problems. Since the principle of beneficence considers only the consequences, direct and indirect, of a particular violation of a moral rule, it often encourages acting in a kind of way which if publicly allowed, would lead to bad consequences. Indeed we suspect that it is because of this tendency of the principle of beneficence to lead to what everyone regards as morally unacceptable conclusions, that the principle of autonomy has attained such prominence in principlism. That is, the principle of autonomy serves to overrule beneficence in all those cases where no rational person would publicly allow the kind of behavior that the principle of beneficence seems to require.

Consider a case in which a physician's breach of confidentiality results in some very good consequences for her patient. Yet, if intuitively it seems clearly wrong to commit the breach, the principle of autonomy can then be brought in as the reason for not following the principle of beneficence. The problem, of course, is that sometimes beneficence should outweigh autonomy, but principlism provides no systematic way of determining which should prevail in any particular conflict. Principlism simply says to weigh or balance the principles against each other without providing any instructions on how to do that weighing or balancing.[14] Common morality has a clear procedure for handing such conflicts: compare the consequences of any proposed violation being publicly allowed with the consequences of its not being publicly allowed. Since the only cases in which an account of morality needs to be invoked explicitly are those in which the principles (or rules and ideals) conflict, it is pointless to have an account of morality which provides no guidance on how to deal with such conflicts.

Summary

The traditional concept of an ethical principle has been one that embodies the moral theory that spawns it. As shorthand for the theory, it is used by itself to enunciate a meaningful directive for action because it has an established, unified theory standing behind it. "Act so as to bring about the greatest good for the greatest number," "Maximize the amount of liberty compatible with a like liberty for all." The thrust of the directive is clear; its goal and intent are unambiguous. Of course there are often ambiguities and differing interpretations with respect to how the principle applies to a particular situation, but the principle itself is never used with other principles that are in conflict with it. Furthermore, if a genuine theory has more than one general principle, the relationship between the principles is clearly stated, as in the case of Rawls's two principles of justice. Unlike principlism, one is not given a number of conflicting principles without being told how to rank them or how to resolve the conflicts between them.

The principles of principlism are quite different. In general, they seem to function more as reminders of topics or concerns which the moral decision maker should review prior to decision. Except for the principle of nonmaleficence, they are not true action guides. The principle of justice is the clearest example of that. The principle of nonmaleficence is acceptable since it simply prohibits the causing of harm, and as such merely summarizes the first four or five moral rules. But since it does not specify what counts as the harms one is prohibited from causing, it is less useful than it might be. Furthermore, since it does not make clear that there are different harms which different people rank differently, it is more misleading than it might be. Nonetheless, insofar as the principle of nonmaleficence is interpreted as "Don't cause harm," it at least meets the criterion of being morally required.

The principles of autonomy and of beneficence are more complicated. They actually sound like action guides; they seem to tell one how to act. But closer inspection shows that they generate confusion. If the principle of autonomy were an action guide, like nonmaleficence, simply telling one not to deprive of freedom, then of course we have no objection to it because it is now synonymous with that moral rule. But unhappily the principle of autonomy goes beyond that clear and defensible rule. It injects confusion because there is confusion and disagreement over the proper meaning of "autonomous action." Another troubling feature, as shown earlier, is that the principle also requires that moral agents promote each other's autonomy. That move, which fails to recognize the crucial moral distinction between moral rules and moral ideals means that the principle cannot be taken seriously as a moral requirement. If the principle is interpreted loosely to mean simply "Respect persons" (the original principle from which the principle of autonomy seems to have been derived), it is still not clear what that entails. At best it might mean, "Morality forbids you from treating others simply as you please. Some ways are acceptable and some are not. Think about it." So then one is back to interpreting the principles as a list of concerns.

The principle of beneficence also has an action-guide appearance. It seems to be saying one has a duty to prevent harm as well as to help others "further their important and legitimate interests." Besides the conceptual confusion over the notion of duty, this principle seems to be concerned primarily with what we call utilitarian ideals. It is certainly not a moral rule, for a person cannot possibly follow this principle impartially, all the time. It is not even a clear moral ideal, for the charge to confer benefits (unlike prevention

of harms) usually cannot be used to justify the violation of a moral rule. As in the case with utilitarianism, from which this principle is derived, following it might lead to unjustified transgressions of moral rules toward the few in order to confer benefits on the many, thus triggering deployment of the principle of autonomy.

Lastly, we highlighted the more general difficulties with principlism. We noted that even if the individual principles are interpreted as action guides, they often conflict with each other. Since they are not part of a public system, there is no agreed-upon method for resolving these conflicts, or even understanding why a particular conflict cannot be resolved. Since they do not share a common ground, there is no underlying theory to appeal to for help in understanding or resolving conflicts. Indeed, each of the principles in effect seems to be a surrogate for the theory from which it is derived. The use of the principles seems to be an unwitting effort to allow the use of whatever ethical theory seems best suited to the particular problem one is considering. It is simply a sophisticated technique for dealing with problems ad hoc.

The appeal of principlism is that it makes use of some features of standard ethical theories that seem to have popular support. But there is no attempt to see how these different features can be blended together as integrated parts of a single adequate theory, rather than disparate features derived from several competing theories. So in effect principlism tells agents to pick and choose as they see fit, as if one can sometimes be a Kantian and sometimes a Utilitarian and sometimes something else, without worrying about consistency or whether the theory one is using is adequate or not. Principlism does not recognize that for a moral decision to be correct it must be one that can be publicly allowed. It not only does not recognize the unified and systematic nature of morality, it does not recognize that the moral system, or morality, must be public.

The upshot of having principles with an unclear content which are not part of any unified public system is that an agent is not aware of the real grounds for his moral decision. Because the principles are not clear and direct imperatives at all, but simply a collection of suggestions and observations, occasionally conflicting, the agent cannot know what is really guiding his action. Nor do these principles tell him what facts are morally relevant, such that a change in them may change what he should do; thus he is not able to propose better alternatives. Though the language of principlism suggests that the agent has applied a principle which is morally well established, a closer look shows that in fact he has looked at and weighed many diverse moral considerations, which may be only superficially interrelated, having no unified, systematic underlying foundation. Principles seem to be involved in complex decisions only in a purely verbal way; the real guiding influences on the moral decision are not the ones the agent believes them to be. Rather, the agent is, in fact, guided by his basic understanding of common morality, and only later cites principles when stating his conclusions, giving the illusion of theoretical support.

Concerning Specification

Our critiques of principlism have led those espousing it to search for a method of transforming the principles into actual action guides instead of a checklist of concerns.[15] The most prominent of these methods is known as "specification." Several articles put this method forth as the solution to some problems of principlism that we have pointed out.[16] Beauchamp and Childress incorporate the notion in their most recent revision of *The Principles of Biomedical Ethics*.[17] Indeed that may be part of the reason that the reviewer of this edition proclaimed it the death of principlism.[18]

Although the addition of "specification" to principlism might be indicative of its demise (no longer being the atheoretical principlism we have known and criticized), there is no doubt that specification is a move in the right direction. The notion of specification and its refinement seems to have originated with the work of Henry S. Richardson in his article, "Specifying Norms as a Way to Resolve Concrete Ethical Problems."[19] Richardson's attempt to make principlism more systematic is certainly a move in the right direction, but it is just a beginning. Richardson states that specification qualifies the norm "by substantive means ... by adding clauses indicating what, where, when, why, how, by what means, by whom or to whom the action is to be, is not to be, or may be done ..."[20] These clauses certainly encompass some of the morally relevant features of a situation or problem, but his questions (what, where, when, why, and so forth) do not help to determine what features are morally relevant, or why they are relevant. Nor does he provide any kind of theory which identifies which "substantive means" should be used to determine that any particular feature is morally relevant.

We applaud the embracing of specification by principlism, for it shows that those supporting principlism recognize the need for a theory to explain and support it. However, as far as we know, neither Richardson nor those who embrace his modification of principlism provide any theory. There is no explanation of where the appropriate specifications come from or how the narrowing of the application of the norms takes place. The theory that we describe in Chapter 2 can explain and support how norms are specified, and also provides a list of the features that are morally relevant. Our theory does not, however, as Richardson assumes that specification of norms does, eliminate all disagreement. We not only acknowledge but indeed emphasize that equally informed, impartial, rational persons can differ, not only in how they specify a norm, but also in how they apply the same specified norm. Richardson recognizes that in applying a norm to a situation, one must identify its morally relevant features, but, having no theory, he provides no clue about how one determines what those morally relevant features are.

One of Richardson's problems is his identification of "universal" with "absolute."[21] However, a norm can be universal without being absolute. The rejection of absolute norms, that is, the recognition that all moral rules have exceptions, is completely compatible with the claim that moral rules are universal, that is, that they apply to all rational persons. Richardson does not recognize that in order to make norms culturally sensitive, it is necessary to allow for some degree of interpretation of the norms. Perhaps most important, Richardson, like all principlists, does not appreciate a central feature of morality, that it is a public system. This explains why he cannot formulate criteria for, or develop a list of, morally relevant features.[22] Finally, his failure to realize that some moral disagreements are not resolvable, makes understandable his failure to formulate any procedure for dealing with conflicts between specified norms.

We conclude that specification helps principlism move in the right direction, namely, toward our account of morality. But if it moves far enough in that direction, it will no longer be appropriate to call it "principlism." So far, however, specification has not moved principlism very far; it has simply pointed it in the right direction and made it clear that it has a lot farther to go. Specification still fails to make critically important moves: listing and defending the morally relevant features of situations, relating those features to a moral theory, and incorporating the requirement that morality be a public system. Specification shows the need for these accomplishments, but does not achieve them.

One article, describing several approaches to bioethical theory, criticizes our account of morality, describing it as "deductivism," and concludes that "specified principlism" is "the most promising model—though it requires development."[23] What the author of that article does not realize is that if specified principlism develops properly, it will become our account. In most cases, our theory is deductivist in that the immorality of an action can be deduced from its description. For example, a clear case of harmful, self-serving deception is seen to be immoral by "deduction" from the moral rule prohibiting deception. However, although that is the most

common and frequent kind of application of a moral rule to a situation, it is almost never discussed because there is no practical or theoretical reason to discuss it. No one doubts that the action is immoral, and because of this there is no point in discussing it. But an adequate moral theory must account for the common and uninteresting cases as well as the uncommon and interesting ones.

For these uncommon and interesting cases, the ones that are described in the medical ethics case books and discussed in all of the medical ethics anthologies and textbooks, our account of morality is not deductivist. What our critics do not appreciate is that we recognize that morality is an informal public system. Like sandlot baseball, there is unspoken agreement on the point of the game and all of the fundamental rules. What causes problems is how one interprets the rules in the nonobvious cases. But without overwhelming agreement on most matters, the game would never even get started. Similarly, there is overwhelming agreement on the point of morality, the lessening of the suffering of evil or harm, and on all of the fundamental rules. But equally informed, rational, impartial persons can disagree on almost all interesting, nonobvious cases.

Our account of the moral system explains how this can happen; for example, people can disagree on the ranking of harms to be avoided, they can disagree on the consequences of publicly allowing a kind of violation, or they can disagree on the interpretation of the particular moral rule. We do not believe, and the moral system does not require, that one and only one solution exists for each moral problem. We do not criticize principlism because it does not provide a unique answer to every moral problem, but rather because it does not explain in any useful way what is responsible for the disagreement and, hence, provides no help in resolving the disagreement.

Like principlism, we borrow from all of the classical theories. Unlike principlism, we do not merely formulate principles which call attention to the insights from these theories. We integrate the best features of each of these theories into a new theory, one that eliminates those features of the previous theories that result in so many devastating counterexamples. Our theory, like all theories, still has problems, but for the most part these are the result of a poor statement of the theory. We look forward to legitimate criticisms of the theory and its applications that we put forward in this book, so that we may continue to revise and improve our statement of it.

Notes

1. K. Danner Clouser and Bernard Gert, "A Critique of Principlism," *The Journal of Medicine and Philosophy* 15 (1990), pp. 219–236, and "Morality vs. Principlism," in *Principles of Health Care Ethics*, ed. Raaman Gillon (New York: John Wiley and Sons, Inc., 1994), pp. 251–266. See also K. Danner Clouser, "Common Morality as an Alternative to Principlism," *Kennedy Institute of Ethics Journal*, 5 (1995), pp. 219–236.

2. Tom L. Beauchamp and James F. Childress, *Principles of Biomedical Ethics* (New York: Oxford University Press, 1979; 2d ed., 1983; 3d ed., 1989, 4th ed., 1994).

3. Ezekiel J. Emanuel, "The Beginning of the End of Principlism," *Hastings Center Report*, 25 (1995), pp. 37–38.

4. Ibid., p. 38.

5. This section is based on the *Federal Register*, Vol. 44, No. 76 (Wednesday, April 18, 1979), pp. 23192–23197.

6. Ibid., p. 23193.

7. John Rawls, *A Theory of Justice* (Cambridge, Mass.: Harvard University Press, 1971), p. 115, see also p. 334.

8. For further discussion of Rawls on this point, see Bernard Gert, *Morality* (New York: Oxford University Press, 1988), ch. 13.

9. Beauchamp and Childress, *Principles*, 3d ed., pp. 122–125.

10. For a more detailed account of the problems caused by autonomy in genetic counseling, and of the way in which using the common moral system can help deal with these problems, see Chapter 6 of Bernard Gert, Edward M. Berger, George F. Cahill Jr., K. Danner Clouser, Charles M. Culver, John B. Moeschler, and George H. S. Singer, *Morality and the New Genetics: A Guide for Students and Health Care Providers* (Sudbury, Mass.: Jones and Bartlett Publishers, 1996).

11. Beauchamp and Childress, *Principles*, 2d ed., pp. 148–149.

12. Ibid., p. 156.

13. Ibid., 3d ed., p. 204.

14. Specified principlism attempts to resolve this problem, but it is not well worked out. Indeed it seems to be merely a way station on the path of principlism to our more complex and systematic account of morality, which does have a procedure for resolving conflicts. See the last section of this chapter for a fuller discussion.

15. See K. Danner Clouser and Bernard Gert, "A Critique of Principlism," *The Journal of Medicine and Philosophy*, 15 (1990), pp. 219–236, and "Morality versus Principlism," *Principles of Health Care Ethics*, ed. Raanan Gillon (New York: John Wiley and Sons, 1994), pp. 251–266.

16. For example, David DeGrazia, "Moving Forward in Bioethical Theory: Theories, Cases, and Specified Principlism," *The Journal of Medicine and Philosophy* 17 (1992): 511–539.

17. Beauchamp and Childress, *Principles*, 4th ed., 1994.

18. See note 3.

19. Henry S. Richardson, "Specifying Norms as a Way to Resolve Concrete Ethical Problems," *Philosophy and Public Affairs* 19 (1990), pp. 279–310.

20. Ibid., pp. 295–296.

21. See ibid., pp. 292 ff.

22. For the connection between morality being a public system that applies to all rational persons and morally relevant features, see Chapter 2.

23. DeGrazia, op. cit., p. 512.

Individual Good and Common Good: A Communitarian Approach to Bioethics

Daniel Callahan

Whe the field of bioethics began to emerge in the late 1960s and early 1970s, one of the first questions to surface was that of its ethical foundation. The earlier, historical field of medical ethics rested either on a theological base, stemming from various religious perspectives, or, much further back in time, on the professional obligations of the physician to the patient and to the profession, embodied in what we think of as the Hippocratic tradition.

The new bioethics, however, needed to find a way to speak in a secular culture, drawing on nonreligious premises, and to encompass a far wider range of medical and biotechnology issues than that of the doctor-patient relationship. The question then became: what ought to be the foundational principles, premises, and perspectives of this new venture? Two answers were quickly forthcoming. One was that the ethical foundations of the field should not be idiosyncratic to its particular issues but should be understood simply as an arena for the application of more general ethical principles and analysis. The other was just the opposite: bioethics should have its own moral basis, suitable to its particular subject matter.

That debate sputtered out by the end of the 1970s, never formally resolved but de facto influenced by the growing number of philosophers drawn to bioethics and prone to import into it the modes of reasoning common to the moral philosophy of the era. Most textbooks and classroom readers in bioethics came to open with an introduction to philosophical ethics, which usually turned out to be an inventory of the familiar philosophical theories of utilitarianism, deontology, natural law thinking, and the like. The idea that there is distinctive biomedical ethic all but disappeared from the inventory.

Two important developments since that time bear on the foundations of bioethics. The first is a general decline of interest in foundational matters—even though, for those who remain interested, there have been new theoretical models added to the older ones, such as feminist and narrative ethics. By "foundational matters," I mean broadly comprehensive theories of a kind symbolized by the arguments between utilitarians and deontologists. There nonetheless remains, at a somewhat lower level, a lively interest in the place of rules and principles, the balancing of universality and contextuality, and the virtues pertinent to patient care.

Although textbooks and readers still have introductions to ethical theory, it is striking how the majority of articles selected for inclusion in the readers are in fact devoid of the direct employment of any of those theories. They may be there tacitly, but it is rare to find them openly used to solve ethical problems. An examination of, say, the case studies carried for over 30 years now in the *Hastings Center Report* reveals a similar phenomenon. In both instances, the main characteristic is the lack of a conspicuous theory. The articles and case studies are, in that respect, all over the place in their analysis, marked by many strengths and charms (if any good at all), but theory is rarely prominent. While "principlism" (the view that four moral principles—autonomy, nonmaleficence, beneficence, and justice—are sufficient to deal with most moral problems in medicine) still raises its head now and then, its numerous critics have taken much of the wind out of its sails (Beauchamp and Childress 2001).

The second development is not unrelated to the first, but moves in a different direction. It might best be characterized as the almost complete triumph of liberal individualism in bioethics. I call this an ideology rather than a moral theory because it is a set of essentially political and social values brought into bioethics, not as formal theory but as a vital background constellation of values. If it does not function as a moral theory as philosophers have understood that concept, it is clearly present and pervasive as a litmus test of the acceptability of certain ideas and ways of framing issues. As a familiar constellation it encompasses a high place for autonomy, for biomedical progress with few constraints, for procedural rather than substantive solutions to controverted ethical problems, and for a strong antipathy to comprehensive notions of the human good.

As a practical matter, the triumph of liberal individualism has led to a systematic marginalization of religious and conservative perspectives, often treated with disdain and hostility; and it has brought to bioethics the cultural wars from which it had earlier been spared. Bioethicists are increasingly labeled as "liberal" or "conservative," and the nastiness and partisanship of the broader political scene has begun to make its appearance (though mainly from the conservative side; liberals seem too indifferent to conservatives to care what they say). It is exceedingly rare to find ethical conferences or symposia that are not dominated by one side or the other, usually unwittingly (our congenial crowd), but sometimes consciously.

Many liberals were distressed that a conservative, Leon R. Kass, was appointed in 2001 to direct President Bush's Council on Bioethics, and that most of the Council members were of a similar persuasion. But each of the three earlier national bioethics commissions had liberal directors and predominantly liberal members, though that had been hardly noticed in the press, much less complained about, presumably because it was taken for granted. As it turned out, the Bush Council showed far more ethical variety and lack of consensus in its work on cloning than had been true of any of the other commissions; more than lip service has been paid to diversity (President's Council on Bioethics 2002). I was not proud of my field when I heard the first question of a prominent science reporter who called me in the summer of 2001 about the stem cell debate. "Why is it," she asked, "that everyone in bioethics is in lock step on stem cells?" A good question, to which I had no ready answer—at least none I was prepared to be quoted on.

I have tried to briefly lay out this historical background in order to set the stage for the two central points I want to make in this paper. The first is the contention that bioethics needs no formal foundations, if for no other reason than that it is, and ought to be, an interdisciplinary field, drawing upon many disciplines for its intellectual resources. No one discipline, whatever its foundation, can claim a privileged place. Of course, it is the lack of formal foundations that dooms interdisciplinary fields to the frowns of disciplinary purists, but that can be survived if some other traits are in place. The traits I believe are most important for bioethical inquiry are, on the one hand, determining the right set of questions to ask and issues to pursue; and, on the other, pursuing them with rationality, imagination, and insight. If that is done, people will listen and progress can be made.

My second contention is that liberal individualism needs a strong competitive voice, one that can be found in communitarianism. In addition to fomenting cultural wars, liberal individualism does not have the intellectual strength or penetration to deal effectively with the most important bioethical issues. Its "thin theory" of the good is a thin gruel for the future of bioethics.

Asking the Right Questions

Contemporary bioethics took its rise from the advances in biomedical knowledge and technological innovation that marked the postwar years and that showed the inadequacy of the older medical ethics to encompass the new issues. I have found it helpful to categorize the issues into three parts, reflecting the impact of the new developments. Each category suggests some fundamental questions for bioethics.

First, scientific knowledge and its practical applications have forced a change in our vision of the goals and purposes in medicine, not simply moving from care to cure, and from palliation to the saving of life, but also showing the possibility of using medical knowledge and techniques only indirectly related, if at all, to the preservation of health traditionally understood; and, at the outer edge, bringing the possibility of an enhancement of human nature and traits into view. That has left us with the question: what are the proper goals and uses of medicine?

Second, scientific knowledge and its applications have led us to reexamine the meaning of health. As a concept, "health" has always had a descriptive component, referring to various biological characteristics of the body and mind and the pathologies that can affect them, and a normative component, referring to the human desire for good health and the related fear of illness and disease. While it would be stretching things to say that health has been redefined recently (debates about its meaning are old and well developed), it does seem evident that the practical standards for what counts as good health, and the attendant expectations for it, have considerably escalated of late.

What was tolerable health earlier—or if intolerable, then fatalistically accepted—is increasingly often now rejected. Why should we suffer from old age, or cancer, or heart disease, or simply a less than perfect face? If research can be brought to bear on what ails us, or even just displeases us, then it ought to be pursued; and, best of all, past research success is taken to guarantee future success (exactly the opposite of the Security and Exchange Commission's required warning on the purchase of stocks and bonds). Since the reality of, and expectations about, health are a significant determinant of our overall sense of well-being, we are then left with the question: what are realistic expectations for our health and what kind of research should we support to achieve it?

Third, the technological developments have led us to what seems to me the most important matter of all: we have been led to reconsider, in the light of biomedical progress, what it means to live a life and to think about the nature of our human nature. Effective contraception has helped change the role of women, the procreation of children, and the significance of sexuality. Advances in the health of the elderly have meant changes in the place of old age in the individual life cycle (and what counts as "old") and in the place of the elderly in our social order. Genetic technologies open up new prospects for choosing the traits of our children, and thus affect both the parent-child relationship and the meaning of parenthood. What do we want to make of ourselves as human beings, and what kinds of lives ought we aspire to live?

I don't mean to suggest here that biomedical developments will be the sole determinants of how we may shape our ideas of medicine, health, and the ordering of our lives. Not only will those three categories interact with and affect each other, but they will also take place in the context of developments in information theory, environmental trends, bioterrorism and new natural pathogens, economic and urban life, and so on. Predicting the outcome of so complex a mix is next to impossible, and predicting the mix of moral, social, and political values that will animate them is no less difficult.

At the same time, it is not a threat to liberty to say that liberal individualism is poorly equipped to help us as human communities develop the moral perspectives to deal with the resulting complexity. Liberal individualism's greatest weakness is what is often thought its greatest strength: eschewing a public pursuit of comprehensive ways of understanding the human good and its future. But it takes an act of arbitrary imagination to see how the principle of autonomy, at the core of individualism, or that of market values as its ideological conservative twin, can provide any helpful guidance. Only if one believes in some version of an "invisible hand" shaping our individual goods into a common good, can that view be made plausible. The inescapable reality of the kinds of changes that biomedical progress introduce is that they affect our collective lives, our social and educational and political institutions, as well as those tacitly shared values that push our culture one way or the other.

As an individual, I need to make choices about how I will respond to those changes. But more important, *we* have to make political and social decisions about which choices will, and will not, be good for us as a community, and about the moral principles, rules, and virtues that ought to superintend the introduction of new technologies into the societal mainstream. Only if we believe that there will be no socially coercive or inadvertent culture-shaping consequences of present and forthcoming medical technologies can we deny the need to take common, and not just individual, responsibility for the deployment of a biomedicine that can change just about everything in our lives.

Analytical Virtues

Bioethics can survive and even flourish in the absence of any formal or agreed-upon foundations. But it cannot do without a set of intellectual skills that will enable its leading questions to be approached in the richest and deepest way possible. My list of such skills would include rationality, imagination, and insight. Rarely will any one of them be adequate by itself; typically, each should come into play to enhance the possibility of a comprehensive judgment. Although I cannot do justice to each of those skills here, I will try to indicate a general direction for each of them.

Rationality

While rationality is obviously important for those of us who think of ourselves as rational animals, it is a complex idea. Nothing is less helpful, I have observed, than moralistically urging people to be rational, as if that is the definitive answer to prejudice and wayward emotions. Rationality is often, of course, taken to be synonymous with the use of scientific knowledge (positivism, long moribund, never quite dies); or with being objective (more easily said than done, and almost always morally contestable); or with thinking consistently (as if that guarantees anything other than consistency); or with making logical moves from premises to conclusions (which anyone of ordinary intelligence can do).

The great problem in bioethics as elsewhere is getting the right premises and points of rational departure, and no one has ever proposed good procedures for doing that. In any case, it is by no means easy to think well, especially about those bioethical issues that are new and whose understanding cannot readily draw on accumulated human experience. Nor is it easy for any of us to see how our tacit political and social ideologies, lurking just below the surface, are pulling the strings of our "rational" thought. Being right and being rational are not necessarily synonymous. The careful and painstaking analysis characteristic of good philosophical work is no guarantee of reasonable outcomes, though it can certainly (and sometimes misleadingly) give that impression. Some very bad ideas have been elegantly argued. Nonetheless, with all those qualifications in mind, rationality remains important. Reason can, on occasion, cut through to some truths not reducible to the passions.

Imagination

I reveal myself as a consequentialist by holding that any form of reasoning that does not reflect on the possible consequences and implications of a chain of reasoning is likely to be blind and illusory. Unfortunately, in bioethics it is often almost impossible to know the likely consequences of new technologies or even, at the clinical level, the likely medical outcome of many procedures with individual patients. That is where imagination comes in. We will have to project a future that is little grounded in past experience, or one in which the experience is too limited to be wholly reliable. Nonetheless, if we must act, we will have nothing better to go by. A comprehensive imagination is needed, beginning with the question of the kind of world we want to live in, and how the various imagined scenarios or alternatives will or won't contribute to that world. If a scenario will not contribute, then there should be a presumption against it, not to be overridden because some individuals, or some market considerations, might make it appear attractive. Knowledge of the outcomes

of other technologies can be helpful in that exercise.

Insight

In using the term *insight*, I have two dimensions in mind. One of them is self-insight, attempting to understand one's biases and proclivities and how either might interfere with good judgment by pushing our reasoning and emotions one way rather than another. The other dimension is that of insight into the context of, and cultural background of, the ethical problem. Where did it come from; how is context shaping it; what is its cultural meaning?

While careful personal observation can sometimes do the necessary work here, the social sciences provide a useful source of insight. A memorable instance of that for me, while working on the care of the dying, was an anthropological study of their care by medical residents. The study concluded that patients "died" for the residents when therapy was no longer effective. Death was a function of the available technology, not something that happened to bodies (Muller and Koenig 1988). That insight helped me to grasp the meaning of the "technological imperative" in a clearer way.

A Communitarian Predilection

While I believe that liberal individualism is, in excessively large doses, a poor ideological base for bioethics, it is too much a valuable part of our culture to simply throw out in favor of an alternative ideology, even communitarianism. Instead, the challenge is to put them in tension with each other, understanding that on some occasions prudence and good judgment will decisively go one way or the other, and on other occasions there will be a compromise blend. The main point though is that communitarianism must be allowed to be a strong competitor—permitted, in fact, to make the opening bid in framing the issues. By the "opening bid" I simply mean that the *first* ethical question always to be raised should bear on the potential societal and cultural impact of a possible decision. While this approach is most evidently important with new technologies that can have major social implications (e.g., germ line therapy), it is no less applicable with the classical problems of individual patient choices and doctor-patient relationships. The fact that they present themselves as individual problems does not mean that they do not, in reality, have social implications. Those implications should always be sought out. Moreover, it is important to be able to interpret some principles assumed to be individualist in a communitarian way, as I will shortly try to show with "principlism."

Let me define what I mean by *communitarianism*. In fashioning a definition, the dominant image is one I take from ecology. The important question for ecologists when new species are introduced into an existing environment is not just how well they will flourish individually, but what they will do to the network of other species. Will they live in harmony with them, perhaps improving the whole ensemble, or will they prove destructive? Or will they perhaps do a little of both? The function of communitarianism is to force us to ask the ecology question, now brought into the realm of ethics. While I will use the example of new technologies and their dissemination as my main examples, a more extended analysis would encompass the full range of the ethical problems of contemporary medicine.

Communitarianism, as I construe the term, is meant to characterize a way of thinking about ethical problems. It is not meant to provide a formula or a set of rigid criteria for solving them. That is why I opened this essay with an emphasis on "analytical virtues" and on asking the right questions rather than on ethical theory

as ordinarily understood. Communitarianism might best be understood as a stance or a way of framing issues. Thereafter, the analytic virtues I sketched above will come into play, offering no sure guide to good decisions, but instead the ingredients of a prudential richness that the mainline philosophical theories usually overshadow.

Here are some key categories to flesh out my understanding of communitarianism.

Human nature. Human beings are social animals. They always exist in a network of other people and within the social institutions and culture of their society.

The public and the private. No sharp distinction can be drawn between the public and private spheres. The private sphere is a fluctuating social construct with few if any intrinsic contents of its own. Although it is important that there be a private sphere, to protect against undue encroachments of public pressure and to acknowledge the diversity of human tastes, values, and ways of life, what counts as private will be a societal decision.

The welfare of the whole. Just as a sensitive ecologist will take the whole of a natural environment or landscape as the point of departure, so too a communitarian will begin with the welfare of a society as a whole as the analogous starting point—understanding "welfare" in the broadest sense, as encompassing the traditions, political institutions, characteristic practices and values, and culture commitments of a society.

Human rights. Every society needs a set of recognized individual rights, both negative and positive. They are imperative as a solid source of resistance to the power of government or public opinion when it goes awry. They also establish the moral standing of individuals, and thus serve to provide a sense of security in their thoughts and actions. At the same time, few human rights are unlimited. They can come in conflict with each other, requiring a choice or efforts at achieving some kind of reasonable balance. For example, some claims of reproductive rights, such as cloning, can threaten the right of a child to its own genetic future. A right to health care without limits in the face of scarce resources can threaten the health needs of others.

Democratic participation. When biomedical developments, theoretical or applied, are likely to affect the community as a whole, including its traditional values, then it is appropriate to initiate a community discussion of the human good, understood comprehensively. A society that avoids confronting the nature of the human good sets itself up to be influenced by the biomedical developments in ways beyond its control and direction. Every member of the community ought to have a part in these discussions, and be allowed to speak the language most congenial to their religious or secular values. The notion that "public reasons" only should count in the public square amounts to empowering groups whose culture easily make that possible at the expense of those which don't. In any case, wholly sectarian positions, though they should have an accepted place in democratic decision-making, are not likely to be efficacious in pluralistic societies.

Individual good and common good. The relationship between individual good and common good is an old issue. When analyzing the introduction of new technologies or the deployment of old ones, a communitarian predilection will require that the very first questions be asked from a communitarian perspective. What will the technology mean for all of us together? The next questions will address what the technology's meaning for individuals will be, and whether (1) the technology is sufficiently compatible with the common good to permit its use, and (2) if the technology is not wholly compatible, whether it should nonetheless be permitted on the grounds that a good society may on occasion permit potential harms to itself in the name of accommodating the special needs of some of its citizens.

Such an approach to biomedical technology would effectively turn upside down the working presumption of liberal individualism when evaluating technology. That presumption can be formulated as a general if not always articulated rule: if a new technology is desired by some individuals, they have a right to that technology unless hard evidence (not speculative possibilities) can be advanced showing that it will be harmful; since no such evidence can be advanced with technologies not yet deployed and in use, therefore the technology may be deployed.

This rule in effect means that the rest of us are held hostage by the desires of individuals and by the overwhelming bias of liberal individualism toward technology, which creates a presumption in its favor that is exceedingly difficult to combat. Such an argument has been used by some supporters of reproductive cloning, who invented heart-wringing scenarios designed to show that it would help some infertile people or help make up for the death of a loved one. Speculative objections were at first put aside, and it was only with the appearance of considerable evidence of harm to animals that even early proponents gave way. At no point, however, was a case advanced that cloning would make a contribution to the overall welfare of our society or any other—only the supposed good of some would-be parents was at stake, and not even their children.

Converting Individualistic Principles to Communitarian Principles

I want to propose, in closing, that many well-accepted principles reflecting a commitment to liberal individualism can be converted into communitarian principles, and that they will be the richer for it. Principlism, for example, has been one of the most widely used methodological tools for the resolution of ethical dilemmas. It has been presented as a set of middle-level principles, of more utility than high-level principles, such as deontology and utilitarianism. While much criticized over the years, principlism has managed to survive, and it has been particularly popular with clinicians and others who want a relatively clear and simple way of thinking through ethical problems. Principlism has seemed to meet those needs, and it is usually presented as a non-ideological methodology.

In practice, however, principlism is an expression of liberal individualism. Its four principles are meant to cover the major ethical considerations that should bear on clinical and policy-making decisions. In reality, autonomy turns out to be king: all the other principles lead back to it, and the interpretation of the principles is classically liberal. Autonomy as interpreted by principlism enshrines the right to make one's own decisions, but assiduously avoids specifying a means of evaluating the ethical content of those decisions; nonmaleficence, aiming to protect patients from harm, is a variant of the autonomy principle, emphasizing negative liberty, the right of bodily noninterference; the point of justice as a principle is to ensure a sufficiently fair share of social and medical resources, such that individuals are free to make efficacious autonomous judgments in living their lives, unhampered by social inequities; and beneficence comes down to assisting people to be treated fairly and empowered to live their autonomous lives. It is no wonder that of all the principles, beneficence is the most neglected. For it to be taken with full seriousness would require coming to some judgment about what is actually beneficial to people. And that would mean crossing the brightest of all liberal lines, moving into the taboo territory of "the human good," about which too many bad things cannot be said.

Each of these principles admits of a communitarian translation. Autonomy should be broadened to encompass an analysis of what constitutes morally good and bad free choices. The claim that so-called private choices should be exempt from moral analysis is the death of ethics. Private choices can be right and wrong, good and bad, and at the least, we benefit from the moral counsel and judgment of our fellow citizens. How ought I to live? That question is

an ancient part of ethics, not to be neutered by designations of private choice. Those private choices will determine in great part our view of how we ought to live together.

Non-maleficence should encompass an analysis of those harms other than physical that can be done to people, threats to their values and social relationships, for instance—that is, the making of judgments about what truly harms people in the broadest sense of "harms." Beneficence should include an effort, requiring community reflection and support, to determine just what constitutes the good of individuals, even if that means trespassing into the forbidden territory of comprehensive theories of the human good. Justice, finally, requires a judgment not only about what constitutes a fair distribution of health care resources but must—in the face of scarce resources—also determine just what constitutes appropriate resources, among those already available for distribution or those that could be created by research advances. If, for instance, we are interested in a fair allocation of future resources, what kind of a research agenda for what kind of medical progress would most promote it?

As these suggestions should make clear, I understand communitarianism to include a social rather than individual starting point for ethical analysis, but also a solid place for substantive reflection and judgment about ends and goals—and that is its greatest strength. Liberal individualism works overtime to avoid substantive analysis and judgment. Communitarianism goes in just the opposite direction, embracing the hardest and deepest questions about the right uses of medical knowledge and technology. Given their power to change the way we live our lives, and to understand our own nature, nothing else will suffice.

The greatest fear of liberal individualism is authoritarianism. But that fear, reasonable enough, fails to take account of the fact that the power of technology, and the profit to be made from it, can control and manipulate us even more effectively than authoritarianism. Moral dictators can be seen and overthrown, but technological repression steals up on us, visible but with an innocent countenance, and is just about impossible to overthrow, even as we see it doing its work on us. Liberal individualism makes this scenario more easily possible, and that is why it is not a tolerable guide to the sensible use of medical knowledge and technology.

It is just possible as well that a stronger place for communitarianism in our society will help to dampen the cultural war that has broken out in bioethics. A well-formulated communitarianism will not be indifferent to the rights and values of individuals; it will make room for them. In that respect, it need not worry political liberals as much as it does. A stronger appreciation of communitarianism could also hope to open up a stronger dialogue with conservative thought. Conservative thought is willing to take seriously the notion of a human good and of the need for substantive inquiry into the nature of good and evil in scientific progress and technological innovation. The liberal individualism of much contemporary bioethics needs to take seriously that way of thinking. Without it, bioethics risks being empty and leaving everyone else at the mercy of biomedical developments that will have their way with us. It should be the other way around.

References

Beauchamp, T., and J. Childress. 2001. *Principles of biomedical ethics*, 5th ed. New York: Oxford Univ. Press.

Muller, J. H., and B. Koenig. 1988. On the boundary of life and death: The definition of dying by medical residents. In *Biomedicine examined*, ed. M. Lock and D. Gordon. Dordrecht: Kluwer Academic; 351–374.

President's Council on Bioethics. 2002. *Human cloning and human dignity.* New York: Public Affairs.

7. Principles of Biomedical Ethics

Beauchamp and Childress identify the following principles of biomedical ethics: Respect for Autonomy, Nonmaleficence, Beneficence and Justice.

Respect for Autonomy

(Originally *Autonomy*) Protects every human being's right to act or allow acting on it, fully informed of potential risks, consequences and damage that such action might implicate. However, at the same time, autonomy states the obligation to respect that right, which will become a difficult problem for principlism.

Beauchamp and Childress say:

> Although we begin our discussion of principles of biomedical ethics with respect for autonomy, our order of presentation does not imply that this principle has moral priority over other principles. We do not hold, as some critics suggest, that the principle for respect for autonomy overrides all other

moral considerations. Furthermore, we attempt to show that, in a properly structured theory, respect for autonomy is not excessively individualistic (thereby neglecting the social nature of individuals and the impact of individual choices and actions on others), not excessively focused on reason (thereby neglecting the emotions) and not unduly legalistic (thereby highlighting legal rights and downplaying social practices and responsibilities).[1]

Thus, we can see in this principle two basic requirements of freedom which are shared by several doctrinal currents: individual autonomy and intentionality. Autonomy implies a power and an appetite; namely, the ability to make decisions and the will to do it. This means that autonomy require a certain understanding on the value of choice. On the other hand, intentionality involves a deliberative consciousness and the capacity for self-determination. Hence, according to Beauchamp and Childress, autonomy also means the right to hold views,

---

1   Beauchamp, T. and Childress, J., *Principles of Biomedical Ethics,* 7th Edition, New York-Oxford, Oxford University Press, 2012, p. 101.

make choices and take actions based on personal values and beliefs.

The authors identify seven rules of autonomy: Information, Intentionality, Understanding, Consciousness, Voluntariness, No external coercion, and Surrogate decision. These rules, procedurally speaking, become real conditions of possibility to meet what the principle of respect for autonomy orders. When these seven rules are specified, we can observe more concrete norms that point out positive and negative obligations. Among the positive obligation we have rules such as respectful treatment, disclosure, foster autonomous decision making, tell the truth, respect the privacy of others, protect confidential information, obtain consent for interventions with patients, when asked, help others make important decisions, and know and consider patient's personal history. As negative obligations we can recognize no external constraints and no external intervention.

Now, the renaming of this principle deserves some consideration. Beauchamp and Childress realized that the original principle of autonomy led to many controversies, mainly since it could be understood as the absolute freedom of the patient to decide and impose his/her decision. However, that does not happen in practice because of the paternalistic culture of science and medicine. Many times the decisions of patients, when they were inconsistent with the decisions of scientists and doctors, are not taken into account. Thus, to establish a greater consistency between theory and the actual application of the principle, Beauchamp and Childress narrowed the epistemological and procedural scope of principle by renaming it "Respect for Autonomy."

Therefore, the authors argue that we should not understand individual autonomy as an absolute and unilateral power, but as a capability or competence characterized by detailed information, understanding of the essential things and absence of coercion. Thereby, respect for autonomy does not only establish a binding obligation (which the authors call a positive obligation) but also the individual right of the patient to be independent in his decisions, implicit in what Beauchamp and Childress call negative obligation.

The fundamental requirement is to respect a particular person's autonomous choices, whatever they may be. Respect for autonomy is not a mere *ideal* in health care; it is a professional *obligation*. Autonomous choice is a *right*—not a *duty*—of patients. However, obligations to respect autonomy do not extend to persons who cannot act in sufficiently autonomous manner (and those who cannot be rendered autonomous), because they are immature, incapacitated, ignorant, coerced, or exploited, for instance, infants, suicidal individuals, and drug-dependent patients.

Nonmaleficence

This principle superimposes the moral obligation of not doing harm over doing good. Moreover, it shows that duty is to never hurt, either physically or morally, human beings, and to avoid, at all costs, actions that may involve some damage to them.

The first point is very important, and Beauchamp and Childress stress it:

> Obligations not to harm others are sometimes more stringent than obligations to help them, but the reverse is also true. If in a particular case a health care provider inflicts a very minor injury (swelling from a needlestick, say), then we consider the obligation of beneficence to take priority over the obligation of nonmaleficence. The point is that causing some risks of surgical harm, introducing social costs to protect the public health, and placing burdens on some research subjects can all be justified by the benefits of the actions.[2]

---

2   Ibid., p. 151.

Based on the thesis of Frankena, Beauchamp and Childress make a distinction between Nonmaleficence and Beneficence, because they think the two principles should not be understood as one. Frankena divides the principle of beneficence into four general obligations (which in some cases may be ranked depending of the specific situation):

1. One ought not to inflict evil or harm (what is bad).
2. One ought to prevent evil or harm.
3. One ought to remove evil.
4. One ought to do or promote good.[3]

Beauchamp and Childress agreed with the enunciation of these obligations, but they do not believe that all of them mean beneficence. Their main reason is that the obligation of doing good is not morally equivalent with the obligation of not doing harm, so in a medical and clinical context, the first obligation would be more binding than the other three, because it implies the duty of never inflicting harm or hurting someone; namely, to respect the maxim *primum non nocere*. Therefore, they rearranged the obligations as follows:

Nonmaleficence

1. One ought not to inflict evil or harm.

Beneficence

2. One ought to prevent evil or harm.
3. One ought to remove evil or harm.
4. One ought to do or promote good.

The obligation of not doing harm implies a moral correctness criterion, which is morally higher than the obligation of simply doing good. However, the intention of Beauchamp and Childress is not to support a superiority of the principle of nonmaleficence over beneficence but to explain that the obligation of doing good is epistemologically and procedurally related to the obligation of not doing evil. In my view, this creates a complex problem and a clear contradiction. Let's see.

Sometimes, the obligation of doing good may be tragically contradicted with the obligation of not doing evil since both involve principles that are *prima facie*. Therefore, we lack, at least in theory, some plausible criterion to rank them. Can we force the patient to bear the heavy burden of treatment (nonmaleficence) to preserve his life (beneficence), at the cost of an acute and constant suffering and relentless deterioration? Is there a contradiction between the right to dignity (dignified life) and the duty to protect, preserve and promote life? Should physicians continue that kind of treatment, at any cost, regardless of the patient's wishes? Is a disproportionate medical treatment that only prolongs the agony of terminally ill patients, legitimate? If the therapeutic means are useless or ineffective and their application causes the patient acute suffering, must we continue with them until the end? Is death always harmful? If we respond to these questions affirmatively, we would have to accept that nonmaleficence is, *a priori* and by definition, superior to beneficence since the obligation of not harming would imply a greater moral objectivity than doing good, because it would protect higher values like life. However, in some circumstances, and in the name of beneficence, these values could be transformed into abstract concepts whose dogmatic and intolerant defense could cause great suffering to a person. Only when the detriment is minor, the obligation of beneficence should take precedence over the obligation of nonmaleficence. We can see this clearer if we consider the negative rules of nonmaleficence: 1. Never hurt; 2. Do no harm patients either physically or psychologically; 3. Do not impose the risk of harm; 4. Do not kill; 5. Do not cause pain or suffering; 6. Do not incapacitate; 7. Do

---

3 Frankena, William, *Ethics*, Second Edition, New Jersey, Prentice Hall, 1973, p. 47.

not cause offense; 8. Do not deprive others of the goods of life.

Therefore, nonmaleficence and beneficence could only be justified as separate principles if we understand the former as a duty, and the latter as an individual right. Thus, the collision between them could be resolved by imposing nonmaleficence over beneficence, because nonmaleficence implies binding obligations which are grounded in the protection and promotion of universally accepted values, eg, life. Therefore, under certain circumstances, an individual could be required to waive his right to beneficence because his particular understanding about what good is cannot prevail over what has been socially agreed as such. Otherwise, if we consider both nonmaleficence and beneficence as duties, it will be very difficult to find plausible criteria to rank them when they come into conflict.

Beneficence

Beneficence implies that every person is ensured to receive appropriate care. For Beauchamp and Childress the essence of morality is contained in this principle: doing good. This duty is not only a conventional obligation but part of human nature and an essential tendency of human beings. However, beneficence, besides being a personal option, is also an obligation. In this sense, these authors attempt to separate the concept of beneficence from benevolence, understanding the former not merely as an act of charity or an ideal of virtue, but as the positive duty to:

1. Protect and defend the rights of others.
2. Prevent harm from occurring to others.
3. Remove conditions that will cause harm to others.
4. Help persons with disabilities.
5. Rescue persons in danger.

Nevertheless, these obligations are not absolute, because each individual could only partially fulfill them; that is, no one is capable of doing all the good that is possible to do. Beauchamp and Childress emphasize this ambiguous character of Beneficence and recognize that "the line between an obligation and moral ideal is often unclear". The case of rule number (1) is eloquent. To protect and defend the rights of others means to defend their autonomy and will. This implies to defend their individual and inalienable right of following a particular life project based on what each person understands by good. However, in the case of principlism we have to understand individual rights as a heteronomous concept; that is, as a prerogative that people cannot perform nor choose by themselves because beneficence is a right that is determined by other criteria, which do not necessarily match with the involved person. This situation is justified by the paternalism doctrine since, in certain cases, when a patient is in an evident risk of suffering harm, it could be warranted to restrict his autonomy and to contradict his personal understanding of beneficence in order to protect him and to respect the duty of always doing good for the patient. In this sense, the principle of beneficence stresses its status of duty over its category of right.

Beauchamp and Childress also distinguish between *Positive beneficence* and utility. *Positive beneficence* requires the action to produce benefits and the presence of an agent who benefits others.

Utility beneficence requires a reasonable balance between risks and benefits involved. However, this distinction shows us that Beauchamp and Childress consider two principles of beneficence where the agent is more important than the patient: *Positive beneficence* requires agents to provide benefits to others. *Utility beneficence* requires that agents balance benefits, risks, and costs to produce the best overall results.

Therefore, we find here a very transcendental problem to bioethical deliberation, which can be posed as a question: Who decides what the good is, the patient or the agent? Is Paternalism acceptable in all cases? Does every human being have the right to freely consider what is good for him, and believe, practice and hold a truth from his cultural and religious identity?

In my view, the obligation to do good must be linked to the obligation of protecting and promoting the legitimate interests of the affected person. It is clear that we cannot force an alive and healthy person to donate his heart to another individual to save his/her life. Nor is it plausible to force someone to give all their property to help many more people who live in poverty. In the same way, it should be clear that in certain circumstances, we should not force individuals to go beyond what they consider good for themselves. That would imply the imposition of supererogatory obligations, which are not always legitimate. Thereby, there are circumstances in which is much more reasonable to respect what each person considers to be good and not to objectify in a paternalistic way the principle of beneficence. Otherwise, the intrinsic definition of the principle of beneficence would reveal a kind of sophism, or at least, a paraconsistent argumentation.

Beneficence implies an altruistic act; namely, thinking about the other, and thus means to do the good for the patient where the good is sometimes what the patient thinks is good for him/her. Therefore, the simple fact of accepting beneficence as a kind of altruism can show us the ambiguity of this principle. Sometimes, paternalism is morally justified. Sometimes, it is not.

Justice

This principle emphasizes the duty to protect a human being from any kind of discrimination that violates his identity, dignity and status as an end in himself, and thus always treats him as an equal. The main orientation of this principle must be to recognize the equality among human beings and provide a fair, equitable and appropriate distribution of benefits and burdens.

However, it is necessary to clarify the requirements of this equality, recognizing, at least, three basic rights that involve the duty to respect them: 1. The right to a physically and psychologically healthy life; 2. The right of access to a proper, adequate and timely medical attention; and 3. The right to have equal opportunities to access the healthcare system.

Nevertheless, and due to the absence of a social consensus about diverse theories of justice, the analysis becomes very complicated. The authors recognize, at least, six kinds of distributive justice:

1. To each person an equal share.
2. To each person according to need.
3. To each person according to effort.
4. To each person according to contribution.
5. To each person according to merit.
6. To each person according to free-market exchanges.

Many theories accept these six principles as valid. Beauchamp and Childress also do so, noting that each of them identifies a *prima facie* obligation but, at the same time, no one has pre-eminence over one another. The problem then is to determine which one has precedence over one another in certain circumstances. Beauchamp and Childress do not consider it possible to accomplish this task without reviewing some classical theories in order to specify and balance these obligations. Thus, they complete a cursory analysis of Utilitarian, Libertarian, Communitarian and Egalitarian theories. While they clarify that they are using these theories as a methodological resource and claim to seek a complementation between these theoretical approaches, they probably have a predilection for Rawl's theory of justice, which implies, according to the authors, two main principles: 1. Each individual's liberty must be compatible, in a similar measure, with the liberty of others, and 2. The fair equality of opportunity must be assured to can accept inequalities in social primary goods. However, Rawls's conception, whatever is its theoretical value, does not resolve the practical problem of balancing the different principles of distributive justice. In this way, the criterion to rank those diverse obligations and rights keep its relative character.

I think that the model chosen by Beauchamp and Childress to support the principle of justice is unable to provide a ranking of the rules that come into play to resolve a conflict. This model only allows us to establish provisional conclusions regarding rights and depending on each particular case; namely, it leads us to an extreme casuistry.

Readings

Beauchamp, Tom L.; Childress, James F., "Respect for Autonomy," in *Principles of Biomedical Ethics*, 7th Edition, Oxford University Press, 2012: **101–120.**

Beauchamp, Tom L.; Childress, James F., "Nonmaleficence," in *Principles of Biomedical Ethics*, 7th Edition, Oxford University Press, 2012: **150–169.**

Beauchamp, Tom L.; Childress, James F., "Beneficence," in *Principles of Biomedical Ethics*, 7th Edition, Oxford University Press, 2012: **202-212.**

Beauchamp, Tom L.; Childress, James F., "Justice," in *Principles of Biomedical Ethics*, 7th Edition, Oxford University Press, 2012: **249-262.**

Study Questions

1. Explain why the principle of respect for autonomy imply rights and obligations.
2. Why does nonmaleficence point out a negative obligation?
3. Identify and explain the main aspects of beneficence.
4. Explain why both nonmaleficence and beneficence imply professional obligations.
5. Why are the rules of justice hard to apply as deliberative criteria?
6. Which principle of biomedical ethics is, according to you, the most important and why.

Respect for Autonomy

Tom L. Beauchamp and James F. Childress

This theory needs more than a convincing account of second-order preferences: It needs a way for ordinary persons to qualify as deserving respect for their autonomy even when they have not reflected on their preferences at a higher level. Few choosers and few choices would be autonomous if held to the standards of higher order reflection in this theory, which presents an aspirational ideal of autonomy. An appropriate test of the adequacy of any theory of autonomy is whether it coheres with the moral requirement that we respect the ways in which we govern our lives, such as the ways we take care of our health and take care of our children, as well as our everyday choices, such as opening bank accounts, purchasing goods in stores, and authorizing repair of an automobile. A theory of autonomy should be kept consistent with pretheoretical assumptions implicit in the principle of respect for autonomy (as analyzed later on pp. 103–05). No theory of autonomy is acceptable if it presents an ideal beyond the reach of normal agents and choosers.

Instead of depicting an ideal of this sort, our analysis of autonomy focuses on nonideal conditions that fit with the moral requirements of "respect for autonomy." We analyze autonomous action in terms of normal choosers who act (1) intentionally, (2) with understanding (see pp. 119–20, 127ff later), and (3) without controlling influences that determine their action (see pp. 132ff later). The first of these three conditions of autonomy is not a matter of degree: Acts are either intentional or nonintentional. However, acts can satisfy both the conditions of understanding and absence of controlling influences to a greater or lesser extent. Actions therefore can be autonomous by degrees, as a function of satisfying these two conditions to different degrees. For both conditions, a broad continuum exists on which autonomy stretches from being fully present to being wholly absent. Many children and many elderly patients, for example, exhibit various degrees of understanding and independence found on this continuum and thus varying degrees of autonomous action.

For an action to qualify as autonomous in our account, it needs only a substantial degree of understanding and freedom from constraint, not a full understanding or a complete absence of influence. To restrict adequate decision making by patients and research subjects to the ideal of fully or completely autonomous decision making strips their acts of any meaningful place in the practical world, where people's actions are rarely, if ever, fully autonomous. A person's appreciation of information and independence from controlling influences in the context of health care need not exceed, for example, a person's information and independence in making a financial investment, hiring a new employee, buying a new house, or deciding to attend a university. Such consequential decisions must be *substantially* autonomous, but being *fully* autonomous is a mythical ideal.

The line between what is substantial and what is insubstantial may appear arbitrary. However, thresholds marking substantially autonomous decisions can be carefully fixed in light of specific objectives such as meaningful decision making. Patients and research subjects can achieve substantial autonomy in their decisions, just as substantially autonomous choice occurs in other areas of life such as buying a car. The appropriate criteria for substantial autonomy are best addressed in a particular context.

Autonomy, Authority, and Community

Some theorists argue that autonomous action is incompatible with the authority of governments, religious organizations, and other communities that prescribe behavior. They maintain that autonomous persons must act on their own reasons and can never submit to an authority or choose to be ruled by others without losing their autonomy.[5] We believe, however, that no fundamental inconsistency exists between autonomy and authority if individuals exercise their autonomy in choosing to accept an institution, tradition, or community that they view as a legitimate source of direction.

Choosing to follow medical authority is a prime example. Other examples are a Jehovah's Witness who accepts the authority of that tradition and who refuses a recommended blood transfusion, and a Roman Catholic who accepts the authority of the church and chooses against an abortion. That persons share moral principles

with authoritative institutions does not prevent these principles from being autonomously accepted, even when these principles derive from cultural tradition and institutional authority. If a Jehovah's Witness who insists on adhering to the doctrines of his faith in refusing a blood transfusion is deemed nonautonomous, and therefore unworthy of respect, many of our choices based on our confidence in institutional authority will be deemed unworthy of respect. In our judgment, a theory of autonomy that takes this course is morally unacceptable.

We encounter many problems of autonomy in medical contexts because of the patient's dependent condition and the medical professional's authoritative position. On some occasions authority and autonomy are incompatible, but not because the two *concepts* are incompatible. Conflict arises because authority has not been properly delegated or accepted. In these circumstances, the patient's autonomy is sometimes compromised because the physician has assumed an unwarranted degree of authority, as in certain paternalistic actions.

Some critics of the prominent role played by autonomy in biomedical ethics question the model of an independent, rational will that is inattentive to emotions, communal life, reciprocity, and the development of persons over time. They charge that such an account of autonomy focuses too narrowly on the self as independent and rationally controlling. For instance, some feminist critics fault theories that place an overriding value on autonomy or fail to see communal relationships involved in acting autonomously.[6]

Some feminists have sought to affirm autonomy but to interpret it through relationships. These conceptions of "relational autonomy" derive from the conviction that persons' identities are shaped through social relationships and complex intersecting social determinants, such as race, class, gender, ethnicity, and authority structures. These accounts see persons as interdependent, but they also caution that "oppressive socialization and oppressive social relationships" can impair autonomy, for instance, through forming an agent's desires, beliefs, emotions, and attitudes and through thwarting the development of the capacities and competencies essential for autonomy.[7] Such a relational conception of autonomy is illuminating and defensible as long as it does not neglect or obscure the main features of autonomy that we analyze in this chapter.

The Principle of Respect for Autonomy

To respect autonomous agents is to acknowledge their right to hold views, to make choices, and to take actions based on their personal values and beliefs. Such respect involves respectful *action*, not merely a respectful *attitude*. It requires more than noninterference in others' personal affairs. It includes, in some contexts, building up or maintaining others' capacities for autonomous choice while helping to allay fears and other conditions that destroy or disrupt autonomous action. Respect, in this account, involves acknowledging the value and decision-making rights of persons and enabling them to act autonomously, whereas disrespect for autonomy involves attitudes and actions that ignore, insult, demean, or are inattentive to others' rights of autonomous action.

Why is such respect owed to autonomous persons? In Chapter 9, we examine the theories of two philosophers who have powerfully influenced contemporary interpretations of respect for autonomy: Immanuel Kant and John Stuart Mill. Kant argued that respect for autonomy flows from the recognition that all persons have unconditional worth, each having the capacity to determine his or her own moral destiny.[8] To violate a person's autonomy is to treat that person merely as a means; that is, in accordance with others' goals without regard to that person's own goals. Mill concerned himself primarily with the "individuality" of autonomous agents. He argued that society should permit individuals to

develop according to their own convictions, as long as they do not interfere with a like expression of freedom by others or unjustifiably harm others; but he also insisted that we sometimes have an obligation to persuade others when they have false or ill-considered views.[9] Mill's position requires both not interfering with and actively strengthening autonomous expression, whereas Kant's position entails a moral imperative of respectful treatment of persons as ends in themselves. In their different ways, these two philosophers both support a principle of respect for autonomy (although Kant is largely concerned with *morally* correct autonomous choices).

The principle of respect for autonomy can be stated as a negative obligation and as a positive obligation. As a *negative* obligation: Autonomous actions should not be subjected to controlling constraints by others. This demand asserts a broad, abstract obligation that is free of exceptive clauses such as "We must respect individuals' views and rights so long as their thoughts and actions do not seriously harm other persons." Of course, the principle of respect for autonomy needs specification in particular contexts to function as a practical guide to conduct, and appropriate specification will incorporate valid exceptions. This process of specification will affect rights and obligations of liberty, privacy, confidentiality, truthfulness, and informed consent (several of which receive sustained attention in subsequent chapters).

As a *positive* obligation, this principle requires both respectful treatment in disclosing information and actions that foster autonomous decision making. Many autonomous actions could not occur without others' material cooperation in making options available. Respect for autonomy obligates professionals in health care and research involving human subjects to disclose information, to probe for and ensure understanding and voluntariness, and to foster adequate decision making. As some contemporary Kantians declare, the demand that we treat others as ends requires that we assist them in achieving their ends and foster their capacities as agents, not merely that we avoid treating them solely as means to our ends.[10]

Temptations arise in health care for physicians and other professionals to foster or perpetuate patients' dependency, rather than to promote their autonomy. But discharging the obligation to respect patients' autonomy requires enabling patients to overcome their sense of dependence and to achieve as much control as they desire. These positive obligations of respect for autonomy derive in part from the special fiduciary obligations that health care professionals have to their patients and researchers to their subjects.

These negative and positive sides of respect for autonomy are capable of supporting many more specific moral rules. (Other principles, such as beneficence and nonmaleficence, help justify some of these same rules.) Examples include the following:

1. Tell the truth.
2. Respect the privacy of others.
3. Protect confidential information.
4. Obtain consent for interventions with patients.
5. When asked, help others make important decisions.

Respect for autonomy has only prima facie standing, and competing moral considerations sometimes can override this principle. Examples include the following: If our choices endanger the public health, potentially harm innocent others, or require a scarce resource for which no funds are available, others can justifiably restrict our exercises of autonomy. The principle of respect for autonomy does not by itself determine what a person ought to be free to know or do or what counts as a valid justification for constraining autonomy. For example, a patient with an inoperable, incurable carcinoma once asked, "I don't have cancer, do I?" The physician lied, saying, "You're as good as you were ten years ago." This lie denies the patient information that he may need to determine his future course of action, thereby infringing the principle of respect for autonomy. Although the matter is controversial,

the lie may be justified (by a principle of beneficence) if we posit certain major benefits to the patient. (See our discussions of paternalism in Chapter 6 and veracity in Chapter 8.)

Our obligations to respect autonomy do not extend to persons who cannot act in a sufficiently autonomous manner (and who cannot be rendered autonomous) because they are immature, incapacitated, ignorant, coerced, or exploited. Infants, irrationally suicidal individuals, and drug-dependent patients are examples.

The Triumph or Failure of Respect for Autonomy?

Some writers lament the "triumph of autonomy" in American bioethics. They charge that autonomy's proponents sometimes disrespect patients by forcing them to make choices, even though many patients do not want to receive information about their condition or to make decisions. Carl Schneider claims that proponents of autonomy, whom he labels "autonomists," concern themselves less with what patients *do want* than with what, from the point of view of autonomy, they *should want*. He attempts to correct these views by appealing to human experience and empirical research. He concludes that, "while patients largely wish to be informed about their medical circumstances, a substantial number of them [especially the elderly and the very sick] do not want to make their own medical decisions, or perhaps even to participate in those decisions in any very significant way."[11]

The duty of respect for autonomy that we defend has a correlative *right* to choose, not a mandatory *duty* to choose. Several empirical studies of the sort cited by Schneider seem, like him, to misunderstand how autonomous choice functions in a theory such as ours and how it should function in clinical medicine. In one study, UCLA researchers examined the differences in the attitudes of elderly subjects (sixty-five years or older) from different ethnic backgrounds toward (a) disclosure of the diagnosis and prognosis of a terminal illness, and (b) decision making at the end of life. The researchers summarize their main findings, based on 800 subjects (200 from each ethnic group): "Korean Americans (47%) and Mexican Americans (65%) were significantly less likely than European Americans (87%) and African Americans (88%) to believe that a patient should be told the diagnosis of metastatic cancer. Korean Americans (35%) and Mexican Americans (48%) were less likely than African Americans (63%) to believe that a patient should be told of a terminal prognosis and less likely to believe that the patient should make decisions about the use of life-supporting technology (28% and 41% vs. 60% and 65%). Korean Americans and Mexican Americans tended to believe that the family should make decisions about the use of life support." Investigators in this study stress that "belief in the *ideal* of patient autonomy is far from universal" (italics added), and they contrast that ideal with a "family-centered model" focused on an individual's web of relationships and "the harmonious functioning of the family."[12]

However, this statement is misleading in light of the actual data. The investigators themselves conclude that "physicians should ask their patients if they wish to receive information and make decisions or if they prefer that their families handle such matters." Far from abandoning or supplanting the moral demand that we respect individual autonomy, this recommendation accepts its central condition that the choice is rightly the patient's. Even if the patient delegates that right to someone else, the choice to delegate can itself be autonomous.

In a second study, this time of Navajo values and ways of thinking regarding the disclosure of risk and medical prognoses, two researchers sought to determine how health care providers "should approach the discussion of negative information with Navajo patients" to provide "more culturally appropriate medical care." Frequent conflicts emerge, these researchers report, between autonomy and the traditional

Navajo conception that "thought and language have the power to shape reality and to control events." According to the traditional conception, telling a Navajo patient who has recently been diagnosed with a disease the potential complications of that disease may actually produce those complications, because "language does not merely describe reality, language shapes reality." Traditional Navajo patients may tend to process negative information as potentially harmful to them. They expect a "positive ritual language that promotes or restores health.

One middle-aged Navajo nurse reported that a surgeon explained the risks of bypass surgery to her father in such a way that he refused to undergo the procedure: "The surgeon told him that he may not wake up, that this is the risk of every surgery. For the surgeon it was very routine, but the way that my Dad received it, it was almost like a death sentence, and he never consented to the surgery." The researchers therefore found "ethically troublesome" those policies that, in compliance with the Patient Self-Determination Act, attempt to "expose all hospitalized Navajo patients to the idea, if not the practice, of advance care planning."[13]

These two studies and numerous others enrich our understanding of diverse cultural beliefs and values that affect what particular communities and individuals believe and do. However, several studies reflect a misinterpretation of what the principle of respect for autonomy and many laws and policies require. They mistakely view their results as opposing rather than enriching the principle of respect for autonomy. A fundamental obligation exists to ensure that patients have the right to choose, as well as the right to accept or to decline information. Forced information and forced choice are inconsistent with this obligation. From this perspective, a tension exists between the two studies just discussed. One study recommends inquiring in advance to ascertain patients' preferences regarding information and decision making, whereas the other suggests (tenuously) that even informing certain patients of a right to decide may cause harm.

The practical question is whether it is possible to inform patients of their rights to know and to decide without compromising their systems of belief and values and without otherwise disrespecting them.

Health professionals should always inquire in general terms about their patients' wishes to receive information and to make decisions, and they should never assume that because a patient belongs to a particular community or culture, he or she affirms that community's worldview and values. The fundamental requirement is to respect a particular person's autonomous choices, whatever they may be. Respect for autonomy is not a mere *ideal* in health care; it is a professional *obligation*. Autonomous choice is a *right*—not a *duty*—of patients.

Complexities in Respecting Autonomy

Varieties of autonomous consent. The basic paradigm of autonomy in health care, research, politics, and other contexts is *express* consent. However, this paradigm captures only one form of consent. Another form is *tacit* consent, which people express silently or passively by omissions. For example, if the staff of a long-term care facility asks residents whether they object to having the time of dinner changed by one hour, a uniform lack of objection constitutes consent (assuming the residents understand the proposal and the need for their consent). Similarly, *implicit* or *implied* consent is often inferable from actions. Consent to a medical procedure may be implicit in a specific consent to another procedure, and providing general consent to treatment at a teaching hospital may imply consent to various roles for physicians, nurses, and others in training. *Presumed* consent reduces to either implied or express consent if consent is presumed on the basis of what we know about a particular person's choices or values. By contrast. presuming consent on the basis of a general theory of human goods or of the rational will is morally perilous. Consent should refer to an individual's actual choices, not to presumptions about the choices the individual would or should make.

Nonmaleficence

Tom L. Beauchamp and James F. Childress

Different conceptions of consent have appeared in teaching medical students how to perform intimate examinations, especially pelvic and rectal examinations.[14] Often medical students have learned and practiced on anesthetized patients, many of whom have not given their explicit informed consent. For instance, many teaching hospitals have allowed one or two medical students to participate in the examination of women who are under anesthesia in preparation for surgery. Anesthetized patients have been considered ideal for teaching medical students how to perform a pelvic examination because the patients are relaxed and would not feel any mistakes. When questioned, some directors of obstetrics and gynecology programs have pointed to the patient's general consent provided on entering a teaching hospital. Such general consent typically authorizes medical students and residents to participate in patients' care for teaching and learning purposes. However, this consent does not specify which procedures might involve participation by medical students.

It is debatable whether general consent is sufficient or whether specific, express, informed consent is necessary in these circumstances. We often seek specific informed consent when a procedure is invasive, as in the case of surgery, or when it is risky. Although pelvic examinations are not invasive by comparison to surgery, or particularly risky, patients may object to the invasion of their bodies for others' purposes, in this case for education and training. Some women readily consent to the participation of medical students in such examinations, but others view it as a violation of their dignity and privacy. One commentator rightly stresses that "the patient must be treated as the student's teacher, not as a training tool."[15]

Determining appropriate consent in particular circumstances may require giving different weights to the different values. Using anesthetized women with general consent may be efficient, but, in view of the importance of respect for autonomy, there are ethically preferable alternatives, such as using anesthetized patients who have given informed consent or using healthy volunteers who are willing to serve as trainers or models. Either of these alternatives respects personal autonomy and avoids negative medical education. A study of medical students in the Philadelphia area found that the practice of conducting pelvic exams on anesthetized patients without specific informed consent desensitized physicians to the need for patients to give their consent before medical students undertake such procedures. For students who had finished an obstetrics/gynecology clerkship, consent was significantly less important (51%) than for students who had not completed a clerkship (70%). The authors conclude that "to avoid this decline in attitudes toward seeking consent, clerkship directors should ensure that students perform examinations only after patients have given consent explicitly."[16]

William Frankena, for example, divides the principle of beneficence into four general obligations, the first of which we identify as the obligation of nonmaleficence and the other three of which we refer to as principles and obligations of beneficence:

1. One ought not to inflict evil or harm.
2. One ought to prevent evil or harm.
3. One ought to remove evil or harm.
4. One ought to do or promote good.[3]

If we bring the ideas of benefiting others and not injuring them under a single principle, we will be forced to note, as does Frankena, the several distinct obligations embedded in this general principle. In our view, conflating nonmaleficence and beneficence into a single principle obscures important distinctions. Obligations not to harm others (e.g., those prohibiting theft, disablement, and killing) are distinct from obligations to help others (e.g., those prescribing the provision of benefits, protection of interests, and promotion of welfare).

Obligations not to harm others are sometimes more stringent than obligations to help them, but the reverse is also true. If in a particular case a health care provider inflicts a very minor injury (swelling from a needlestick, say), but simultaneously provides a major benefit (a lifesaving intervention, say), then we consider the obligation of beneficence to take priority over the obligation of nonmaleficence.[4] The point is that causing some risks of surgical harm, introducing social costs to protect the public health,

and placing burdens on some research subjects can all be justified by the benefits of the actions.

One might try to reformulate the idea of nonmaleficence's increased stringency as follows: Generally, obligations of nonmaleficence are more stringent than obligations of beneficence, and, in some cases, nonmaleficence overrides beneficence, even if the best utilitarian outcome would be obtained by acting beneficently. If a surgeon, for example, could save two innocent lives by killing a prisoner on death row to retrieve his heart and liver for transplantation, this outcome would have the highest net utility (in the circumstances), but the surgeon's action would be morally indefensible. This formulation of the stringency of nonmaleficence has an initial ring of plausibility, especially if the act of benefiting involves committing a moral wrong. Again, however, we should be cautious about constructing axioms of priority. A beneficial action does not necessarily take second place to an act of not causing harm. Nonmaleficence typically overrides other principles, but the weights of these moral principles vary in different circumstances. In our view, no rule in ethics favors avoiding harm over providing benefit in *all* circumstances. The claim that an order of priority exists among elements 1 through 4 in Frankena's scheme mentioned earlier is therefore unsustainable.

Rather than attempting to structure a hierarchical ordering, we group the principles of nonmaleficence and beneficence into four norms that (a priori) lack hierarchical ordering:

Nonmaleficence

1. One ought not to inflict evil or harm.

Beneficence

2. One ought to prevent evil or harm.
3. One ought to remove evil or harm.
4. One ought to do or promote good.

Each of the three principles of beneficence requires taking action by *helping*— preventing harm, removing harm, and promoting good— whereas nonmaleficence preventing requires only *intentionally refraining* from actions that cause harm. Rules of nonmaleficence therefore take the form "Do not do X." Some philosophers accept only principles or rules that take this proscriptive form. They even limit rules of respect for autonomy to rules of the form "Do not interfere with a person's autonomous choices." These philosophers reject all principles or rules that require helping, assisting, or rescuing other persons (although they recognize these norms as legitimate *moral ideals)*. Mainstream moral philosophy, however, does not accept such a *sharp* distinction between obligations of refraining from harming and obligations of helping and, instead, recognizes and preserves the relevant distinctions in other ways. We take this same path, and in Chapter 6 we explain further the nature of the distinction.

Legitimate disagreements arise about how to classify actions under categories 1 through 4, as well as about the nature and stringency of the obligations that arise from them. Consider the following case: Robert McFall was dying of aplastic anemia, and his physicians recommended a bone marrow transplant from a genetically compatible donor to increase his chances of living one additional year from twenty-five percent to a range of forty to sixty percent. The patient's cousin, David Shimp, agreed to undergo tests to determine his suitability as a donor. After completing the test for tissue compatibility, he refused to undergo the test for genetic compatibility. He had changed his mind about donation. Robert McFall's lawyer asked a court to compel Shimp to undergo the second test and donate his bone marrow if the test indicated a good match.[5]

Public discussion focused on whether Shimp had an obligation of beneficence toward McFall in the form of an obligation to prevent harm, to remove harm, or to promote McFall's welfare. McFall's lawyer contended (unsuccessfully) that even if Shimp did not have a legal obligation of beneficence to rescue his cousin, he did have a legal obligation of nonmaleficence, which required that he not make McFall's situation worse. The lawyer argued that when Shimp agreed to undergo the first test and then backed out, he caused a "delay of critical proportions" that constituted a violation of the obligation of nonmaleficence. The judge ruled that Shimp did not violate any legal obligations but also held that his actions were "morally indefensible."[6]

This case illustrates difficulties of identifying specific obligations under the principles of beneficence and nonmaleficence. Again we see the importance of *specifying* these principles to handle circumstances such as donating organs or tissues, withholding life-sustaining treatments, hastening the death of a dying patient, and biomedical research involving both human and animal subjects.

The Concept of Harm

The concept of nonmaleficence has been explicated by the concepts of *harm* and *injury*, but we confine our analysis to harm. This term has both a normative and a nonnormative use. "X harmed Y" sometimes means that X wronged Y or treated Y unjustly, but it sometimes means only that X's action had an adverse effect on Y's interests. As we use these notions, *wronging* involves violating someone's rights, but *harming* need not signify such a violation. People are harmed without being wronged in attacks by disease, natural disasters, bad luck, and acts by others to which the harmed person has consented.[7] People can also be wronged without being harmed. For example, if an insurance company improperly refuses to pay a patient's hospital bill and the hospital shoulders the full bill, the insurance company wronged the patient without harming him or her.

We construe harm exclusively in the second and nonnormative sense of thwarting, defeating, or setting back some party's interests. Therefore, a *harmful* action by one party may not be wrong or unjustified, although acts of harming in general are prima facie wrong. The reason for their prima facie wrongness is that they set back the interests of the persons affected. Harmful actions that involve *justifiable* setbacks to another's interests are not wrong. They include cases of justified punishment of physicians for incompetence or negligence, justified demotion of an employee for poor performance in a job, and some forms of research involving animals.

Some definitions of harm are so broad that they include setbacks to interests in reputation, property, privacy, and liberty. So broad is the term *harm* in some writings that it seems to include causing discomfort, humiliation, offense, and annoyance. Such a broad conception can still distinguish trivial harms from serious harms by the magnitude of the interests affected. Other accounts with a narrower focus view harms exclusively as setbacks to physical and psychological interests, such as those in health and survival.

Whether a broad or a narrow construal is preferable is not a matter we need to decide. Although *harm* is a contested concept, everyone agrees that significant bodily harms and other setbacks to significant interests are paradigm instances of harm. We concentrate on physical harms, especially pain, disability, suffering, and death, while still affirming the importance of mental harms and other setbacks to one's interests. In particular, we concentrate on intending, causing, and permitting death or the risk of death.

Rules Specifying the Principle of Nonmaleficence

The principle of nonmaleficence supports several more specific moral rules (although principles other than nonmaleficence help justify some of these rules).[8] Examples of more specific rules include the following:[9]

1. Do not kill.
2. Do not cause pain or suffering.

3. Do not incapacitate.
4. Do not cause offense.
5. Do not deprive others of the goods of life.

Both the principle of nonmaleficence and its specifications in these moral rules are prima facie, not absolute (see pp. 14–16).

Negligence and the Standard of Due Care

Obligations of nonmaleficence include not only obligations not to inflict harms, but also obligations not to impose *risks* of harm. A person can harm or place another person at risk without malicious or harmful intent, and the agent of harm may or may not be morally or legally responsible for the harms. In some cases agents are causally responsible for a harm that they did not intend or know about. For example, if cancer rates are elevated at a chemical plant as the result of exposure to a chemical not previously suspected as a carcinogen, the employer has placed its workers at risk by its actions or decisions, although the employer did not intentionally or knowingly cause the harm.

In cases of risk imposition, both law and morality recognize a standard of due care that determines whether the agent who is causally responsible for the risk is legally or morally responsible as well. This standard is a specification of the principle of nonmaleficence. Due care is taking sufficient and appropriate care to avoid causing harm, as the circumstances demand of a reasonable and prudent person. This standard requires that the goals pursued justify the risks that must be imposed to achieve those goals. Grave risks require commensurately momentous goals for their justification. Serious emergencies justify risks that many nonemergency situations do not justify. For example, attempting to save lives after a major accident justifies, within limits, the dangers created by speeding emergency vehicles. A person who takes due care in this sense does not violate moral or legal rules, even in imposing great risk on other parties.

Negligence is the absence of due care. In the professions negligence involves a departure from the professional standards that determine due care in given circumstances. The term *negligence* covers two types of situations: (1) intentionally imposing unreasonable risks of harm (advertent negligence or recklessness) and (2) unintentionally but carelessly imposing risks of harm (inadvertent negligence). In the first type, an agent knowingly imposes an unwarranted risk. For example, a nurse knowingly fails to change a bandage as scheduled, creating an increased risk of infection. In the second type, an agent unknowingly performs a harmful act that he or she should have known to avoid. For example, a physician acts negligently if he or she forgets that a patient does not want to receive certain types of information and discloses that information, causing fear and shame in the patient. Both types of negligence are morally blameworthy, although some conditions may mitigate the blameworthiness. Subtle forms of such judgments pervade morality and medical ethics, as well as criminal and civil law.[10]

In treating negligence, we concentrate on conduct that falls below a standard of due care that law or morality establishes to protect others from the careless imposition of risks. Courts must determine responsibility and liability for harm, because a patient, client, or customer seeks compensation for setbacks to interests or punishment of a responsible party, or both. We do not here consider legal liability, but the legal model of responsibility for harmful action suggests a framework that we can adapt to express moral responsibility for harm caused by health care professionals. The following are essential elements in a professional model of due care:

1. The professional must have a duty to the affected party.

2. The professional must breach that duty.
3. The affected party must experience a harm.
4. The harm must be caused by the breach of duty.

Professional malpractice is an instance of negligence that involves not following professional standards of care.[11] By entering into the profession of medicine, physicians accept a responsibility to observe the standards specific to their profession. If their conduct falls below these standards, they act negligently. Conversely, even if the therapeutic relationship proves harmful or unhelpful, malpractice occurs if and only if physicians do not meet professional standards of care. For example, in *Adkins v. Ropp* the Supreme Court of Indiana considered a patient's claim that a physician acted negligently in removing foreign matter from the patient's eye:

> When a physician and surgeon assumes to treat and care for a patient, in the absence of a special agreement, he is held in law to have impliedly contracted that he possesses the reasonable and ordinary qualifications of his profession and that he will exercise at least reasonable skill, care and diligence in his treatment of him. This implied contract on the part of the physician does not include a promise to effect a cure and negligence cannot be imputed because a cure is not effected, but he does impliedly promise that he will use due diligence and ordinary skill in his treatment of the patient so that a cure may follow such care and skill. This degree of care and skill is required of him, not only in performing an operation or administering first treatments, but he is held to the same degree of care and skill in the necessary subsequent treatments unless he is excused from further service by the patient himself, or the physician or surgeon upon due notice refuses to further treat the case.[12]

The line between due care and inadequate care (that which falls below what is due) is often difficult to draw. Increased safety measures in epidemiological and toxicological studies, educational or health promotional programs, and other training programs can sometimes reduce health risks. A substantial question, however, remains about the lengths to which physicians, employers, and others must go to avoid or lower risks—a problem in determining the scope of obligations of nonmaleficence.

Distinctions and Rules Governing Nontreatment

Religious traditions, philosophical discourse, professional codes, and the law have developed several guidelines to specify the requirements of nonmaleficence in health care, particularly with regard to treatment and nontreatment decisions. Some of these guidelines are helpful, but others need revision or replacement. Many draw heavily on at least one of the following distinctions:

1. *Withholding* and *withdrawing* life-sustaining treatment
2. *Extraordinary* (or heroic) and *ordinary* treatment
3. Sustenance technologies and medical treatments
4. *Intended* effects and *merely foreseen* effects
5. *Killing* and *letting die*

Although at times influential in medicine and law, these distinctions are all outmoded and untenable. The venerable position that these traditional distinctions have occupied in professional codes, institutional policies, and writings in biomedical ethics provides no warrant for retaining them, and some of these distinctions are morally dangerous.

Withholding and Withdrawing Treatments

Debate about the principle of nonmaleficence and forgoing life-sustaining treatments has centered on the omission–commission distinction, especially the distinction between withholding (not starting) and withdrawing (stopping) treatments. Many professionals and family members feel justified in withholding treatments they never started, but not in withdrawing treatments already initiated. They sense that decisions to stop treatments are more momentous and consequential than decisions not to start them. Stopping a respirator, for example, seems, to some, to cause a person's death, whereas not starting the respirator does not seem to have this same causal role.

In one case, an elderly man suffered from several major medical problems with no reasonable chance of recovery. He was comatose and unable to communicate. Antibiotics to fight infection and an intravenous (IV) line to provide nutrition and hydration kept him alive. No evidence indicated that he had expressed his wishes about life-sustaining treatments while competent, and he had no family member to serve as a surrogate decision maker. The staff quickly agreed on a "no code" or "do not resuscitate" (DNR) order, a signed order not to attempt cardiopulmonary resuscitation if a cardiac or respiratory arrest occurred. In the event of such an arrest, the physicians would allow the patient to die. The staff felt comfortable with this decision because of the patient's overall condition and prognosis, and because they could view not resuscitating the patient as withholding rather than withdrawing treatment.

Questions arose about whether to continue the interventions in place. Some members of the health care team thought that they should stop all medical treatments, including antibiotics and artificial nutrition and hydration, because they were "extraordinary" or "heroic measures." Others thought it wrong to stop these treatments once they had been started. A disagreement erupted about whether it would be permissible not to insert the IV line again if it became infiltrated; that is, if it broke through the blood vessel and began leaking fluid into surrounding tissue. Some who had opposed stopping treatments were comfortable with not inserting the IV line again, because they viewed the action as withholding rather than withdrawing. They emphatically opposed reinsertion if it required a cutdown (an incision to gain access to the deep large blood vessels) or a central line. Others viewed the provision of artificial nutrition and hydration as a single process and felt that inserting the IV line again was simply continuing what had been interrupted. For them, not restarting was equivalent to withdrawing and thus (unlike withholding) morally wrong.[13]

In many similar cases caregivers' discomfort about withdrawing life-sustaining treatments appears to reflect the view that such actions render them causally responsible for a patient's death, whereas they are not responsible if they never initiate a life-sustaining treatment. The conviction that starting a treatment often creates valid claims or expectations for its continuation frequently serves as another source of caregiver discomfort. Only if patients waive the claim for continued treatment does it seem legitimate to many caregivers to stop procedures. Otherwise stopping procedures appears to breach expectations, promises, or contractual obligations to the patient, family, or surrogate decision maker. Patients for whom physicians have not initiated treatments seem to hold no parallel claim.[14]

Feelings of reluctance about withdrawing treatments are understandable, but the distinction between withdrawing and withholding treatments is morally irrelevant, and can be dangerous. The distinction is unclear, inasmuch as

Beneficence

Tom L. Beauchamp and James F. Childress

The Obligation to Rescue

Some circumstances eliminate discretionary choice regarding beneficiaries of our beneficence; these circumstances render *specific* actions obligatory Consider the stock example of a passerby who observes someone drowning, but stands in no special moral relationship with the drowning person. The obligation of beneficence is not strong enough, in our view, to require a passerby who is a very poor swimmer to risk his or her life by trying to swim a hundred yards to rescue someone drowning in deep water. Nonetheless, there is still a critical moral relationship between the victim and the passerby, because the passerby is well-placed at that moment to help the victim. As such, a specific obligation of beneficent action does arise in this circumstance. If the passerby does nothing (e.g., fails to alert a nearby lifeguard or fails to call out for help), the failure is morally culpable.

Apart from very close moral relationships, such as contracts or the ties of family or friendship, we suggest that a person X has a determinate obligation of beneficence toward a person Y if and only if each of the following conditions is satisfied (assuming that X is aware of the relevant facts):[10]

1. Y is at risk of significant loss of or damage to life or health or some other major interest.
2. X's action is necessary (singly or in concert with others) to prevent this loss or damage.
3. X's action (singly or in concert with others) has a very high probability of preventing it.[11]
4. X's action would not present very significant risks, costs, or burdens to X.[12]
5. The benefit that Y can be expected to gain outweighs any harms, costs, or burdens that X is likely to incur.

Although it is difficult to specify in the abstract "very significant risks, costs, or burdens," the implication of the fourth condition is clear: Even if X's action would probably save Y's life and would meet all of the conditions except the fourth, the action would still not be *obligatory* on grounds of beneficence.

We now test these theses about the demands of beneficence with two cases. The first is a borderline case of specific obligatory beneficence, involving rescue, whereas the second presents a clear-cut case of specific obligatory beneficence. In the first case, originally introduced in Chapter 5, Robert McFall was diagnosed as having aplastic anemia, which is often fatal, but his physician believed that a bone marrow transplant from a genetically compatible donor could increase his chances of surviving. David Shimp, McFall's cousin, was the only relative willing to undergo the first test, which established tissue compatibility. However, Shimp then refused to undergo the second test for genetic compatibility. When McFall sued to force his cousin to undergo the second test and to donate bone marrow if he turned out to be compatible, the judge ruled that the *law* did not allow him to force Shimp to engage in such acts of positive beneficence, but the judge added that Shimp's refusal was *"morally* indefensible."

Conditions 1 and 2 given earlier were met for an obligation of specific beneficence in this case, but condition 3 was not clearly satisfied. McFall's chance of surviving one year (at the time) would have only increased from 25% to between 40% and 60%. These contingencies make it difficult to determine whether principles of beneficence demanded a particular course of action. Although most medical commentators agreed that the risks to the donor were minimal, Shimp was especially concerned about what we call condition 4. Bone marrow transplants, he was told, require 100 to 150 punctures of the pelvic bone. These punctures can be painlessly performed under anesthesia, and the major risk is a one-in-10,000 chance of death from anesthesia. Shimp, however, believed that the risks were greater ("What if I become a cripple?" he asked) and that they outweighed the probability and magnitude of benefit to McFall. This case, then, is a borderline case of obligatory specific beneficence.

In the *Tarasoff* case (the first case in Chapter 1), a therapist, on learning of his patient's intention to kill an identified woman, notified the police but not the intended victim, because of constraints of confidentiality. Suppose we modify the actual circumstances in this case to create the following hypothetical situation: A psychiatrist has informed his patient that he does not believe in keeping information confidential. The patient agrees to treatment under these conditions and subsequently reveals a serious intention to kill an identified woman. The psychiatrist may now either remain aloof or take measures to protect the woman (by notifying her or the police). What does morality—and specifically beneficence—demand of the psychiatrist in this case?

Only a remarkably narrow account of moral obligation would assert that the psychiatrist is under no obligation whatever to protect the woman by contacting her or the police. The psychiatrist is not at risk and, moreover, will suffer virtually no inconvenience or interference with his life plans. If morality does not demand this much beneficence, it is hard to see how morality imposes any positive obligations at all. Even if a competing obligation exists, such as protection of confidentiality, requirements of beneficence will in some cases override it. Sometimes, for example, health care professionals have a moral obligation to warn spouses or lovers of HIV-infected patients who refuse to disclose their status and who refuse to engage in safer sex practices (see Chapter 8).

What, now, is the morally relevant difference between these rescue cases involving individuals and those discussed in the previous section involving global poverty and public health? We suggested that rescuing a drowning person involves a special obligation not present with global poverty, because the rescuer is "well-placed at that moment to help the victim." But we are all placed well enough to help people in poverty by giving modest sums of money, as we can easily do so at little risk to ourselves and with a high probability of some degree of success. One possible response is that in the drowning case there is a specific individual toward whom we have an obligation, whereas in the poverty cases we seem to have vast obligations toward entire populations of people, only a very few of whom we can hope to help through a gift. Perhaps we are obligated only when there are specific individuals whom we can help, not when there is a whole group and we can only help some of the members.

However, this line of argument has implausible implications, particularly when the size of groups is smaller in scale. Suppose an epidemic breaks out in a reasonably small community, calling for immediate quarantine, and hundreds of persons who are not infected cannot return to their homes where there are infected persons. But they are also not allowed to leave the city limits, and all hotel rooms are filled. Authorities project that you could prevent the deaths of approximately twenty noninfected persons by offering them your house to stay in. Conditions would become unsanitary if more than twenty persons were housed in one home, but there are enough homes to house every stranded person if each house in the community takes twenty persons. It seems very implausible to say that no person in any household is morally obligated to open their houses to these people for the weeks needed to control the epidemic, even though no one person has an obligation to any one of the stranded people as specific individuals. The hypothesis might be offered that this obligation arises only because they are all members of the community, but even this principle is implausible because it would arbitrarily exclude visitors who got caught. Accordingly, it does seem that we have obligations beyond those to specific individuals. Any other conclusion is morally unacceptable, and likely would be judged unacceptable across cultures that share the common morality.

In light of these considerations, common-morality beneficence requires people who are well off to provide at least some level of aid to people in extreme poverty. From this perspective Singer's weaker principles become very plausible, as we hinted earlier they might. However, we do not think that the duty to rescue, as we have now developed it, plausibly supports Singer's strong principle of beneficence. We return to this issue, focusing on global poverty and public health, in the chapter on justice (Chapter 7, pp. 264–66, during a discussion of cosmopolitan

ethical theories). We also return, in Chapter 9, to the importance of *practicability* in a normative theory (pp. 22, 77–8). We do not believe that Singer's strong principle can be made practicable, whereas the weaker principles can.

To conclude, it is doubtful that ethical theory or practical deliberation can set precise, determinate conditions of obligations of beneficence. Any attempt to do so will almost certainly be a revisionary line in the sense that it will draw a sharper boundary for our obligations than exists in the common morality. Although beneficence is unclear at its heart, it should not be concluded that we can never fix or specify obligations of beneficence with any clarity.

Role Obligations and Special Relations

Obligations of specific beneficence usually rest on special moral relations (e.g., in families and friendships) or on special commitments, such as explicit promises and acceptance of roles with accompanying responsibilities. These special moral relationships and role relationships may not appear to generate the problems about specifying the limits of obligatory beneficent risk-taking and cost-bearing that we have encountered thus far. However, there are related limits. For instance, how far are parents obligated to go in providing expensive care for their severely ill children?[13] Are physicians and other health care professionals obligated to accept extraordinary risks while caring for abusive or contagious patients?

At this stage in the discussion, we note only that there is an implicit assumption of beneficence in all medical and health care professions and their institutional contexts: Promoting the welfare of patients—not merely avoiding harm—embodies medicine's goal, rationale, and justification. Preventive medicine and public health interventions have also long embraced concerted social actions of beneficence, such as vaccination programs and health education, as obligatory, not merely optional.

A Reciprocity-Based Justification of Obligations of Beneficence

Several justifications can be proposed for obligations of general and specific beneficence. One is a reciprocity-based account, which is particularly well-suited to biomedical ethics.

David Hume argued that the obligation to benefit others arises from social interactions: "All our obligations to do good to society seem to imply something reciprocal. I receive the benefits of society, and therefore ought to promote its interests."[14] Reciprocity is the act or practice of making an appropriate and often proportional return—for example, returning benefit with proportional benefit, harm with proportional criminal sentencing, and friendly actions with gratitude. Hume's reciprocity account rightly maintains that we incur obligations to help or benefit others at least in part because we have received, will receive, or stand to receive beneficial assistance from them.

Reciprocity is a pervasive feature of social life, although not so pervasive that we can reduce all of the moral life to obligations of reciprocity. Nonetheless, many obligations of beneficence to society (as distinct from those to identified individuals) typically derive from some form of reciprocity. It is implausible to maintain that we are largely free of, or can free ourselves from, a broad range of indebtedness to our parents, to researchers in medicine and public health, to educators, and to social institutions such as schools. The claim that we make our way independent of our benefactors is as unrealistic as the idea that we can always act autonomously without affecting others.[15]

Codes of medical ethics have sometimes inappropriately viewed physicians as independent, self-sufficient philanthropists whose beneficence is analogous to generous acts of giving. The Hippocratic oath states that physicians' obligations to patients represent philanthropic service, whereas obligations to their teachers represent debts incurred in the course of becoming physicians. However, today many physicians and health care professionals owe a large debt to society (e.g., for education and privileges) and to their patients, past and present (e.g., for research and "practice"). Because of this indebtedness, the medical profession's role of beneficent care of patients is misconstrued if modeled primarily on philanthropy, altruism, and personal commitment. This care is rooted in a reciprocity of giving after having received.[16]

Obligations of specific beneficence, by contrast, typically derive from special moral relationships with persons, frequently through institutional roles and contractual arrangements. These obligations arise from implicit and explicit commitments, such as promises and roles, as well as from the acceptance of specific benefits. Both our "station and its duties" and our promises impose obligations. When a patient contracts with a physician for services, the latter assumes a role-specific obligation of beneficent treatment that would not be present apart from the relationship. Although physicians in private practice typically have no legal obligation to see patients in emergencies or to help those injured in an automobile accident, moral obligations of beneficence do, on occasion, require such acts. The obligation to render assistance in extraordinary circumstances, such as an automobile accident, is not limited to physicians or to health care professionals. Anyone who falls under our five-condition analysis of the specific obligation of beneficence has an obligation to provide such assistance, as he or she is able.

Of course, physicians are typically able to lend more assistance in a medical emergency than other citizens, and we can therefore ask whether the physician has a specific obligation of assistance unique to persons with such skills and training. Here we encounter a gray area between a role-specific obligation and a non-role-specific obligation. The physician at the scene of an accident is obligated to do more than the lawyer or student to aid the injured, to the degree there is a need for medical skills. Yet a physician-stranger is not morally required to assume the same level of commitment and risk that a prior contractual relationship with a patient or hospital would morally require.

Paternalism: Conflicts Between Beneficence and Autonomy

The idea that beneficence expresses the primary obligation in health care is ancient. Throughout the history of health care, the professional's obligations and virtues have generally been interpreted as commitments of beneficence. We find perhaps the most celebrated expression in the Hippocratic work *Epidemics:* "As to disease, make a habit of two things—to *help, or at least to do no harm.*"[17] Traditionally, physicians relied almost exclusively on their own judgments about their patients' needs for information and treatment. However, over the last few decades, medicine has increasingly confronted assertions of patients' rights to make independent judgments. As assertions of autonomy rights increased, the problem of paternalism loomed larger.

for autonomy has grounded several rights for patients, including rights to receive information, to consent to and refuse procedures, and to have confidentiality and privacy maintained. Others ground such obligations on the health care professional's primary obligation of beneficence, which is to act for the patient's medical benefit.

Proponents of the autonomy model and proponents of the beneficence model—as we refer to these two contrasting paradigms—sometimes fail to carefully distinguish between the principles of beneficence and respect for autonomy. For example, beneficence could be construed to *incorporate* the patient's autonomous choices in the sense that the patient's preferences help to determine what counts as a medical benefit. Along these lines, two defenders of the beneficence model, Edmund Pellegrino and David Thomasma, argue that "the best interests of the patients are intimately linked with their preferences," from which "are derived our primary duties toward them."[18] This formulation of the beneficence model simply restates the autonomy model. If the patient's preferences alone determine the content of the physician's obligation to act beneficently, respect for autonomy rather than pure medical beneficence has triumphed, and the problem of paternalism evaporates.

However, we argued earlier that beneficence provides the primary goal and rationale of medicine and health care and that it can directly conflict with respect for autonomy. This creates a serious and pervasive problem of paternalism. We now begin to address it by considering critical conceptual issues.

Disputes about the Primacy of Beneficence

Whether respect for the autonomy of patients should have priority over professional beneficence directed at those patients is a central problem in biomedical ethics. The principle of respect

The Nature of Paternalism

What is paternalism? The *Oxford English Dictionary (OED)* dates the term *paternalism* to the 1880s, giving its root meaning as "the principle and practice of paternal administration; government as by a father; the claim or attempt to supply 's or to regulate the life of a nation or community in the same way a father does those of his children." The analogy with the father presupposes two features of the paternal role: that the father acts beneficently (i.e., in accordance with his conception of the interests of his children) and that he makes all or at least some of the decisions relating to his children's welfare, rather than letting them make those decisions. In health care relationships, the analogy is this: A professional has superior training, knowledge, and insight and is thus in an authoritative position to determine the patient's best interests. From this perspective, a health care professional is like a loving parent with dependent and often ignorant and fearful children.

Paternalistic acts often use such forms of influence as deception, lying, manipulation of information, or nondisclosure of information, as well as coercion and force. However, they may simply involve a refusal to carry out the other's wishes. According to some definitions in the literature, paternalistic actions by definition restrict *autonomous* choices, and thus restricting nonautonomous conduct is not paternalistic. Although one author of this text prefers this conception,[19] we here accept and build on the broader definition suggested by the *OED:* intentional nonacquiescence or intervention in another person's preferences, desires, or actions with the intention of either preventing or reducing harm to or benefiting the person. Even if a person's desires, intentional actions, and the like are *not substantially autonomous,* overriding them can still be paternalistic under this definition.[20] For example, if a man ignorant of his fragile, life-threatening condition and sick with a raging fever attempts to leave a hospital, it is paternalistic to detain him, even if his attempt to leave does not derive from a substantially autonomous choice.

Accordingly, we define "paternalism" as *the intentional overriding of one person's preferences or actions by another person, where the person who overrides justifies this action by appeal to the goal of benefiting or of preventing or mitigating harm to the*
person whose preferences or actions are overridden. This definition is normatively neutral—it does not presume that paternalism is either justified or unjustified. Although the definition assumes an act of beneficence analogous to parental beneficence, it does not prejudge whether the beneficent act is justified, obligatory, misplaced, and so forth.

Problems of Medical Paternalism

Throughout the history of medical ethics both the principles of nonmaleficence and beneficence have been invoked as a basis for paternalistic actions toward patients. For example, physicians have traditionally held that disclosing certain kinds of information can cause harm to patients under their care and that medical ethics obligates them not to cause such harm. Consider a typical case: A man brings his father, who is in his late sixties, to his physician because he suspects that his father's problems in interpreting and responding to daily events may indicate Alzheimer's disease. The man also makes an "impassioned plea" that the physician not tell his father if the tests suggest Alzheimer's. Tests subsequently indicate that the father probably does have the disease. The physician now faces a dilemma, because of the conflict between demands of respect for autonomy (assuming that the father has substantial autonomy and is competent at least some of the time) and demands of beneficence. The physician first considers the now widely recognized obligation to inform patients of a diagnosis of cancer. This obligation typically presupposes accuracy in the diagnosis, a relatively clear course of the disease, and a competent patient—none of which is clearly present in this case. The physician also notes that disclosure of Alzheimer's disease adversely affects patients' coping mechanisms, and thus could harm the patient, particularly by causing further decline, depression, agitation, and paranoia.[21] (See also our discussion of veracity in Chapter 8.)

Some patients—for example, those who are depressed or addicted to potentially harmful drugs—are unlikely to reach adequately reasoned decisions, at least not likely under certain conditions or mental states. Other patients who are competent and deliberative may make poor choices, judged by the courses of action that their physicians recommend. When patients of either type choose harmful courses of action, some health care professionals respect autonomy (in the case of stated preferences that are autonomous) by not interfering beyond attempts at persuasion, whereas others act beneficently by attempting to protect patients against the potentially harmful consequences of their own stated preferences. Discussions of medical paternalism focus on how to specify these principles, which principle to follow under which conditions, and how to intervene in the decisions and affairs of such patients when intervention is warranted.

Insofar as depression, drug addiction, and the like substantially interfere with the exercise of a patient's autonomy, beneficent acts to protect the patient and promote his or her interests represent soft paternalism. Here there is generally no troublesome conflict between autonomy and beneficence because of the absence of substantial autonomy. Because the beneficiary lacks substantial autonomy, the intervention is much easier to justify than it would be if a comparable preference or action were substantially autonomous. However, in contrast to much of the literature on paternalism, we also argue that beneficence sometimes provides grounds for justifiably restricting substantially autonomous actions.

Justice

Tom L. Beauchamp and James F. Childress

Lotteries of social and biological life do not provide grounds for morally acceptable discrimination between persons in social allocations if people do not have a fair chance to acquire or overcome these properties.

The attempt to supply all citizens with a basic education raises moral problems analogous to those in health care. Imagine a community that offers a high-quality education to all students with basic abilities, regardless of gender or race, but does not offer a comparable educational opportunity to students with reading difficulties or mental deficiencies. This system is unjust. The students with disabilities lack basic skills and need special training to overcome their problems. They should receive an education suitable to their needs and opportunities, even if it costs more. The fair-opportunity rule requires that they receive the benefits needed to ameliorate the unfortunate effects of life's lottery. By analogy, persons with functional disabilities lack capacity and need health care to reach a higher level of function and have a fair chance in life. If they are responsible for their disabilities, they might not be entitled to health care services. But if they are not responsible, the fair-opportunity rule demands that they receive that which will help them reduce or overcome the unfortunate effects of life's lottery of health.

Mitigating the Negative Effects of Life's Lotteries

Numerous properties might be disadvantageous and undeserved—for example, a squeaky voice, an ugly face, inarticulate speech, an inadequate early education, malnutrition, or disease. But which undeserved properties create a right *in justice* to some form of assistance?

One hypothesis is that virtually all abilities and disabilities are functions of what Rawls calls the natural lottery and the social lottery. "Natural lottery" refers to the distribution of advantageous and disadvantageous genetic properties, and "social lottery" refers to the distribution of assets or deficits through family property, school systems, government agencies, and the like. It is possible that all talents and disabilities result from heredity, natural environment, family upbringing, education, inheritance, and the like, in some combination. From this perspective, even the ability to work long hours, the ability to compete, and a warm smile are biologically, environmentally, and socially engendered. If so, talents, abilities, and successes are not to our credit, just as genetic disease is acquired through no fault of the afflicted person.

Rawls uses fair opportunity as a rule of redress. To overcome disadvantaging conditions (whether from biology or society) that are not deserved, the rule demands compensation for disadvantages. The full implications of this approach are uncertain, but his conclusions are challenging:

> [A free-market arrangement] permits the distribution of wealth and income to be determined by the natural distribution of abilities and talents. Within the limits allowed by the background arrangements, distributive shares are decided by the outcome of the natural lottery; and this outcome is arbitrary from a moral perspective. There is no more reason to permit the distribution of income and wealth to be settled by the distribution of natural assets than by historical and social fortune. Furthermore, the principle of fair opportunity can be only imperfectly carried out, at least as long as the institution of the family exists. The extent to which natural capacities develop and reach fruition is affected by all kinds of social conditions and class attitudes. Even the willingness to make an effort, to try, and so to be deserving in the ordinary sense is itself dependent upon happy family and social circumstances.[14]

At a minimum, current social systems of distributing benefits and burdens would undergo massive revision if this approach were accepted. Rather than allowing broad inequalities in social distribution based on effort, contribution, and merit, justice is achieved only if radical inequalities are reduced. Inequalities are permissible only if disadvantaged persons benefited more from them than from an equal distribution of benefits.

At some point the process of reducing inequalities introduced by life's lotteries must stop, and at that point persons who are disadvantaged will lose meaningful protection by the fair-opportunity rule.[15] Libertarians rightly stress that limited resources will constrain the implementation of this rule, but they draw the line at a different place. Some disadvantages are merely *unfortunate*, they argue, whereas others are *unfair*, and therefore obligatory in justice to correct. Tristram Engelhardt has argued that society should call a halt to claims of fairness or justice precisely at the point of this distinction between the unfair and the unfortunate.[16]

However, we argue that the problems addressed in this chapter create a need for criteria other than the distinction between the unfortunate and the unfair, a criterion that may only beg the central questions of what is fair. We will see that no bright lines distinguish the unfair from the unfortunate or fair from unfair allocation schemes. Nevertheless, if one accepts the fair-opportunity rule, as we do, it will deeply affect moral reflection about health policy and other areas.

Racial, Ethnic, and Gender Disparities in Health Care

Disparities in health care based on racial and gender properties are social problems that fall under the fair-opportunity rule. Health care has often been covertly distributed on the basis of these properties, resulting in a differential impact in many countries on the health of racial and ethnic minorities as well as women.[17] Many studies in the United States indicate that blacks and women have poorer access to various forms of health care in comparison to white males. For example, gender and racial inequities in employment have an impact on job-based health insurance; and the race and gender of physicians often play a role in the quality of patient-physician interaction.[18]

In the face of apparent disparities, studies conducted in various parts of the health care system have led to efforts, partially successful but largely unsuccessful, to overcome racial and ethnic disparities.[19] One controversy centers on the rates of coronary artery bypass grafting (CABG) between white and black Medicare patients, as well as between male and female Medicare patients. Differences have been evident since the mid-1980s in many parts of the United States.[20] Differences in need cannot entirely account for the variance, and it remains unclear to what extent the rates can be explained by physician supply, poverty, awareness of health care opportunities, reluctance among blacks and women to undergo surgery, and racial prejudice. One study found that, after controlling for age, payer, and appropriateness and necessity for CABG, African American patients in New York State had significant access problems unrelated to patient refusals.[21] Disparities also appear in the management of acute myocardial infarction[22] and in the care of chronic conditions such as glucose control for patients with diabetes or cholesterol control among patients with cardiovascular disorders.[23]

A major report from the Institute of Medicine on racial and ethnic disparities in health care identifies several "unacceptable" racial and ethnic disparities across a wide range of medical conditions and health care services, leading to "worse health outcomes."[24] While insurance status, income, and level of education are important in access, the report stresses that other, independent factors are also significant. These include the broader context of historic and continuing social and economic inequality; patient-level variables such as cultural preferences and some biological differences; system-level factors, such as language barriers, time constraints in health care, geographic availability; and care process-level variables, including bias, stereotyping, and uncertainty based in part on racial and ethnic differences and on the clinician's need to

make medical decisions under the pressure of time and with limited information.[25]

Renal transplantation provides another informative case study because financial barriers play a less significant role in kidney transplantation than in most other areas of health care. The federal End-Stage Renal Disease (ESRD) Program ensures coverage for kidney dialysis and transplantation for virtually everyone who needs them if their private insurance does not provide the coverage. However, concerns about costs can still be a factor because immunosuppressant medications needed for life are not covered under the ESRD program after three years. Evidence suggests that discrimination against blacks, other minorities, and women occurs leading up to and at the point of referral to transplantation centers and admission to waiting lists, where criteria may vary considerably. For instance, blacks are much less likely than whites to be referred for evaluation at transplant centers and to be placed on a waiting list or to receive a transplant.[26] Factors include minority distrust of the system (in part based on prior experience), delayed or limited access to health care, and inadequate guidance through the system by health care professionals.

Once patients are admitted to the waiting list, the criteria for selecting recipients of donated cadaveric organs are public and are, to a significant extent, represented through point systems. Disputes continue about how much weight to give to different factors in the distribution of kidneys for transplantation, with particular attention to human lymphocyte antigen (HLA) matching. The degree of HLA match between a donor and a recipient affects the long-term survival of the transplanted kidney. However, assigning priority to tissue matching—and giving less weight to time on the waiting list and other factors—has been shown to produce "disparate effects" for minorities. Most organ donors are white; certain HLA phenotypes are different in white, black, and Hispanic populations; and the identification of HLA phenotypes is less complete for blacks and Hispanics. Yet nonwhites have a higher rate of end-stage renal disease and are also disproportionately represented on dialysis rolls. Blacks on the waiting list also, on average, wait much longer than whites to receive a first kidney transplant, if they receive one at all.

In an interim report on one policy change, analysts predicted that eliminating the relevant HLA matching (HLA-B) as a priority would increase the number of kidney transplantations among nonwhites by 6.0% while reducing the number for whites by 4.0% and, at the same time, increasing the rate of graft loss by 2.0%. They conclude that, "Such a change would reduce the tension inherent in the current allocation policy by improving equity without sacrificing utility."[27] Normatively, the tension between utility and providing fair opportunity persists, and critics have challenged the use of "disparate impact tests" to shift from policies that seek to maximize the number of quality-adjusted life-years per organ to trying to increase the access of racial or ethnic groups to transplantation.[28]

The problems plaguing minority patients are similar to those facing women patients. Several years ago, the Council on Ethical and Judicial Affairs of the American Medical Association examined data that raised concerns about whether women are disadvantaged because of inadequate attention to research, diagnosis, and treatment of their health problems.[29] The Council found gender disparities, for example, in the diagnosis and treatment of cardiac disease. Biological differences do not account for these disparities. The Council notes that gender bias need not be manifest in an overt manner. Social attitudes involving stereotypes, prejudices, and gender-role attributions may be present, including the attribution of women's health complaints to emotional rather than physical causes. In the use of diagnostic and therapeutic procedures for patients with coronary heart disease, for example, evidence exists that men and women are treated differently for reasons that appear unrelated to their medical conditions.

In a review of studies of cardiovascular disease, the leading cause of women's death, women were less aggressively screened and treated for cholesterol problems than men.[30] However, in a sign of progress beginning in 2004, virtually the same percentage of women and men with Medicare received recommended care in the hospital following a heart attack.[31] In another area, HIV-infected women were less likely than HIV-infected men to be placed on highly active antiretroviral therapy and to receive medications to prevent possible opportunistic infections.[32]

In short, while some disparities in health care for women and men have declined, others persist. The best available interpretations of known causal factors suggest many violations of the fair-opportunity rule.

Vulnerability and Exploitation

We turn now to some quite different problems of fair opportunity. These are not problems of health care distribution, but problems about the vulnerability of human research subjects at risk of exploitation. We concentrate on the recruitment and enrollment in clinical research (primarily pharmaceutical trials) of the economically disadvantaged, who are often disadvantaged by the social lottery.

By "economically disadvantaged," we mean persons who are impoverished, may lack significant access to health care, may be homeless, may be malnourished, and so forth, and yet possess mental capacity to "volunteer" in, for example, safety and toxicity (phase I) drug studies. Thus, we are considering only persons who possess a basic competence to reason, deliberate, decide, and consent. Data indicate that somewhere between 50% and 100% of research subjects who are healthy volunteers self-report that financial need or financial reward is their primary motive for volunteering.[33] We know that such persons are involved in some research in North America, but we do not know the full extent of their involvement, just as we do not know the scope of the use of poor persons as research subjects in other parts of the world, including developing countries.[34]

Vulnerability and Vulnerable Groups

It should not be assumed that there is a straightforward connection between economically disadvantaged groups and vulnerability or between vulnerability and exploitation by researchers. The connections are subtle and the concepts complicated. The literature has sometimes viewed the class of the economically disadvantaged who are vulnerable as narrow, at other times broad. Those so classified may or may not include individuals living on the streets, low-income persons who are the sole financial support of a large family, persons desperately lacking access to health care, persons whose income falls below a certain threshold level, and so forth. Their situation of economic distress could be long-term or only temporary.

The notion of a "vulnerable group" was considered very significant in bioethics and health policy between the 1970s and the early 1990s. However, over the years it has suffered from overexpansion because so many groups have now been declared vulnerable—from the infirm elderly, to the undereducated, to those with inadequate resources, to whole countries whose members lack rights or are subject to exploitation.[35] The language of "vulnerable groups" suggests that all members of a vulnerable group—for example, all prisoners, all poor people, and all pregnant women—are by category vulnerable. The problem is that for many groups a label covering all members of the group serves to overprotect, stereotype, and even disqualify members capable of making their own decisions.[36] "Vulnerable" is an inappropriate label for any class of persons when some members of the class are not vulnerable in the relevant respects. For example, pregnant women as a class are not vulnerable, although some pregnant women are. Accordingly, we do not speak of the economically disadvantaged as a categorically vulnerable group. Instead, we speak of *vulnerabilities*. Ideally, research ethics can supply a schema of forms and conditions of vulnerability, rather than a list of vulnerable groups.[37]

The concept of vulnerability. In biomedical ethics, the notion of vulnerability often focuses on a person's susceptibility, whether as a result of internal or external factors, to inducement or coercion, on the one hand, or to harm, loss, or indignity, on the other.[38] The economically disadvantaged may be vulnerable in several ways to influences that introduce a significant risk of harm. Their situation may leave them lacking in critical resources and forms of social powers that might have been created on their behalf. Hence, they may not be able to resist or refuse acceptance of the risk involved, requiring trade-offs among their interests.[39]

Categorical exclusion of the economically disadvantaged? A tempting strategy to protect their interests is to exclude economically disadvantaged persons categorically, even if they are not categorically vulnerable. This remedy would eliminate the problem of their unjust exploitation, but it would deprive them of the freedom to choose and would often be harmful to their financial interests. Nothing about economically disadvantaged persons justifies their exclusion, as a group, from participation in research, just as it does not follow from their status as disadvantaged that they should be excluded from participation in any legal activity. To be sure, there is an increased risk of taking advantage of the economically distressed, but to exclude them categorically would be an inexcusable, paternalistic form of discrimination and deprivation of fair opportunity that may only serve to further marginalize, deprive, stigmatize, or discriminate against them.

Consider the weakly analogous case of what has long been the paradigm of competent persons who are categorically excluded from phase I clinical trials— namely, prisoners. The right to volunteer as a research subject has been denied to prisoners in most nations on grounds of the potential for manipulation or coercion in penal institutions.[40] Were this same potential to exist for economically disadvantaged persons, the same categorical exclusion might be appropriate. However, this problem needs to be examined in each context to determine if competent persons, whatever their vulnerabilities, are able to consent freely in that circumstance.

We turn now to the major moral problems about enrolling the economically disadvantaged in research: undue inducement, undue profit, and exploitation.

Undue Inducement, Undue Profit, and Exploitation

Some persons report feeling heavily pressured to enroll in clinical trials, even though their enrollment is correctly classified as voluntary.[41] These individuals are in desperate need of money. Attractive offers of money and other goods can leave a person with a sense of having no meaningful choice but to accept research participation. Such a person feels constrained by influences that many individuals easily resist.

Constraining situations. In these constraining situations—sometimes misleadingly termed *coercive* situations—there is no coercion, strictly speaking, because no one has intentionally issued a threat to gain compliance. (See our discussion of coercion in Chapter 4.) A person feels controlled by the constraints of a situation, such as severe illness or lack of food and shelter, rather than by the design or threat of another person. Sometimes people unintentionally make other persons feel "threatened" by their actions, and sometimes illness, powerlessness, and lack of resources are perceived as harms that a person

feels compelled to prevent or ameliorate. These situations significantly constrain choices, even though they do not involve threats. The prospect of another night on the streets or another day without food can constrain a person to accept an offer of research participation, just as such conditions could constrain a person to accept an unpleasant or risky job that the person would otherwise not accept. A person can rightly report in both cases, "I had no choice; it was unthinkable to refuse the offer."

Undue inducement. In constraining situations, monetary payments and related offers such as shelter or food give rise to questions of *undue inducement,* on the one hand, and *undue profit,* on the other. The "Common Rule" in the United States requires investigators to "minimize the possibility of" coercion and undue inducement, but it does not define, analyze, or explain these notions.[42] The bioethics and public policy literatures also do not adequately handle issues of exploitation, undue inducement, and undue profit.

Monetary payments seem unproblematic if the payments are welcome offers that persons do not want to refuse and the risks are at the level of everyday activities.[43] But inducements become increasingly problematic as (1) risks are increased, (2) more attractive inducements are introduced, and (3) the subjects' economic disadvantage is increased. The problem of exploitation centers on whether solicited persons are situationally disadvantaged and without viable alternatives, feel forced or compelled to accept attractive offers that they otherwise would not accept, and assume increased risk in their lives. As these conditions are mitigated, the problem of exploitation diminishes and may vanish. As these conditions are increased, the problem of exploitation looms larger.

The presence of an irresistibly attractive offer is a *necessary* condition of "undue inducement," but this condition is not by itself *sufficient* to make an inducement *undue.* A situation of undue inducement must also involve a person's assumption of a sufficiently serious risk of harm that he or she would not ordinarily assume. We will not try to pinpoint a precise threshold level of risk, but it would have to be above the level of common job risks such as those of unskilled construction work. Inducements are not undue unless they are both above the level of standard risk (hence "excessive" in risk) and irresistibly attractive (hence "excessive" in payment) in light of a constraining situation. Although these offers are not coercive, because no *threat* of excessive risk or of taking money away from the person is involved, the offer can still be manipulative. Indeed, since irresistibly attractive payment is involved, these offers almost certainly should be categorized as manipulative, although not necessarily as unjustifiably manipulative (see analysis of these distinctions in Chapter 4, pp. 133–35).

Undue profit. Undue inducements should be distinguished from *undue profits,* which occur from a distributive injustice of too small a payment, rather than an irresistibly attractive, large payment. In the undue-profit situation, the subject of research receives an unfairly low payment, while the sponsor of research gets more than is justified. Often, this seems to be what critics of pharmaceutical research believe happens: Those approached are in a weak to nonexistent bargaining situation, constrained by their poverty, and are given a pitifully small amount of money and unjust share of the benefits, while companies reap unseemly profits. If this is the worry, the basic question is how to determine a nonexploitative, fair payment.

How should we handle these two moral problems of exploitation—undue inducement (unduly large and irresistible payments) and undue profit (unduly small and unfair payments)? One possible answer is that if the research involves excessive risk, it should be prohibited categorically, even if a good oversight system is in place. This answer is appealing, but we would still need to determine what constitutes excessive risk, irresistibly attractive payment, unjust underpayment, and constraining situations—all difficult and unresolved problems.

The moral dilemma can be very challenging here: To avoid undue inducement, payment schedules must be kept reasonably low, approximating an unskilled labor wage, or possibly even lower. Even at this low level, payment might still be sufficiently large to constitute an undue inducement for some research subjects. As payments are lowered to avoid undue inducement, research subjects (in some circumstances) will be recruited largely or entirely from the ranks of the economically disadvantaged. Somewhere on this continuum the amount of money paid will be so little that it is exploitative by virtue of undue profits yielded by taking advantage of a person's misfortune. If the payment scales were increased to avoid undue profit, they would at some point become high enough to attract persons from the middle class. At or around this point, the offers would be declared excessively attractive and judged undue inducements for impoverished persons interested in the payments.[44] This dilemma becomes a profound problem of potential injustice if the pool of research subjects is comprised more or less exclusively of the economically disadvantaged.

There may be situations in which payments that are too high (creating undue inducements) are, *at the same time,* payments that are too low (creating undue profits). To the desperate, $.25/hr. or $10/hr. might be irresistibly attractive, while distributively unfair. Critics charge that pharmaceutical companies routinely take advantage of such situations, but insufficient information is available at present for a definite judgment. However, from what we know, at least some contexts of research conducted in North America do not seem to involve either undue inducement or undue profit. Whatever the actual situation in North America or elsewhere, we have attempted to locate the moral problems that must be addressed and to consider possible paths to their resolution.

Finally, some brief comments are in order that should help frame discussion of these issues: An important reason for caution about prohibiting research or about encouraging pharmaceutical companies to pull out of poor communities is that payments for studies are a vital source of needed funds for the economically disadvantaged and a way to build an infrastructure and jobs in these communities.[45] One of the few readily available sources of money for some economically distressed persons are jobs such as day labor that expose them to more risk and generate less money than the payments generated by participation in phase I clinical trials.[46] To deny these persons the right to participate in clinical research on grounds of the potential exploitation already discussed can be paternalistic and demeaning, as well as economically distressing.

It is often unclear when a practice becomes a way to exploit the disadvantaged for the benefit of the privileged. This question of justice can be answered only by specifying and defending the precise conditions under which an arrangement is unfair—a task beyond the scope of this chapter. However, we ought not to assume that a fair system of incentives for research subjects cannot be constructed, including one with effective committee and regulatory oversight.

National Health Policy and the Right to Health Care

Questions about who shall receive what share of a society's resources have generated many controversies about appropriate national health policies, unequal distributions of health advantages, and rationing of health-related goods and services. The primary economic barrier to health care access in many countries—most visibly the United States—is the lack of adequate insurance.

Close to 50 million U.S. citizens (approximately 18% of the nonelderly population) lack health insurance of any kind.[47] Inadequate insurance affects persons who are uninsured, uninsurable, underinsured, or only occasionally insured. In many other countries the primary barriers to both health and health care are poverty and limited government resources. Problems of justice are very different in different parts of the world.

Some problems of unfairness arise in the United States because of the extraordinary reliance on employers for financing the system. Persons with medium to large size employers are not only better covered, but are also subsidized by tax breaks in the system. When employed persons who are not covered become ill, taxpayers rather than free-riding employers usually pick up the bill. The financing of health care is also regressive. Low-income families pay premiums comparable to and often higher than the premiums paid by high-income families, and many individuals who do not qualify for group coverage pay dramatically more for the same coverage than those who qualify in a group.

Despite various controversies, a social consensus appears to be emerging in the United States that all citizens should be able to secure equitable access to health care, including insurance coverage. The problem with this consensus is its content-thinness: Citizens and politicians disagree sharply on a range of solutions proffered to improve access, on the role of government in these solutions, and on methods of financing them. It is unclear whether such a fragile consensus can generate a secondary consensus about how to implement equitable access in public policy.

Part Two
Practice

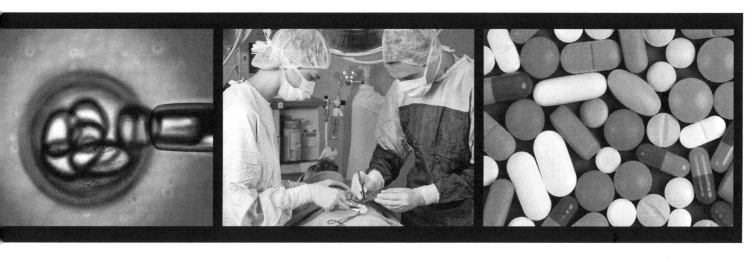

Introduction

Principles and rules enjoy a privileged theoretical status in ethics. They are widely regarded as being "exhaustive of ethics, that is, as though all that moral understanding requires is a commitment to some code of rules, which can be accepted as authoritative."[1] In this sense, ethical problems are solved by adhering to a determined set of rules or values and adjusting our actions to it. According to Jonsen and Toulmin, such approach to moral deliberation is incomplete. Principles and rules are not to be understood as the beginning and end of moral decision makings, instead, they urge us to think the possibility of facing moral quandaries with a different approach in mind—the "casuistic approach—," so that we may be set free of the "tyranny of principles."

To completely grasp the idea of "casuistry vs. principles" the authors present an excellent example. A young woman, who was struggling with her rent and food in order to help herself reach the end of the month afloat, started working in a telephone answering service. This job got her the money she needed to pay for her expenses. There was only one problem: she was also receiving social security payments (which were insufficient to cover all her needs, hence she started the phone service). Once the Social Security Office found out of this activity, which she did not inform to the Office, they ceased all payment for concepts of social security and made her even repay money for she was classified as a case of "welfare fraud." A male news reporter who was covering her story said about this case "There should be a rule to prevent this kind of thing from happening." Jonsen and Toulmin stressed that he did not say there should be more "discretion", more "equity" or more "flexibility" in the application of rules he outright said there should be a rule for covering such a case. This kind of thinking implies that "Justice [...] is ensured only by establishing an adequate system of rules, so as to prevent such inequities from happening again in the future." Actually, the authors note, principles can only do so much for moral deliberation, as seen in this example, where it is clear that what was needed was more wisdom rather than more rules. All decision making moral cases are in need of "perceptiveness" and "discernment," "and the more problematic the situations become, the greater is the need

---

1 Jonsen and Toulmin, *The Abuse of Casuistry: A History of Moral Reasoning*, Berkeley, University of California Press, 1988.

for such discernment." Thereby, principles by themselves cannot suffice in moral practical decision-making for rules cover only unique situations contemplated expressly in them. Therefore, when cases depart from the paradigmatic case contained in the rule or law, the rule or law proves unhelpful since it does not contain a solution for a case that it does not contemplate.

As an answer to this central problem in ethics, Jonsen and Toulmin try to revitalize an old tradition, that is, the tradition of "casuistry," which has been in disrepute for hundreds of years, especially since the attacks Pascal fired unto Casuists in the mid-seventeenth century. "Casuistry" is described succinctly by the authors as "a reasonable and effective set of practical procedures for resolving the moral problems that arise in particular real-life situations."

But what happened to this centuries-old tradition? Why did casuistry suddenly fall into oblivion? Why does it suffer such a bad reputation among contemporary intellectuals? Jonsen and Toulmin set forward to answer these questions, and subsequently, clean the name of "case ethics" or "casuistics." As an interesting fact, these authors note that the Oxford English Dictionary has an accurate definition of casuistry but, it does also comment that the word's use was "apparently at first contemptuous" and it cites as relevant quotations three sources which question its value.

As said, it was Blaise Pascal that delivered the finishing blow of casuistry with his Provincial Letters. Being the influential intellectual he was at his time, his pen would prove the end of casuistry as his influence on readers was all it took to disrepute casuistry completely. On the Letters, Pascal directly addressed the problems of the abuse of casuistry, since, at that time, he argued, casuistry was used by the French Jesuits for justifying unduly and partial treatment to those of their penitents that were wealthy or highborn. Interestingly enough, the authors hold, Pascal

is obscure in this point, for it is not quite clear if he intended to attack "bad" casuistry only (the abuse of casuistry for the benefit of some privileged group or individual) or to attack the casuistic system as a whole.

Another important historical blow to casuistry was delivered by philosopher Henry Sidgwick in his book *The Methods of Ethics* in 1874. Herein Sigwick proposed the departure from case analysis in ethics to a more general and theoretical approach to ethical and "meta-ethical" theory.

However it may be particular case-analysis keeps intact today in daily life decision-makings. Jonsen and Toulmin maintain that although in highly-intellectual circles casuistry has been almost completely disdained—except for some two noteworthy examples, Sissela Bok's book Lying and Michael Walzers's book Just and Unjust wars—, we have not forgotten its use in our regular lives. Therefore, casuistry is not dead, it is only sleeping.

Bioethics is not a neutral discipline in the context of the current technologized and globalized world. Despite the impossibility of achieving complete consensus on what bioethics' task exactly should be, today more than ever before, the need for deliberative procedures to address and resolve moral quandaries arisen by virtue of biotechnological empowerment and the emergence of brand new biomedical techniques has become an urgent claim and an unavoidable call for bioethicists. Being princier the back-bone of bioethics it is still not clear how it should be applied. What do exactly people do when they apply principlism? How could we make principlism more practical? In the following pages we will explore the methodological strengths and weaknesses of the applicability of principlism through relevant readings and analysis of practical scenarios.

Students are encouraged to think objectively and impartially in order to resolve the ethical dilemmas that stem from biotechnological empowerment and biomedical techniques. Impartiality means that each individual's interests are equally important, and that moral judgments and arguments must be based on and backed by good reasons. Impartiality is a requirement of moral deliberation and decision-making processes since the best decision possible is usually the most objective and impartial one.

Readings

Gordon, John-Stewart, Rauprich, Oliver, Vollmann, Jochen, "Applying the Four-Principle Approach," in *Bioethics*, Jul; 25(6), UK, Blackwell Publishing, 2011: **293–300.**

Beauchamp, Tom L., "Making Principlism Practical: A Commentary on Gordon, Raupich, and Vollmann," *Bioethics*, Jul; 25(6), UK, Blackwell Publishing, 2011: **301–303.**

Applying The Four-Principle Approach

John-Stewart Gordon, Oliver Raupich and Jochen Vollman

Keywords

principlism, four principles, specification, balancing, common morality, applying principlism

Abstract

The four-principle approach to biomedical ethics is used worldwide by practitioners and researchers alike but it is rather unclear what exactly people do when they apply this approach. Ranking, specification, and balancing vary greatly among different people regarding a particular case. Thus, a sound and coherent applicability of principlism seems somewhat mysterious. What are principlists doing? The article examines the methodological strengths and weaknesses of the applicability of this approach. The most important result is that a sound and comprehensible application of the four principles is additionally ensured by making use of the organizing meta-principle of common morality, which is the starting point and constraining framework of moral reasoning.

Introduction

The *Journal of Medical Ethics* 2003, a festschrift edition in honour of Raanan Gillon, includes articles on the question of how to apply the four principles—autonomy, nonmaleficence, beneficence, and justice—to different cases in biomedical ethics. Although the essays are interesting, they seem too perfunctory with regard to a thorough application of the principles to different cases. It is striking that there is hardly any literature that is thorough on the question of how to apply the four-principles approach to a special case. This might be for two different reasons: first, the authors pay, in general, rather little attention to presenting a detailed case study, or secondly, there is a systematic weakness in this approach.

Beauchamp and Childress hold a common morality approach, which can be roughly described as follows:

> The common morality is the set of norms shared by all persons committed to morality. The common morality is not merely *a* morality, in contrast to other moralities. The common morality is applicable to all persons in all

places, and we rightly judge all human conduct by its standards.[1]

Furthermore, the justification of the four universal prima facie principles rests on the shared considered judgements of persons who are serious about morality. Common morality is the starting point and the constraining framework of moral reasoning. Particular moralities contain non-universal moral norms, which are due to cultural, religious, or institutional sources. These norms are concrete and rich in substance, unlike the universal principles, which are abstract and content-thin. The method of specification and the method of balancing are the main tools for enriching the abstract and content-thin universal principles with empirical data that come from the particular moralities. That is, people from different particular moralities may specify and balance the principles differently by virtue of differing empirical data and sources. Some particular moralities, such as the *Pirates' Creed of Ethics*, lie outside the boundaries of the common morality and, hence, are deficient. Beauchamp and Childress seem to claim that the other particular moralities strive for perfection and try to come as close as possible to the common morality. The most developed particular morality is closest to the common morality.

In this article we present a case study using the method of principlism in order to analyze methodological strengths and weaknesses with regard to the applicability of this particular approach. The first part of the article contains the case description, which will be the starting point for the present case study. The second part offers a systematic application of the four-principles approach by presenting different specifications in order to grasp the moral conflict. The third part deals with the issue of how a principlist can deal with a given moral problem after discovering that it cannot be solved by a simple application of the four principles. The fourth part examines the methodological question of whether principlists (can) make use of an organizing or guiding principle in order to decide between conflicting principles. The last part contains some closing remarks.

1. The Case of Maria[2]

Maria was a woman from Athens who died at the age of 82. She was seriously incapacitated by arthritis for over two years prior to her death and was also virtually blind following unsuccessful cataract and glaucoma treatment. Maria had been cared for at home by her family, who never complained. Maria's condition deteriorated drastically when she suffered a severe stroke and was admitted to hospital where she fell into a 'semi-coma'. There, Maria was provided with artificial nutrition and hydration by means of a nasogastric tube. According to the physician, no other treatment was appropriate as Maria was very unlikely to recover.

Maria's family visited her at the hospital regularly but they found these visits very upsetting. Maria found it extremely difficult to speak and was very distressed. Right from the beginning, Maria found her situation intolerable and during the first six weeks of her hospitalization she repeatedly expressed her wish to be allowed to die. She did this through the use of signs and hard-fought words, even though this was itself extremely difficult and distressing for her. Maria became increasingly frustrated and made several repeated attempts to remove her feeding tube.

Maria's family knew that their mother had a lifelong aversion to hospitals and medicine. They also felt a duty to respect her wish to die. After discussing this among themselves, Maria's

1   T. Beauchamp & J. Childress. 2009. *Principles of Biomedical Ethics*. Oxford: Oxford University Press: 3.

2   M. Parker & D. Dickenson. 2005. *The Cambridge Medical Ethics Workbook: Case Studies, Commentaries and Activities*. Cambridge: Cambridge University Press (abridged version): 4–5.

children decided to approach her physician about the possibility of withdrawing treatment and allowing her to die. The physician made it very clear that he would not consider acceding to such a request. He emphasized that the request would contravene his responsibilities as a physician. Further, he argued that Maria's request should not be taken at face value since Maria had a recent history of mild depression. Maria's family were unhappy with this decision and with the physician's reasoning; they thought that they had no other choice but to accept it.

One week later, Maria fell into a full and irreversible coma. After further discussion with the family, the physician agreed to withdraw nutrition but refused to withdraw hydration. Maria had no complications during the next two weeks; she then died suddenly when she suffered a second stroke.

After Maria's death, her son complained bitterly to the physician about the way his mother had been dealt with. He argued that his mother would have died sooner and would have suffered a great deal less if the physician had agreed with the family's request to withdraw all kinds of treatment when this was originally requested. He claimed that when it is clear that a patient will die soon, the physician's duty is to alleviate the patient's suffering; this means that it can sometimes be wrong to keep a patient alive for as long as possible and at all costs.

The physician responded that hydration was not simply another 'form of treatment' but, in fact, the most fundamental form of care. It was his duty as a physician to provide this fundamental care to any patient. Although he would not unnecessarily prolong a dying patient's life, he strongly believed that allowing a patient to die from lack of hydration could not be considered a dignified and peaceful death. This would, in fact, contravene his duty of care as a physician. Additionally, he argued that such action would be against any Greek medical or religious tradition and against his personal beliefs.

2. Applying the Four-Principle Approach

The following analysis is an attempt to apply the four-principle approach thoroughly to a particular case and may be helpful for the examination of other cases as well. In the case of Maria, we detected two main differing views: (i) the principle of nonmaleficence (as interpreted from Maria's and her relatives' view) and the principle of beneficence (as interpreted from the physician's view) are conflicting, and (ii) the persons concerned interpret the principle of autonomy differently. Both points are addressed in order.

(i) Nonmaleficence and Beneficence

Both Maria and the physician agree that there is no chance Maria will recover and that she will die soon; hence the goal is not to prolong life but to provide appropriate care at the end of her life. However, according to Maria, nutrition/hydration is harmful because it prolongs suffering, and therefore a dignified and peaceful death means—with regard to her present situation—allowing her to die by withdrawing treatment. According to the physician, artificial nutrition and hydration is not just another form of medical treatment but the most fundamental form of care which a terminally ill patient should receive by any means. It is a necessary condition for a dignified and peaceful death. To withdraw hydration and nutrition would undermine the patient's dignity. This conflict can be specified as follows:

Maria
1. Do respect the principle of nonmaleficence.
2. Do respect the principle of nonmaleficence by not harming another person.
3. Do not harm another person by violating another person's dignity.

4. Do not violate another person's dignity by preventing a patient who will die soon from dying in a dignified and peaceful manner.

5. Do not prevent a patient who will die soon from dying in a dignified and peaceful manner by providing life-sustaining treatments which prolong suffering.

6. Do not sustain the life of a suffering patient who will die soon by providing artificial nutrition and hydration.

Physician

1. Do respect the principle of beneficence.
2. Do respect the principle of beneficence by promoting good.
3. Do promote good by promoting/enabling dignity.
4. Do promote/enable dignity by letting a patient die in a dignified and peaceful manner.
5. Do let a patient die in a dignified and peaceful manner by (still) providing fundamental care.
6. Do provide fundamental care for a patient by providing artificial nutrition and hydration.

(ii) The Principle of Autonomy

As we saw, the principle of nonmaleficence (as specified from Maria's viewpoint) and the principle of beneficence (as specified by the physician's viewpoint) are in conflict with one another. The core of the conflict seems to be that artificial nutrition and hydration is a precondition for a dignified death, according to the physician, while Maria believes that it is incompatible with a dignified death. How can we decide this issue? Whose view should prevail? Could the principle of autonomy solve the case? The following analysis concerns the principle of autonomy and presents in detail the differing readings of the persons concerned. Maria wants to die through the withdrawal of treatment and she wants her wish to be respected. The physician, however, denies her request, in part because

he thinks that Maria's recent diagnosis of mild depression calls her competence into question. Further, and more important, he stresses the traditional duties and commitments of his profession, that is, his professional autonomy.

Maria

1. Do respect the principle of autonomy.
2. Do respect the principle of autonomy by respecting the concept of informed consent.
3. Do respect the concept of informed consent by respecting individual informed consent.
4. Do respect individual informed consent by giving the patient the right to decide what is in his or her best interest.
5. Do respect the patient's right to decide what is in his or her best interest by respecting his or her refusal of artificial nutrition and hydration.

Physician

1. Do respect the principle of autonomy.
2. Do respect the principle of autonomy by respecting the physician's right to self-determination.
3. Do respect the physician's right to self-determination by respecting his or her personal and professional belief that nutrition and hydration is the most fundamental form of care all terminally ill patients should receive.
4. Do respect the physician's personal and professional belief that nutrition and hydration is the most fundamental form of care all terminally ill patients should receive by respecting his decision to refuse Maria's wish to withdraw artificial nutrition and hydration.

Evaluation 1: Where Is the Moral Conflict?

The first step of principlism (and any other ethical theory) is to detect and determine the moral conflict of a given case by using the power of judgement. In the case of Maria, two vital conflicts have been examined: (i) the conflict between the principle of nonmaleficence (Maria) and the principle of beneficence (physician), and (ii) the different specifications of the principle of autonomy, i.e. autonomy as respect for informed refusal (Maria) and as respect for conscious objection (physician). At first sight, the analysis of the moral conflict above seems successful, although we should say something more about this below. One should always keep in mind, however, that there is no absolute certainty that one is able to determine all the issues of a given case by one single method; good work is done when the core problems of a case are identified and a solution presented.

It is obvious that the physician does not need to deny that nutrition or hydration prolong Maria's suffering but he can still argue that dying through the withdrawal of treatment is even worse because it undermines Maria's dignity. Hence, it is better to suffer physically and psychologically at the end of one's life than to die without dignity. Whether it is possible that Maria acknowledges the physician's point of view but nevertheless adheres to her wish to die is questionable for logical reasons if the manner of her death undermines her concept of dignity. The deep conflict between the principle of nonmaleficence (Maria) and the principle of beneficence (physician) in the present case is challenging and should be further examined. There is no (absolute) certainty that all central aspects of a given case are always properly reconstructed. Case analysis rests for large parts on experience and the ethical power of judgement irrespective of the particular method applied, although different methods, of course, generally determine the outcome. We hold the view that the central issues have

been discovered, but it seems to us that we need more information in order to make a sound principlist decision. This can be done by adding missing facts and by examining the assumptions of the conflicting views.

Deepening the Analysis

First, from what does Maria suffer? Maria suffers from severe pain which is both physical (problems with swallowing) and psychological (total dependency on others);[3] she has made it clear, by signs, hard-fought words, and repeated attempts to remove her feeding tube, that she wants to die. She is distressed and frustrated, has great difficulty in speaking, is handicapped and solely dependent on other people, and has had a lifelong aversion to hospitals and medicine. In addition, she will die soon and wants no further nutrition or hydration because she supposes that this will quicken her death, which in turn will end her suffering.

Secondly, given that Maria has mild depression, as the physician diagnosed, which affects her capacity for decision-making, what follows from this? The decisive question is whether the depression rests on her increasing frustration because of the physician's refusal to let her die by withdrawing nutrition and hydration, or whether it rests on her initial ill-health so that she was already incompetent when she first expressed her wish to die after being admitted to hospital. According to us, it seems more likely, with regard to the case description, that her mild depression rests on the physician's refusal to let her die; and thus her initial wish to die should be respected. To put it in a nutshell, it may be, of course, that Maria's condition is getting worse during her illness but it seems somewhat inappropriate to question her initial decision to be

---

3 Unfortunately, the case description offers no other details about Maria's pain, which could help us to determine issues with important consequences for the evaluation of the case.

allowed to die by virtue of her later, deteriorated condition; this would be putting the cart before the horse.

Thirdly, is artificial hydration just another 'form of treatment' or is it the 'most fundamental form of care that [...] a physician feels is his duty to provide to any patient'? This point seems somewhat controversial: On the one hand, it is certainly true that artificial hydration is, of course, a form of medical treatment. On the other hand, we acknowledge the fact that the physician wants to make a distinction between other forms of treatment and providing a patient with hydration, which he claims to be 'the most fundamental form of care'. Losing a patient because he or she dies of thirst seems to be like having to bite the bullet against the background of probably the most important medical credo, *primum nil nocere*. According to other people, however, providing hydration is seen in some cases as a futile treatment, which only prolongs the patient's suffering, and hence patients should be allowed to die through the withdrawal of treatment. We think that there is no ultimate solution to this issue; one has to examine each case in order to find its suitable solution.

Fourthly, should the medical tradition of a given country always prevail over the patient's personal beliefs? To justify his decision to refuse Maria's demand to die, the physician claims that acceding to this request would contravene the medical tradition of his country. Maria is also Greek but she may not be absolutely devoted to the rules of the predominant medical tradition of her country. The decisive question is whether this should play any vital role in the process of ethical decision-making. Who decides which tradition is the predominant one and how many people should support it? Should it be 51%, 75%, or over 90% of the people in the country, or just the highest number of supporters in comparison to other groups (30%, 28%, 22%, 10% etc.)? Should the predominant tradition be allowed to influence the lives of other people who live according to

different standards? There seems to be no one tradition or culture; there are always different ways of being devoted to a country's tradition and culture.

Fifthly, should the religious beliefs of the physician play any decisive role? According to principlism, the country's religious traditions are part of the particular morality. The particular morality provides the empirical data for the specification and balancing of the four principles of the common morality. Regarding the religious tradition and the physician's religious beliefs, one may question whether either should play any vital part in the decision-making process. It is difficult to assess whether the specific religious beliefs of a given country or idiosyncratic convictions (ever) lead to valid specifications of universal principles. Religious beliefs may well explain why one holds a special view but they seem less good at justifying particular specifications or forming a reasonable and reliable guide for solving conflicts by meeting universal demands.

The main result is that the abovementioned facts[4] are additional determinants in the process of decision-making. They provide us with additional information on issues related to the main conflicts of the case in question and are meant to broaden our minds to be more case-sensitive.

3. How Can a Principlist Deal with the Present Moral Problem?

There are two different ways, at least, to enrich the moral analysis of a particular case with

---

4   (i) The kind of harm Maria suffers, (ii) the assessment of Maria's competence with respect to her capacity to make informed decisions, (iii) whether artificial nutrition is a form of treatment or the most fundamental form of care, (iv) the issue of whether the medical tradition of the country should play a vital role in the process of decision making, and (v) whether the personal and religious beliefs of the physician should be acknowledged.

regard to the principlist strategy: (i) to make additional specifications, and (ii) to make use of the method of balancing.

(i) Additional Specifications

By making additional specifications, the principlist tries to solve the conflicts between (a) differing principles (e.g. nonmaleficence and beneficence) or (b) different interpretations of one principle (e.g. autonomy). Conflicting principles and interpretations should be reconciled against the background of new facts and assumptions in order to solve the moral conflict.

(a) Beneficence

The following specification of the principle of beneficence (physician) can solve the conflict between the differing principles of Maria and the physician. The line of argumentation is as follows: Dying through the withdrawal of treatment (nutrition/hydration) is an undignified death if and only if it expresses disrespect for the person in question (Maria). However, withdrawing treatment and, at the same time, providing high-quality palliative care and personal attention to Maria would certainly not express disrespect, and hence it should not be seen as an undignified death.

(b) Autonomy

The principle of autonomy was initially directed against the more paternalistic reasoning of physicians who cared little about patients' wishes. In the present case, however, the line of argumentation concerning Maria's mild depression can be specified as follows: Maria has the right to decide what is in her best interest if and only if her decision is based on her informed consent. At the time of her decision, she must be competent and her decision voluntary; her initial decision must not be conditioned by a state of depression (or maybe mild depression), in order to be sure that she is able to make sound decisions. It seems plausible to us, then, that Maria's initial wish can be seen as an oral advance directive, assuming that she was competent, which functions as her present living will in cases of incompetence. Thus, the physician should acknowledge and accept this as legally binding. This means that he is committed to her initial wish that artificial nutrition and hydration should be withdrawn.

The additional specifications support the general line of argumentation that Maria should be allowed to have her treatment withdrawn. High-quality palliative care and her initial will, which can be seen as an oral advance directive, seem to be appropriate reasons for her justified decision. It is hard to see how the physician can argue in another well-justified way with regard to principlism, given the prior examination of the principles concerning the case in question. Therefore, it seems that no sound alternative specifications are available for the physician that could justify his view. The analysis is determined in form and content by the method of principlism.

(ii) Balancing: Personal Autonomy Trumps Professional Autonomy

The principle of autonomy can be specified in different ways; in Maria's case two rival but valid specifications (personal autonomy and professional autonomy) conflict with each other. One systematic way for the four-principle approach to deal with such conflicts is to balance the conflicting specifications.[5] We hold the view

---

5 Balancing is, according to Beauchamp and Childress, 'especially important for reaching judgments in individual cases' (T. Beauchamp & J. Childress. 2001. *Principles of Biomedical Ethics*. Oxford: Oxford University Press: 18), i.e. balancing is 'the process of finding reasons to support beliefs about which moral norms should prevail' (Beauchamp & Childress, *op. cit.* note 1, p. 20). This means that balancing has something to do with providing good

that personal autonomy trumps professional autonomy in the present case because the six conditions given by Beauchamp and Childress seem to justify the former in a more appropriate way. Professional duties and traditions, that is, professional autonomy, should play an important role in daily medical practice but they are improper when they undermine the personal autonomy of a patient who prefers treatment to be withdrawn because he or she will not recover, is suffering greatly, and will die soon.

In order to show why we think that personal autonomy trumps professional autonomy with regard to this particular case we would like to focus on the third condition, 'the infringement is morally preferable', in more detail. We have seen that the physician's position of preferring to provide fundamental care causes severe physical and mental harm to Maria. Given that she is an old woman who has lived her life and will die soon it seems somewhat inappropriate to refuse her initial wish (i.e. her oral advance directive) for treatment to be withdrawn against the background that high-quality palliative care could be provided. Professional autonomy is certainly very important in health care, but there are cases where the personal autonomy of the patient should prevail. It seems morally preferable to us that personal autonomy prevails in the present case and, therefore, to treat Maria according to her initial will, which will give her dignity, at least in her view.

Evaluation 2: Solving the Moral Problem

The opponents of principlism such as Gert and Clouser claim that principlists do not use a guiding principle and hence are unable to make a justified decision with regard to opposing specifications in a particular case. The reason is that Beauchamp and Childress' conception of principlism, in their view, does not contain an organizing meta-principle such as Kant's Categorical Imperative or the Utilitarian principle that decides which of the four principles or particular specifications should prevail when people are faced with a deep moral conflict, such as in the case of Maria. This also holds against the background of the method of balancing, which is helpful, as we saw above, but still not sufficient.[6] At first sight, this (standard) objection seems to have some plausibility if people only consider the differing specifications without making any attempt to reconcile them in a second step. At second glance, however, one acknowledges that the common morality itself is a principle that organises the specifications, at least, to some extent. The next section examines this promising way of principled reasoning.

4. Common Morality as an Organizing Principle

First, we would like to begin with a clarification with regard to ethical theories that apply a single

---

reasons for justified acts. The following six conditions meet the important objection that balancing seems too intuitive and open-ended: (1) the overriding norm is more reasonable, (2) the infringement's justifying objective must be achievable, (3) the infringement is morally preferable, (4) the infringement must be in accord with the primary goal of action, (5) the infringement's possible negative effects must be minimized, and (6) there must be impartiality in action (Ibid: 23). That is why Beauchamp and Childress make the conciliatory claim that 'in some circumstances we will not be able to determine which moral norm to follow' (Ibid: 24).

---

6   One may gain the impression that there is still no really sufficient solution to the case in question; but this is somewhat misleading. One has to distinguish two levels in this issue: the practical level and the theoretical level. Practically speaking, the results at stake seem sufficient for solving the problem but still lack the theoretical constraining framework. That is, the theoretical level should be examined in more detail in order to help us see how it can enrich the practical level by providing more methodological certainty.

organizing or guiding principle, such as is provided by classical Kantianism (the Categorical Imperative) or Utilitarianism (the greatest good for the greatest number). Proponents of these classical theories usually argue that their theories are superior to other theories that have no single organizing principle but several independent principles. This is so, according to their view, because the other theories are simply unable to solve moral problems in a clear and comprehensible way (e.g. principlism). This can be called the standard objection. It remains unclear, however, whether this is really the case; Kantianism and Utilitarianism usually have greater problems when they are applied to complex cases in applied ethics because of their lack of case sensitivity. These ethical theories adhere to the deductive model of justification (theory–principle–rules–judgement), which seems to be less sufficient in the area of applied ethics, in particular, bioethics.

Even one of the most vehement opponents of principlism, Bernard Gert, acknowledges in his work, *Common Morality. Deciding What to Do*:

> But the claim that morality is based solely on human nature does not mean that common morality provides a unique correct answer to every moral question. It is impossible to provide a description of morality that will both resolve every moral disagreement and also be endorsed by all rational persons. Common morality is a framework or system that can help individuals decide what to do when faced with a moral problem, but within limits, it allows for divergent answers to most controversial questions.[7]

His considerations are certainly true, but what is most interesting concerning his criticism of principlism is that he seems to accept plausible divergent answers to controversial

issues for his own theory, but denies the same right to Beauchamp and Childress. In the following, however, we would like to show how one could conceive of common morality as an organizing or guiding principle.

Common morality not only concerns certain particular moralities by being their starting point and constraining framework, but also applies to concrete situations, in which, for example, one knows not to lie, not to steal property, to keep promises, to respect the rights of others, not to kill or cause harm to innocent persons, and the like.[8] This is important because common morality can, then, function as a guiding principle in situations where diverse principles and rules may conflict. Of course, we do not hold the view that common morality is able to provide a unique correct answer,[9] but it can be seen as a constraining framework that, first, separates ethical from unethical answers, and secondly, indicates which ethical answer seems more appropriate with regard to the ideal of common morality without saying that this is the only correct available answer. However, if the regulative idea of common morality can be seen as the proposed meta-principle of principlism, then we should be able to apply this meta-principle to the present case in order to provide a well-justified solution for the moral conflict.

What then are the particular weighting considerations that can be derived from the common morality in order to solve the particular conflict? An appropriate response to this important question concerns the notion of common morality itself and how the common morality is justified. In recent years, Beauchamp and Childress have

---

7 B. Gert. 2007. *Common Morality. Deciding What to Do.* Oxford: Oxford University Press: 4.

8 Beauchamp & Childress. *op.cit.* note 1.

9 The view that there is only 'one' best solution to a moral problem has been held by various well-known philosophers such as Aristotle (virtue ethics), Kant (deontology), and Bentham (Utilitarianism). Other philosophers, however, e.g. Beauchamp and Childress (principlism) or Gert (common morality approach), believe instead that there can be different and equally good solutions to moral problems. To 'solve a moral problem', then, means to provide a well-justified solution for a particular moral conflict without necessarily claiming that this is the only acceptable answer.

offered three main ways to determine the common morality: (i) by appealing to morally serious persons,[10] (ii) by appealing to persons committed to the objectives of morality,[11] or (iii) by appealing to persons committed to morality.[12]

In the first approach, common morality is defined as a set of norms shared by all morally serious persons. In the second approach, common morality is defined as a set of norms shared by all persons committed to the objectives of morality, which are those 'of promoting human flourishing by counteracting conditions that cause the quality of people's lives to worsen'.[13] In the third approach the notion of common morality is based neither on morally serious persons nor on the objectives of morality but on the idea that common morality— as a set of norms shared by all persons committed to morality—is applicable to all persons in all places and judges all human conduct.

We believe that the first approach (morally serious persons) is the best one to use in applying common morality to particular cases. Although considered judgements are moral convictions of the highest grade of confidence and the lowest level of bias, Rawls[14] claims that considered judgements should be accepted 'provisionally as fixed points' but that they are 'liable to revision'. For Beauchamp and Childress the aim of reflective equilibrium is to match, prune, and adjust considered judgements in order to make them coherent with the premises of the most general moral commitments concerning human conduct. Furthermore, the powerful methods of specification and balancing provide further 'weighting considerations' in order to solve the moral conflict, as we have thoroughly demonstrated by our detailed analysis of how to apply principlism in the present case of Maria.

To put it in a nutshell, the appeal to common morality suggests the following main line of argumentation: Morally serious persons agree that the wishes of competent adult persons with regard to medical treatments should be respected unless they are not in their best interest. Maria experiences suffering from a serious health condition and will die soon, hence she should be allowed to die by the withdrawal of nutrition and hydration. To prolong the process of dying by acting against her expressed wish seems not to be in her best interest. Given the many details of this case, her request to be allowed to die seems reasonable and in accord with common morality. To act otherwise, that is, to continue the medical treatment, would be unjustified and would undermine her initial autonomous decision.

Evaluation 3: Does the Organizing Principle Do any Good?

By applying the meta-principle of common morality in the above-mentioned way as a constraining framework, it seems that Maria's wish should be respected and that high-quality palliative care and personal attention must be provided to her. To act otherwise would harm Maria and deprive her of her initial autonomous decision to arrange the way in which her life should end. Maria's deliberations should be respected even if it means that the physician in charge has serious doubts; and if he is not willing to comply with her wishes, he should refer the case to another colleague. The latter point is of great importance because not to offer Maria the opportunity to see another physician would severely undermine her autonomy and right to self-determination. This would harm Maria in addition to her current situation.

Elderly people who suffer from a severe illness and will die soon are not living puppets

10 Beauchamp & Childress, *op. cit.* note 5.
11 T. Beauchamp. Defense of Common Morality. *Kennedy Inst Ethics J* 2003: 13(3): 259–274.
12 Beauchamp & Childress, *op. cit.* note 1.
13 Beauchamp, *op. cit.* note 11, p. 260.
14 J. Rawls. 1971. *A Theory of Justice.* Cambridge MA: Harvard University Press.

in the medical theatre of end-of-life decisions; their wishes should be respected as a form of showing final respect toward them. Human well-being can fall victim to wrong paternalistic and idiosyncratic reasoning when we do not act in the patient's best interest. End-of-life decisions should be made by mutual consent; that is, both parties—the patient and the physician—should act in concert. In complex cases, however, this does not always happen and the important question is, what should then be done. Although the physician, by virtue of his understanding of his medical profession, is no simple handmaid who fulfils all patients' wishes without question, he nevertheless has a duty not to give the patient feelings of helplessness and loneliness by simply acting against the patient's wishes. It seems that, depending on the particular situation, but particularly in hopeless end-of-life cases, physicians should simply accept that their patients might be permitted to do what they want to do.

5. Conclusions

We have seen that applying the method of principlism is not an easy task. Our analysis showed that principlism is not a mere 'checklist' method when it is done properly. The application of principlism is a challenging way to solve moral conflicts in biomedical ethics; it follows certain procedures to achieve the best solution it can. The analysis has shown, however, that the most important feature, in addition to the methods of specification and balancing, is the guiding meta-principle of common morality, which functions as a regulative idea to solve deep conflicts between rival principles. The four-principles approach, properly used, is a powerful tool for bioethical decision-making.

Making Principlism Practical: A Commentary on Gordon, Raupich, and Vollman

Tom L. Beauchamp

In their article in this issue, John-Stewart Gordon, Oliver Raupich, and Jochen Vollman examine the justifiability and practicality of principlist theory. The authors show a solid grasp of the theoretical foundations of principlism, and they make an original contribution to literature on the use of case studies in the four-principle approach. I substantially agree with the authors' conclusions and the path taken to reach those conclusions. Nonetheless, I will raise questions that need more attention than they receive in this article. One problem is whether their analysis is applicable only to principlism or is applicable more broadly to other areas of practical ethics. Another problem concerns whether they need to make modifications in their conception of how moral reasoning should proceed when principles come into contingent conflict.

Section 1 in the article treats the main case of a seriously compromised and mildly depressed patient, Maria; and Section 2 concentrates on how to think through this and other cases, that is, how to apply the four-principle approach. The authors omit discussion of moral directives that are less general than principles such as moral rules, guidelines, codes, and regulations (which can themselves be assessed for adequacy on a principlist account). However, this omission does not detract from the methodological thrust of the article, because contingent conflict situations occur at all levels of generality, and principlist *methods* are invariant across the levels of generality in conflict situations.

A related problem is whether the methods of handling contingent conflict and the application of general norms—as presented by Gordon, Rauprich, and Vollmann—affect only principlist theory. Their arguments can without difficulty be interpreted as general lessons in 'applied ethics', despite the fact that the methods under discussion are those that have been proposed in the literature by principlists. As long as the focus is solely on the four principles and their application, then nonprinciplist alternative moral theories or frameworks (e.g. Bernard Gert and Danner Clouser's theory) will not come under discussion. But other accounts could easily be included in the scope of the arguments in this article. Nothing is unique to principlism when it comes to contingent conflict, balancing, and specification of general norms. Put another way, Gordon, Rauprich, and Vollmann could make the claim that the methods they identify are the methods required for any successful applied ethics, or at least required for any account that starts from norms of obligation. This claim is defensible, and I would like to see them head their arguments in this direction.

When discussing decision-making in the case of Maria, the authors invoke the method of specification. They are right to say that the 'method of specification and the method of balancing are the main tools for enriching the abstract and content-thin universal principles' proposed in principlist theory. Since the authors do not explain what specification is, a short explanation of it here may prove helpful. Specification is a methodological tool that adds content to abstract principles, ridding them of their indeterminateness and providing action-guiding content for the purpose of coping with complex cases. Many already specified norms will need further specification to handle new circumstances of indeterminateness and conflict. Incremental specification can progressively reduce circumstances of conflict to more manageable dimensions. This increase of substance is essential for decision-making in clinical and research ethics. Otherwise, abstract principles cannot be carried to the ground and will not be serviceable for the resolution of cases.

Specifying norms is achieved by narrowing their scope, not by interpreting the meaning of terms in the general norms (such as 'autonomy'). The scope is narrowed, as Henry Richardson puts it in his pioneering work on the subject, by 'spelling out where, when, why, how, by what means, to whom, or by whom the action is to be done or avoided.'[1] A definition of 'respect for autonomy' (as, say, 'allowing competent persons to exercise their liberty rights') clarifies the meaning of a moral notion, but it does not narrow the scope of the norm or render it more specific and practical. The definition is therefore not a specification.

The authors' treatment of the conflict at work in the case of Maria's desperate circumstance

conforms to this conception of specification. The authors say that specification has the potential to enrich moral analysis of, and even 'solve', the problems in the case. I agree with the general direction of their argument, and in particular I support their attempt to reconcile the different points of view that arise in the case. I also agree with their resolution of this case: 'It is hard to see how the physician can argue in another [i.e. any other such] well-justified way with regard to principlism.'

Nonetheless, their analysis needs additional clarity regarding which norms are in contingent conflict and how the several norms are specified. They claim that the principles of nonmaleficence and beneficence are in conflict, and they also suggest that the patient's point of view in invoking these principles and the physician's point of view in invoking these principles are in conflict. They even speak of 'the differing principles of Maria and the physician'. These claims seem to derive from their view that *Maria* accepts the principle 'Do respect the principle of nonmaleficence,' whereas the physician accepts the principle 'Do respect the principle of beneficence.' However, this confluence of claims and arguments is confusing. The principles in the physician's outlook are not different from the principles in the patient's outlook. They both accept the principles of nonmaleficence and beneficence. They simply have different *specifications* of these principles. That is, the patient does not have *principles* that differ from the physician's principles. Differences arise only because the principles are competitively specified (and with some differences in the interpretation of central concepts).

The conflict in the case of Maria is between the physician's perspective (which by itself coherently appeals, free of contingent conflict, to both nonmaleficence and beneficence and their specification) and the patient's perspective (which also by itself coherently appeals, without contingent conflict, to the principles of nonmaleficence and beneficence and their specification). The conflicting directives reached by the

1   Henry S. Richardson. 2005. Specifying, Balancing, and Interpreting Bioethical Principles. In *Belmont Revisited: Ethical Principles for Research with Human Subjects*. J.F. Childress, E.M. Meslin & H.T. Shapiro, eds. Washington DC: Georgetown University Press: 205–227.

physician and the patient do call for what the authors call a 'deeper analysis' that impartially assesses how to handle the deeper type of conflict at work in the case, and they are right to say that resolution can only be achieved by further specification and/or balancing in light of careful attention to the details of the case.

The authors could have claimed that there is a conflict between respect for autonomy and either beneficence or nonmaleficence (thus highlighting the conflict between patient decision-making and professional beneficence), and I suspect this perspective would have improved the analysis. However, this seems not to be the claim made. They say only that a vital conflict occurs between two competitive specifications of the principle of respect for autonomy. In focusing on Maria's mild depression and her specification of the principle of respect for autonomy, the authors say that 'the line of argumentation concerning Maria's mild depression can be specified as follows: Maria has the right to decide what is in her best interest if and only if her decision is based on her informed consent.' This specification is clearly central to the case, but the claim made is questionable in this form. The more appropriate formulation of the idea is that Maria has the right to decide what is in her best interest if and only if she is acting voluntarily and is competent to make such a decision. This norm descends, by specification, from the more general norm 'respect the autonomy of voluntary and competent patients by following their voluntary and informed decisions about their care.'

The condition of competence is not identical to the condition of informed consent. If Maria is competent, she has the right to decide whether to consent, to refuse, to waive her right by designating a surrogate, and the like. Consent need not be involved in an exercise of the right. This framework allows the principlist to move to the conclusion that Gordon, Rauprich, and Vollmann in fact ultimately reach in the case: 'Maria should be allowed to have her treatment withdrawn.' If Maria is not a competent

decision-maker, then another body of principles or specifications would be needed.

The authors next argue that, in Maria's case, 'personal autonomy trumps professional autonomy.' This claim is correct, but at times their formulations suggest that they might be using a general trumping strategy to the effect that whenever genuine exercises of patient autonomy conflict with professional autonomy in decision-making, patient autonomy trumps. However, these authors do *not* make the implausible claim that autonomy is a privileged principle having priority over other principles. They mean to assert only that, all things considered, personal autonomy overrides professional autonomy *in the particular case* of Maria. They do not give any higher place to the principle of respect for autonomy.

This conclusion is exactly in line with the principlist claim that respect for autonomy is not an a priori trump over other moral principles and is simply one principle in a framework of prima facie principles. A theory cannot be principlist while claiming that autonomy always has a privileged priority in circumstances of contingent conflict with professional beneficence. The principle of respect for autonomy has never been treated in principlism as a privileged, overriding principle. Although autonomy is not privileged in this way, it does not follow that a *valid refusal* of treatment by a patient is not a trumping consideration in cases of contingent conflict. Whether valid refusals always trump professional beneficence and authority is a difficult problem of medical ethics that cannot be considered here. I note only that on the final page of their article (in the conclusion to 'Evaluation 2'), the authors suggest that they might in fact support this particular strong trumping thesis regarding valid refusals, but they do not pause to argue either for or against it.

I am unsure how to categorize and understand the authors' various appeals, throughout their article, to 'dignity' and what is 'undignified'–categories often associated with autonomy, especially in Kant's philosophy. The first three appearances of this notion in their article have to do with a 'dignified death.' Shortly thereafter, the authors shift to the dignity of patients and persons—and from there they shift to a focus on Maria's dignity. Dignity is one of the most frequently mentioned moral notions in the article, yet 'dignity' is not defined or analysed, and it is a moral notion that has never played a role in principlist theory. I suspect that the authors have not made up their mind about either the meaning of the notion or how it might function in their analysis of applied principlism. Most important would be to decide whether dignity is coming through the back door in this article as a fifth principle (in which case we would no longer have a four-principle framework) or whether dignity is to somehow be situated under one or more of the four principles. I think the notion is expendable without loss.

I particularly appreciate the concluding section of this article on 'Common Morality as an Organizing Principle.' I am reluctant to speak of the common morality as a *principle* (rather, it is a collection of principles and rules). However, the authors propose the interesting and promising thesis that common morality can be interpreted as a *meta-principle* rather than a moral principle in the moral framework of principles. This novel idea leads the authors to a provocative contribution of the still thin literature on the common morality and its role in practical ethics. I highly commend the points made about the need for a constraining meta-principle of this sort.

1. Paternalism and Self-Determination

The term paternalism has been around since ancient times. Etymologically, it means father-like and points out a decision made for a person by someone else who is deemed wiser or eventually has the power to make decisions.

The Greeks and Romans used to live in a mostly patriarchal system so it was common (and natural) that physicians did not feel the obligation to disclose information to their patients. It was trusted and assumed that the physicians were able to make the best decision for their patient without telling them anything.

The fact of acting paternalistically can be morally justified. For instance, sometimes in the clinical field, a true act of paternalism may be plausible if implies the attempt to benefit the patient and also has the goal of helping him/her to feel better and recover. Paternalism is not necessarily supposed to undermine the patient's self-determination to get better, as it is precisely the patients' self-determination that has led them to the doctor. Beauchamp and Childress affirm that for an act to be paternalistic this must restrict the decision of a person who has made an autonomous choice. In their book *Principles of Biomedical Ethics*, these authors recognize this as the "intentional overriding of one person's preferences or actions by another person, where the person who overrides justifies this action by appeal to the goal of benefiting or of preventing or mitigating harm to the person whose preferences or actions are overridden."

Throughout the history of medicine, physicians have always had a certain silence so as not to burden the patient with information that was not deemed necessary for the patient know or have a say in or panic over. Before the conflict that freedom of choice was being taken by the doctors, the silence was considered as part of protecting the patient and doing their job. The sharing of decision-making, and the idea of self-determination, were seen as alien and subjective to the physicians who were being thrust this obligation that differed from the history of care.

Throughout the history of health care, paternalism has long been seen as a commitment of that physician or health worker to beneficence. Observing this principle does not necessarily means to follow or uphold all the rights laid out in the principle of respect for autonomy. However, if doctors are asked to perform their job, then they as physicians have a moral obligation, which does not undermine rights but uphold them.

Self-determination is deciding to seek the available help or not. Deciding on whether to go through treatment or not. Self-determination is the desire to do something or make that particular decision and can also be applied to doctors in both a negative and positive obligation. A negative obligation implies not to coerce patients when they are in the process of decision-making. The positive obligation is equally relevant. Physicians have the obligation to inform thoroughly and take into consideration the background and beliefs of the patient.

Paternalism is not balanced when persons' self-determination is completely ignored. Strong overbearing paternalistic attitudes are how the Nazis justified the concentration camps, sustaining that cleaning the country from those deemed unhealthy and unworthy, such as the Jews and minorities, was the way breed the perfect humans. Self-determination in decisions needs to be considered by those in an authority position. The Tuskegee case is an example where paternalism was used to make research decisions. The study started out as a "study in nature" when 399 African-American men were identified as having syphilis and were just observed. There were not any written protocol and no one was noted as being in charge. To determine the stage of the disease a painful and potentially dangerous spinal tap was performed on the "volunteers." They were offered free transportation, hot lunch, medicine for any disease (other than syphilis), and free burials in exchange for spinal taps and, later, autopsies. Deception was used as well, when the "volunteers" were told about their "Bad blood" and how the spinal taps were "treatment," and the result of not being treated was broadcasted. The doctors used their knowledge over others to take away the choices of those infected. The study violated every human right and was just running on paternalistic decisions. This shows why self-determination should be present in decision-making processes. The question is can paternalism and self-determination coexist in that process?

The Concept of Autonomy[1]

Consent and refusal are both *actions*, actions, which can be performed by either autonomous or non-autonomous *agents* (in exceptional cases). This distinction between actions and agents is relevant to deepen the concepts of paternalism and self-determination. As we shall see, sometimes, autonomous individuals with the capacity to give informed consent, actually act constrained, due to error, ignorance or other reasons. On the contrary, although exceptionally, non-autonomous individuals can in fact act autonomously and consent or refuse without constraints.

Of course, the concept of what it means to act autonomously is not an easy one to define. Theories of autonomy are related to theories of autonomous persons, but we must be cautious when defining autonomous persons for some definitions can be too stringent and render the whole idea of an autonomous being unrealistic. "Theories of the autonomous person need not to be so demanding," in the sense that they should be restricted to the basic, the just necessary. Hence requirements for autonomous actions need to be stated in this fashion too. So, the focus is to examine autonomous actions (of refusal or consent) in order to set the basic requirements for such an action to be called so.

There are three basic conditions for autonomous actions:

X acts autonomously only if X acts:

1. - Intentionally
2. - With Understanding
3. - Without Controlling Influences

The first condition is "not a matter of degree," you whether have the intention to act (and are potentially autonomous) or you do not (and are non-autonomous). The other two conditions are subject to scaling and can be satisfied

---

1   This paragraph is based upon Faden, R., Beauchamp, T., *A History and Theory of Informed Consent*, Oxford University Press, 1986.

to certain degrees, they "may be placed on a broad continuum from fully present to wholly absent." Continuing with the idea of degrees of understanding and control (requisites 2 and 3) there is a point in which enough understanding and non-control renders an action substantially autonomous, which is equivalent to say that it is an action performed with sufficient freedom in order for it to be binding, but "if any one of the three conditions is unsatisfied, the act is non-autonomous."

The idea behind a limit that marks substantially autonomous actions is based on the understanding that complete or fully autonomous actions are nonexistent. Nowhere in real life are we expected to consent with complete understanding and completely uncontrolled, thus, the substantial standard aims to give informed consent in research and treatment ethics a similar approach inspired in other instances of life. The limit of substantially autonomous actions may seem at first arbitrary, but when dealing with specific goals in medicine and research it can be effectively defined and located for the case.

The condition of intentionality refers to the question of "what does it mean to act intentionally?" It does not merely mean to intend to do something, like "I intend to do work", intentionality presupposes that an action must occur preceded by the intention to perform such action, only then can it be said it is an intentional action. Furthermore, an intentional action must be an action in accordance to a plan; the actor must have planned an action in order to perform it (even when the outcomes were not foreseen). So, we can define intentionality simply as "an action willed in accordance with a plan, whether the act is wanted or not." In this sense, an act that is not wanted is still intentional, at least in the minimal sense that it is not accidental, habitual or similar. The case of a man that puts his arm out of the window to signal a turn and gets his shirt wet is a good example. He did not want to get his shirt wet, but the action of sticking his hand out of the car was completely intentional. In this case, the not wanting to get the shirt

wet was not enough to stop him from doing it because he wanted more to signal the turn. This kind of unwanted but intentional acts can be simply called "tolerated" acts.

The Condition of understanding is central to avoid unnecessary paternalism (and to understand informed consent), it goes hand in hand with the information that we are given for in order for us to make a decision based on that information we must "understand" it. Now, no agreement exists on psychology or philosophy about what it means to understand. We use this word in diverse ways, for example, 'I understand how to play football', where understand means competence or "know how". We may also use it as 'I understand you love me', used here as knowing (I understand that proposition X is true). Another way of using understanding is exemplified when we say 'I understand your arguments', in this case, one is not saying that one think those arguments are true (as a matter of knowledge), one is just saying that one "apprehends what has been said." In informed consent, the use of the word understand entails that patients or subjects need to "come to understand *that* they must consent or refuse a particular proposal by understanding *what* is communicated in an informational exchange with a professional."

The general definition would be, then:

> "A person has full or complete understanding of an action when there is a fully adequate apprehension of all the relevant propositions or statements (those that contribute in any way to obtaining an appreciation of the situation) that correctly describe (1) the nature of the action, and (2) the foreseeable consequences and possible outcomes that might follow as a result of performing and not performing the action."[2]

---

2   Faden, R., Beauchamp, T., *A History and Theory of Informed Consent*, Oxford University Press, 1986, p. 252.

So, when an action is executed with less understanding than the required by these criteria, that action is logically less autonomous. When dealing with this idea of full understanding several problems emerge. The fact that someone fails to understand any amount of act-descriptions does not necessarily mean that individual fails to fully understand. "Some act-descriptions are irrelevant", and even when someone is able to understand all possible act-descriptions involved in the case *but one*, let us say, the *vital one* to form his consent, we have a lack of understanding. Deciding which act-descriptions are relevant and which ones are not is a complicated task in itself. There is also a problem emerging from ignorance and false beliefs. If a person bases his actions on false beliefs, whether he is accountable for them or not, and if that false belief is vital to an understanding of the action, that person is then acting in a less than fully autonomous manner. Moreover, some action are probabilistic, their effectiveness is variable in nature. If a treatment turns out to be ineffective in a special case, it is not a false belief to think it is effective in general just because it was ineffective in particular. It is the duty of individuals to understand the probabilistic nature of certain actions, when it is not understood *then* it can be said a false belief has held. Standards of evidence for this kind of beliefs are needed in order to assess their acceptability. Is a person justified in his belief, that is, justified in believing that it is true? Several epistemological questions rise from such a problem, since we have not yet agreed what is a *sufficient justification* for beliefs we can hardly expect to agree on what constitutes a justified belief. In the end, the most efficient way of understanding is effective communication, which will lead to accurate interpretation of what has been said.

The condition of non-control is here understood as a negative condition of "not being controlled by others," it is a logical synonym to autonomy or self-governance. Control is exerted through influences, but not all influences are necessarily controlling, some influences are trivial and some others can even be resisted. Since not all influences are controlling, we can then argue that some are more controlling than others, there degrees of control (or non-control). In this sense, control can be illustrated in a "continuum of influences." In fact, some influences may even facilitate choices. There are three main forms of influence in this analysis: coercion, manipulation and persuasion. Coercion by nature is always controlling and persuasion, on the other hand, is always non-controlling. The degrees of manipulation as influence is correlative to the idea of degrees of autonomy, here too we see that a theoretical threshold separates substantially non-controlling influences from the rest of the continuum (and the theoretical ambiguous area), illustrating that control can be substantial or not when affecting the autonomy of an individual.

A condition of authenticity has been proposed as necessary for a complete account of autonomous actions. Authenticity would broadly be understood as actions in accordance with our character—stable or consistent actions—, actions that seem "authentically ours." A condition of authenticity as such would necessarily narrow the scope of autonomous actions in the sense that many times acts are done specifically against our usual character, maybe to try new experiences, like the old man who rides a roller coaster who never had done it before, or just to purposely act against what others expect of us. These actions of course are autonomous, even though they do not seem authentic to our character. What about a condition of authenticity understood as actions that are not repudiated by the agent? In other words, "values and motives are authentic if and only if the agent does not reflectively repudiate or abjure them." Cases like drug addictions can fall under this category as agents seem to be non-controlled when performing them but still they seem to be non-autonomous. If we take this idea and place it in less extreme examples it starts to lose its appeal. Can we say that, for example, a student of Medicine that dislikes studying, waking up early, going to class, memorizing, et cetera, is non-autonomous when engaging in these activities on a daily basis? It seems rather unlikely. Theories of authenticity rely on practically unknown facts, like what actually *belongs* to the self and what not (as theories of identity) and on the examination of motives in human behavior, its causes and underlying reasons.

Coercion, Manipulation and Persuasion

One final analysis must be completed in order to secure the notions of paternalism and self-determination here presented; namely, the condition of non-control. This condition has to be analyzed from the perspective of three concepts: coercion, manipulation and persuasion.

Coercion is, of the three concepts, the least controversial. No coerced act can ever be autonomous and therefore constitute informed consent, however, the situation changes when we deepen paternalism. What does coercion actually mean? "If one party intentionally and successfully influences another by presenting a credible threat of unwanted and avoidable harm so severe that the person is unable to resist acting to avoid it." This definition has three critical features:

1. The agent of influence must intend to influence the other person by presenting a severe threat,
2. There must be a credible threat, and
3. The threat must be irresistible.

In using this definition we find that offers are not, in fact, forms of coercion. It does not matter how appealing the offer may be, how exaggeratedly attractive the offer may result for a person, for, if we accepted exaggerated offers as forms of coercion, some real life situations like "fat contracts" for athletes would end up being coercive.

Also, not all threats are coercive, only those strong enough so as to make it impossible for the threatened individual to resist acting to avoid them. Then again, by which standard do we measure the resistance? Because threats may perfectly well coerce some individuals and not others, a subjective standard is needed. In some hard cases, where a subjective standard would me impracticable, an objective standard should be used (cases of public or institutional policies of general application, for example).

The case of coercive situations is also in need of analysis. Sometimes situations are so pressing that the psychological effect is similar, if not the same, as that of regular coercion. In this sense, people acting by pressure of coercive situations are not acting freely, but it does not follow that they are not acting autonomously. Basically, a coercive force has to come from the will of another individual, if there is lack of intent to threat there is of course a threat, but an unwilled one. Following this line of thought, not just any force or pressure through threat is coercive it must be a willed threat.

Persuasion, on the other hand, is a rational process, which intends to "successfully induce a person, through appeals to reason, to freely accept—as his or her own—the beliefs, attitudes, values, intentions, or actions advocated by the persuader." Persuasion, then, is a rational reasoning with which you want to influence another individual, these reasons must exist "independent of the persuader." Hence, warning and predictions as arguments must be clearly distinguished from threats and offers. If the persuader controls information, he may choose to disclose certain possible consequences—negative or positive—which he does not in fact control, but has knowledge of. This constitutes persuasion and not manipulation or coercion.

Reasons in persuasion must be good reasons, and by this we must not understand that any reason is good just because an individual holds it, this would make reasons all too subjective.

Good reasons to persuade must be actually believed by the persuader to be true, arguing for a treatment by using a lie amounts to manipulation because the persuaded may believe what he was told, but not the persuader. Persuaders must believe that what they are saying about X is true, or at least demonstrable by evidence.

Manipulation is a "label for a class of influence strategies whose common feature is that they are neither instances of persuasion nor instances of coercion." Manipulative actions can be arranged in a spectrum of influence, according to the model previously discussed, ranging in different degrees of control. It can be defined as "any intentional and successful influence of a person by noncoercively altering the actual choices available to the person or by nonpersuasively altering the other's perception of those choices."[3]

There are three kinds of Manipulative actions: Manipulation of Options, Manipulation of Information, and Psychological Manipulation.

Manipulation of Options "involves the direct modification of the options available for a person with the intent, which is successful, of modifying the person's behavior or belief." It can be an increase or decrease in the number of options or it can be an increase or decrease in the attractiveness of certain options, as when giving incentives or threats for taking those options. The point here is to know which of all the possible manipulations of options can be deemed substantially non-controlling and compatible with sense one informed consent.

Threats, on one hand, can be deemed non-controlling if the "influence" can in fact resist the threat, but chooses not to. Coercion and threats vary only in degrees, as already stated, coercion presents harms so pressing that the influence cannot possibly resist acting to avoid them, in non-coercive threats the degree of harm can be actually resisted.

Offers, on the other hand, pose more trouble when dealing with informed consent. As long as an offer is welcomed, in other words, wanted or willed by the influence, it is always compatible with autonomy and informed consent in sense one. The offer may very well seem hard to resist, but because the influence wants it, welcomes it, it is in accordance and compatible with autonomy because there is no control by others. A harder case is presented by "unwelcomed offers" or situations of desperate need. When considering cases of desperate need, autonomy is compromised in "function of the ease or difficulty the manipulate finds in attempting to resist the offer." This means that any unwelcomed offer will be compatible with informed consent in sense one as long as it is "reasonably easily resisted by the person manipulated." This is nothing more than a subjective criterion for assessing resistance levels.

Manipulation of Information "is a deliberate act that successfully influences a person by nonpersuasively altering the persons understanding of the situation, thereby modifying perceptions of the available options." It is important no understand that there is no actual change in the options available, just a change in perception of those options. Informational Manipulation can be compatible to informed consent in sense one if the requisites of substantial understanding are met; namely, the core disclosure of information, the objective criterion, and the subjective criterion of meeting all relevant information material to the individual's decision for authorization. The case of deception is important for it is the "the most common form of informational manipulation." Deception consists basically of using certain strategies to "cause a person to believe what is false," which inevitably renders deception incompatible with informed consent in sense one.

Psychological manipulation is a broad term for any sort of psychological tactic meant to successfully influence the response of individuals by causing changes in their mental processes "other than those involved in understanding."

---

3 Ibid, p. 354.

It is evidently a hard task to assess if certain psychological manipulation is in a particular case controlling, thus, as a general rule psychological manipulation should be avoided in clinical scenarios.

Readings

Goldman, Alan, "The Refutation of Medical Paternalism," in *The Moral Foundations of Professional Ethics* by Alan Goldman, New Jersey, Rowman & Littlefield, 1980: **173–195.**

Ackerman, Terrence F., "Why Doctors Should Intervene," in *Hastings Center Report*, vol. 12, no. 4 (August 1982): **14–17.**

Practical Scenarios

Instructions for analysis:

1. Explain, in general terms, why the case is morally relevant and controversial.
2. Identify the central moral issue. Justify.
3. Identify and explain the main facts to be considered in your analysis.
4. Identify and explain the principles and theories useful in analyzing the case. Justify why those principles and theories are relevant in the case. Specify conflicts between them.
5. Identify and raise arguments to support the conflicting options/decisions/actions that are evident in the case (Specifications and balancing of rules are necessary at this stage).
6. Identify and weigh alternative courses of action and then decide. Justify your decision. Answer the question(s) posed by the author as part of your conclusion.

Scenario 1

Too Old to Make Decisions?

Sally, a 90 year old woman living alone and independently, is described as spry and mentally "with it." She presents to the emergency room with gastrointestinal bleeding. Her surgeon advises her that, without surgery for what is presumed to be colon cancer, she will bleed to death. She refuses, stating she realizes that her "time has come." The surgeon is alarmed that this very active person is refusing the proposed treatment. He is concerned that she is "too old" to decide for herself.[4]

Question

Should in this case the physician act paternalistically? Why?

Scenario 2

Dilemma at the Emergency Room

Brandon is a 16-year-old single male with cystic fibrosis. He is brought into the emergency room in respiratory crisis. His girlfriend accompanies him. He refuses to be intubated and his girlfriend supports his decision. She states that his condition has been steadily worsening; they both know he is dying, and he is adamant about not wanting to die in a hospital. When his mother appears she demands that he be intubated in no uncertain terms.[5]

Question

Should physicians act paternalistically and intubate Brandon to save his life? Justify your answer.

---

4 Adapted from, *Fletcher's Introduction to Clinical Ethics*, 3rd Edition, University Publishing Group, 2005.
5 Adapted from Taylor, Carol, *Health Care Ethics Course*, Georgetown University School of Medicine, AY 2010-2011.

Scenario 3

The "Retarded" Patient

Frank is a 40 years old man who is unemployed and unsophisticated. He is admitted to the hospital with severe dehydration and impending shock following 36 hours of vomiting. Evaluation reveals a possible small bowel obstruction. After intravenous rehydration, he feels much improved and wants to leave. His family agrees with him. His physician, who is concerned that Frank may still have a bowel obstruction, obtains a court order to treat on the grounds that the patient is "retarded."[6]

Question

Is Frank's physician's decision morally justified? Why?

Scenario 4

The Physician Who Favored "The Moral Health"

In 1970 Doctor Robert Browne was a kindly, 63-year-old British general practitioner. He had been the family physician of a 16-year-old woman since this young woman's birth. This young woman thought she should get some contraceptive counseling. She realized that Dr. Browne might not look to favorably upon this plan, so she went to a place called the Birmingham Brook Advisory Center. This was a local birth control counseling clinic. She got contraceptive counseling, a physical examination and a prescription for oral contraceptives. It is standard medical practice to inform a family physician if one writes a prescription for someone who normally sees another physician. The clinic's physician asked if he could notify her physician, Dr. Browne. Perhaps without thinking, she gave her approval.

Dr. Browne received in the mail, unsolicited, a letter informing him that his patient was on the pill. Dr. Browne expressed two concerns. First, he was concerned about her pharmacological well-being. In 1970 *had not been on the market very long. Nobody understood what the effects might be, especially in a 16-year-old. But he was also worried about her total well-being: in particular about what he called her "moral health."*

Dr. Browne consulted with some colleagues, got their advice, and finally came out with a plan. One day when the young woman's father was in the doctor's office, Dr. Browne told him the whole story.

The young woman was not pleased with this turn of events. The clinic physician was not pleasant either. Dr. Browne was charged before the General Medical Council in Great Britain, with the violation of patient confidentiality. Dr. Browne in his defense introduced two documents: the Hippocratic Oath and the British Medical Association code. The Oath says that the physician should not disclose "that which should not be spread abroad." That, in turn, has traditionally been interpreted as confirming the core Hippocratic principle, that his moral duty is to do what he thinks will benefit the patient. Likewise, the BMA code explicitly permits disclosures when doing so is believed to be for the benefit of the patient. Dr. Browne, having struggle with his conscience and consulted with colleagues, claimed he did what he thought was best for his patient. He may have had a somewhat archaic view about what would benefit her, but he really believed that this was the most beneficial course.[7]

Question

Should the General Medical Council exonerate Dr. Browne? Why?

---

6 Adapted from Taylor, Carol, *Health Care Ethics Course*, Georgetown University School of Medicine, AY 2010-2011.

7 Extracted from, Veatch, Robert, *The Basis of Bioethics*, 3rd Edition, USA, Pearson, 2012.

The Refutation of Medical Paternalism

Alan Goldman

Refutation of Medical Paternalism

There are two ways to attack an argument in favor of paternalistic measures (while accepting our criteria for justified paternalism). One is to argue that honoring rather than overriding the right of the person will not in fact harm him. The other is to admit that the satisfaction of the person's right may harm in some way, but argue that the harm does not merit exception to the right, all things considered. The first is principally an empirical, the second a moral counterargument.

The latter is not a perfectly clear-cut distinction, either in general or in application to the question of paternalism. For one thing, the most inclusive notion of harm is relative to the values and preferences of the particular individual. (This point will be important in the argument to follow.) A person is harmed when a state of affairs below a certain level on his preference scale is realized rather than one higher up. Our notion of harm derives what objectivity it has from two sources, again one principally empirical and the other more purely moral. The first

is the fact that certain states of affairs are such that the vast majority of us would wish to avoid them in almost all conceivable contexts: physical injury, hastened death, or depression itself for example. It is an empirical question whether these states of affairs result from certain courses of conduct, hence, when they are predicted results, principally an empirical question whether harm ensues. The second source of a concept of harm independent of individual differences in subjective preferences is ideal-regarding: when the development of an individual capable of freely and creatively formulating and acting to realize central life projects is blocked, that person is harmed, whether or not he realizes it, and whether or not any of his present desires are frustrated.

The first argument against paternalistic interference holds that allowing an individual free choice is not most likely to result in harm taken in its objective sense. The second argument is somewhat more complex. It admits likely harm in the objective sense—worsened health, depression, or even hastened death in the examples we are considering—but holds that even greater harm to the individual is likely to ensue from the interference, harm in the more inclusive sense that takes account of his whole range of value orderings and the independent value of his integrity as an individual. In this latter situation there is one sense in which the individual is likely to suffer harm no matter what others do, since a state of affairs will be realized that he would wish to avoid, other things being equal, a state of affairs well below the neutral level in his preference orderings. But from the point of view of others, they impose harm only by interfering, since only that action results in a state of affairs lower on his scale of preferences than would otherwise be realized. In this sense harm is a relative notion, first because it is relative to subjective value orderings, and second because it is imposed only when a situation *worse* that what would otherwise occur is caused. We appeal to this second more inclusive notion in the second type of argument against paternalism.

Empirical Arguments

Returning to the medical context, other philosophers have recently questioned the degree of truth in the empirical premise that patients are likely to be harmed when doctors fully inform them. Sissela Bok, for example, has noted that in general it appears to be false that patients do not really want bad news, cannot accept or understand it, or are harmed by it. Yet she does not deny that information can sometimes harm patients, can cause depression, prolong illness, or even hasten death; and she explicitly allows for concealment when this can be shown in terminal cases.[10] Allen Buchanan questions the ability of the doctor to make a competent judgment on the probability of harm to the patient, a judgment that would require both psychiactric expertise and intimate knowledge of the patient himself. Doctors are not generally trained to judge long-term psychological reactions, and even if they were, they would require detailed psychological histories of patients in order to apply this expertise in particular

cases. As medical practices tend to become more impersonal, certainly a trend in recent years, such intimate knowledge of patients, even on a nontheoretical level, will normally be lacking. Physicians would then have to rely upon loose generalizations, based on prior impressions of other patients and folklore from colleagues, in order to predict the effect of information on particular patients.

Buchanan appears to consider this point sufficient to refute the argument for paternalism, eschewing appeal to paitents' rights.[11] But unless we begin with a strong presumption of a right of the patient to the truth, I do not see why the difficulties for the doctor in judging the effect of information on the patient recommends a practice of disclosure. If the decision is to be based upon risk-benefit calculation (as it would be without consideration of rights), then, just as in other decisions regarding treatment, no matter how difficult to make, it seems that the doctor should act on his best estimate. The decision on what to say must be made by him one way or the other; and without a right-based presumption in favor of revealing the truth, its difficulty is no argument for one outcome rather than the other. In fact, the difficulty might count against revelation, since telling the truth is generally more irreversible than concealment or delay.

One could, it is true, attempt to make out a case for full disclosure on strict risk-benefit grounds, without appeal to rights. As we have seen in earlier chapters, utilitarians can go to great lengths to show that their calculations accord with the intuitive recognition of particular rights. In the case of lying or deceiving, they standardly appeal to certain systematic disutilities that might be projected, e.g. effects upon the agent's trustworthiness and upon the trust that other people are willing to accord him if his lies are discovered. In the doctor's case, he might fear losing patients or losing the faith of patients who continue to consult him, if he is caught in lies or deceptions. A utilitarian could argue further that, even in situations in which these disutilities appear not to figure, this appearance tends to be misleading, and that potential liars should therefore resist the temptation on this ground. One problem with this argument, as pointed out in the chapter on political ethics, is that it is empirically falsified in many situations. It is not always so difficult to foretell the utilitarian effects of deception, at least no more difficult than is any other future-looking moral calculation. In the case of terminally ill patients, for example, by the time they realize that their doctors have been deceiving them, they will be in no condition to communicate this fact to other patients or potential patients, even if such communication were otherwise commonplace. Thus the doctor has little to fear in the way of losing patients or patients' faith from his policy of disclosure or concealment from the terminally ill. He can safely calculate risks and benefits with little regard for such systematic disutilities. Again we have little reason to prefer honoring a right, in this case a right to be told the truth, without appealing to the right itself. The only conclusion that I would draw from the empirical points taken in themselves is that doctors should perhaps be better trained in psychology in order to be better able to judge the effects of disclosure upon patients, not that they should make a practice of full disclosure and of allowing patients full control over decisions on treatment. These conclusions we must reach by a different rights-based route.

I shall then criticize the argument for paternalistic strong role differentiation on the more fundamental moral ground. To do so I shall restrict attention to cases in which there is a definite risk or probability of eventual harm (in the objective sense) to the patient's health from revealing the truth about his condition to him, or from informing him of all risks of alternative treatments and allowing him a fully informed decision. These cases are those in which the high probability of harm can be supported or demonstrated, but in which the patient asks to know the truth. Such cases are not decided by the points of Bok or Buchanan, and they are the crucial ones for the question of strong role differentiation.

The issue is whether such projected harm is sufficient to justify concealment. If the patient's normal right to self-determination prevails, then the doctor, in having to honor this right, is acting within the same moral framework as the rest of us. If the doctor acquires the authority to decide for the patient, a normally competent adult, or to withhold the truth about his own condition from him, then he has special professional license to override otherwise obtaining rights, and his position is strongly differentiated.

Before presenting the case against strong role differentiation on this basis, I want to dispense quickly with a possible conceptual objection. One might claim that the justification of medical paternalism would not in itself satisfy the criteria for strong role differentiation as defined. Since paternalism is justified as well in other contexts, the exceptions to the rights in question need not be seen to derive from a special principle unique to medical ethics, but can be held simply to instantiate a generally recognized ground for restricting rights or freedoms. If serious harm to a person himself generally can be counted as overriding evidence that the projected action is contrary to his own true preferences or values, and if this generally justifies paternalistic interference or delegation of authority for decisions to others, if, for example, legislators assume authority to apply coercive sanctions to behavior on these grounds, then the authority to be paternalistic would not uniquely differentiate doctors.

The above may be true in so far as paternalism is sometimes justified in other than medical contexts, but that does not alter the import of the argument for medical paternalism to our perception of the doctor's role. If the argument were sound, the medical profession might still be the only one, or one of only a few, paternalistic in this way. This would differentiate medical ethics sufficiently. I argued earlier that legislators must in fact honor normal moral rights. While paternalistic legislation is sometimes justified, as in the requirement that motorcycle riders wear helmets, such legislation is so relatively small a part of the legislator's concerns, and the amount of coercion justified itself so relatively light, that this does not alter our perception of the legislator's general moral framework. If the paternalist argument were sound in relation to doctors, on the other hand, this would substantially alter the nature of their practice and our perception of their authority over certain areas of our lives. We can therefore view the paternalist argument as expressing the underlying moral purposes that elevate the Hippocratic principle and augment the doctor's authority to ignore systematically rights that would obtain against all but those in the medical profession. The values expressed and elevated are viewed by doctors themselves as central to their role, which again distinguishes this argument from claims of justified paternalism in other contexts. Furthermore, viewing the argument in this way brings out the interesting relations between positions of doctors and those in other professions and social roles. It brings out that doctors tend to assume broader moral responsibility for decisions than laymen, while those in certain other professions tend to assume less. In any case, while I shall not in the end view the doctor's role as strongly differentiated, I do not want to rely upon this terminological point, but rather to refute the argument for overriding patients' rights to further the medical goal of optimal treatment.

The Moral Argument

In order to refute an argument, we of course need to refute only one of its premises. The argument for medical paternalism, stripped to its barest outline, was:

1. Disclosure of information to the patient will sometimes increase the likelihood of depression and physical deterioration, or result in choice of medically inoptimal treatment.
2. Disclosure of information is therefore sometimes likely to be detrimental to the patient's health, perhaps even to hasten his death.
3. Health and prolonged life can be assumed to have priority among preferences for patients who place themselves under physicians' care.
4. Worsening health or hastening death can therefore be assumed to be contrary to patients' own true value orderings.
5. Paternalism is therefore justified: doctors may sometimes override patients' prima facie rights to information about risks and treatments or about their own conditions in order to prevent harm to their health.

The Relativity of Values: Health and Life

The fundamentally faulty premise in the argument for paternalistic role differentiation for doctors is that which assumes that health or prolonged life must take absolute priority in the patient's value orderings. In order for paternalistic interference to be justified, a person must be acting irrationally or inconsistently with his own long-range preferences. The value ordering violated by the action to be prevented must either be known to be that of the person himself, as in the train example, or else be uncontroversially that of any rational person, as in the motorcycle helmet case. But can we assume that health and prolonged life have top priority in any rational ordering? *If* these values could be safely assumed to be always overriding for those who seek medical assistance, then medical expertise would become paramount in decisions regarding treatment, and decisions on disclosure would become assimilated to those within the treatment context. But in fact very few of us act according to such an assumed value ordering. In designing social policy we do not devote all funds or efforts toward minimizing loss of life, on the highways or in hospitals for example.

If our primary goal were always to minimize risk to health and life, we should spend our entire federal budget in health-related areas. Certainly such a suggestion would be ludicrous. We do not in fact grant to individuals rights to minimal risk in their activities or to absolutely optimal health care. From another perspective, if life itself, rather than life of a certain quality with autonomy and dignity, were of ultimate value, then even defensive wars could never be justified. But when the quality of life and the autonomy of an entire nation is threatened from without, defensive war in which many lives are risked and lost is a rational posture. To paraphrase Camus, anything worth living for is worth dying for. To realize or preserve those values that give meaning to life is worth the risk of life itself. Such fundamental values (and autonomy for individuals is certainly among them), necessary within a framework in which life of a certain quality becomes possible, appear to take precedence over the value of mere biological existence.

In personal life too we often engage in risky activities for far less exalted reasons, in fact just for the pleasure or convenience. We work too hard, smoke, exercise too little or too much, eat what we know is bad for us, and continue to do all these things even when informed of their possibly fatal effects. To doctors in their roles as doctors all this may appear irrational, although they no more act always to preserve their own health than do the rest of us. If certain risks to life and health are irrational, others are not. Once more the quality and significance of one's life may take precedence over maximal longevity. Many people when they are sick think of nothing above getting better; but this is not true of all. A person with a heart condition may decide that important unfinished work or projects must take priority over increased risk to his health; and his priority is not uncontroversially irrational. Since people's lives derive meaning and fulfillment from their projects and accomplishments, a person's risking a shortened life for one more fulfilled might well justify actions detrimental to his health.

This question of the meaning and value of life, one of the classic questions of philosophy, is raised directly by our issue in medical ethics. We cannot avoid a brief plunge into such deep waters, if we are to come to grips with the doctor's claim to be justified in acting above all else to protect the life and health of his patients. We have seen that this claim presupposes an ultimate value to life itself, but this is called into question once we begin to ponder life's meaning, the sources of its value and significance beyond mere physical existence. We noted above that in both social policy and individual activity we appear willing to trade near certainty of shorter life for the chance of accomplishments and even small enjoyments. The same value ordering is manifest in our varying attitudes toward different forms of life.[12] Not all biological life is considered sacred: lower forms of animal life, for example certain insects, are held to have little if any value at all. Nor is it simply a matter of human life versus all other forms; we recognize a continuum in which some forms of animal life are due greater respect and even granted rights, against cruel treatment for example. It also seems clear that not only humans could qualify for full scale moral status as persons, i.e. beings with a full battery of moral rights. Extra-terrestrial forms of life might so qualify if they met certain criteria. This suggests that it is on the basis of such criteria that humans too deserve full moral respect, a point of great relevance here. These criteria might include self-motivativation, the ability to have desires and feelings, make plans, enjoy satisfactions and suffer frustrations, and to respect the autonomy and rights of others. Thus the value of life, as this is measured by the respect shown it by other valuing persons, is connected to the fundamental right of self-determination, the ability to create and realize value in activities. Respect for individual lives is connected to respect for individual moral agency.

From the personal point of view as well, life has meaning when it has value for the subject himself; and the value it has derives from the value that the subject finds in his activities and satisfactions. What gives life meaning for the individual are the goals and projects he sets for himself, in terms of which particular means acquire significance and hence derive value. These goals and projects may of course vary in dimension, ranging from life-long plans to immediate desires for pleasurable sensations. They may be more or less biologically determined. Those more so are not necessarily less significant for it, since they are a source of natural enjoyments, from the satisfactions of sating physical appetites to those of interpersonal relations. But such natural enjoyments themselves derive whatever greater significance they may have from their place in longer-term relationships and longer-range goals and projects. The latter stand in various nesting and subordinate relations to each other, giving to life as a whole its timbre and significance for the person whose life it is.

This view is of course sharply in contrast with the predominant religious view, in terms of which an individual life derives ultimate meaning from without, from its place in God's plan and its relation to the afterlife. These radically different orientations toward life entail different stances toward death as well. The religious stance appears to me somewhat schizophrenic: on the one hand the demand to preserve life is nearly absolute, since one is not to choose death before one's appointed time (the influence of the clergy on medical ethics is clear here); on the other hand, the arrival of death cannot be conceived as an unmitigated evil, at least for those religions in which belief in afterlife is central. The common thread is the idea that the manner of death is never to be a matter of individual choice or purely human intervention. This idea reflects the other-worldly perspective from which one's life is not truly one's own, nor its significance one's own creation. The secular stance toward death is less ambivalent. Nevertheless, the evil of death is clearly relative to the quality of life in question on this view.

If living has meaning and value for the individual only in terms of his capacity to plan, act, desire and value, then it follows that when these capacities are lost, the value of continuing to live is lost as well, and death is no longer an evil. For most of us desires are constant and goals and projects follow automatically. But, in terminal illness for example, when significant desires can no longer be fulfilled, and when pain robs its victim of simple enjoyments and even the power of thought, life may lose all positive value for the individual. (Despite their radical differences, the religious and secular views may share implications regarding heroic life-prolonging medical strategies in the context of terminal illness, but from different premises.) In other less drastic circumstances as well the sources of value in life may rationally take precedence over minimizing risks to longevity.

The upshot of these ruminations for our issue in medical ethics is that questions such as whether a person has affairs to be arranged, projects to be completed, or simply desires a peaceful death, will affect the rationality of various courses of treatment, not all of which will be optimal for curing, prolonging life, or avoiding depression. Certainly the rationality of such decisions has an important bearing on the right to be informed of risks or incapacitating side effects of various treatments, or of a terminal disease. Furthermore, where a diseased condition is not likely to be immediately fatal if not optimally treated, different attitudes toward risk itself become significant. The doctor is likely to assume that his own neutral attitude should be that of the patient as well, giving equal weight to all degrees of probability for benefit and harm. He is likely to dismiss other attitudes toward risk as expressions of understandable but irrational fear; but again, there is no uniquely rational attitude under any noncontroversial definition of rationality.

Of course to be neutral toward risks is not to be indifferent towards them. It is rather to be averse toward more serious risks in strict proportion to their increasing seriousness. The latter is to be measured in terms of the disutility attached to a particular outcome discounted by the probability of its occurring or not occurring. More precisely, the risk-neutral agent performs an approximation to a Bayesian calculation. He considers the products of the utilities (positive or negative) of each possible outcome of each alternative action and the probabilities of their occurrence, totals these for each possible action, and then performs the action that maximizes expected utility.[13] But this model, which the doctor is likely to assume when he puts himself paternalistically in his patient's place, amounting to a utilitarian calculation applied to the individual self-regarding agent, is only one model of rational behavior.

The patient may have a different reaction toward risks, and, given his reaction, it may be rational to opt for a less than optimal treatment, if optimality is defined as above, strictly in terms of percentage chance of cure versus chance of harmful side effects or death. The doctor may view the patient's reaction to risk as emotional and irrational, as itself justifying the withholding of information regarding risks of various treatments in order to avoid it. But the reaction may be more deeply engrained in other value orderings; it may reflect values that can be realized except if the worst risk is actualized. It may again reflect, in other words, discontinuities or lexical priorities among outcomes that are not expressed in the normal Bayesian calculation, which takes utilities as in principle continuous. The patient with an important project to complete, for example, may be rationally unwilling to risk even minimal chance of death or prolonged incapacitation, even for a good chance to correct an extremely unpleasant condition, an attitude that is likely to appear irrational to his doctor. We encounter here once more the point about value orderings that resulted (along with ideal-regarding considerations) in the recognition of rights and in the inability of utilitarians to account for them. In the medical context the further point here is that the doctor may be unaware not only of facets of the patient's personal life that affect his assignment of utilities and disutilities to medical outcomes, but also of the discontinuous ways in which these assignments may be affected. What is dismissed as an overly emotional reaction toward risk may not be irrational given the patient's own preferences. He may not even be able to express these

preferences well except in light of his reactions to various proposals. Certain patients may indeed react in ways inconsistent with their true long-range preferences, but the doctor will be in no position to know this without approaching full disclosure. If he can estimate harm at all from disclosure, it will only be in the narrow objective sense, insufficient ground on which to base decision.

To doctors in their roles as professionals whose ultimate concern is the health or continued lives of patients, it is natural to elevate these values to ultimate prominence. The death of a patient, inevitable as it is in many cases, may appear as an ultimate defeat to the medical art, as something to be fought by any means, even after life has lost all value and meaning for the patient himself. The argument in the previous section for assuming this value ordering was that health, and certainly life, seem to be necessary conditions for the realization of all other goods or values. But this point, even if true, leaves open the question of whether health and life are of ultimate, or indeed any, intrinsic value, or whether they are valuable *merely* as means. It is plausible to maintain that life itself is not of intrinsic value, since surviving in an irreversible coma seems no better than death. It therefore again appears that it is the quality of life that counts, not simply being alive. Although almost any quality might be preferable to none, it is not irrational to trade off quantity for quality, as in any other good.

Even life with physical health and consciousness may not be of intrinsic value. Consciousness and health may not be sufficient in themselves to make the life worth living, since some states of consciousness are intrinsically good and others bad. Furthermore, if a person has nothing before him but pain and depression, then the instrumental worth of being alive may be reversed. And if prolonging one's life can be accomplished only at the expense of incapacitation or ignorance, perhaps preventing lifelong projects from being completed, then the instrumental value of longer life again seems overbalanced. It is certainly true that normally life itself is of utmost value as necessary for all else of value, and that living longer usually enables one to complete more projects and plans, to satisfy more desires and derive more enjoyments. But this cannot be assumed in the extreme circumstances of severe or terminal illness. Ignorance of how long one has left may block realization of such values, as may treatment with the best chance for cure, if it also risks incapacitation or immediate death.

Nor is avoidance of depression the most important consideration in such circumstances, as a shallow hedonism might assume. Hedonistic theories of value, which seek only to produce pleasure or avoid pain and depression, are easily disproven by our abhorrence at the prospect of a "brave new world," or our unwillingness, were it possible, to be plugged indefinitely into a "pleasure machine." The latter prospect is abhorrent not only from an ideal-regarding viewpoint, but, less obviously, for want-regarding reasons (for most persons) as well. Most people would in fact be unwilling to trade important freedoms and accomplishments for sensuous pleasures, or even for the illusion of greater freedoms and accomplishments. As many philosophers have pointed out, while satisfaction of wants may bring pleasurable sensations, wants are not primarily *for* pleasurable sensations, or even for happiness more broadly construed, per se. Conversely, the avoidance of negative feelings or depression is not uppermost among primary motives. Many people are willing to endure frustration, suffering, and even depression in pursuit of accomplishment, or in order to complete projects once begun. Thus information relevant to such matters, such as medical information about one's own condition or possible adverse effects of various treatments, may well be worth having at the cost of psychological pain or depression.

The Value of Self-Determination

We have so far focused on the inability of the doctor to assume a particular value ordering for his patient in which health, the prolonging of life, or the avoidance of depression is uppermost. The likelihood of error in this regard makes it probable that the doctor will not know the true interests of his patient as well as the patient himself. He is therefore less likely than the patient himself to make choices in accord with that overall interest, and paternalistic assumption of authority to do so is therefore unjustified. There is in addition another decisive consideration mentioned earlier, namely the independent value of self-determination or freedom of choice. Personal autonomy over important decisions in one's life, the ability to attempt to realize one's own value ordering, is indeed so important that normally no amount of other goods, pleasures or avoidance of personal evils can take precedence. This is why it is wrong to contract oneself into slavery, and another reason why pleasure machines do not seem attractive. Regarding the latter, even if people were willing to forego other goods for a life of constant pleasure, the loss in variety of other values, and in the creativity that can generate new sources of value, would be morally regrettable. The value of self-determination explains also why there is such a strong burden of proof upon those who advocate paternalistic measures, why they must show that the person would otherwise act in a way inconsistent with his own value ordering, that is irrationally. A person's desires are not simply evidence of what is in his interest—they have extra weight.

Especially when decisions are important to the course of our lives, we are unwilling to relinquish them to others, even in exchange for a higher probability of happiness or less risk of suffering. Even if it could be proven, for example, that some scientific method of matching spouses greatly increased chances of compatibility and happiness, we would insist upon retaining our rights over marriage decisions. Given the present rate of success in marriages, it is probable that we could in fact find some better method of matching partners in terms of increasing that success rate. Yet we are willing to forego increased chances of success in order to make our own choices, choices that tend to make us miserable in the long run. The same might be true of career choices, choices of schools, and others central to the course of our lives. Our unwillingness to delegate these crucial decisions to experts or computers, who might stand a better chance of making them correctly (in terms of later satisfactions), is not to be explained simply in terms of our (sometimes mistaken) assumptions that we know best how to satisfy our own interests, or that we personally will choose correctly, even though most other people do not. If our retaining such authority for ourselves is not simply irrational, and I do not believe it is, this can only be because of the great independent value of self-determination. We value the exercise of free choice itself in personally important decisions, no matter what the effects of those decisions upon other satisfactions. The independent value of self-determination in decisions of great personal importance adds also to our reluctance to relinquish medical decisions with crucial effects on our lives to doctors, despite their medical expertise.

Autonomy or self-determination is independently valuable, as argued before, first of all because we value it in itself. But we may again add to this want-regarding or utilitarian reason a second ideal-regarding or perfectionist reason. What has value does so because it is valued by a rational and autonomous person. But autonomy itself is necessary to the development of such valuing individual persons or agents. It is therefore not to be sacrificed to other derivative values. To do so as a rule is to destroy the ground for the latter. Rights in general not only express and protect the central interests of individuals (the raison d'être usually emphasized in their exposition); they also express the dignity and inviolability of individuality itself. For this reason the most fundamental right is the right to control the course of one's life, to make

decisions crucial to it, including decisions in life-or-death medical contexts.[14] The other side of the independent value of self-determination from the point of view of the individual is the recognition of him by others, including doctors, as an individual with his own possibly unique set of values and priorities. His dignity demands a right to make personal decisions that express those values.

Refutation of Other Arguments Against Informing

These considerations destroy the analogies used in support of the argument for medical paternalism. One such analogy attempted to equate lying to one person in order to prevent more serious harm to another with lying to a person to prevent his causing harm to himself, and the latter with lying to or withholding information from a patient to prevent harm to his health. The criterion that morally distinguishes such cases is whether the person who requests the information has a right to acquire it. To decide this, one has to weigh the individual interests on opposing sides. Normally a person will not have this right when serious harm may befall another from his acquiring the information in question; and normally a person will have the right when the information concerns him alone, and when important decisions vital to the conduct of his life may depend upon the information acquired. Thus lying to prevent harm to a third party and lying to a medical patient about his condition or about alternative treatments cannot in general be equated, and cases in which the former is justified do not help to justify the latter. While rights are recognized in order to benefit individuals, and while we therefore generally do not recognize them if this will cause only harm to their prospective bearers, acknowledging a right of patients to be fully informed is more likely to prevent harm to them in the fullest moral sense.

The second analogy in support of the initial argument was to the legal profession, to the assumption of responsibility by lawyers for courtroom strategies and tactics. The disanalogy between that delegation of authority to lawyers and the assumption by doctors of responsibility for decisions regarding treatments and information given to patients consists in the importance of differences in value orderings among patients. Such differences, we pointed out, may falsify doctors' assumptions of the absolute priority of health and prolonged life. Trial strategies, on the other hand, generally lack side effects upon clients: the choice of particular strategies and tactics normally has import only as it contributes to winning or losing the trial. Hence clients can be assumed generally to desire those tactics to be chosen that will maximize chances for winning. Choosing tactics for them is not normally a matter of overriding their rights, hence does not amount to strong role differentiation for lawyers. Where such choices do reflect upon the clients themselves, apart from the question of winning or losing their cases, as in opting for pleas of insanity, for the use of morally questionable tactics, or tactics harmful to the interests of persons close to the clients, they should be expected to have a say in the choices. Turning back to informed choices of medical treatments, these are likely to produce side effects that may be more important to the patients themselves than even the degree of medical success of the treatments. The effects, if incapacitating, will relate directly to the quality of the patients' lives. Thus the right to choice in this area is a matter crucial to self-determination. In addition, medical treatment involves invasion of the patient's body, again a violation of a fundamental right in the absence of consent. Once more the analogy with the legal profession breaks down.

A third supposed analogy in the previous section was to other cases of justified paternalism in medicine. I accepted there that licensing of physicians and requirement of prescriptions for many drugs are justified on grounds that

laymen would otherwise make choices out of ignorance contrary to their own true preferences. It can now be seen that such cases support the argument for full disclosure to patients by their doctors, rather than supporting the opposing paternalistic position. Nondisclosure results in ignorance that blocks free choice, as would deception by drug companies or unqualified physicians in the absence of controls. Disclosure is therefore required on these very same grounds.

Reiterating the main argument of this section: because it is not patently irrational to decide against a course of treatment with optimal chances of cure or of prolonging life, because neither health nor longevity can be assumed to be of utmost value, and because self-determination is of independent and indeed of more fundamental value, the Hippocratic principle of maximizing benefits to the health of patients cannot override their rights to make decisions or know the truth in medical contexts. Nor do other excuses for withholding information when decisions regarding treatment depend upon it have force in the context of this broader argument. That a patient will not be able to understand his condition, possible courses of treatment, risks and prognoses, that he will be more likely than his doctor to make wrong decisions because of misunderstanding, must be dismissed. Given the argument of this section, the harm that might result to a patient from his own wrong decision is of less moral consequence than that which might result from a wrong decision of his doctor, which the doctor had no right to make in the first place.

The adoption of a rule that bars doctors from withholding information from patients on the basis of judgments that disclosure will result in harm to them may well occasionally result in overall harm to a patient. Some doctors operating under such a rule may forget that even bad news can be divulged kindly and sympathetically; some may tend to be unnecessarily blunt and brutal. But even statements of patients' conditions or of risks associated with treatments that are properly made can occasionally be harmful, all things considered. It is our inability to predict correctly every time that raises the moral issue of authority to act as one sees fit in the first place, the issue with which this book is primarily concerned. That our powers of predicting human reactions and the full consequences of our actions are limited means that we must grant rights and adopt rules that do not operate optimally in every circumstance. The harm that may occasionally result from granting patients rights to medical information concerning them whenever they request it is parallel in this sense to the unnecessary offense sometimes caused when people exercise their rights to free speech. We need not deny that the harm may be genuine in both cases in order to hold that the rights nevertheless ought to be granted. For the harm that results from granting them is less serious (nonaggregatively) than that which would be caused to individuals (and individuality) if we did not grant them. Obviously, if we demand full disclosure from doctors, we cannot hold them morally or legally liable for the distress or harm caused to patients who exercise their rights to information. We can expect them to divulge the information in an intelligible and reasonably humane way, however.

If the right to decide remains with the patient, then it becomes part of a doctor's competence to be able to explain these matters in clear and intelligible terms,[15] just as a lawyer must be able to explain legal rights or lines of defense, or an accountant the financial condition of his client. Regarding decisions about treatments, routine disclosure consists in recommended procedures, projected risks and benefits (including magnitudes of harm and benefit and rough probabilities of their occurring), as well as degrees of uncertainty in these estimates, monetary costs, and alternative treatments with their probable risks and benefits. This explanation should of course be followed by a request for questions. Sometimes arguments against disclosure appeal to the possibility of mistaken diagnosis, but surely the patient can be made to understand the degree of uncertainty of a

prognosis or degree of likelihood of a risk. One need not understand the underlying biological causes of a disease in order to be able to grasp the likelihood of recovery and possible side effects of alternative treatments when these are explained. The claim that the demand for full disclosure assumes knowledge or intellectual capacity on the part of the patient comparable to that of the doctor is nonsense. The patient is asked to comprehend only the likely gross effects of a few alternative courses of action. Surely it is presumptuous of a doctor to assume that a normally competent patient's mental capacity is so far below his own that the patient cannot comprehend when told this tiny fraction of what the doctor is expected to remember routinely without even consulting his texts.

It is not credible either that a doctor could fully comprehend the prognosis and yet be unable to explain it in English. If there is an epistemological factor in a doctor's unwillingness to disclose, it more likely relates to an unwillingness to reveal his uncertainties or ignorance. But there is no moral reason to keep these hidden. Whether a very unlikely or uncertain risk need be reported depends upon the importance of its potential effect on the patient and its possible effect upon his decision. That such detailed explanation takes time is also no excuse for withholding it. How much time a doctor should spend in informing depends upon the decision to be made and the centrality of those values likely to be involved.[16] Many patients will not want detailed explanations; if those who do want them require the doctor to see fewer patients, then the answer is to loosen the present restrictions on the number of doctors.

Finally, when a patient asks to know the truth or the possible risks from treatment, his doctor must assume that he really wants the information requested. While a right may be waived or not exercised by the rightholder, in the absence of explicit waiver, he must be assumed to desire to have it honored. Psychological hypothesis regarding possible insincerity is therefore out of place here. There is first of all in this regard a real question whether the doctor has the competence as a psychologist to judge insincerity or hidden motive from subtle intonations in the patient's phrasing of his questions. And for those accustomed to withholding truth, there may be perceptual set to detect such lack of desire despite the questions. After all, discussing possible or actual disaster for the patient may be very unpleasant. Given an expectation on the part of the doctor that a patient would rather avoid such discussion, a genuine uneasiness natural for the patient may be misinterpreted as a hidden desire to be deceived.

Second, when doctors find it legitimate to engage in such psychological speculation, there exists a difference in recourse available to the patient who wants to know the truth versus the one who wants to avoid the anguish of a dire prognosis. If a patient can be assumed not to want the truth despite asking for it, then he is helpless to have his right honored; whereas a person who wants to relegate responsibility to his doctor or avoid hearing bad news can simply indicate this explicitly in advance. (I discuss the honoring of this request below.) Of course, if a patient who does not want to know the worst must request explicitly that such information be withheld, then by doing this he foregoes the possible satisfaction of a good prognosis known to be truthful. But this requirement is necessary to protect the more important right of others to self-determination.

The fact that there is a right to the truth here also destroys the distinction, to which appeal is sometimes made, between lying and simply withholding information. Normally our duty not to lie to people is both broader and stronger than our duty to disclose truthfully whatever information they may request. Lying is an expression of disrespect to the person who is deceived. In many circumstances, however, persons do not have rights to information we possess, and we therefore have the right to remain silent or change the subject when they request it. But when a person does have the right to information, as I have claimed that patients have rights to medical information concerning them, remaining silent has the same moral effect as lying and cannot be distinguished. The former, as the latter, prevents informed decision-making. I have not appealed to the intrinsic wrongness of lying in the course of this argument. It has not been a question of opposing the value of truth or of truth-telling to that of kindness or the minimization of suffering, although many doctors who deceive patients undoubtedly see it that way. Rather, lying to a patient has been seen as shifting the power to make decisions central to his life away from him and toward his doctor. It is his ignorance that debilitates him here, and this ignorance results equally from lack of information as from outright deception. The right violated is that to self-determination, and this is the right now shown to override the Hippocratic principle for doctors, the principle of maximizing benefits and minimizing risks to health or life.

The Principle of Patients' Choice

The principle of patients' rights for which I am arguing does not imply that information ought never to be withheld. I maintain only that when a right to the truth, deriving from a more fundamental right of self-determination, would otherwise obtain, it may not be overridden by the rule to do no harm to patients' health, or to provide the best treatments possible. The principle implied by the dismissal of strong role differentiation does not demand that the truth always be told, but neither does it allow withholding truth whenever its probable effect is harm rather than benefit to the patient's health and happiness. It demands telling the truth or providing information whenever the patient has a right to it that he does not explicitly waive. He will have this right whenever the information is relevant to his control over decisions affecting his life, when the information concerns himself in a way that affects what he does or can do.

Of course if the information relates to the patient's condition at all, then it ought to be open to him in the absence of strong reason to withhold it. Medical records and charts should be routinely open for patients' inspection. It is only when a serious threat to health or psychological well-being is seen to be posed that the question of concealment arises at all. When it does, the right to self-determination, the possible relevance of the information to decisions of the patient, becomes the criterion for whether or not to disclose.

When that right becomes relevant, the doctor cannot argue that he would be able to convince the patient to accept his recommended treatment or procedure even after full disclosure of risks, uncertainties and alternatives, and that disclosure would therefore have no effect on the final decision. Although after the fact, when the doctor has convinced the patient, it may appear that the process of disclosure only caused needless

Why Doctors Should Intervene

Terrence F. Ackerman

Patient autonomy has become a watchword of the medical profession. According to the revised 1980 AMA Principles of Medical Ethics,[1] no longer is it permissible for a doctor to withhold information from a patient, even on grounds that it may be harmful. Instead the physician is expected to "deal honestly with patients" at all times. Physicians also have a duty to respect the confidentiality of the doctor-patient relationship. Even when disclosure to a third party may be in the patient's interests, the doctor is instructed to release information only when required by law. Respect for the autonomy of patients has given rise to many specific patient rights—among them the right to refuse treatment, the right to give informed consent, the right to privacy, and the right to competent medical care provided with "respect for human dignity."

While requirements of honesty, confidentiality, and patients rights are all important, the underlying moral vision that places exclusive emphasis upon these factors is more troublesome. The profession's notion of respect for autonomy makes noninterference its essential feature. As the Belmont Report has described it, there is an obligation to "give weight to autonomous persons' considered opinions and choices while refraining from obstructing their actions unless they are clearly detrimental to others."[2] Or, as Tom Beauchamp and James Childress have suggested, "To respect autonomous agents is to recognize with due appreciation their own considered value judgments and outlooks even when it is believed that their judgments are mistaken." They argue that people "are entitled to autonomous determination without limitation on their liberty being imposed by others."[3]

When respect for personal autonomy is understood as noninterference, the physician's role is dramatically simplified. The doctor need be only an honest and good technician, providing relevant information and dispensing professionally competent care. Does noninterference really respect patient autonomy? I maintain that it does not, because it fails to take account of the transforming effects of illness.

Terrence F. Ackerman *is director of the Program on Human Values and Ethics, at the University of Tennessee Center for the Health Sciences and an adjunct member in medical ethics at St. Jude Children's Research Hospital.*

"Autonomy," typically defined as self-governance, has two key features. First, autonomous behavior is governed by plans of action that have been formulated through deliberation or reflection. This deliberative activity involves processes of both information gathering and priority setting. Second, autonomous behavior issues, intentionally and voluntarily, from choices people make based upon their own life plans.

But various kinds of constraints can impede autonomous behavior. There are physical constraints—confinement in prison is an example—where internal or external circumstances bodily prevent a person from deliberating adequately or acting on life plans. Cognitive constraints derive from either a lack of information or an inability to understand that information. A consumer's ignorance regarding the merits or defects of a particular product fits the description. Psychological constraints, such as anxiety or depression, also inhibit adequate deliberation. Finally, there are social constraints—such as institutionalized roles and expectations ("a woman's place is in the home," "the doctor knows best") that block considered choices.

Edmund Pellegrino suggests several ways in which autonomy is specifically compromised by illness:

> In illness, the body is interposed between us and reality—it impedes our choices and actions and is no longer fully responsive. ... Illness forces a reappraisal and that poses a threat to the old image; it opens up all the old anxieties and imposes new ones—often including the real threat of death or drastic alterations in life-style. This ontological assault is aggravated by the loss of ... freedoms we identify as peculiarly human. The patient ... lacks the knowledge and skills necessary to cure himself or gain relief of pain and suffering. ... The state of being ill is therefore a state of "wounded humanity," of a person

compromised in his fundamental capacity to deal with his vulnerability.[4]

The most obvious impediment is that illness "interposes" the body or mind between the patient and reality, obstructing attempts to act upon cherished plans. An illness may not only temporarily obstruct long-range goals; it may necessitate permanent and drastic revision in the patient's major activities, such as working habits. Patients may also need to set limited goals regarding control of pain, alteration in diet and physical activity, and rehabilitation of functional impairments. They may face considerable difficulties in identifying realistic and productive aims.

The crisis is aggravated by a cognitive constraint—the lack of "knowledge and skills" to overcome their physical or mental impediment. Without adequate medical understanding, the patient cannot assess his or her condition accurately. Thus the choice of goals is seriously hampered and subsequent decisions by the patient are not well founded.

Pellegrino mentions the anxieties created by illness, but psychological constraints may also include denial, depression, guilt, and fear. I recently visited an eighteen-year-old boy who was dying of a cancer that had metastasized extensively throughout his abdomen. The doctor wanted to administer further chemotherapy that might extend the patient's life a few months. But the patient's nutritional status was poor, and he would need intravenous feedings prior to chemotherapy. Since the nutritional therapy might also encourage tumor growth, leading to a blockage of the gastrointestinal tract, the physician carefully explained the options and the risks and benefits several times, each time at greater length. But after each explanation, the young man would say only that he wished to do whatever was necessary to get better. Denial prevented him from exploring the alternatives.

Similarly, depression can lead patients to make choices that are not in harmony with their life plans. Recently, a middle-aged woman with a history of ovarian cancer in remission returned to the hospital for the biopsy of a possible pulmonary metastasis. Complications ensued and she required the use of an artificial respirator for several days. She became severely depressed and soon refused further treatment. The behavior was entirely out of character with her previous full commitment to treatment. Fully supporting her overt wishes might have robbed her of many months of relatively comfortable life in the midst of a very supportive family around which her activities centered. The medical staff stalled for time. Fortunately, her condition improved.

Fear may also cripple the ability of patients to choose. Another patient, diagnosed as having a cerebral tumor that was probably malignant, refused life-saving surgery because he feared the cosmetic effects of neurosurgery and the possibility of neurological damage. After he became comatose and new evidence suggested that the tumor might be benign, his family agreed to surgery and a benign tumor was removed. But he later died of complications related to the unfortunate delay in surgery. Although while competent he had agreed to chemotherapy, his fears (not uncommon among candidates for neurosurgery) prevented him from accepting the medical intervention that might have secured him the health he desired.

Social constraints may also prevent patients from acting upon their considered choices. A recent case involved a twelve-year-old boy whose rhabdomyosarcoma had metastasized extensively. Since all therapeutic interventions had failed, the only remaining option was to involve him in a phase 1 clinical trial. (A phase 1 clinical trial is the initial testing of a drug in human subjects. Its primary purpose is to identify toxicities rather than to evaluate therapeutic effectiveness.) The patient's course had been very stormy and he privately expressed to the staff his desire to quit further therapy and return home. However, his parents denied the hopelessness of his condition, remaining steadfast

in their belief that God would save their child. With deep regard for his parents' wishes, he refused to openly object to their desires and the therapy was administered. No antitumor effect occurred and the patient soon died.

Various social and cultural expectations also take their toll. According to Talcott Parsons, one feature of the sick role is that the ill person is obligated "... to seek *technically competent* help, namely, in the most usual case, that of a physician and to *cooperate* with him in the process of trying to get well."[5] Parsons does not describe in detail the elements of this cooperation. But clinical observation suggests that many patients relinquish their opportunity to deliberate and make choices regarding treatment in deference to the physician's superior educational achievement and social status ("Whatever you think, doctor!"). The physical and emotional demands of illness reinforce this behavior.

Moreover, this perception of the sick role has been socially taught from childhood—and it is not easily altered even by the physician who ardently tries to engage the patient in decision making. Indeed, when patients are initially asked to participate in the decision-making process, some exhibit considerable confusion and anxiety. Thus, for many persons, the institutional role of patient requires the physician to assume the responsibilities of making decisions.

Ethicists typically condemn paternalistic practices in the therapeutic relationship, but fail to investigate the features that incline physicians to be paternalistic. Such behavior may be one way to assist persons whose autonomous behavior has been impaired by illness. Of course, it is an open moral question whether the constraints imposed by illness ought to be addressed in such a way. But only by coming to grips with the psychological and social dimensions of illness can we discuss how physicians can best respect persons who are patients.

Returning Control to Patients

In the usual interpretation of respect for personal autonomy, noninterference is fundamental. In the medical setting, this means providing adequate information and competent care that accords with the patient's wishes. But if serious constraints upon autonomous behavior are intrinsic to the state of being ill, then noninterference is not the best course, since the patient's choices will be seriously limited. Under these conditions, real respect for autonomy entails a more inclusive understanding of the relationship between patients and physicians. Rather than restraining themselves so that patients can exercise whatever autonomy they retain in illness, physicians should actively seek to neutralize the impediments that interfere with patients' choices.

In *The Healer's Art*, Eric Cassell underscored the essential feature of illness that demands a revision in our understanding of respect for autonomy:

> If I had to pick the aspect of illness that is most destructive to the sick, I would choose the loss of control. Maintaining control over oneself is so vital to all of us that one might see all the other phenomena of illness as doing harm not only in their own right but doubly so as they reinforce the sick person's perception that he is no longer in control.[6]

Cassell maintains, "The doctor's job is to return control to his patient." But what is involved in "returning control" to patients? Pellegrino identifies two elements that are preeminent duties of the physician: to provide technically competent care and to fully inform the patient. The noninterference approach emphasizes these factors, and their importance is clear. Loss of control in illness is precipitated by a physical or mental defect. If technically competent therapy can fully restore previous health, then

the patient will again be in control. Consider a patient who is treated with antibiotics for a routine throat infection of streptococcal origin. Similarly, loss of control is fueled by lack of knowledge—not knowing what is the matter, what it portends for life and limb, and how it might be dealt with. Providing information that will enable the patient to make decisions and adjust goals enhances personal control.

If physical and cognitive constraints were the only impediments to autonomous behavior, then Pellegrino's suggestions might be adequate. But providing information and technically competent care will not do much to alter psychological or social impediments. Pellegrino does not adequately portray the physician's role in ameliorating these.

How can the doctor offset the acute denial that prevented the adolescent patient from assessing the benefits and risks of intravenous feedings prior to his additional chemotherapy? How can he deal with the candidate for neurosurgery who clearly desired that attempts be made to restore his health, but feared cosmetic and functional impairments? Here strategies must go beyond the mere provision of information. Crucial information may have to be repeatedly shared with patients. Features of the situation that the patient has brushed over (as in denial) or falsely emphasized (as with acute anxiety) must be discussed in more detail or set in their proper perspective. And the physician may have to alter the tone of discussions with the patient, emphasizing a positive attitude with the overly depressed or anxious patient, or a more realistic, cautious attitude with the denying patient, in order to neutralize psychological constraints.

The physician may also need to influence the beliefs or attitudes of other people, such as family members, that limit their awareness of the patient's perspective. Such a strategy might have helped the parents of the dying child to conform with the patient's wishes. On the other hand, physicians may need to modify the patient's own understanding of the sick role. For example, they may need to convey that the choice of treatment depends not merely upon the physician's technical assessment, but on the quality of life and personal goals that the patient desires.

Once we admit that psychological and social constraints impair patient autonomy, it follows that physicians must carefully assess the psychological and social profiles and needs of patients. Thus, Pedro Lain-Entralgo insists that adequate therapeutic interaction consists in a combination of "objectivity" and "cooperation." Cooperation "is shown by psychologically reproducing in the mind of the doctor, insofar as that is possible, the meaning the patient's illness has for him."[7] Without such knowledge, the physician cannot assist patients in restoring control over their lives. Ironically, some critics have insisted that physicians are not justified in acting for the well-being of patients because they possess no "expertise" in securing the requisite knowledge about the patient.[8] But knowledge of the patient's psychological and social situation is also necessary to help the patient to act as a fully autonomous person.

Beyond Legalism

Current notions of respect for autonomy are undergirded by a legal model of doctor-patient interaction. The relationship is viewed as a typical commodity exchange—the provision of technically competent medical care in return for financial compensation. Moreover, physicians and patients are presumed to have an equal ability to work out the details of therapy, *provided that* certain moral rights of patients are recognized. But the compromising effects of illness, the superior knowledge of physicians, and various institutional arrangements are also viewed as giving the physician an unfair power advantage. Since the values and interests of patients may conflict with those of the physician, the emphasis is placed upon noninterference.[9]

This legal framework is insufficient for medical ethics because it fails to recognize the impact of illness upon autonomous behavior. Even if the rights to receive adequate information and to provide consent are secured, affective and social constraints impair the ability of patients to engage in contractual therapeutic relationships. When people are sick, the focus upon equality is temporally misplaced. The goal of the therapeutic relationship is the "development" of the patient—helping to resolve the underlying physical (or mental) defect, and to deal with cognitive, psychological, and social constraints in order to restore autonomous functioning. In this sense, the doctor-patient interaction is not unlike the parent-child or teacher-student relationship.

The legal model also falls short because the therapeutic relationship is not a typical commodity exchange in which the parties use each other to accomplish mutually compatible goals, without taking a direct interest in each other. Rather, the status of patients as persons whose autonomy is compromised constitutes the very stuff of therapeutic art. The physician is attempting to alter the fundamental ability of patients to carry through their life plans. To accomplish this delicate task requires a personal knowledge about and interest in the patient. If we accept these points, then we must reject the narrow focus of medical ethics upon noninterference and emphasize patterns of interaction that free patients from constraints upon autonomy.

I hasten to add that I am criticizing the legal model only as a *complete* moral framework for therapeutic interaction. As case studies in medical ethics suggest, physicians and patients *are* potential adversaries. Moreover, the disability of the patient and various institutional controls provide physicians with a distinct "power advantage" that can be abused. Thus, a legitimate function of medical ethics is to formulate conditions that assure noninterference in patient decision making. But various positive interventions must also be emphasized, since the central task in the therapeutic process is assisting patients to reestablish control over their own lives.

n the last analysis, the crucial matter is how we view the patient who enters into the therapeutic relationship. Cassell points out that in the typical view "... the sick person is seen simply as a well person with a disease, rather than as qualitatively different, not only physically but also socially, emotionally, and even cognitively." In this view, "... the physician's role in the care of the sick is primarily the application of technology ... and health can be seen as a commodity."[10] But if, as I believe, illness renders sick persons "qualitatively different," then respect for personal autonomy requires a therapeutic interaction considerably more complex than the noninterference strategy.

Thus the current "Principles of Medical Ethics" simply exhort physicians to be honest. But the crucial requirement is that physicians tell the truth in a way, at a time, and in whatever increments are necessary to allow patients to effectively use the information in adjusting their life plans.[11] Similarly, respecting a patient's refusal of treatment maximizes autonomy only if a balanced and thorough deliberation precedes the decision. Again, the "Principles" suggest that physicians observe strict confidentiality. But the more complex moral challenge is to use confidential information in a way that will help to give the patient more freedom. Thus, the doctor can keep a patient's report on family dynamics private, and still use it to modify attitudes or actions of family members that inhibit the patient's control.

At its root, illness is an evil primarily because it compromises our efforts to control our lives. Thus, we must preserve an understanding of the physician's art that transcends noninterference and addresses this fundamental reality.

References

[1]American Medical Association, *Current Opinions of the Judicial Council of the American Medical Association* (Chicago, Illinois: American Medical Association, 1981), p. ix. Also see Robert Veatch, "Professional Ethics: New Principles for Physicians?," *Hastings Center Report* 10 (June 1980), 16–19.

[2]The National Commission for the Protection of Human Subjects of Biomedical and Behavioral Research, *The Belmont Report: Ethical Principles and Guidelines for the Protection of Human Subjects of Research* (Washington, D.C.: U.S. Government Printing Office, 1978), p. 58.

[3]Tom Beauchamp and James Childress, *Principles of Biomedical Ethics* (New York: Oxford University Press, 1980), p. 59.

[4]Edmund Pellegrino, "Toward a Reconstruction of Medical Morality: The Primacy of the Act of Profession and the Fact of Illness," *The Journal of Medicine and Philosophy* 4 (1979), 44–45.

[5]Talcott Parsons, *The Social System* (Glencoe, Illinois: The Free Press, 1951), p. 437.

[6]Eric Cassell, *The Healer's Art* (New York: Lippincott, 1976), p. 44. Although Cassell aptly describes the goal of the healer's art, it is unclear whether he considers it to be based upon the obligation to respect the patient's autonomy or the duty to enhance the well-being of the patient. Some parts of his discussion clearly suggest the latter.

[7] Pedro Lain-Entralgo, *Doctor and Patient* (New York: McGraw-Hill, 1969), p. 155.

[8]See Allen Buchanan, "Medical Paternalism," *Philosophy and Public Affairs* 7 (1978), 370–90.

[9]My formulation of the components of the legal model differs from, but is highly indebted to, John Ladd's stimulating analysis in "Legalism and Medical Ethics," in John Davis et al., editors, *Contemporary Issues in Biomedical Ethics* (Clifton, NJ: The Humana Press, 1979), pp. 1–35. However, I would not endorse Ladd's position that the moral principles that define our duties in the therapeutic setting are of a different logical type from those that define our duties to strangers.

[10]Eric Cassell, "Therapeutic Relationship: Contemporary Medical Perspective," in Warren Reich, editor, *Encyclopedia of Bioethics* (New York: Macmillan, 1978), p. 1675.

[11]Cf. Norman Cousins, "A Layman Looks at Truthtelling," *Journal of the American Medical Association* 244 (1980), 1929–30. Also see Howard Brody, "Hope," *Journal of the American Medical Association* 246 (1981), 1411–12.

2. Truth-Telling

Truth-telling or Veracity comes into play in the context of the physician (professional)-patient relationship.[1] It essentially refers to comprehensive and objective transmission of information as well as the way the physician encourages the patient's understanding and ability of self-determination.

According to Beauchamp and Childress, three elements support obligations of veracity: 1. Respect for persons beyond informed consent; 2. Obligations of fidelity, promise-keeping, and contract; and 3. Trust in relationships between physicians and patients.

Like other obligations pointed out by principlism, veracity is prima facie binding but it does not represent an absolute mandate. Physicians have a plausible range to manage information given determined circumstances. Limited disclosure, deception and even lying can be justified when veracity conflicts with other obligations such as those of beneficence.

It is clear that the professional obligation of veracity consists in telling the truth and no lying the patients. This rule, hence, has an objective or descriptive level (True or false information), and one intentional or subjective (interpretation of information and possible consequences). Thus, veracity can be based upon deontological and utilitarian criteria. In other words, it can be understood as an unconditional obligation to respect the autonomy of persons, or as a relative obligation conditioned by circumstances.

Veracity is a rule derived from the principle of respect for autonomy. Not telling the truth a patient is incompatible with that rule since it limits his/her ability of self-determination and undermines his/her right to be full informed to make autonomous decisions. However, the issue becomes more complicated when this rule collides with rules of beneficence. For instance, when the information given to the patient may cause a severe and immediate deterioration of his/her mental and physical state, the stuff does not only consider the patient' somatic condition but also and very specially his/her mental state, morality, beliefs, projects, interests, and ideals.

What kind of information does a patient demand? What are the limits of disclosure, privacy and right to know the truth? Who should define the epistemological and procedural scopes of veracity? Under the principle of respect for autonomy, telling always the truth seems to

---

1 The principle of veracity does not only acquire relevance in clinical practice but also in research involving human subjects, and public health.

be morally plausible and an obligatory ethical mandate for physicians. However, it is also true that telling everything may often negatively impact the patient by causing even more harm and suffering. In this case, and by following the principle of beneficence, physicians should be prudent and administrate the transmission of information to avoid worse consequences.

As veracity is related to autonomy, self-determination, privacy, confidentiality, and even integrity and inviolability, is still a controversial procedural field in bioethics. The criteria to interpret and apply this rule are epistemologically prima facie but methodologically opposing. The discussion is open.

Readings

Kant, Immanuel, "On a Supposed Right to Lie from Altruistic Motive," in Vaughn, Lewis, *Bioethics. Principles, Issues and Cases*, Oxford University Press, Second Edition, 2010: **121-122.**

Thomasma, David C., "Telling the Truth to Patients: A Clinical Ethics Exploration," in *Cambridge Quarterly of Healthcare Ethics*, vol. 3, no. 3 (1994): **372-382.**

Siegler, Mark, "Confidentiality in Medicine—A Decrepit Concept," in *The New England Journal of Medicine*, vol. 307, no. 24, 1982: **1518-1521.**

Practical Scenarios

Instructions for analysis:

1. Explain, in general terms, why the case is morally relevant and controversial.
2. Identify the central moral issue. Justify.
3. Identify and explain the main facts to be considered in your analysis.
4. Identify and explain the principles and theories useful in analyzing the case. Justify why

those principles and theories are relevant in the case. Specify conflicts between them.
5. Identify and raise arguments to support the conflicting options/decisions/actions that are evident in the case (Specifications and balancing of rules are necessary at this stage).
6. Identify and weigh alternative courses of action and then decide. Justify your decision. Answer the question(s) posed by the author as part of your conclusion.

Scenario 1

The Case of the Fat Patient

Jim Sullivan in his early thirties comes to Dr. Tom Wordsworth's office for a routine exam in conjunction with a new job. Dr. Wordsworth starts taking the history. It is obvious that Mr. Sullivan is grossly overweight. He tells the physician that he does not get any exercise, smokes two packs of cigarettes a day, and has done so since he was fourteen. He drinks a lot and generally does not take very good care of himself.

Dr. Wordsworth feels that he should encourage his patient to change his lifestyle. He realizes he is not very likely to change anything simply by telling the patient that he should not drink as much and should quit smoking. This is a man who is not likely to take up an exercise routine simply because this physician says so.

Dr. Wordsworth contemplates another approach. He decides to do a chest x-ray, suspecting that some opacity will appear that will do the trick. He sees nothing terribly alarming on the x-ray, but notices some spots that would serve his purpose: to shock his patient into changing his lifestyle. With an air of great alarm he brings the x-ray to his patient saying that the spots indicate precancerous developments. He says that if Mr. Sullivan stops smoking now, there is a good chance he can stop this development. But if he keeps smoking he is headed for lung cancer. Intentionally overstating, Dr. Wordsworth rationalizes that it is true that Sullivan's chances of developing lung cancer are higher if he continues to smoke and that it is an innocent, benevolent stretching of the truth to point to the meaningless spots and exaggerate the probability that the smoking would cause cancer. He believes that overstating the risk will benefit his patient. It is the only thing he can think of that will shock him into a new lifestyle.[2]

Question

Is, in this case, the physician's lie morally justified? Why?

Scenario 2

Prudence or Disclosure?

A woman originally from the Middle East calls the doctor and tells him that her 16-year old son has both HIV-infection and is recovering from chemotherapy for lymphoma at NIH. He is no longer on protocol and needs a new Peds Infectious Disease Specialist to follow him. Her son knows about the cancer but not the HIV infection acquired by transfusion as newborn in the US.[3]

Question

Should the physician treat this patient without telling him he is HIV infected? Justify your answer.

Scenario 3

A Little White Lie?

Donald Robertson, a 46 year old father of three being treated in employee health for high blood pressure and diabetes, schedules a visit with Elizabeth Collins, the nurse practitioner he generally sees. He tells Ms. Collins that his wife, who is currently deployed to Afghanistan, is scheduled for leave next week and he desperately wants to take at least two days off to

maximize their time together. Finances are a huge issue for the Robertson family. Mr. Robertson needs this job and can't just call in sick without a note. He begs Ms. Collins to write a note documenting medical need for the absence.

She knows and likes Mr. Robertson and has great sympathy for his situation and understands his wanting to spend as much time as possible with his wife. She knows that trying to hold the family together during her absence has not been easy for Mr. Robertson.[4]

Question

Should Ms. Collins lie to the company to help Mr. Robertson? Justify your answer.

---

2   Extracted from, Veatch, Robert, *The Basis of Bioethics*, 3rd Edition, USA, Pearson, 2012.
3   Adapted from Taylor, Carol, *Health Care Ethics Course*, Georgetown University School of Medicine, AY 2010-2011.

---

4   Ibid.

On a Supposed Right to Lie from Altruistic Motives

Immanuel Kant

n the work called *France*, for the year 1797, Part VI., No. 1, on Political Reactions, by *Benjamin Constant*, the following passage occurs, p. 123:—

"The moral principle that it is one's duty to speak the truth, if it were taken singly and unconditionally, would make all society impossible. We have the proof of this in the very direct consequences which have been drawn from this principle by a German philosopher, who goes so far as to affirm that to tell a falsehood to a murderer who asked us whether our friend, of whom he was in pursuit, had not taken refuge in our house, would be a crime."

The French philosopher opposes this principle in the following manner, p. 124:—"It is a duty to tell the truth. The notion of duty is inseparable from the notion of right. A duty is what in one being corresponds to the right of another. Where there are no rights there are no duties. To tell the truth then is a duty, but only towards him who has a right to the truth. But no man has a right to a truth that injures others." The here lies in the statement that *"To tell the truth is a duty, but only towards him who has a right to the truth."*

It is to be remarked, first, that the expression "to have a right to the truth" is unmeaning. We should rather say, a man has a right to his own *truthfulness* (*veracitas*), that is, to subjective truth in his own person. For to have a right objectively to truth would mean that, as in *meum* and *tuum* generally, it depends on his *will* whether a given statement shall be true or false, which would produce a singular logic.

Now, the *first* question is whether a man—in cases where he cannot avoid answering Yes or No—has the *right* to be untruthful. The *second* question is whether, in order to prevent a misdeed that threatens him or some one else, he is not actually bound to be untruthful in a certain statement to which an unjust compulsion forces him.

Truth in utterances that cannot be avoided is the formal duty of a man to everyone, however great the disadvantage that may arise from it to him or any other; and although by making a false statement I do no wrong to him who unjustly compels me to speak, yet I do wrong to men in general in the most essential point of duty, so that it may be called a lie (though not in the jurist's sense), that is, so far as in me lies I cause that declarations in general find no credit, and hence that all rights founded on contract should lose their force; and this is a wrong which is done to mankind.

If, then, we define a lie merely as an intentionally false declaration towards another man, we need not add that it must injure another; as the jurists think proper to put in their definition (*mendacium est falsiloquium in praejudicium alterius*). For it always injures another; if not another individual, yet mankind generally, since it vitiates the source of justice. This benevolent lie *may*, however, by *accident* (*casus*) become punishable even by civil laws; and that which escapes liability to punishment only by accident may be condemned as a wrong even by external laws. For instance, if you have *by a lie* hindered a man who is even now planning a murder, you are legally responsible for all the consequences. But if you have strictly adhered to the truth, public justice can find no fault with you, be the

unforeseen consequence what it may. It is possible that whilst you have honestly answered Yes to the murderer's question, whether his intended victim is in the house, the latter may have gone out unobserved, and so not have come in the way of the murderer, and the deed therefore have not been done; whereas, if you lied and said he was not in the house, and he had really gone out (though unknown to you), so that the murderer met him as he went, and executed his purpose on him, then you might with justice be accused as the cause of his death. For, if you had spoken the truth as well as you knew it, perhaps the murderer while seeking for his enemy in the house might have been caught by neighbours coming up and the deed been prevented. Whoever then *tells a lie*, however good his intentions may be, must answer for the consequences of it, even before the civil tribunal, and must pay the penalty for them, however unforeseen they may have been; because truthfulness is a duty that must be regarded as the basis of all duties founded on contract, the laws of which would be rendered uncertain and useless if even the least exception to them were admitted.

To be *truthful* (honest) in all declarations is therefore a sacred unconditional command of reason, and not to be limited by any expediency

Telling the Truth to Patients: A Clinical Ethics Exploration

David C. Thomasma

In this essay I will examine why the truth is so important to human communication in general, the types of truth, and why truth is only a relative value. After those introductory points, I will sketch the ways in which the truth is overridden or trumped by other concerns in the clinical setting. I will then discuss cases that fall into five distinct categories. The conclusion emphasizes the importance of truth telling and its primacy among secondary goods in the healthcare professional-patient relationship.

Reasons for Telling the Truth

... In all human relationships, the truth is told for a myriad of reasons. A summary of the prominent reasons are that it is a right, a utility, and a kindness.

It is a right to be told the truth because respect for the person demands it. As Kant argued, human society would soon collapse without truth telling, because it is the basis of interpersonal trust, covenants, contracts, and promises.

The truth is a utility as well, because persons need to make informed judgments about their actions. It is a mark of maturity that individuals advance and grow morally by becoming more and more self-aware of their needs, their motives, and their limitations. All these steps toward maturity require honest and forthright communication, first from parents and later also from siblings, friends, lovers, spouses, children, colleagues, co-workers, and caregivers.[1]

Finally, it is a kindness to be told the truth, a kindness rooted in virtue precisely because persons to whom lies are told will of necessity withdraw from important, sometimes life-sustaining and life-saving relationships. Similarly, those who tell lies poison not only their relationships but themselves, rendering themselves incapable of virtue and moral growth.[2] ... When we stop and think of it, there are times when, at least for the moment, protecting us from the truth can save our egos, our self-respect, and

From *Cambridge Quarterly of Health care Ethics*, vol. 3, no. 3 (1994), pp. 372–82. Copyright © 1994 Cambridge University Press. Reprinted with permission of Cambridge University Press.

even our most cherished values. Not all of us act rationally and autonomously at all times. Sometimes we are under sufficient stress that others must act to protect us from harm. This is called necessary paternalism. Should we become seriously ill, others must step in and rescue us if we are incapable of doing it ourselves. ...

In General Relationships

In each of the three main reasons why the truth must be told, as a right, a utility, and a kindness, lurk values that may from time to time become more important than the truth. When this occurs, the rule of truth telling is trumped, that is, overridden by a temporarily more important principle. The ultimate value in all instances is the survival of the community and/or the well-being of the individual. Does this mean for paternalistic reasons, without the person's consent, the right to the truth, the utility, and the kindness, can be shunted aside? The answer is "yes." The truth in a relationship responds to a multivariate complexity of values, the context for which helps determine which values in that relationship should predominate.

Nothing I have said thus far suggests that the truth may be treated in a cavalier fashion or that it can be withheld from those who deserve it for frivolous reasons. The only values that can trump the truth are recipient survival, community survival, and the ability to absorb the full impact of the truth at a particular time. All these are only temporary trump cards in any event. They only can be played under certain limited conditions because respect for persons is a foundational value in all relationships.

In Healthcare Relationships

It is time to look more carefully at one particular form of human relationship, the relationship between the doctor and the patient or sometimes between other healthcare providers and the patient.

Early in the 1960s, studies were done that revealed the majority of physicians would not disclose a diagnosis of cancer to a patient. Reasons cited were mostly those that derived from nonmaleficence. Physicians were concerned that such a diagnosis might disturb the equanimity of a patient and might lead to desperate acts. Primarily physicians did not want to destroy their patients' hope. By the middle 1970s, however, repeat studies brought to light a radical shift in physician attitudes. Unlike earlier views, physicians now emphasized patient autonomy and informed consent over paternalism. In the doctor–patient relation, this meant the majority of physicians stressed the patient's right to full disclosure of diagnosis and prognosis.

One might be tempted to ascribe this shift of attitudes to the growing patients' rights and autonomy movements in the philosophy of medicine and in public affairs. No doubt some of the change can be attributed to this movement. But also treatment interventions for cancer led to greater optimism about modalities that could offer some hope to patients. Thus, to offer them full disclosure of their diagnosis no longer was equivalent to a death sentence. Former powerlessness of the healer was supplanted with technological and pharmaceutical potentialities.

A more philosophical analysis of the reasons for a shift comes from a consideration of the goal of medicine. The goal of all healthcare relations is to receive/provide help for an illness such that no further harm is done to the patient, especially in that patient's vulnerable state.[3] The vulnerability arises because of increased dependency. Presumably, the doctor will not take advantage of this vulnerable condition by adding to it through inappropriate use of power or the lack of compassion. Instead, the vulnerable person should be assisted back to a state of human equality, if possible, free from the prior dependency.[4]

First, the goal of the healthcare giver–patient relation is essentially to restore the patient's autonomy. Thus, respect for the right of the patient to the truth is measured against this goal. If nothing toward that goal can be gained by telling the truth at a particular time, still it must be told for other reasons. Yet, if the truth would impair the restoration of autonomy, then it may be withheld on grounds of potential harm. Thus the goal of the healing relationship enters into the calculus of values that are to be protected.

Second, most healthcare relationships of an interventionist character are temporary, whereas relationships involving primary care, prevention, and chronic or dying care are more permanent. These differences also have a bearing on truth telling. During a short encounter with healthcare strangers, patients and healthcare providers will of necessity require the truth more readily than during a long-term relation among near friends. In the short term, decisions, often dramatically important ones, need to be made in a compressed period. There is less opportunity to maneuver or delay for other reasons, even if there are concerns about the truth's impact on the person.

Over a longer period, the truth may be withheld for compassionate reasons more readily. Here, the patient and physician or nurse know one another. They are more likely to have shared some of their values. In this context, it is more justifiable to withhold the truth temporarily in favor of more important long-term values, which are known in the relationship.

Finally, the goal of healthcare relations is treatment of an illness. An illness is far broader than its subset, disease. Illness can be viewed as a disturbance in the life of an individual, perhaps due to many nonmedical factors. A disease, by contrast, is a medically caused event that may respond to more interventionist strategies.[5]

Helping one through an illness is a far greater personal task than doing so for a disease. A greater, more enduring bond is formed. The strength of this bond may justify withholding the truth as well, although in the end "the truth will always out."

Clinical Case Categories

The general principles about truth telling have been reviewed, as well as possible modifications formed from the particularities of the healthcare professional–patient relationship. Now I turn to some contemporary examples of how clinical ethics might analyze the hierarchy of values surrounding truth telling.

There are at least five clinical case categories in which truth telling becomes problematic: intervention cases, long-term care cases, cases of dying patients, prevention cases, and nonintervention cases.

Intervention Cases

Of all clinically difficult times to tell the truth, two typical cases stand out. The first usually involves a mother of advanced age with cancer. The family might beg the surgeon not to tell her what has been discovered for fear that "Mom might just go off the deep end." The movie *Dad*, starring Jack Lemmon, had as its centerpiece the notion that Dad could not tolerate the idea of cancer. Once told, he went into a psychotic shock that ruptured standard relationships with the doctors, the hospital, and the family. However, because this diagnosis requires patient participation for chemotherapeutic interventions and the time is short, the truth must be faced directly. Only if there is not to be intervention might one withhold the truth from the patient for a while, at the family's request, until the patient is able to cope with the reality. A contract about the time allowed before telling the truth might be a good idea.

The second case is that of ambiguous genitalia. A woman, 19 years old, comes for a checkup because she plans to get married and has not yet had a period. She is very mildly retarded. It turns out that she has no vagina, uterus, or ovaries but does have an undescended testicle in her abdomen. She is actually a he. Should she be told this fundamental truth about herself? Those who argue for the truth do so on grounds that she will eventually find out, and more of her subsequent life will have been ruined by the lies and disingenuousness of others. Those who argue against the truth usually prevail. National standards exist in this regard. The young woman is told that she has something like a "gonadal mass" in her abdomen that might turn into cancer if not removed, and an operation is performed. She is assisted to remain a female.

More complicated still is a case of a young Hispanic woman, a trauma accident victim, who is gradually coming out of a coma. She responds only to commands such as "move your toes." Because she is now incompetent, her mother and father are making all care decisions in her case. Her boyfriend is a welcome addition to the large, extended family. However, the physicians discover that she is pregnant. The fetus is about 5 weeks old. Eventually, if she does not recover, her surrogate decision makers will have to be told about the pregnancy, because they will be involved in the terrible decisions about continuing the life of the fetus even if it is a risk to the mother's recovery from the coma. This revelation will almost certainly disrupt current family relationships and the role of the boyfriend. Further, if the mother is incompetent to decide, should not the boyfriend, as presumed father, have a say in the decision about his own child?

In this case, revelation of the truth must be carefully managed. The pregnancy should be revealed only on a "need to know" basis, that is, only when the survival of the young woman becomes critical. She is still progressing moderately towards a stable state.

Long-Term Cases

Rehabilitation medicine provides one problem of truth telling in this category. If a young man has been paralyzed by a football accident, his recovery to some level of function will depend upon holding out hope. As he struggles to strengthen himself, the motivation might be a hope that caregivers know to be false, that he may someday be able to walk again. Yet this falsehood is not corrected, lest he slip into despair. Hence, because this is a long-term relationship, the truth will be gradually discovered by the patient under the aegis of encouragement by his physical therapists, nurses, and physicians, who enter his life as near friends.

Cases of Dying Patients

Sometimes, during the dying process, the patient asks directly, "Doctor, am I dying?" Physicians are frequently reluctant to "play God" and tell the patient how many days or months or years they have left. This reluctance sometimes bleeds over into a less-than-forthright answer to the question just asked. A surgeon with whom I make rounds once answered this question posed by a terminally ill cancer patient by telling her that she did not have to worry about her insurance running out!

Yet in every case of dying patients, the truth can be gradually revealed such that the patient learns about dying even before the family or others who are resisting telling the truth. Sometimes, without directly saying "you are dying," we are able to use interpretative truth and comfort the patient. If a car driver who has been in an accident and is dying asks about other family members in the car who are already dead, there is no necessity to tell him the truth. Instead, he can be told that "they are being cared for" and that the important thing right now is that he be comfortable and not in pain. One avoids the awful truth because he may feel responsible and guilt ridden during his own dying hours if he knew that the rest of his family were already dead.

Prevention Cases

A good example of problems associated with truth telling in preventive medicine might come from screening. The high prevalence of prostate cancer among men over 50 years old may suggest the utility of cancer screening. An annual checkup for men over 40 years old is recommended. Latent and asymptomatic prostate cancer is often clinically unsuspected and is present in approximately 30% of men over 50 years of age. If screening were to take place, about 16.5 million men in the United States alone would be diagnosed with prostate cancer, or about 2.4 million men each year. As of now, only 120,000 cases are newly diagnosed each year. Thus, as Timothy Moon noted in a recent sketch of the disease, "a majority of patients with prostate cancer thatis not clinically diagnosed will experience a benign course throughout their lifetime."[6]

The high incidence of prostate cancer coupled with a very low malignant potential would entail a whole host of problems if subjected to screening. Detection would force patients and physicians to make very difficult and life-altering treatment decisions. Among them are removal of the gland (with impotence a possible outcome), radiation treatment, and most effective of all, surgical removal of the gonads (orchiectomy). But why consider these rather violent interventions if the probable outcome of neglect will overwhelmingly be benign? For this reason the U.S. Preventive Services Task Force does not recommend either for or against screening for prostate cancer. Quality-of-life issues would take precedence over the need to know.

Nonintervention Cases

This last example more closely approximates the kind of information one might receive as a result of gene mapping. This information could tell you of the likelihood or probability of encountering a number of diseases through genetic heritage, for example, adult onset or type II diabetes, but could not offer major interventions for most of them (unlike a probability for diabetes).

Some evidence exists from recent studies that the principle of truth telling now predominates in the doctor-patient relationship. Doctors were asked about revealing diagnosis for Huntington's disease and multiple sclerosis, neither of which is subject to a cure at present. An overwhelming majority would consider full disclosure. This means that, even in the face of diseases for which we have no cure, truth telling seems to take precedence over protecting the patient from imagined harms.

The question of full disclosure acquires greater poignancy in today's medicine, especially with respect to Alzheimer's disease and genetic disorders that may be diagnosed in utero. There are times when our own scientific endeavors lack a sufficient conceptual and cultural framework around which to assemble facts. The facts can overwhelm us without such conceptual frameworks. The future of genetics poses just such a problem. In consideration of the new genetics, this might be the time to stress values over the truth.

Conclusion

Truth in the clinical relationship is factored in with knowledge and values.

First, truth is contextual. Its revelation depends upon the nature of the relationship between the doctor and patient and the duration of that relationship.

Second, truth is a secondary good. Although important, other primary values take precedence over the truth. The most important of these values is survival of the individual and the community. A close second would be preservation of the relationship itself.

Third, truth is essential for healing an illness. It may not be as important for curing a disease.

That is why, for example, we might withhold the truth from the woman with ambiguous genitalia, curing her disease (having a gonad) in favor of maintaining her health (being a woman).

Fourth, withholding the truth is only a temporary measure. *In vino, veritas* it is said. The truth will eventually come out, even if in a slip of the tongue. Its revelation, if it is to be controlled, must always aim at the good of the patient for the moment.

At all times, the default mode should be that the truth is told. If, for some important reason, it is not to be immediately revealed in a particular case, a truth-management protocol should be instituted so that all caregivers on the team understand how the truth will eventually be revealed.

Notes

1. Bok S. *Lying: Moral Choice in Public and Personal Life.* New York: Vintage Books, 1989.
2. Pellegrino E. D., Thomasma D. C. *The Virtues in Medical Practice.* New York: Oxford University Press, 1993.
3. Cassell E. The nature of suffering and the goals of medicine. *New England Journal of Medicine* 1982; 306(11):639–45.
4. See Nordenfelt L., issue editor. Concepts of health and their consequences for health care. *Theoretical Medicine* 1993; 14(4).
5. Moon T. D. Prostate cancer. *Journal of the American Geriatrics Society* 1992; 40:622–7 (quote from 626).
6. See note 5. Moon. 1992; 40:622–7.

Confidentiality in Medicine—A Decrepit Concept

Mark Siegler

Medical confidentiality, as it has traditionally been understood by patients and doctors, no longer exists. This ancient medical principle, which has been included in every physician's oath and code of ethics since Hippocratic times, has become old, worn-out, and useless; it is a decrepit concept. Efforts to preserve it appear doomed to failure and often give rise to more problems than solutions. Psychiatrists have tacitly acknowledged the impossibility of ensuring the confidentiality of medical records by choosing to establish a separate, more secret record. The following case illustrates how the confidentiality principle is compromised systematically in the course of routine medical care.

A patient of mine with mild chronic obstructive pulmonary disease was transferred from the surgical intensive-care unit to a surgical nursing floor two days after an elective cholecystectomy. On the day of transfer, the patient saw a respiratory therapist writing in his medical chart (the therapist was recording the results of an arterial blood gas analysis) and became concerned about the confidentiality of his hospital records. The patient threatened to leave the hospital prematurely unless I could guarantee that the confidentiality of his hospital record would be respected.

This patient's complaint prompted me to enumerate the number of persons who had both access to his hospital record and a reason to examine it. I was amazed to learn that at least 25 and possibly as many as 100 health professionals and administrative personnel at our university hospital had access to the patient's record and that all of them had a legitimate need, indeed a professional responsibility, to open and use that chart. These persons included 6 attending physicians (the primary physician, the surgeon, the pulmonary consultant, and others); 12 house officers (medical, surgical, intensive-care unit, and "covering" house staff); 20 nursing personnel (on three shifts); 6 respiratory therapists; 3 nutritionists; 2 clinical pharmacists; 15 students (from medicine, nursing, respiratory therapy, and clinical pharmacy); 4 unit secretaries; 4 hospital financial officers; and 4 chart reviewers (utilization review, quality assurance review, tissue review, and insurance auditor). It is of interest that this patient's problem was straightforward, and he therefore did not require many other technical and support services that the modern hospital provides. For example, he did not need multiple consultants and fellows, such specialized procedures as dialysis, or social workers, chaplains, physical therapists, occupational therapists, and the like.

Upon completing my survey I reported to the patient that I estimated that at least 75 health professionals and hospital personnel had access to his medical record. I suggested to the patient that these people were all involved in providing or supporting his health-care services. They were, I assured him, working for him. Despite my reassurances the patient was obviously distressed and retorted, "I always believed that medical confidentiality was part of a doctor's code of ethics. Perhaps you should tell me just what you people mean by 'confidentiality'!"

Two Aspects of Medical Confidentiality

Confidentiality and Third-Party Interests

Previous discussions of medical confidentiality usually have focused on the tension between a physician's responsibility to keep information divulged by patients secret and a physician's legal and moral duty, on occasion, to reveal such confidences to third parties, such as families, employers, public-health authorities, or police authorities. In all these instances, the central question relates to the stringency of the physician's obligation to maintain patient confidentiality when the health, well-being, and safety of identifiable others or of society in general would be threatened by a failure to reveal information about the patient. The tension in such cases is between the good of the patient and the good of others.

Confidentiality and the Patient's Interest

As the example above illustrates, further challenges to confidentiality arise because the patient's personal interest in maintaining confidentiality comes into conflict with his personal interest in receiving the best possible health care. Modern high-technology health care is available principally in hospitals (often, teaching hospitals), requires many trained and specialized workers (a "health-care team"), and is very costly. The existence of such teams means that information that previously had been held in confidence by an individual physician will now necessarily be disseminated to many members of the team. Furthermore, since health-care teams are expensive and few patients can afford to pay such costs directly, it becomes essential to grant access to the patient's medical record to persons who are responsible for obtaining third-party payment. These persons include chart reviewers, financial officers, insurance auditors, and quality-of-care assessors. Finally, as medicine expands from a narrow, disease-based model to a model that encompasses psychological, social, and economic problems, not only will the size of the health-care team and medical costs increase, but more sensitive information (such as one's personal habits and financial condition) will now be included in the medical record and will no longer be confidential.

The point I wish to establish is that hospital medicine, the rise of health-care teams, the existence of third-party insurance programs, and the expanding limits of medicine all appear to be responses to the wishes of people for better and more comprehensive medical care. But each of these developments necessarily modifies our traditional understanding of medical confidentiality.

The Role of Confidentiality in Medicine

Confidentiality serves a dual purpose in medicine. In the first place, it acknowledges respect for the patient's sense of individuality and privacy. The patient's most personal physical and psychological secrets are kept confidential in order to decrease a sense of shame and vulnerability. Secondly, confidentiality is important in improving the patient's health care—a basic goal of medicine. The promise of confidentiality permits people to trust (i.e., have confidence) that information revealed to a physician in the course of a medical encounter will not be disseminated further. In this way patients are encouraged to communicate honestly and forthrightly with their doctors. This bond of trust between patient and doctor is vitally important both in the diagnostic process (which relies on an accurate history) and subsequently in the treatment phase, which often depends as much on the patient's trust in the physician as its does on medications and surgery. These two important functions of confidentiality are as important now as they were in the past. They will not be supplanted entirely either by improvements in medical technology or by recent changes in relations between some patients and doctors toward a rights-based, consumerist model.

Possible Solutions to the Confidentiality Problem

First of all, in all nonbureaucratic, noninstitutional medical encounters—that is, in the millions of doctor–patient encounters that take place in physicians' offices, where more privacy can be preserved–meticulous care should be taken to guarantee that patients' medical and personal information will be kept confidential.

Secondly, in such settings as hospitals or large-scale group practices, where many persons have opportunities to examine the medical record, we should aim to provide access only to those who have "a need to know." This could be accomplished through such administrative changes as dividing the entire record into several sections—for example, a medical and financial

section—and permitting only health professionals access to the medical information.

The approach favored by many psychiatrists—that of keeping a psychiatric record separate from the general medical record—is an understandable strategy but one that is not entirely satisfactory and that should not be generalized. The keeping of separate psychiatric records implies that psychiatry and medicine are different undertakings and thus drives deeper the wedge between them and between physical and psychological illness. Furthermore, it is often vitally important for internists or surgeons to know that a patient is being seen by a psychiatrist or is taking a particular medication. When separate records are kept, this information may not be available. Finally, if generalized, the practice of keeping a separate psychiatric record could lead to the unacceptable consequence of having a separate record for each type of medical problem.

Patients should be informed about what is meant by "medical confidentiality." We should establish the distinction between information about the patient that generally will be kept confidential regardless of the interest of third parties and information that will be exchanged among members of the health-care team in order to provide care for the patient. Patients should be made aware of the large number of persons in the modern hospital who require access to the medical record in order to serve the patient's medical and financial interests.

Finally, at some point most patients should have an opportunity to review their medical record and to make informed choices about whether their entire record is to be available to everyone or whether certain portions of the record are privileged and should be accessible only to their principal physician or to others designated explicitly by the patient. This approach would rely on traditional informed–consent procedural standards and might permit the patient to balance the personal value of medical confidentiality against the personal value of high-technology, team health care. There is no reason that the same procedure should not be used with psychiatric records instead of the arbitrary system now employed, in which everything related to psychiatry is kept secret.

interrogated concerning their complaint in a tone of voice which cannot be overheard."[1] We in the medical profession frequently neglect these simple courtesies.

Afterthought: Confidentiality and Indiscretion

There is one additional aspect of confidentiality that is rarely included in discussions of the subject. I am referring here to the wanton, often inadvertent, but avoidable exchanges of confidential information that occur frequently in hospital rooms, elevators, cafeterias, doctors' offices, and at cocktail parties. Of course, as more people have access to medical information about the patient the potential for this irresponsible abuse of confidentiality increases geometrically.

Such mundane breaches of confidentiality are probably of greater concern to most patients than the broader issue of whether their medical records may be entered into a computerized data bank or whether a respiratory therapist is reviewing the results of an arterial blood gas determination. Somehow, privacy is violated and a sense of shame is heightened when intimate secrets are revealed to people one knows or is close to—friends, neighbors, acquaintances, or hospital roommates—rather than when they are disclosed to an anonymous bureaucrat sitting at a computer terminal in a distant city or to a health professional who is acting in an official capacity.

I suspect that the principles of medical confidentiality, particularly those reflected in most medical codes of ethics, were designed principally to prevent just this sort of embarrassing personal indiscretion rather than to maintain (for social, political, or economic reasons) the absolute secrecy of doctor–patient communications. In this regard, it is worth noting that Percival's Code of Medical Ethics (1803) includes the following admonition: "Patients should be

Conclusion

The principle of medical confidentiality described in medical codes of ethics and still believed in by patients no longer exists. In this respect, it is a decrepit concept. Rather than perpetuate the myth of confidentiality and invest energy vainly to preserve it, the public and the profession would be better served if they devoted their attention to determining which aspects of the original principle of confidentiality are worth retaining. Efforts could then be directed to salvaging those.

University of Chicago–
Pritzker School of Medicine
Chicago, IL 60637

MARK SIEGLER, M.D.

---

1 Leake CD, ed. Percival's medical ethics. Baltimore: Williams & Wilkins, 1927.

Supported by a grant (OSS-8018097) from the National Science Foundation and by the National Endowment for the Humanities. The views expressed are those of the author and do not necessarily reflect those of the National Science Foundation or the National Endowment for the Humanities.

3. Futility

I n "The Problem with Futility" by Robert Truog, Joel Frader and Allan Brett, the authors offer a short historical account of what has been considered medical futility, starting from the Hippocratic Oath until the recent court decisions and policy statements in the U.S.

It asserts, "The fact that this concept has appeared in law and policy may seem to indicate that is clearly understood and widely accepted. In reality however, the notion of futility hides many deep and serious ambiguities that threaten its legitimacy as a rationale for limiting treatment."[1]

The discussion is led by discussing the so-called three major "paradigms in contemporary discussion of futility."[2] These cases are; Patients in Persistent Vegetative State, Cases involving use of CPR (Cardiopulmonary Resurrection) and cases involving Organ-Replacement Technology. As an example of a controversial case dealing with Patients with Persistent Vegetative State the authors cite the famous case of Helga Wanglie, a 86 year old woman who was in a persistent vegetative state, sustained by a respirator and artificial nutrition and hydration. The hospital decided that further medical treatment was futile, unnecessary and inappropriate, besides, that hospital was struggling with financial issues which this case didn't help to solve. Helgas physician sought her husband's consent in order to remove the respirator, to which Mr. Wanglie completely refused, arguing Helga was a Christian and that she would want to go whenever god said so. Thus, both parties went to court to settle their differences. In the end, the judges decided in favor of Mr. Wanglie.

Medical Futility involving CPR is explained by the circumstances in which it is used and its usefulness. Finally, Organ-Replacement technology is cited as a technology that could possibly prolong the life of virtually any dying patient. Hence, the authors note, because physicians do not offer this technology to terminally ill patients, it is a matter of judging futility in medical treatments.

"Futility" is an ambiguous and dark concept with no general acceptance or definition, as such, the authors suggest that those problems might be grouped better as "value problems" and "probability problems".

---

1   Monagle, John F. and Thomasma, David C. *Health Care Ethics: Critical Issues for the 21st Century*, rg, MD: Aspen, 1998. P. 323.
2   Ibid.

Value Problems are those described by the questions: "What value does X treatment have?" or in other words "Which valuable goal is being pursued by X treatment?" In a pluralistic society where values are as different as they are abundant there has been no way to agree upon the goals of medicine and, especially in medical futility, the goals of treatments. According to the authors, a relatively successful approach in defining Medical Futility has been the "value-free" approach reached by the Hastings Center. This approach was called "physiologic futility" and it basically means that "if a treatment is clearly futile in achieving its physiological objective and so offers no physiological benefit to the patient, the professional has no obligation to provide it."[3] As always, problems arise and, defining what the actual physiological objective of a treatment is, is a matter of debate. Also, this definition of futility seems to be of little use in real life, for it applies to only a marginal number of cases in real life. We have to consider that many end-of-life situations are more complex than just consisting of one mere procedure for facing them, they involve several procedures and parallel goals and the gravity of cases is ample.

On the other hand, probability problems in futility are related to the judging of treatments as futile not because of their over-all value but because of the low probabilistic chance of success. Questions are immediately done, "What statistical cutoff point should be chosen as the threshold for determining futility?", in other words, "What probability of success is *enough success* when judging medical treatments?", "Who decides?"

Moreover, the authors state that physicians are "highly unreliable in estimating the likelihood of success," this is mostly due to the nature of the human mind, the tendency to remember mostly unique cases (whether miraculous or tragic) and the fact that, theoretically speaking, what can be said statistically of one group (of

patients) cannot be predicted to another group (of patients).

Some have considered Medical futility as feasible way of understanding and implementing resource allocation in health care, but the authors reject this view with a short critique of Futility as Resource allocation. It is based mainly on the fact that Futility is not sufficient to actually matter in macroeconomic terms when dealing with resource allocations. Medically Futile treatments are not applied enough to make a difference in the global scheme of resources.

Also, the authors note that Resource Allocation issues make explicit the value and probabilistic problems implicit in Medical Futility issues, so we shouldn't need to mask the subject of resource allocation with another name, since the problem of resources has to be addressed too. Finally, the authors propose a departure from the concept of "futility", which they regard as not useful. This departure is based on the confidence that there can be a professional ideal and a social consensus guiding the practices of supposedly futile treatments.

Professional ideals deal with the "duties" (in a general sense) physicians as professionals have with patients. Not only do they have to respect their autonomy, but they also have to act compassionately and minimize their suffering. Communication is seen as one of the key aspects in which physicians and patients should engage in order to resolve their differences, this, because "inadequate or insensitive communication by providers probably accounts for a substantial proportion of unrealistic requests, such discussions will successfully resolve many conflicts. Empirical studies of ethics consultations have demonstrated precisely this point."[4]

When communication is not enough, because of the deep differences in values and beliefs, we should, according to the authors, resort to social deliberation on the topic. A social consensus should establish the legal framework for physicians when dealing with

---

3   Ibid. p. 325.

4   Ibid. p. 328.

medically futile treatments and it should determine the scope of actions for physicians. Institutional mechanisms that somehow represent the general point of view of society's members, such as courts and ethics committees, should be the ones to hold the last words when differences cannot be solved privately.

The problem with an approach based on such ideas of societal agreement or social contracting, is that it is too general (does not provide actual guidelines to solve the issues), leaving the actual answer to the futility problem in a hypothetical future in which members of society will actually reflect and deliberate on such issues, thus leaving us with no answers *today*. Needless to say, such a contractual decision does not attend the morality of the issue itself; it merely leaves the answer to majorities, legitimizing whatever decision the members of this society agree upon by whichever reasons they want (religious or philosophical, well-founded or ignorant). These procedural laws the authors have in mind may very well solve the problems in practice, in other words, whenever such a clash of values arises the courts can and will utilize their jurisdictional powers to solve the differences, but such laws do not necessarily assure an ethical answer to every case (or to any case).

Another relevant exploration on futility can be found in *The Patient as Person, Exploration in Medical Ethics* by Paul Ramsey. In Chapter 3 "On (Only) Caring for the Dying," the author starts up with a reflection over practical cases of painful deaths and life-sustaining means, the author identifies quickly the problematic behind end-of-life treatment, amongst many questions done; one is especially eloquent, "Is there no end to the doctor's vocation to maintain life until the matter is taken out of his hands?" This question encompasses a serious of moral issues that must be addressed in order to be answered, issues such as: What means should be used to maintain life and why? Where do we draw the line between saving a life and merely prolonging death? Is it the same to kill than to let a patient die? Questions of "Futility", "Ordinary

and Extraordinary means of treatment" and "Defining Death" are all taken care of.

Ramsey suggests that means of treatments can be classified as ordinary and extraordinary, but this classification must be understood not as absolute, but rather as principles that have to be applied in practice. Hence, the distinction is a practical one, case by case. As a general principle, the author notes, Ordinary means of treatment would be those easily available, routine, standard, common treatments, those that are *not* expensive, hard, rare or exceptional. Extraordinary means would be those means that prove to be excessively expensive, painful, and inconvenient or of low probable benefit to the patient.

This distinction is then used in order to examine some main questions: Can patients morally refuse an ordinary treatment? Can physicians morally refuse to give ordinary treatment? And is it possible for ordinary means to become extraordinary given the circumstances of the case? To the three questions presented the answer is yes, although the limits are not set clearly.

Ramsey supposes that extraordinary means of treatment are *per se* not obligatory, so the focus of the matter is on the ordinary means.

Ordinary means are examined by doing an analysis of Gerald Kelly's *The Duty of Using Artificial Means of Preserving Life*, which has proven to be a foundational work on ordinary and extraordinary means of treatments. Ramsey shows the argumentation given by Kelly on the subject and agrees with the general conclusion drawn; namely, "that there is no duty to use useless means, however natural or ordinary or customary in practice."[5] This conclusion rests on the notion that, given, the circumstances, treatments *can* be useless to the patient, "One is excused from using a proposed remedy if it does not offer a reasonable hope of success; it is then, not a *remedy*." Here he proposes a sort of objective criteria for judging treatments, a

---

5   For full argumentation, see: Ramsey, P., *The Patient as Person: Exploration In Medical Ethics*, New Haven, CT: Yale University Press, 2002. 283, p. 132.

rather technical-medical criterion. It also rests on the idea of "process of dying" which entails that dying patients should be treated as such, much like live patients should be treated as living, dying patients should be treated with treatments according to dying, hence, no treatments that deny or ignore this end-of-life stage are obligatory for it is inherent to the medical profession and the human nature to care for others and not further their pain and agony.

In a sense, identifying the limits of living and dying and the course of treatment is a physician's duty not only because of his medical profession but because of his humanity (this is what Ramsey calls the *Medical Imperative* and the *Moral Imperative*, the first is to act leaning towards his medical expertise to keep options open for the patient and the second means to make room for the patient to judge according to his own whether he desires life-sustaining treatment or not).

Readings

Brody, Howard, "Medical Futility: A Useful Concept?" in Zucker, Marjorie B.; Zucker, Howard D., *Medical Futility and the Evaluation of Life-Sustaining Intervention*, Cambridge University Press, 1997: **1–14.**

Prip, William; Moretti, Anna, "Medical Futility: A Legal Perspective," in Zucker, Marjorie B.; Zucker, Howard D., *Medical Futility and the Evaluation of Life-Sustaining Intervention*, Cambridge University Press, 1997: **136–154.**

Practical Scenarios

Instructions for Analysis:

1. Explain, in general terms, why the case is morally relevant and controversial.
2. Identify the central moral issue. Justify.
3. Identify and explain the main facts to be considered in your analysis.
4. Identify and explain the principles and theories useful in analyzing the case. Justify why those principles and theories are relevant in the case. Specify conflicts between them.
5. Identify and raise arguments to support the conflicting options/decisions/actions that are evident in the case (Specifications and balancing of rules are necessary at this stage).
6. Identify and weigh alternative courses of action and then decide. Justify your decision. Answer the question(s) posed by the author as part of your conclusion.

Scenario 1

The Case of the "Murderer" Father

Tracy Latimer was born November 23, 1980. An interruption in Tracy's supply of oxygen during the birth caused cerebral palsy leading to severe mental and physical disabilities including seizures that were controlled with seizure medication. She had little or no voluntary control of her muscles, and could not walk or talk. Her doctors described the care given by her family as excellent.

Despite having a hip that had been dislocated for many months Tracy could not take painkillers because she was on anti-seizure medication which, in combination with painkillers, could lead to renewed seizures, stomach bleeding, constipation, and aspiration pneumonia. Robert Latimer reported that the family was not aware of any medication other than Tylenol that could be safely administered to Tracy. Considering it too intrusive, the Latimers did not wish a feeding tube to be inserted, though it might have allowed more effective pain medication to be administered, as well as improve her nutrition and health.

During her life, Tracy underwent several surgeries, including surgery to lengthen tendons and release muscles, and surgery to correct scoliosis in which rods were inserted into her back. People who knew Tracy described her smile, love of music and reaction to horses at the circus. According to the Crown prosecutors' brief presented at the second trial, "She also responded to visits by her family, smiling and looking happy to see them. There is no dispute that through her life, Tracy at times suffered considerable pain. As well, the quality of her life was limited by her severe disability. But the pain she suffered was not unremitting, and her life had value and quality." In October 1993, her doctor recommended further surgery on November 19, 1993 in the hope that it would lessen the constant pain in Tracy's dislocated hip. Depending on the state of her hip joint, the procedure might have been a hip reconstruction or it might have involved removing the upper part of her thigh bone, leaving the leg connected to her body only by muscles and nerves. The anticipated recovery period for this surgery was one year. The Latimers were told that this procedure would cause pain, and the doctors involved suggested that further surgery would be required in the future to relieve the pain emanating from various joints in Tracy's body." Her doctor reported that "the post-operative pain can be incredible", and described the only useful short-term solution being the use of an epidural to anesthetize the lower part of the body and help alleviate pain while Tracy was still in hospital.

On October 24, 1993, Laura Latimer found Tracy dead. She had died under the care of her father while the rest of the family was at church. At first Robert Latimer maintained that Tracy had died in her sleep; however, when confronted by police with autopsy evidence that high levels of carbon monoxide were found in Tracy's blood, Latimer confessed that he had killed her by placing her in his truck and connecting a hose from the truck's exhaust pipe to the cab. He said he had also considered other methods of killing Tracy, including Valium overdose and "shooting her in the head."

The Supreme Court judgment of 1997 noted, "It is undisputed that Tracy was in constant pain." In her medical testimony Dr. Dzus, Tracy's orthopedic surgeon, noted "the biggest thing I remember from that visit is how painful Tracy was. Her mother was holding her right leg in a fixed, flexed position with her knee in the air and any time you tried to move that leg Tracy expressed pain and cried out".

Robert Latimer said his actions were motivated by love for Tracy and a desire to end her pain. He described the medical treatments Tracy had undergone and was scheduled to undergo as "mutilation and torture." "With the combination of a feeding tube, rods in her back, the leg cut and flopping around and bedsores, how can people say she was a happy little girl?" Latimer asked.[6]

Scenario 2

The Dying Child

You find it hard to accept that the parents of a child actively dying of cancer refuse to accept your recommendation to transition to purely palliative goals and refuse to authorize a Do Not Resuscitate order. You believe they are painfully prolonging their child's dying. If the child is extubated you can concentrate on a peaceful dignified death. You believe that continuing to ventilate the child is disproportionately burdensome. You are evaluating whether or not to medically manage the child to prevent unnecessary suffering and a prolonged period of dying by changing the ventilator settings without telling the parents. This would result in the child's death.[7]

Question

What should you do in this case? Justify your arguments.

Scenario 3

Baby Theresa

In March 1992, in a Florida hospital, Theresa Ann Campo Pearson was born with anencephalia, a rare condition in which most of the upper skull and brain

6 Extracted from Rachels. James; Rachels, Stuart, *The Elements of Moral Philosophy*, Sixth Edition, McGraw-Hill, 2010.
7 Adapted from Taylor, Carol, *Health Care Ethics Course*, Georgetown University School of Medicine, AY 2010-2011

cortex are missing, but in which the partially developed brain stem can still produce breathing and a heartbeat. In the United States, most cases of anencephaly are detected during pregnancy and aborted. Of those not aborted, half are stillborn. About 300 each year are born alive, and they usually die within a few days.

Knowing that their baby could not live long, and that, even if she could, she would never have a conscious life, Baby Theresa's parents volunteered her organs for transplant. They thought her kidneys, liver, heart, lungs, and eyes should go to other children who could benefit from them.

The physicians agreed that this was a good idea. At least 2000 infants need transplants each year, and there are never enough organs available.

But the organs were not taken, because Florida Court does not allow the removal of organs until the donor is dead. Circuit Court Judge Estella Moriarty ruled that a Florida statute does not allow a person to be declared dead while any part of the brain is functioning. The judge told the parents: "I can't authorize someone to take your baby's life, however short, however unsatisfying, to save another child." When Baby Theresa died of respiratory failure nine days later, it was too late for the other children—her organs could not be transplanted because they had deteriorated too much. [8]

Question

Would it have been right to remove Theresa's organs, thereby causing her immediate death, to help other children?

---

8 Extracted from Rachels. James; Rachels, Stuart, The Elements of Moral Philosophy, Sixth Edition, McGraw-Hill, 2010

Medical Futility: A Useful Concept?

Howard Brody

The problem of medical futility involves two questions.

1. Are there medical interventions in a specific patient with a particular disease that we can label *futile* or *useless* because we are sufficiently confident that they will not be beneficial?
2. If so, are physicians entitled, or indeed obligated, to refuse to provide those interventions to the patient in question even if the treatment is requested or demanded by the patient or appropriate surrogate?

Those who argue that futility is a dangerous or unhelpful concept that should be abandoned rest their case on the observation that these two questions are extremely hard to answer. I agree that attempting to answer these questions leads us into a thicket of a peculiarly vexing nature, the like of which has seldom been encountered in medical ethics. However, I argue that the concept of futility is unavoidable or can be avoided only by paying far too high a price. We have no choice but to enter the thicket and seek whatever compasses and machetes will best allow us to navigate.

In this chapter, I review some of the arguments commonly raised against the concept of medical futility and then indicate why I think that futility judgments are unavoidable nonetheless. Next, I argue that futility is so closely bound up with critical concepts of professional integrity that medicine risks losing its moral bearings if it ignores the issue. Finally, I suggest that arguments that seem perplexing in the abstract are more resolvable at the level of practical policy. Thus, it may be at the practical level—particularly by asking what sorts of discussions we want to take place within health care institutions—that we will eventually come to understand what futility means and what its appropriate limitations are.

Anti-Futility Arguments

Bernard Lo (1995) has carefully reviewed arguments against permitting physicians to make unilateral futility judgments. Lo argues for a moderate position—that futility judgments can sometimes be justified but that the concept is "fraught with confusion, inconsistency, and controversy" (1995:73). However, the arguments that he reviews have been used by more skeptical authors as reasons to dispense entirely with the concept of futility in medical ethics. Hence, for our purposes, Lo's list of concerns summarizes the anti-futility position.

Lo starts by granting that there are some senses of the word "futility" that appear to justify a unilateral decision to withhold a treatment. These include the following: the treatment has no pathophysiologic rationale, the patient is not responding even when treatment is at its maximal level, the treatment has already been given to the patient and the patient has not responded, and it is nearly certain that the treatment will not achieve the goals that the patient has specified. (An example of the fourth category might be the patient's stated desire to leave the hospital to return home, whereas the treatment would only succeed, at best, in keeping the patient alive in the intensive care unit dependent on machines.)

Lo distinguishes these more legitimate senses of futility from other commonly encountered usages of the term today: the likelihood of success is very small but not zero, the goals that the physicians perceive to be worthwhile cannot be achieved, the patient's quality of life is unacceptable, and the prospective benefit is not worth the resources required. It is easy to find examples of futility being used in each of Lo's questionable senses, both in the hallways of hospitals and even in the medical literature. This highlights Lo's point that the term may simply be too slippery to be allowed into the vocabulary of ethical discourse.

Besides this inconsistency in the use of the term "futility," Lo sees other problems with the concept. Futility judgments may be mistaken. We lack precise data on the usefulness of common treatments for many conditions, and it is easy for physicians to confuse either their frustration that the patient is not responding better to treatment or their distaste for the patient's present quality of life with scientific assessments of the likelihood of improvement. This leads directly to Lo's next problem: value judgments may be mistaken for factual or

scientific expertise. It has become commonplace in today's medical ethics to distinguish between issues of technical knowledge, in which the physician legitimately claims expertise, and questions of value, in which physicians are duty bound to respect the wishes of the autonomous patient. With that model, unilateral physician futility judgments can easily slide into what Robert Veatch (1973) called "generalization of expertise," with physicians illegitimately claiming authority over the value judgments that patients ought to be allowed to make. Lo adds that one may not need to employ the specific language of futility to commit this ethical error. For instance, a decision that a treatment is "not medically indicated" may mask an illegitimate value judgment.

After reading Lo's list of concerns, many would conclude that medical ethics would be much better off without any appeals to futility (just as many have tried to eliminate appeals to the distinction between ordinary and extraordinary care as being more likely to mislead than to illuminate). The anti-futility camp fears that futility judgments may turn the clock back to the bad old days of physician paternalism by granting physicians unilateral powers to make treatment decisions. Moreover, the slipperiness of the concept assures us that if we allow physicians to make such decisions in the clearest cases, they will easily slide into making unjustified decisions in the muddier cases. To borrow a concept from Jay Katz (1984), we have been trying during the modern era of medical ethics to encourage a special sort of conversation between physician and patient, which invites the patient to become an active, informed participant in therapeutic decisions. Now, the futility supporters would replace conversation with silence, as physicians conclude that they can resolve these knotty questions without discussing the issues with patients or families.

The nature of the debate is further illustrated by one specific definitional dispute. Schneiderman and Jecker (1995) have suggested that a treatment should be considered futile when it has not worked once in the last 100 times it was tried. Waisel and Truog (1995) attack this definition by noting that the criterion is statistically equivalent to saying that a therapy is futile if physicians are 95% confident that it would be successful no more than 3 in 100—a mathematical truism that Schneiderman et al. (1990) had themselves admitted in an earlier publication. Waisel and Truog find this an unacceptably loose definition and argue instead for a definition of strict physiologic futility—that is, a treatment is futile only when it is unable to achieve its physiologic objective. Cardiopulmonary resuscitation (CPR), for instance, would be futile if it failed to restore heartbeat and circulation but not if it kept the patient alive for an hour before suffering a second cardiac arrest and dying. Although these authors believe that their physiologic definition is superior because it avoids controversial value judgments, in fact it makes a value judgment that physicians ought to find especially controversial—that when we administer therapy, we care only what happens to the organs, and we do not care what happens to the patient.

CPR: Are Futility Judgments Avoidable in Practice?

No matter how powerful the arguments for throwing the term "futility" out of the lexicon may seem, they fail if it can be shown that physicians must make value-laden futility judgments whether they like it or not. To make the case that this is so, I take a somewhat lengthy detour into the practice of CPR in hospitals.

It is standard practice in U.S. hospitals and emergency care settings to attempt CPR if a patient is discovered without pulse or respiration from a recent cardiac arrest. CPR was developed in the early 1960s to address a new opportunity for intervention—the coronary care unit with electronic monitoring of otherwise healthy patients who had recently sustained serious heart

damage. This new setting allowed for the concentration of highly trained personnel near the patient's bedside and instantaneous notification of the onset of a potentially fatal rhythm disturbance of the heart. In this setting, CPR soon was shown to be successful about 50% of the time. Later, similar success rates were shown when CPR was used in patients with drug overdoses and in patients who suffered cardiac arrest or arrhythmias during general anesthesia.

The success of CPR led to a phenomenon fairly typical of American medicine—the uncritical use of technology that has proved beneficial to a small number of patients for treating other patients who have not been shown to benefit. CPR soon became the standard reaction to any patient in any U.S. health care setting who suffered a cardiac arrest. It was not until the late 1980s that research showed that although CPR still had about a 50% success rate in the populations of patients for whom it was initially designed, its success rate rapidly fell to 20% or less when it was applied to patients in other settings. There were even subpopulations in which the success rate was so close to zero that the label "futile" seemed appropriate. In general terms, CPR seems uniformly to be unsuccessful in patients who suffer a cardiac arrest in the face of concomitant failure of one or more major organ systems, overwhelming infection, or metastatic cancer (Moss 1989).

The debate over futility has focused on the decision to write a "do not attempt resuscitation" (DNAR)[1] order in the patient's chart. If this order appears, CPR will not be performed if a serious arrhythmia or cardiac arrest occurs. If no such order appears, in the event of an arrest, a CPR team applies a combination of external chest compression, mechanical ventilation by mask or endotracheal tube, cardiac drugs, and electroshock according to well-recognized protocols. Heartbeat may be restored within 5 or 10 minutes, but, more commonly, after about

---

1 A common but less precise usage is do not resuscitate (DNR). All the other authors in this volume use DNR rather than DNAR.

30 minutes of intense effort—perhaps 45 or even 60 minutes if the patient is young or previously healthy—the physician in charge of the team will decide that further efforts are pointless, and the code will be terminated.

The pro-futility side argues that in situations in which CPR is predictably without benefit (because of near zero success rates in scientific studies) and the patient or family will not agree to a DNAR order despite full explanations of these facts, physicians should be empowered to enter a DNAR order unilaterally. The rebuttal from the anti-futility side is that any decision to enter a DNAR order is fraught with value-laden assumptions—what counts as a benefit and what counts as sufficient evidence of lack of benefit, to mention just two. According to this line of argument, physicians can never ethically impose their values on patients without patients' consent, especially when life and death may hang in the balance.

I have gone into this much detail about CPR to make one critically important point. To my knowledge, all of the discussion about unilateral decision making, value judgments, and futility relates to the decision whether or not to start CPR. I am aware of no serious policy consideration ever being given to demanding the consent of the patient or family as to when to stop CPR. In principle, however, these two decisions seem equally value laden. After all, no one can say with total certainty that the patient could not have responded if a code that was stopped at 45 minutes had continued for another 15 minutes, or that the extra 15 minutes of effort might not have provided some benefit (even if only psychologic comfort) to some party in the case. No one on the anti-futility side of the debate, however, seems upset that physicians are allowed to make reasonable judgments about what is working or not working and unilaterally decide to stop the code based on those judgments.

The reason it does not bother them and does not bother the vast majority of patients and families is obvious—when one considers all aspects of the practical situation, no other

policy makes any sense. This feature of how CPR decisions are made in the real world illustrates conclusively to me that those on the anti-futility side of the debate are caught in a logical contradiction. If they are so worried about unilateral physician decision making whether to start CPR, they should be equally worried about unilateral physician decision making when to stop CPR. If they are not, I allege that they must be confused. I suggest that they cannot logically defend a patient's right to demand CPR when the patient is 87 and has widely metastatic cancer and pneumonia yet fail to defend the right of a patient or family to demand that the code team continue CPR for at least 12 hours.

Although I have claimed that the anti-futility position ultimately cannot succeed, the strong arguments raised by Lo and others ought to cause us considerable unease when we contemplate physicians who misuse the futility concept or refuse to discuss critical decisions with patients. I argue that we should take those concerns very seriously but that we can do so within a framework that admits the occasional justification for physician determination of futility. However, we first have to be very clear on what ethical concerns are at stake in physician futility judgments. This, in turn, forces us to undertake a discussion of professional integrity. Furthermore, we must address practical policy matters to ensure that appeals to futility and to physician integrity are used to start and not to stop useful conversations between physicians and patients.

Futility and professional integrity

The ethical principle of patient autonomy seems to require that value-laden medical decisions be discussed with the patient and that the patient be allowed the last word. If, in futility cases, the physician's determination is supposed to carry more weight than the patient's own choice, we need to appeal to some countervailing ethical principle to explain why. I propose that the relevant principle is respect for professional integrity (Brody 1994).

The principle of professional integrity has been (sadly) little discussed in recent work on medical ethics, compared with such principles as autonomy, beneficence, and justice. This chapter is not the place for an extended analysis, but a few critical points can be offered.

Professional integrity appears as an ethical principle if we start with the assumption that medical practice has some sort of core moral content and that physicians make a moral commitment of some sort when they profess to practice medicine. As Pellegrino and Thomasma (1981) have argued, medicine is not defined either as a science or as an application of science. Instead, it is best understood as the application of scientific principles to individual cases with the goal of promoting a right and good healing action. Therefore, at least some ethical standards are defined by the nature of the practice of medicine itself, and physicians of integrity are required to adhere to those standards.

Consider some commonplace examples of things we typically expect of physicians of integrity.

1. Not to perform surgery for people who do not have the disease for which the surgery is usually indicated
2. Not to prescribe anabolic steroids for teenage body-builders
3. Not to engage in sexual relationships with their patients

Notice two important things about this list. First, we do not specify anything about the patient's level of autonomy or information. We do not, for example, say that if the teenage bodybuilder has exhaustively read all available scientific articles on the benefits and risks of anabolic steroids, it would be all right to prescribe them. We assume that since the appeal here is to the standards that define medicine as a type of practice, physicians as a group have legitimate say over those standards, even though physicians do not practice in a social

vacuum and even if professional–public dialogue and negotiation are ultimately critical in formulating ethically defensible standards.

Second, this list is independent of the physician's personal value system. Consider two physicians, one with religious views strongly opposing sterilization, the second with different philosophical views. If the first physician were to perform sterilizations, we would hold that he lacked personal integrity because one crucial aspect of his behavior stood opposed to values that he claimed to be important in defining his moral identity. We would not say this of the second physician were he to perform sterilizations. We would hold, however, that both physicians were equally lacking in professional integrity if they prescribed anabolic steroids or surgically removed gallbladders known in advance to be healthy.

It is important to see that medicine may have internal ethical standards that define its legitimate practice, even when these standards are subject to heated controversy. Consider the debate over physician-assisted suicide and euthanasia. Some argue that these actions would be permissible for physicians in extreme cases, as when a competent patient was suffering terribly and had no other available means to relieve suffering. Others would argue that such actions are contrary to the internal moral standards of physicians, who should always strive to be healers and never to be agents of death. Some would conclude from the vigorous and unresolved debate over this question that medicine cannot have any internal, defining ethical standards, or we would expect near unanimity on such a critical issue. I claim instead that this debate shows that it makes good sense to talk about internal ethical standards because there would be no point to the debate if medicine did not have such standards.

What does this have to do with futility? The example of unnecessary surgery suggests that physician integrity includes an injunction not to perform actions that predictably fail to offer benefit (and that could, in some cases, cause harm). With a more detailed analysis of the elements of professional integrity (Miller and Brody 1995), the following reasons emerge.

1. The ethical goals that define medical practice include healing and curing disease, promoting health and preventing disease, and relieving suffering caused by disease symptoms. If a treatment can be reasonably predicted not to do any of these, to require that physicians offer it is to require them to act contrary to their goals of practice.

2. Physicians are obligated to adhere to high standards of scientific competence. Employing a treatment that predictably will not work deviates from that standard of competence.

3. Physicians also are obligated to represent standards of scientific knowledge truthfully to the public, claiming neither more nor less than what medicine can actually deliver. Reasonable people will conclude that if a physician offers a treatment, it must have some chance of working. Thus, physicians who employ futile treatments risk becoming quacks or frauds.

4. Physicians are justified in risking harm to patients only when the possible benefit strongly outweighs the risk. If benefit is practically zero, there can be no justification for any risk of harm. Demanding futile treatments, especially those, such as CPR, that can cause pain, forces physicians to become agents of harm, not benefit.

I conclude that physicians should not be forced to provide treatments reliably determined to be futile, as that would force them to violate the dictates of their own professional integrity. We must now ask what practical policies could balance physicians' concerns with maintaining their own integrity against ethical concerns that patients' rights not be trampled in the process.

Toward Practical Futility

Policies

We have seen why the concept of futility has proven so complex and perplexing yet carries so much moral weight that it cannot be dismissed. Let us conclude by asking a final set of questions: does the problem get worse when we stop talking in generalities and start talking about real cases with real persons? Or might it be that the abstraction itself has caused some of the problem, so that once we deal with specifics, the view actually becomes clearer?

Recall that in discussing CPR, I suggested two things: first, that when we looked at the relatively abstract question of whether physicians could unilaterally decide DNAR status, the debate was intense and intractable; and second, that when we looked at an issue with undeniably practical implications—whether physicians should unilaterally decide whether and when to stop CPR—most of the debate melted away. That

Table 1.1 Outline of a Hospital Policy on Futile CPR

1. Definition: *Futile*, provides no meaningful possibility of extended life or other benefit for the patient.
2. Physician (with appropriate specialty consultation) makes preliminary determination that attempted resuscitation would be futile or harmful for a given patient.
3. Attending physician informs competent patient, or surrogate for an incompetent patient, when a preliminary determination of futility has been made. Physician explains reasoning and seeks concurrence with decision not to attempt CPR.
4. If patient or surrogate concurs, physician documents discussion and enters DNAR order.
5. If patient or surrogate does not concur, physician seeks input of ethics committee consultation team to a Evaluate correctness of futility determination, b Aid with communication and negotiation process.
6. If ethics consultation team supports physician, and patient or family continues to disagree, physicians or hospital try to identify another physician within or outside of facility willing to assume care under conditions specified.
7. If transfer of care cannot be arranged, case goes back to full ethics committee for review and final disposition, in concert with legal counsel if needed.
8. Implementation of policy requires extensive and ongoing staff education around futility issues.

Source: Adapted from Tomlinson and Czlonka 1995.

example gives us some hope that the descent from the general to the particular will improve our understanding of futility in practice.

Tomlinson and Czlonka (1995) offer one particularly well-developed approach to a futility policy for a health care institution. A brief summary of the key points of their policy is provided in Table 1.1, but such a synopsis does not really do justice to their insights into how a futility policy actually should work. They understand quite well that in the practical setting, many of the issues that most vex the philosopher or the theoretician recede into the background, and other issues move to center stage.

For instance, it would seem absolutely essential to define futility precisely and consistently before developing a policy on how to deal with it. A good part of the wisdom of Tomlinson and Czlonka's policy lies in refusing to take this approach. To a degree, the response to the demand for a definition is like that of the proverbial baseball umpire, who, on being asked whether the previous pitch was a ball or a strike, replied, "It ain't nothin' till I call it." For practical policy purposes, the question ceases to be "What are the necessary and sufficient conditions for a medical intervention to be said to be futile?" and becomes "How should we resolve disputes over what medical interventions should be deemed futile?" A fair and thoughtful mechanism for dispute resolution turns out to have far more value in the real world than a philosophically elegant definition.

Underlying this aspect of the policy is a deeper insight. Opponents of the concept of futility charge that unilateral futility judgments are an unacceptable abuse of the physician's power over the patient or family. Futility defenders respond by trying to define futility ever more precisely, which in turn leads the opponents to charge that the fancy definitions merely conceal the abuse of power. Tomlinson and Czlonka, by contrast, accept that futility judgments involve the exercise of power by physicians. The question then becomes how to monitor and supervise that use of power and resolve disagreements evenhandedly when abuse is charged.

One way to summarize the wisdom of a practical approach to futility decisions in medicine is to turn to the metaphor of *conversation*. Conversation, in the view of Katz (1984), is useful for better understanding informed consent. What might at first seem a legal fiction unrelated to medicine can be reconceptualized as a vital component of medical practice once physicians realize that informed consent is an invitation to have a certain type of conversation with their patients. Katz deliberately used the homely word "conversation" instead of a more technical term to demystify what had seemed to many an arcane debate: one need not be a lawyer or an ethicist to comprehend what it means for a doctor to talk with a patient about a treatment decision.

Consider situations in which physicians are talking with patients (or surrogates) about what treatment ought to be used. Such a circumstance requires one of at least three different sorts of conversations. One type of conversation will be by far the most common, but occasionally other considerations will require the conversation to assume one of the other two forms.

The physician's side of the first and by far most common form of conversation goes roughly like this.

The autonomy conversation
"You have a disease, and the treatment options for this disease are the following. Each one (including no treatment) has consequences that might be either good or bad for you. I'd like to describe these consequences to you, along with some idea of how likely or unlikely each one is, so that you can decide which treatment option would best promote your overriding values. If you want, I can list the options and their consequences in a neutral fashion and leave the decision totally up to you. Or, if you prefer, I can offer advice and suggestions as we go along. The

goal of this conversation is to allow you to make an informed choice of a treatment option, taking as active a role in the decision as you wish."

This could also be dubbed the "informed consent conversation." It assumes that patient autonomy is the operative principle and generally trumps competing principles.

The other two, less frequent conversations are called for when it appears, at least at first glance, that some other moral principle might outweigh respect for patient autonomy. As we have seen, one such competing principle is respect for professional integrity. Another competing principle, increasingly important in an era of scarce resources and fixed budgets, is justice. Issues of justice have arisen for a long time in deciding who gets to be first in line for transplant organs or who gets the last bed when the intensive care unit is full. Today, these issues also arise commonly in managed care settings, when explicit decisions have to be made about whether a patient will receive a very expensive treatment that offers little if any benefit. Since Lo and others are concerned that resource scarcity will be linked inappropriately to futility, it is critical to distinguish these two conversations carefully. They go roughly as follows.

The futility conversation

"You seem to have settled on a decision to request or demand a certain medical intervention. I have a problem with this choice. As best as I can tell, this particular intervention will not succeed in achieving the goals that I presume you want to pursue with regard to your health. So first I have to explore with you the facts about your present situation, as it appears likely that your choice of this intervention is based simply on not knowing these facts. If we find that the discussion of the facts doesn't cause you to change your mind, our conversation will have to take a

new direction. Perhaps you can show me that you are trying to pursue a goal different from the one I had assumed; or perhaps you reject my facts and want to get another opinion. In either case, I feel obligated to let you know that what you are asking of me seems to require me to do something that I consider to be bad medical practice. Possibly, our ongoing conversation will show me that I am wrong, but I want you to understand why I am raising this issue and why I feel strongly about the matter—not to be disrespectful of you and your choice but rather to fulfill my professional obligations."

The justice conversation

"You seem to have settled on a decision to request or demand a certain medical intervention. I have no problem with this choice insofar as it seems to be a rational choice for you and to offer you some prospect of benefit. But the role I play [for instance, as a primary physician working within an HMO plan] has imposed on me certain obligations—not only to you but also to other patients who might need scarce or expensive treatment. According to the rules or standards of this system [such as an HMO's benefit package], you don't seem to me to qualify. I need to explain to you why I think this, and you might then wish to challenge my reasoning. If you and I can't agree, I need to tell you about the mechanisms for appeal that you may use, especially if you think that any form of inappropriate bias has entered into my decision or that I am not adequately informed about all aspects of the treatment that you want. I'm sorry to have to take this position, but I feel forced into it because the duty I owe to you is balanced against the duty that I owe to other patients."

Four points about these conversations are especially important. First, it is important to understand the difference between the futility (integrity) conversation and the justice conversation, as at least some futility advocates seem to think that they are basically the same (Murphy 1994). Treatment that is of small benefit and that is very costly might appropriately be provided to the patient if for some reason it were to become much cheaper, but treatment that violates the physician's professional integrity does so regardless of its cost. If one is principally concerned about justice, it is important to identify which treatments are futile, as it seems totally unjust to withhold a potentially beneficial treatment from one patient while another patient gets a treatment of no benefit whatsoever. It does not follow, however, that if one is principally concerned about professional integrity, one must consider the cost or relative scarcity of the treatment or make any comparative judgments between the degree of entitlement of different patients.

The second point is that the futility conversation is not the autonomy conversation. Some would argue that futility conversations are never necessary because in almost all cases we could accomplish everything we want by using the autonomy conversation, and by phrasing the futility conversation to indicate where it overlaps partially with autonomy (that is, the hope that a clearer explanation of the facts will lead the patient voluntarily to renounce the treatment originally requested). There is something deceptive about trying to characterize the futility conversation as a form of the autonomy conversation, however, because a different moral principle is at stake. In the futility conversation, the physician accurately informs the patient that there is a conflict. If the futility conversation were replaced with an autonomy conversation, the professional integrity issues would be obscured.

Third, putting futility into conversation form may help to defuse some of the fears of the opponents. To some degree, almost all of the objections to the futility concept come down to the fear that it will provide physicians with a license to do things (or to fail to do things) to patients without bothering to talk to the patients about them. (This is why the term "unilateral" stirs up so much heat.) If calling an intervention "futile" requires that the ethical physician engage in a special sort of conversation with the patient, we seem to have a reasonable safeguard that full and frank discussions will occur. If a futility policy results in conversations of this type within health care institutions whenever physicians feel compelled to refuse treatment on grounds of futility, the policy may offer reasonable protection to the moral values of both physicians and patients.

The fourth point is closely related to the third. The danger in futility determinations is the abuse of physician power. In futility conversations, physicians state clearly what power they propose to exercise, on what authority they feel entitled to exercise it, and what checks and balances ensure that these exercises of power do not constitute abuses. The physicians also remind the patients, as part of the conversation, about the countervailing sources of power they possesses (such as a right to a second medical opinion, ethics committee review, and so on). Under these circumstances, it seems hard to imagine how the power to determine futility could be abused on a regular basis. Of course in some settings, both futility conversations and autonomy conversations might be nonexistent or perfunctory. Up to this point, I have assumed that U.S. health care institutions have learned the autonomy lesson of the last quarter-century and strive to involve patients or surrogates in key decisions about care, including end-of-life issues. Sadly, some data show that this is far from universal (Solomon et al. 1993; SUPPORT Principal Investigators 1995). Inadequate attention to patient autonomy is not a good reason to dismiss the concept of futility, however. Instead, it calls for a more careful distinction of whether autonomy or futility is the basis of the conversation we ought to have. Indeed, better understanding of futility may indirectly spur enhanced respect for autonomy, as the principle of autonomy is both more understandable and more acceptable to physicians once they see its proper limits.

Conclusion

This chapter reviews reasons why the concept of futility has proved so perplexing for medical ethicists. As long as we try to subsume all futility considerations under the principles of autonomy or justice and demand abstract but precise definitions, we are likely to remain muddled. In contrast, once we realize that the ethical principle of professional integrity plays a pivotal role, that futility judgments should start rather than stop conversations among physicians, patients, and families, and that most of the difficult problems are matters of practical policy, we may find ourselves on firm ground.

References

Brody, H. 1994. The physician's role in determining futility. *Journal of the American Geriatrics Society* 42: **875–8.**

Katz, J. 1984. *The Silent World of Doctor and Patient.* New York: Free Press.

Lo, B. 1995. Futile interventions. In *Resolving Ethical Dilemmas: A Guide for Clinicians,* pp. 73–81. Baltimore: Williams & Wilkins.

Miller, F.G., and Brody, H. 1995. Professional integrity and physician-assisted death. *Hastings Center Report* 25(May–June): **8–17.**

Moss, A.H. 1989. Informing the patient about cardiopulmonary resuscitation: when the risks outweigh the benefits. *Journal of General Internal Medicine* 4: **349–55.**

Murphy, D.J. 1994. Can we set futile care policies? Institutional and systemic challenges. *Journal of the American Geriatrics Society* 42: **890–3.**

Pellegrino, E.D., and Thomasma, D.C. 1981. A *Philosophical Basis of Medical Practice.* New York: Oxford University Press.

Schneiderman, L.J., and Jecker, N.S. 1995. *Wrong Medicine: Doctors, Patients, and Futile Treatment.* Baltimore: Johns Hopkins University Press.

Schneiderman, L.J., Jecker, N.S., and Jonsen, A.R. 1990. Medical futility: its meaning and ethical implications. *Annals of Internal Medicine* 112: **949–54.**

Solomon, M.Z., O'Donnell, L., Jennings, B., et al. 1993. Decisions near the end of life: professional views on life-sustaining treatment. *American Journal of Public Health* 83: **14–23.**

SUPPORT Principal Investigators. 1995. A controlled trial to improve care for seriously ill hospital patients. The Study to Understand Prognoses and Preferences for Outcomes and Risks of Treatment (SUPPORT). *Journal of the American Medical Association* 274: **1591–8.**

Tomlinson, T., and Czlonka, D. 1995. Futility and hospital policy. *Hastings Center Report* 25(May–June): **28–35.**

Veatch, R.M. 1973. Generalization of expertise. *Hastings Center Studies* 1(Mar–Apr): **29–40.**

Waisel, D.B., and Truog, R.D. 1995. The cardiopulmonary-resuscitation-not-indicated order. *Annals of Internal Medicine* 122: **304–8.**

Medical Futility: A Legal Perspective

William Prip, M.A., and Anna Moretti, R.N., J.D.

For the past two decades, much of the medical, ethical, and legal discussion about death and dying has focused on the right of individuals to reject treatments that only prolong the dying process. Yet if the volume of literature devoted to medical futility in recent years is any indicator, a significant number of individuals are now clamoring for the very treatments that others fought to reject.

Much of this discussion concerning medical futility comes from a medical or philosophical perspective. On the few occasions that the judicial system has addressed the subject of medical futility, it has applied the law unevenly and often without much reflection about the consequences of its rulings, leaving clinicians and patients with little guidance. Statutes that address medical futility directly are fewer still and have proved ineffective at resolving the hypothetical and real problems that the futility debate creates for clinicians and patients across the country.

In this chapter, we survey the legislation and court decisions that have specifically addressed the issues of medical futility and explore whether the established right to refuse treatment can inform the futility debate and the right to receive treatment, or whether a new set of laws and legal principles is needed.

The Emergence o the Futility Problem

A consensus on what constitutes futile treatment remains elusive. However, conflicts over medical futility are beginning to surface as a new type of end-of-life decision-making case. As medical technology developed over the years, a standard emerged that demanded treatment at all cost without much thought to outcome. One of the consequences of this reflexive standard was the emergence of the right-to-die movement. Patients became more vocal in their refusal of treatment that merely prolonged the dying process, and, eventually, advance directive statutes were enacted in every state. In effect, patients were telling physicians that, from their perspective, treatment that could not return them to an acceptable quality of life was futile.

We now have come full circle; patients and their families are challenging the physician's decision to stop life-sustaining treatment. Today, physicians assert that the treatments being requested are futile and that providing them would be contrary to the accepted standard of care for that medical situation.

Although standards of care may serve as the legal defense in medical malpractice cases, it is unclear what constitutes accepted standards of care or reasonable medical practice in the futility case scenario. Despite the availability of scientifically developed indicators of the efficacy of various medical treatments and procedures, physicians cannot consistently define futility (Curtis et al. 1995). The treatments offered to dying patients with similar prognoses may differ significantly. As there are no standards of practice that say that treatment must stop, physicians decide what is futile on a case by case basis. To date, this ad hoc approach has not been effective in creating standards of care that can be applied uniformly in the clinical setting.[1]

Is Medical Futility a Legal Issue?

Whatever one's position in the futility debate, an important question remains: Does the law offer an effective remedy for the futility problem? If the law indeed becomes the arbiter between patients and physicians in the futility debate, will a formal legal process be constructed for identifying futility, or will the courts rely on an approach similar to Justice Stewart Potter's technique for identifying obscenity: "I know it when I see it"?

Clearly, the law has had considerable influence in effecting a consensus on some contentious social issues concerning medical ethics.[2]

Indeed, the New Jersey Supreme Court's 1976 ruling in the Karen Ann Quinlan case provided the impetus for much of the debate about patient autonomy in end-of-life decision making for the next two decades. Not only did the notoriety of the case provide the catalyst for enactment of the nation's first living will law in California later that year (Glick 1992:53), but it undoubtedly sparked the public's interest in the issue that eventually produced a devolution of power from doctors to patients regarding end-of-life decision making. By 1982, the year the American Medical Association's Judicial Council concluded that "withholding or removing life supporting means is ethical" (President's Commission 1983:299), 13 states and the District of Columbia had already enacted advance directive laws,[3] and six appellate state courts had decided on right-to-die cases.[4] Clearly, the medical profession's standards of care have lagged behind the law in addressing the issue of a patient's right to refuse unwanted care.

However, although it may be convenient and appear expeditious to defer to the law for resolution of the futility debate, we must realize at the outset that the law governing the right of patients to refuse treatment has not been very successful in affecting the behavior of health care providers in the clinical setting. It is important to remember that even after more than two

---

1 The case of Baby Nguyen is evidence that practice variation adds to the tenuous nature of using "accepted medical standards" as the legal basis for stopping treatment. Ryan Nguyen was born with severe medical problems, including kidney failure, bowel obstruction, and brain damage. Although physicians at one hospital argued that continued aggressive treatment would only prolong his suffering, physicians at another facility were more than willing to continue aggressive treatment (Kolata 1994).

2 For example, the consensus today that brain death is a definition of death has its roots in 1970 when the Kansas Legislature enacted a law, sponsored by a physician–legislator, that included an alternative definition to the

common-law and customary method of defining death: a cessation of circulatory or respiratory function (President's Commission 1981:62). Although the new definition still relied on physicians to determine whether death had occurred—specifically, to determine if there was an "absence of spontaneous brain function"—this legal watershed undoubtedly influenced other developments, including model brain death standards issued by the American Bar Association in 1975, the National Conference of Commissioners on Uniform State Laws in 1978, and the American Medical Association in 1979 (President's Commission 1981: 117–19). Eventually, in 1980–81, all three groups settled on the Uniform Law Commissioners' "Uniform Definition of Death Act," which has been enacted in all but three states.

3 Alabama, Arkansas, California, Delaware, Idaho, Kansas, Nevada, New Mexico, North Carolina, Oregon, Texas, Vermont, Washington, and the District of Columbia.

4 Florida, Massachusetts, New Jersey, New York, Tennessee, and Louisiana.

decades of litigation and legislation protecting the right of patients to refuse unwanted care, the preponderance of decision-making conflicts involving critically ill patients still results from the reluctance of the physician or health care institution to permit the forgoing of unwanted life-sustaining measures.

Legal Rights in the Futility Debate

One can argue that the right to demand and receive medical treatment even when it is deemed medically ineffective by the attending physician is a logical extension of the right to patient autonomy.[5] This argument observes roughly the following logic: if one has the right to control one's health care by refusing medical treatment even if that decision is contrary to medical advice, one also retains the right to request and receive health care, again over a physician's objections. In essence, this position contends that the right to patient autonomy would be hollow if it were confined only to the right to refuse care—regardless of the fact that most patient self-determination laws are silent regarding the right to receive treatment. An analogous argument, although applied to effect the reverse conclusion, has been made regarding the common law doctrine of informed consent. That is, if, as in the words of the U.S. Supreme Court, the "logical corollary of the doctrine of informed consent is that the patient generally possesses the right not to consent, that is, to refuse treatment" (*Cruzan v. Director* 1990: 270), the logical corollary of the right to refuse treatment is the right to receive treatment.

Although this logic may be compelling, it is important to realize that the law underlying the right to refuse treatment does not easily transfer to the right to receive treatment. The difference between the demands "don't touch me" and "you must touch me" is dramatic. The law has almost uniformly conceded the former but has only hesitantly recognized the latter, and only in situations related to public health and safety.

The Right to Refuse versus the Right to Receive

The challenge is to determine if the patient autonomy model, as it has evolved over recent years, adequately addresses the futility question. Historically, the public readily accepted the dominance of patient autonomy over the "doctor knows best" approach to medical decision making, although it took well over a decade, beginning in 1976 with the *Quinlan* ruling, for the issue to permeate the American consciousness. Today, the right to refuse treatment is supported by a myriad of laws: all states and the District of Columbia have enacted advance directive legislation. All of the state appellate courts that have addressed the issue have found a legal right of patients to forgo life-prolonging procedures; the U.S. Supreme Court has ruled that patients have a constitutional right to be free of unwanted medical treatments, and the Congress has enacted federal legislation aimed at educating the public about their right to refuse treatment under state law.

However, the right asserted in futility cases is different. As Meisel points out, the right to refuse treatment and the right to receive treatment are, respectively, negative and positive rights (Meisel 1995:546-8). A negative right bestows on individuals a right that is protected by prohibiting others from certain behavior. The right to liberty guarantees personal freedom, for example, by prohibiting incarceration by the state without due process. In contrast, a positive right obliges others to provide a service or expend resources in order for an individual to exercise such right.

---

5 Proponents of the right to assisted suicide argue similarly that the right to autonomy in medical decision making encompasses the right to receive, directly or indirectly, death-inducing medications (*Compassion in Dying v. Washington* 1994).

Certain civil and political rights, as well as rights established by government entitlement programs and consumer protection laws, are positive rights. Thus, both the right to a trial by jury and the right to suffrage require the state to establish and support processes that guarantee these positive rights to all citizens. Similarly, consumer protection laws require that consumers be provided with nutrition information and content labels on all food products sold in the country—that is, the state establishes a positive right (to information) and obliges another private actor to fulfill the right.

Importantly, a positive right to be touched by another is only found in the area of public health and safety and is established exclusively by statute. For example, many cities and states have created rights to certain types of health care under the aegis of sound public policy, such as prenatal care for indigent mothers-to-be and immunization for children. Individuals also have the right to be touched for safety purposes in emergency situations, including the right to receive assistance from rescue squads, fire departments, and emergency medical services.

In applying the concept of negative and positive rights to the issue of patient autonomy, Meisel writes (1995:546)

> A *negative* right embodies the freedom to do what one wants without interference from others. The right to refuse medical treatment is such a right. ... The right being asserted in futility cases, by contrast, is a *positive* right. ... In the context of medical decision making, it is the freedom to have whatever medical treatment one might wish.

As a negative right, the right to refuse medical care, whether life saving or routine, is bolstered by a long legal tradition, rooted in the constitutional right to privacy and liberty and the common law right to be let alone. As early as 1891, the right to be free of unwanted touching was articulated by the U.S. Supreme Court: "No right is held more sacred, or is more carefully guarded, by the common law, than the right of every individual to the possession and control of his own person, free from all restraint or interference of others, unless by clear and unquestionable authority of law" (*Union Pacific R. Co. v. Botsford* 1891:25). Over 20 years later, Justice Benjamin Cardozo applied this thinking to medical treatments: "Every human being of adult years and sound mind has a right to determine what shall be done with his own body; and a surgeon who performs an operation without his patient's consent commits an assault, for which he is liable in damages" (*Schloendorff* v. *Society of New York Hospital* 1914:129–30).

In this respect, the right to refuse treatment dictates that bodily integrity must not be violated without informed consent. Indeed, to trespass upon the person without consent is generally considered a tortious act that is compensable in damages. Over the years, penalties for nonconsensual touching in the medical setting have been articulated in numerous cases.[6] Even when a treatment is beneficial, the courts have frowned on nonconsensual touching. For example, an Ohio appeals court declared, "[a] physician who treats a patient without consent

---

6 See, for example, *Mohr v. Williams* (1905) (allowing recovery of damages for assault and battery against a physician who operated on the left ear of patient who only consented to surgery on the right ear); *Schmeltz v. Tracy* (1935) (permitting assault and battery charges against a physician who removed moles not consented to during a consent to acne procedure); *Chouinard v. Marjani* (1990) (accepting negligence and intentional assault charges for performance of bilateral surgery when patient only consented to surgery on one breast); *Fox v. Smith* (1992) (acknowledging battery claim against a physician for removal of intrauterine device without consent from a patient undergoing another procedure); *Perkins v. Lavin* (1994) (permitting assault and battery claim against a hospital for the administration of a blood transfusion against patient's explicit instructions); *Cohen v. Smith* (1995) (allowing claims of battery and intentional infliction of emotional distress for allowing a male nurse to view and touch an unclothed female patient against patient's wishes).

commits a battery, even though the procedure is harmless or beneficial" (*Leach v. Shapiro* 1984:1051).

In contrast, the right to receive treatment is not supported by a similar historic foundation. Indeed, the federal judiciary has been reluctant to find a constitutional right that requires the state or other individuals to provide services or expend resources or both to safeguard an individual's claim to such right. Even through the various tort remedies in common law that better govern the relations between private actors, the right asserted in futility cases is not firmly settled.

A recent law review note asserted that elements in the theory of negligence, specifically, the concept of a legal duty to act, can be used to penalize physicians who unilaterally deny health care to their patients (Mordarski 1993: 765).

> In a case in which a patient is dependent on a life support system, the physician would have duty to act as a reasonable physician would act when dealing with that patient. If the physician were to terminate the life support system against the wishes of the family, the family would have to convince a jury that a reasonable physician, in the same circumstances, would not have terminated the life support.

This line of argument was put to test in a recent law suit (*Gilgunn* 1995) brought by the daughter of a patient who died as a result of the withdrawal of ventilator support and the withholding of cardiopulmonary resuscitation (CPR). However, a jury refused to find the defendants (the hospital, the physician who wrote the do not resuscitate, DNR, order, and the head of the ethics committee) negligent because the jury believed the treatments requested by the daughter were "futile."

Another approach to the futility debate is to consider the issue of abandonment. In general, a duty is imposed on physicians to continue to care for their patients once the patient–physician

relationship has been established unless the relationship is terminated by the patient or the physician after reasonable notice to the patient. To prove that a physician abandoned a patient, however, it would be necessary to demonstrate that the physician "completely and unilaterally sever[ed] the relationship" with the patient (Meisel 1995:39), an unlikely situation in a futility case, in which a physician, for example, may refuse to provide artificial ventilation but would likely continue various other treatments. Medical abandonment is a complex issue that, to date, has not been applied to medical futility. However, it is possible that a patient may rely on the duty of nonabandonment to request treatment from a physician with whom he or she has had a long-standing patient–physician relationship.[7]

Meisel suggests that perhaps another recourse for patients and their families requesting treatment is to argue that a contractual relationship between a physician and patient requires the patient's wishes to be honored (Meisel 1995:548). This argument, however, has not been tested in the courts.

Perhaps the right to receive treatment, then, must rely solely on statutory law, which is generally the mechanism used to establish positive rights. Indeed, because it is the only method of creating a positive right that compels another individual to touch the person exercising the right, a legal resolution of the futility debate may lie in the hands of the federal and state

---

7 The abandonment argument has been used in two emerging issues in medical ethics: palliative care and assisted suicide. For example, some have called for greater use of palliative care for patients for whom life-sustaining treatments have been withheld or withdrawn: e.g., a physician's duty to care for his or her patient does not end with the cessation of aggressive life-support measures. Similarly, proponents of assisted suicide argue that physicians have a duty to provide the option of physician-assisted suicide to their terminally ill patients and that to withhold that option is tantamount to abandonment. Even further, some argue that if one accepts the legitimacy of physician-assisted suicide (and given the possibility that patients may be alone at the time of suicide and may botch the suicide attempt), "then the norm of nonabandonment supports physician presence at this moment" (Miller and Brody 1995:15).

legislatures, although courts may be forced to rely on creative interpretations of existing statutes in the interim. For example, the federal district and circuit courts in the *Baby K* case (1994) relied on the Emergency Medical Treatment and Active Labor Act (EMTALA)[8] to order a continuation of artificial ventilation that was deemed futile or at least against standard medical practice by the health care providers involved.

Statutes Addressing Medical Futility

To date, only a few statutes refer to futile or medically ineffective treatment. The types of statutes that embody the notion of futility include a federal act, DNR laws, and advance directive statutes governing living wills and medical powers of attorney. Some states go so far as to offer a method by which its citizens may request that all types of treatment be provided. Although it is unlikely that advance directive statutes would be interpreted as creating a positive right to receive any and all treatment, the legislatures that enacted these laws, as well as the individuals who rely on them, most likely believe they are protecting the patient's decision to be kept alive.

Federal Legislation

Through the enactment of the Child Abuse Amendment Act in October 1984, Congress has already articulated a federal policy regarding futility. Although the provisions of the act

apply only to neonates, its definition of futile treatment perhaps can be used to predict the language of any future federal legislation or regulation on the issue. The act may also provide support for a judicial finding of a right to receive treatment.

The Child Abuse Amendment Act ostensibly aims to protect handicapped infants from "discriminatory" behavior on the part of their parents or health care providers or both. This congressional intervention sought to end the controversy that erupted in 1982 when a minor surgical procedure was withheld from an infant born with Down syndrome. (See p. 51 for details about the Bloomington, Indiana, "Infant Doe" case and the futility debate concerning minors in general.) To combat the possibility of future discriminatory decisions, that is, decisions based on the likelihood of an infant surviving as a disabled person, the act requires all "medically indicated treatment" to be provided to neonates unless

(A) the infant is chronically and irreversibly comatose;

(B) the provision of such treatment would

   (i) merely prolong dying,

   (ii) not be effective in ameliorating or correcting all of the infant's life-threatening conditions, or

   (iii) otherwise be futile in terms of the survival of the infant; or

(C) the provisions of such treatment would be virtually futile in terms of the survival of the infant and the treatment itself under such circumstances would be inhumane. (42 U.S.C. 5102(3))

By introducing "futile" twice into the section governing the withholding of medical treatment, Congress apparently expected to introduce reason into the debate about the care of severely handicapped neonates, acknowledging that some neonates suffering extreme distress

---

8 By enacting EMTALA, Congress created a positive right for indigent patients to receive emergency medical care—in effect, a right that compels doctors to touch patients for the purpose of providing medical care during an emergency regardless of their ability to pay for these services. However, it is unlikely that the Congress intended EMTALA to be used to resolve the futility problem.

will not survive even with the application of aggressive care.

In a 1989 report, the U.S. Commission on Civil Rights considered the Child Abuse Amendment Act. It noted that the futility exception to the mandate that requires physicians to treat critically ill neonates is a "cover all bases" approach that "ties futility to the 'survival' of the infant, emphasizing that only the inevitability of death despite treatment, and not the persistence of disability despite treatment, renders the treatment legally futile" (U.S. Commission on Civil Rights 1989:90). Thus, by defining futile treatment as a treatment that does not guarantee survival beyond the immediate crisis, the federal government applies a very narrow definition of futility to cases involving critically ill neonates.[9]

Interestingly, the first and only futility case to come before the federal judiciary (*Baby K* 1994) notably did not refer to the definition of futility in the Child Abuse Amendment Act. It is possible, however, that other federal courts may view the act as an indication of a broader federal policy regarding futility in future cases.

Do Not Resuscitate (DNR) Legislation

One of the more recent trends in the refusal-of-treatment legislation is the enactment of DNR laws. (Currently 27 states have enacted do not resuscitate statutes.) A DNR order is a physician's written order not to attempt CPR on a particular patient. Although CPR was initially developed for unexpected cardiac and respiratory arrests following surgery or accidents, it is now commonly administered to anyone who arrests. It is presumed, unless otherwise indicated, that all patients would want to receive CPR.

Whereas every DNR law requires consent of either the patient or the surrogate before the order can be issued, a few statutes have adopted a futility rationale as a possible basis of withholding CPR in the absence of consent. That is, consent need not be secured to withhold a procedure that, in the opinion of the physician, should not be offered because it cannot benefit the patient.

Recent amendments to Georgia's DNR law may show a trend of introducing the concept of futility into the law. Before the amendment, the law stated (*Ga. Code Ann. §31-39-3[a]*)

> Every patient shall be presumed to consent to the administration of cardiopulmonary resuscitation in the event of cardiac or respiratory arrest, unless there is consent or authorization for the issuance of an order not to resuscitate.

The 1994 Amendment added the following language to the same section: "Such presumption of consent does not presume that every patient shall be administered cardiopulmonary resuscitation, but rather that every patient agrees to its administration unless it is medically futile." Medically futile is defined within the definition of "candidate for nonresuscitation." A candidate in the original statute "is a person for whom cardiopulmonary resuscitation would be medically futile in that such resuscitation will likely be unsuccessful in restoring cardiac and respiratory function or will only restore cardiac and respiratory function for a brief period of time so that the patient will likely experience repeated need for cardiopulmonary resuscitation over a short period of time." The 1994 amendment added, "... or that such resuscitation would be otherwise medically futile."

Tennessee regulations adopted in response to their DNR law have taken a similar

---

9 According to the interpretative guidelines of the Department of Health and Human Services (DHHS), the third exception's requirement that the treatment be "virtually" futile, again in terms of survival, offers a lower threshold for a treatment to be considered futile. The guidelines interpret "virtually futile" to mean treatment that is "highly unlikely to prevent death in the near future" (45 C.F.R. pt. 1340 App. Interpretative Guideline §8 [1987]). However, the law conditions this reduced stringency on the requirement that the treatment also be "inhumane," an undefined qualifier that can be subjectively interpreted by different individuals and, therefore, offers little guidance.

approach. Under the rules promulgated by the Tennessee Department of Health, "CPR may be withheld from the patient if in the judgment of the treating physician an attempt to resuscitate would be medically futile" (Tenn. Hosp. Rules & Regulations §1200-8-4-.05[5](g]). Resuscitation efforts should be considered futile "if they cannot be expected either to restore cardiac function to the patient or to achieve the expressed goals of the informed patient. In the case of the incompetent patient, the surrogate expresses the goals of the patient" (Tenn. Hosp. Rules & Regulations § 1200-8-4.05[3][h]).

New York also has adopted a law that allows physicians to write a DNR order for patients without capacity for whom there is no surrogate. The physician may issue the order, "provided that the attending physician determines, in writing, that, to a reasonable degree of medical certainty, resuscitation would be medically futile ..." (N.Y. Pub. Health L. § 2966[1]). Medically futile is defined to mean that "cardiopulmonary resuscitation will be unsuccessful in restoring cardiac and respiratory function or that the patient will experience repeated arrest in a short time period before death occurs" (N.Y. Pub. Health L. § 2961[12]).

Advance Directive Legislation

Two recently enacted advance directive statutes also address the futility issue. In 1995, both Maine and New Mexico enacted the Uniform Health-Care Decisions Act, a model law created by the National Conference of Commissioners on Uniform State Laws. The Maine act includes the following provision (Me. Rev. Stat. tit. 18-A, §5-807[f]).

> A health-care provider or institution may decline to comply with an individual instruction or health-care decision that requires medically ineffective health care or health care

contrary to generally accepted health-care standards.

The New Mexico version of the same model act adds the following statement to a section that is otherwise identical to Maine's: " 'Medically ineffective health care' means treatment that would not offer the patient any significant benefit" (N.M. Stat. Ann. § 24-7A-7[f]).

Other advance directive statutes use a similar approach by incorporating sections that would "protect" the physician from being forced to render treatment that is "medically inappropriate" (Louisiana), "medically ineffective" (Maryland), "medically unnecessary" (Virginia), "contrary to reasonable medical standards" (Oklahoma), or "not within accepted health care standards" (South Dakota).

At the other end of the spectrum, presumably in an attempt to create a semblance of neutrality, several living will statutes allow individuals to indicate what treatments they wish to receive, even if they become terminally ill, permanently unconscious, or otherwise critically ill without hope of recovery. Eleven living will laws[10] permit individuals to request life-sustaining treatment. Similarly, nine medical power of attorney statutes allow individuals to indicate their preference to receive medical care.[11]

The Indiana law goes as far as authorizing the use of a separate "Life Prolonging Procedures Declaration" as a final expression of one's "legal right to request medical and surgical treatment." (The option to request treatment in North Dakota's living will also includes similar language, explicitly acknowledging a "legal right that medical or surgical treatment be provided.")

Three additional states[12] have distinct provisions for artificial nutrition and hydration in their living will laws, allowing individuals to

---

10   Arizona, Idaho, Indiana, Kentucky, Maryland, Minnesota, North Dakota, Oregon, Pennsylvania, South Dakota, and Wisconsin.
11   Georgia, Illinois, Kentucky, Maryland, Nevada, Oregon, Pennsylvania, South Carolina, and Vermont.
12   Hawaii, Indiana, and Nevada.

reject all other life-sustaining treatments while simultaneously permitting them to indicate a desire to receive artificial nutrition and hydration. Even further, the Indiana law explicitly allows individuals to request artificial nutrition and hydration "even if the effort to sustain life is *futile* or excessively burdensome" (emphasis added).

The existence of statutes that permit patients to request life-sustaining treatment may or may not prove compelling to a court as establishing a state policy requiring physicians to provide treatment that they deem to be futile. In practice, the enactments of wrongful death and survivorship statutes over the years provide a powerful incentive within the medical profession to follow a family's request to treat a patient, even when the procedures involved generally would be considered futile by physicians and laypeople alike.

Judicial Intervention in Medical Futility Cases

The issue of futile treatment has been addressed on numerous occasions by the courts. However, until recently, the issue was approached from the perspective of a patient's right to refuse futile treatment being offered by a physician. Starting with *Quinlan*, numerous courts have relied on a determination that life-sustaining treatment was futile as one of the reasons for ordering the withholding or withdrawal of treatment.[13] Although these rulings relied

primarily on the notion of the right to self-determination as the basis for their conclusions, the implication was that these decisions were especially appropriate because the treatments were considered futile.

The courts have only recently faced the prospect of deciding if an individual's wish to receive medical care should override a doctor's decision to withhold or withdraw that care. Interestingly, each judicial intervention in a futility case, with one exception, has been in favor of continuing medical treatment, perhaps indicating the pervasiveness of the principle of patient autonomy. However, the lack of consistent reasoning in the decisions concerning the three significant cases to be discussed below is illustrative of the lack of consensus on the issue of medical futility within the law (Table 13.1).

The *Wanglie* Case

The case that inaugurated the futility debate in recent years involved Mrs. Helga Wanglie, a patient at Hennepin County Medical Center (HCMC) in 1991 when a conflict developed between her family and her health care providers on the propriety of continuing mechanical ventilation *(In re Conservatorship of Wanglie* 1991). During the previous 18 months, Mrs. Wanglie had been shuffled between several health care facilities and suffered two cardiac arrests. Eventually, she was transferred back to HCMC, where her physicians suggested to Mrs. Wanglie's family a de-escalation of treatments, including the withdrawal of ventilator support. The family refused to consent to the

---

13   The New Jersey Supreme Court noted the following regarding Karen Ann Quinlan's wishes concerning life-sustaining treatment: "She was said to have firmly evinced her wish, in like circumstances, not to have her life prolonged by the otherwise futile use of extraordinary means" (*In re Quinlan* 1976:21). See also, *In re Dinnerstein* (1978:139) ("... prolonged cardiac arrest dictates the futility of resuscitation efforts"); *Barber v. Superior Court* (1983:491) ("... there is no duty to continue its use once it has become futile in the opinion of qualified medical personnel"); *Bartling v.*

Glendale Adventist Medical Center (1986:363) ("... to provide continuous, but futile, life-sustaining treatment"); *In re Westchester County Medical Center* (1988:537) ("... further treatment would not only be futile but painful"); *West hart v. Mule* (1989:646) ("... the effort will probably be futile and merely draw out the process of dying"); *In re Greenspan* (1989:1206) ("... only when those measures would be futile"); *In re Lawrance* (1991:35) ("... continued treatment is futile").

Table 13.1 Court Cases Addressing Futility

The following cases address in some manner the issue of compelling a physician or health care facility to provide care to patients against the former's wishes or judgment. Although none of these cases is a typical futility case (as are *Wanglie, Baby K*, and *Gilgunn*), they may offer some precedential guidance to judges in future futility cases.

Alvarado v. N.Y.C. Health & Hospitals Corp., 145 Misc. 2d 687, 547 N.Y.S. 2d 190 (Sup. Ct. N.Y. Co. 1989).

Health care providers were not obligated to provide life-support measures to brain dead patient despite the family's request for such treatment.

In re Jane Doe, 262 Ga. 389, 418 S.E.2d 3 (1992).

Statutory requirements prohibited the issuance of a DNR order unless both available parents consented. The Georgia Supreme Court also noted that because the minor patient's parents were in agreement that CPR should be provided, the trial court was correct to compel the hospital to provide CPR if Jane Doe suffered cardiac or respiratory arrest.

Dority v. Superior Court, 193 Cal. Rptr. 288 (1983).

Health care providers were not obligated to provide life-support measures to brain-dead patient despite the family's request for such treatment.

Kranson v. Valley Crest Nursing Home, 755 F.2d 46 (3d Cir. 1985).

A state-run nursing facility did not violate patient's constitutional rights by establishing a policy that instructs staff to withhold CPR from patients who suffer cardiac or respiratory arrest. (This policy can be mitigated by specifically requesting CPR in advance of any crisis.) The federal court also ruled that the facility's reliance on this policy and its decision to withhold CPR from a patient after he choked on a piece of meat did not constitute negligence and wrongful death.

Manning v. Twin Falls Clinic & Hosp., 830 P.2d 1185 (Ida. 1992).

Jury awarded compensatory and emotional distress damages against a hospital and nurse (and awarded punitive damages against only the nurse) for withdrawing oxygen support, despite family pleas, during room-to-room transfer that resulted in the patient's death. Although the family had consented to a DNR order, they alleged that the withdrawal of oxygen support caused the patient to suffer during the ordeal.

Moore v. Baker, 989 F.2d 1129 (11th Cir. 1993).

Physician was not required under consent statute to offer an alternative (to surgery) that is not "generally recognized and accepted by reasonably prudent physicians."

Payton v. Weaver, 182 Cal. Rptr. 225 (1982).

There is no legal obligation to provide care to an uncooperative and disruptive patient, even if patient competently requests the treatment. Also, hemodialysis treatment for chronic condition cannot be considered emergency care, and thus the laws that compel the provision of emergency care do not apply.

Polikiff v. United States, 776 F. Supp. 1417 (S.D. Cal. 1991).

Veterans Administration hospital had no duty to provide AIDS testing for a patient and her spouse after it was determined that the patient had contracted hepatitis from her spouse. The court noted, "there is no duty to provide a patient with information regarding a test when the testing is not recommended to the patient and would not be recommended to the patient by physicians of ordinary knowledge and skill."

Strickland v. Deaconess Hosp., 735 P.2d 74 (Wash. App. 1987).

Patient and unrelated individuals' claims of damages were dismissed for various technical matters of law. The merits of the case were not decided. (Footnote 10 suggests that the court was sympathetic to the notion that health care providers should not unilaterally decide to withhold life-saving care.)

withdrawal of mechanical ventilation, asserting that Mrs. Wanglie was a devout Lutheran and that her religious beliefs and those of her family precluded forgoing life-sustaining treatments. Arguing that Mrs. Wanglie's family and, in particular, her husband were not following the advice and counsel of her physicians, Dr. Steven Miles, a member of HCMC's ethics committee, petitioned the courts to replace Mr. Wanglie with a professional conservator as decision maker for Mrs. Wanglie. Finding no evidence that Mr. Wanglie could not make decisions for his wife, the court denied Dr. Miles' petition (*In re Conservatorship of Wanglie* 1991).

This case represented the first instance of a health care professional petitioning a court to order, albeit indirectly through the appointment of an "impartial" conservator, the cessation of life-sustaining care from an incompetent patient against the wishes of the patient's family. Because *Wanglie* was never appealed beyond the trial court level, it offers little precedential value to courts around the country. However, the value of this case is in the discussions it prompted across the nation about the limits of patient autonomy. In particular, it caused health, legal, and ethics professionals to reach a consensus that the issue of futility is no longer merely an academic issue or the meaningless ruminations of judges.[14]

The *Baby K* Case

A more recent case addressing the futility issue involved an anencephalic infant in Virginia, whose physicians petitioned a federal district court to withdraw ventilator care that had been provided since she was admitted to the hospital's emergency department for respiratory distress (*In re Baby K* 1994). The patient's mother insisted that the hospital was obligated to provide the care Baby K needed to continue living, despite a provision in the Virginia Health Care Decisions Act that explicitly permits physicians to withhold "medically or ethically inappropriate" health care. Relying on an expansive interpretation of EMTALA and the Americans

with Disabilities Act, the district court agreed with Baby K's mother that treatment must be provided.

On appeal, the circuit court affirmed the decision but ruled only that EMTALA requires the provision of health care to every patient admitted in an emergency situation until the patient's emergency condition is stabilized. The court disagreed with the hospital's claim that Baby K's reason for admission through the emergency department was anencephaly, not respiratory distress. Instead, it noted that Baby K generally lived without ventilator support and was admitted to the hospital only when suffering respiratory distress. Therefore, the court argued that she was entitled to receive care until her emergency respiratory problems were stabilized, even if these emergency admissions were based on a chronic condition. The circuit court further noted that the federal law precludes a state law from having effect if the two laws conflict, thereby making the provision of the Virginia Health Care Decisions Act inoperable in this situation. Importantly, the court did not review the substance of the hospital's contention—that ventilator care for anencephalic infants was futile and against prevailing medical standards.

In the *Wanglie* and *Baby K* cases, the judiciary has avoided discussing the merits of the futility argument, which is, "Can a physician withhold or withdraw care that is deemed futile, or does a patient's right to autonomy require that futile care be provided?" In both decisions, the courts ruled on narrow matters of law. Neither court ruled explicitly that individuals have the right to receive futile treatment.

14 For example, in 1987, a Washington Court of Appeals noted the following regarding a claim for damages made by a patient and family against a health care provider who unilaterally decided to withdraw ventilator support and issue a DNR order: "Although the issue is ordinarily framed in terms of an individual's decision to *refuse* life sustaining treatment, we adhere to the fundamental common law and constitutional principles that 'competent adults have a right to determine what shall be done to their own bodies.'" *Strickland v. Deaconess Hosp.* (1987) (citations omitted).

The *Gilgunn* Case

In *Gilgunn v. Massachusetts General Hospital*, a jury decided that the doctors were not negligent when they decided to withdraw mechanical ventilation and issue a DNR order despite the objection of the patient's daughter. The case was brought before the court after Mrs. Gilgunn's death. Mrs. Gilgunn's daughter also asked for damages for her own emotional distress in the case. In what was reported to be a two hour deliberation, the jury found that the hospital and doctors were not negligent in removing treatment from Mrs. Gilgunn despite their belief that she would have wanted to continue treatment. The decision was apparently based on the rationale that the treatment was futile (Kolata 1995). This case has been attacked by ethicists, who question the unilateral decision making of the attending physician (Capron 1995). It is interesting to note that the physician who was in charge of Mrs. Gilgunn's care before cessation of treatments revoked the DNR order after noting, "I find it difficult to provide a medical reason to avoid CPR that is as powerful as their desire to have it done."

This jury decision is the only court case to address the merits of the futility argument. It is also the only case that permitted health care providers to withhold and withdraw medical treatments against the patient's and family's wishes, although only retrospectively, based on the rationale that the treatment was futile.

Although *Gilgunn* is the most recent court decision to address medical futility, it would be premature to state that the tide has turned and that physicians are free to withhold or withdraw health care to patients on the basis of their belief that the treatment is futile. This case is unlike either *Wanglie* or *Baby K* not only because these rulings reached the opposite conclusion but also because the legal conflict in *Gilgunn* emerged only after the death of the patient. It is not unreasonable to speculate that a jury, or more likely, a judge might have ordered the continuation of treatment if presented with the case while Mrs. Gilgunn was still alive. Indeed, it is probably not difficult to convince someone—whether a judge or a lay jury member—that it is appropriate to continue treatment for a critically ill patient who is still alive because preventing the withdrawal of even

futile treatment comes at little cost, whereas denying care is a violation of a living patient's desires and will result in the patient's death. It seems more difficult, however, to expect this same person to punish the physicians through a negligence lawsuit after the patient's death when presented with an argument that the treatments were futile and the physicians were making a medical decision in good faith. That is, the harm to an impersonal medical system in providing even futile care to the patient while alive is relatively minor, whereas the harm in punishing the physicians for stopping futile treatment may seem too drastic.

The three cases discussed and the nine cases listed in Table 13.1, demonstrate the lack of a legal consensus concerning medical futility. Moreover, these cases also illustrate the reluctance of the courts to definitively announce the limits, if any, of patient autonomy. Perhaps the courts prefer to have the issue resolved by society at large through the legislative process and the self-governance of health care professionals.

Conclusion

In essence, a futility case, like the refusal-of-treatment case, pits the patient's and family's desire for control over medical care against the physician's discretion in the practice of medicine. Meisel notes that the debate about futility cases, or what he calls "reverse" right-to-die cases, "is likely to occupy as much, if not more, judicial effort in the coming years as conventional right-to-die cases have in the last two decades unless legislation cuts it short" (Meisel 1995:530). Others doubt that this proliferation of cases will occur. Scofield, an outspoken advocate of the patient's right to refuse treatment, noted that, notwithstanding the volume of literature devoted to futility, "when patients are involved in decisions about medically futile treatment, they agree with their physician in more than 9 out of

10 cases" (Scofield 1994:67). He suggests that the futility problem can, in most instances, be preempted by encouraging an honest dialogue between doctors and patients.

There is undoubtedly at least a potential for an increase in the number of futility cases, especially in view of society's desire to curb the rising cost of health care. Although the courts may be able to address these conflicts on a case-by-case basis, such a scattershot approach will only invite further conflicts and litigation. The judiciary offers poor tools for reaching consensus. However, legislatures across the country may be better able to facilitate a consensus between medical professionals and health care consumers.

What is certainly needed, regardless of judicial and legislative activity, is a greater understanding among physicians and other health care providers that patients and families are often capable of rational discussion about their health care and that conflicts about whether to withdraw or to provide treatment can most likely be avoided by simply talking to patients. Similarly, patients and families must take greater responsibility and insist on becoming active participants in decisions concerning their care.

References

Capron A.M. 1995. Abandoning a waning life. *Hastings Center Report.* 24 (July–Aug): **24–6.**

Curtis, J.R., Park, D.R., Krone, M.R., and Pearlman, R.A. 1995. Use of the medical futility rationale in do-not-attempt-resuscitation orders. *Journal of the American Medical Association* 273: **124–8.**

Glick, H.R. 1992. *The Right to Die: Policy Innovation and Its Consequences.* New York: Columbia University Press.

Kolata, G. 1995. Court ruling limits rights of patients. *New York Times.* April 22, p. A6.

Kolata, G. 1994. Battle over a baby's future raises hard ethical issues. *New York Times.* December 27, p. A1.

Meisel, A. 1995. *The Right to Die.* New York: John Wiley & Sons, 2nd ed., vol. 2.

Miller, F.G., and Brody, H. 1995. Professional integrity and physician-assisted death. *Hastings Center Report.* 25 (May–June): **8–17.**

Mordarski, D.R. 1993. Medical futility: has ending life support become the next "pro-choice/right to life" debate? *Cleveland State Law Review* 41: **751–87.**

President's Commission for the Study of Ethical Problems in Medicine and Bio-medical and Behavioral Research. 1983. *Deciding to Forego Life-Sustaining Treatment.* Washington, DC: Government Printing Office.

President's Commission for the Study of Ethical Problems in Medicine and Biomedical and Behavioral Research. 1981. *Defining Death.* Washington DC: Government Printing Office.

Scofield, G.R. 1994. Medical futility: can we talk? *Generations* Winter: **66–70.**

South Carolina Governor's Office, Division on Aging. 1994. *South Carolina State Survey.*

United States Commission on Civil Rights. 1989. *Medical Discrimination Against Children with Disabilities.*

Cases and Statutes

In re Baby K. 16 F.3d 590 (4th Cir.), *cert, denied sub nom Baby K ex rel. Mr. K v. Ms. H,* 115 S. Ct. 91 (1994).

Barber v. Superior Court, 147 Cal. App. 3d 1006, 195 Cal. Rptr. 484 (Ct. App. 1983).

Bartling v. Glendale Adventist Medical Center, 184 Cal. App. 3d 961, 229 Cal. Rptr. 360 (Ct. App. 1986).

Child Abuse Amendments of 1984, 42 U.S.C. 5101 et seq.

Child Abuse Amendments of 1984 Final Rules, 45 C.F.R. pt. 1340 App. Interpretative Guideline § 8 (1987).

Chouinard v. Marjani, 575 A.2d 238 (Conn. Ct. App. 1990).

Cohen v. Smith, 648 N.E.2d 329 (Ill. App. 5 Dist. 1995).

Compassion in Dying v. Washington, 850 F. Supp. 1454 (D. Wash. 1994), *reversed*, 49 F.3d 586 (9th Cir. 1995).

Cruzan v. Director, Missouri Department of Health, 497 U.S. 261, 110 S. Ct. 2841 (1990).

In re Dinnerstein, 6 Mass. App. 466, 380 N.E.2d 134 (Ct. App. 1978).

Fox v. Smith, 594 So. 2d 596 (Miss. 1992).

Georgia act governing do-not-resuscitate orders, Ga. Code Ann. § 31-39-1 et seq.

Gilgunn v. Massachusetts General Hospital, No. 92-4820 (Mass. Super. Ct. Civ. Action Suffolk Co. April 22, 1995).

In re Greenspan, 137 Ill. 2d 1, 558 N.E.2d 1194 (1989).

Indiana Living Wills and Life Prolonging Procedures Act, Ind. Code Ann. § 16-8-4-11.

In re Lawrance, 579 N.E.2d 32 (Ind. 1991).

Leach v. Shapiro, 469 N.E.2d 1047 (Ohio Ct. App. 1984).

Louisiana Life-Sustaining Procedures Act, La. Rev. Stat. Ann. § 40:1299.58.1.

Maine Uniform Health-Care Decisions Act, Me. Rev. Stat. tit. 18-A, § 5-801 et seq.

Maryland Health Care Decision Act, Md. Health-Gen Code Ann. § 5-601.

Mohr v. Williams, 104 N.W. 12 (Minn. 1905).

New Mexico Uniform Health-Care Decisions Act, N.M. Stat. Ann. §§ 24-7A-1 et seq.

New York Orders Not to Resuscitate Act, N.Y. Pub. Health Law § 2961 et. seq.

New York Pub. Health L., § 2961 and 2966.

North Dakota Uniform Rights of the Terminally Ill Act, N.D. Cent. Code § 23-06.4-03.

Oklahoma Rights of the Terminally Ill or Persistently Unconscious Act, Okla. Stat. Ann. tit. 63, § 3101.12.

Perkins v. Lavin, 648 N.E. 839 (Ohio App. 9 Dist. 1994).

In re Quinlan, 70 N.J. 10, 355 A.2d 647, *cert. denied sub nom Garger v. New Jersey*, 429 U.S. 922 (1976).

Schloendorff v. Society of New York Hospital, 211 N.Y. 125, 105 N.E. 92 (1914).

Schmeltz v. Tracy, 177 A. 520 (Conn. 1935).

South Dakota Living Will Act, S.D. Codified Laws Ann. § 34-12D-19.

Strickland v. Deaconess Hosp., 735 P.2d 74 (Wash. App. 1987).

Tennessee regulations governing do-not-resuscitate orders, Tenn. Hosp. Rules & Regulations § 1200-8-4-.05.

Union Pacific R. Co. v. Botsford, 141 U.S. 250 (1891).

Virginia Health Care Decisions Act, Va. Code § 54.1-2990.

In re Conservatorship of Wanglie, No. PX-91-283 (Minn. Dist. Ct. Hennepin Co. July 1991).

In re Westchester County Medical Center, 72 N.Y.2d 517, 531 N.E.2d 607 (1988). *Westhart v. Mule*, 213 Cal. App. 3d 542, 261 Cal. Rptr. 640 (Ct. App. 1989).

4. Informed Consent

nformed Consent has been influenced significantly these recent years by moral philosophy and law. Historically, though, its roots are connected in "multiple disciplines and social contexts including those of the health profession, the law, the social and behavioral sciences, and moral philosophy,"[1] but it has been mainly the law and philosophy, which have given shape to its vocabulary.

Law has focused on informed consent as a means of financial compensation based on the liability of health professionals. This legal approach has been deemed insufficient to establish a definition or requirements for informed consent, which is why it has been regarded increasingly as a philosophical and moral issue rather than legal. As a moral issue, Faden and Childress affirm that informed consent is directly related to "autonomous choices of patients and subjects." Simply put, the legal approach has been one of pragmatic theory, whilst the moral philosophy's approach has been

Moral deliberations and the justifications, which underlie them, are based on "principles, rules and right, which are understood as abstract action-guides". Morality, first of all, has

a wider scope than philosophical contexts or professional ethics codes. In general, Morality refers to the rights and wrongs that govern cultural practices and institutions, which are transmitted through generations, "it has an objective, ongoing status as a body of action guides." On contrast, "moral philosophy" or "ethical theories" refer to the actual reflections over the institution of morality they seek clarity and precision (amongst other goals) of arguments into the area of morality, as a means of improving the social practices "by challenging presuppositions, assessing moral arguments, and suggesting modifications in existing beliefs."[2] In other words, moral philosophy seeks better *justifications* for our moral systems; these justifications are made through rational analysis and defense of theories and principles.

Two moments marked the birth of informed consent, the first, Canterbury vs. Spencer, a landmark in legal theory on the subject, and second, an opinion emitted by the AMA's Judicial Council in the year 1981, which first recognized informed consent as a "basic social policy." Shortly after *The President's Commission for the Study of Ethical Problems in Medicine and Biomedical and Behavioral Research* issued two

---

1   Faden, R., Beauchamp, T., *A History and Theory of Informed Consent*, Oxford University Press, 1986, p. 3.

2   Ibid, p. 4.

reports, one dealing directly with informed consent called *Making Health Care Decisions: The Ethical and Legal Implications of Informed Consent in the Patient-Practitioner Relationship*, and one dealing indirectly with it called *Deciding to Forego Life-Sustaining Treatment*. Through these reports, the commission stated that informed consent was based on the autonomy of free individuals to choose according to their own values and goals, basically what is known as "Self-determination." In this way, informed consent would travel from legal theories of liability into medical ethics and public debate.

Legally, only one major case can be cited before the twentieth century, which dealt with something similar to an informed consent problem, *Slater vs Baker and Stapleton, 1979*. This English case "had little or no precedential effect on informed consent in twentieth-century American Law." The plaintiff had hired the defendants Drs. Baker and Slater to remove some bandages from a leg fracture. Instead of this, the defendants re-fractured the leg and placed it in an experimental apparatus, which was supposed to straighten and stretch it, all this done against the plaintiff's will. The plaintiff claimed breach of contract by the doctors by saying they "ignorantly and unskillfully" broke his leg and injured him. He presented evidence of orthodox practice by appealing to the opinion of expert witnesses in order to prove his demands. The defendants stated that the proper action then, should have been "trespass *vi et armis* (similar to the battery theory), and not ignorant and unskillful practice of medicine. The court, in order to avoid dismissing the action because of it being brought under the wrong "writ" held the defendants liable under the contract theory.

It was not until the early twentieth-century that basic consent was born in Courts.

"Early twentieth-century cases applied a malpractice standard to determine the scope of express and implied consent without intent to contradict the basic principle that to proceed with no consent was a classic instance of battery."[3]

One example of this is the *Mohr vs Williams* Case in 1905. Anna Mohr had consented surgery on her right ear, the physician operating decided, during the operation, that it was in fact her left ear that needed surgery, so he operated the left one instead. The operation went wrong and Anna Mohr sued the physician for operating the left ear without consent. This was a typical case of battery. Even more, not only did the court reflect upon the rights of "free citizens" and the violations of the bodily integrity without permission, they also reflected on what does it mean to give "consent" to an operation and how does the weighing of risks and dangers affect this consent.

Years after, in 1914, the case *Schloendorff vs Society of New York Hospitals*, Justice Benjamin Cardozo would emit one of the most influential and quoted opinions in informed consent literature (even though the court itself did not address the problem). These early cases helped "fill out the battery theory of liability as grounded in a right of self-determination."

The first case to actually use the expression implicit in earlier cases was *Salgo vs Leland Stanford Jr. University Board of Trustees*. Martin Salgo suffered from permanent paralysis after a translumbar aortography. In suing his physician for negligent in his performance he argued too that he had failed to "warn him of the risk of paralysis." The court then stated that physicians have the duty to disclose "any facts which are necessary to form the basis of an intelligent consent by the patient to proposed treatment." It is not clear if the Court based this "informed consent theory" in battery or negligence, or even both, however, not only did it ground informed consent, it also brought "together the two consent liability theories;" namely, as an

---

3 Ibid., p. 120.

independent duty to respect autonomy and as an aspect of good medical care.

After the Salgo case came three major influential cases that would make informed consent flourish in courts. Of the three, the most important one is *Canterbury vs Spence*, in which a patient underwent a laminectomy because of a severe back pain. After the operation, the patient fell of the bed and suffered paralysis. He had not been warned that laminectomy has a 1% chance of paralysis. This case illustrated the need to examine informed consent "over its appropriate expression." It not only stated the patient's rights of decision-making, it went even further as to "put forward the due-care duty to disclose." This meant that *Canterbury* would reject the professional practice standard of disclosure (which meant that medical practice was to determine what information must be disclosed and what not, and was supported by the majority of cases at the time) and would embrace some sort of a "reasonable person standard" for disclosure of material information. Lastly, the *Truman Case* would state that the duty to disclose information was not only due in treatments that patients consent, but also to treatments that patient reject.

Informed Consent in research ethics is a relatively recent phenomenon, "there was in fact no broad interest in consent to research prior to the Second World War." Some occasional evidence can be found that research ethics in fact existed before World War II, but it is scarce and barely influential to contemporary research ethics. Russian physician V. Smidovich is an example of this, he wrote a critique to medical research in 1901 called *The Confessions of a Physician* which gained some respect in intellectual circles in Russia and was actually translated to English in 1904.

It was not until the Nazi experiments during the Second World War that concern for research ethics gained prominence. The famous Nuremberg Code, prescribed in 1948, was a result of the Nuremberg trial in which Nazi physicians were accused of "murder, torture, and other atrocities committed in the name of medical

science." This code would then prove to be highly influential as many professional codes and governmental codes would draw from it to formulate its rules. Principle one of the Code states that "the primary consideration in research is the subject's voluntary consent which is 'absolutely essential.'" There is, though, no explicit rule as to how the subject's consent can be secured or how are we to limit the risks in experimentation.

The Nuremberg Code was not enough to settle the ethical debates in research ethics, it was to broad and had a limited scope, so the World Medical Association took it in its own hands to create a code that would suffice and cover all the possible situations that the Nuremberg Code was not able to cover. The result of this endeavor was the Helsinki Code adopted in the year 1964. Much like the Nuremberg Code, the Declaration of Helsinki made informed consent a central aspect of research ethics. It would distinguish between therapeutic and non-therapeutic research, informed consent would be required in all non-therapeutic research except for incompetent subjects (in which guardian consent is needed) and it wouldn't be required in therapeutic research if it is not "consistent with patient psychology."

Influenced by these codes and the general interest in medical ethics, individual scholars took on the enterprise of writing their own books and performing their own research on the subject. Henry K. Beecher would publish in 1959 a monography called *Experimentation in Man*, in which he analyses many issues relative to research ethics; "the necessity of human experimentation, relationship between subject and investigator, the justification for clinical trials, and permissible risk"[4] while offering reviews of existing codes in research ethics. Beecher also wrote an influential article in the New England Journal of Internal Medicine in which details of research cases violating ethical considerations were exposed. Through this and other article and editorial entries Beecher brought attention to research ethics when attention was needed.

---

4   Ibid, p.157.

In the year 1972 psychiatrist Jay Katz published *Experimentation with Human Beings*, which is "still today, the most thorough collection of materials on research ethics and law ever assembled between two covers."[5]

On its way, consent grew as an issue in Behavioral Sciences. Psychology has, amongst all of them, the richest and most illustrative history in relation to informed consent. Interest in informed consent in this discipline can be traced back to 1938 when the American Psychological Association created a "Special Committee on Scientific and Professional Ethics." The job of this committee was to consider if the APA should develop an ethics code for its members. At first, it was thought that there was no need for a formal codification, then in the year 1947, the committee changed its mind, considering the years of experience in investigation and the rapid growth of the discipline. Finally, in the year 1951, the draft of the section about ethics in research was published. In no part did "informed consent" appear as a concept, however, it did make a reference to "protecting the subject's welfare" in the section 4.31. Soon after, the first published code of ethics in behavioral sciences appeared, named "Principles of Professional Ethics." This code has stricter consent requirement than the APA's Code.

Controversial cases were present too in the development of research ethics in behavioral sciences. Milgram's Experiment, Zimbardo's Prison Experiment, The Wichita Jury Study and the Tearoom Trade Research, they all left a mark in the debate and controversy. In the Wichita Jury study, professors of the University of Chicago set out to record the discussions of six different juries in order to obtain empirical data of frequently voiced criticisms of the jury system in American Law. This experiment raised questions about the need for information disclosure in experiments. The jurors were never notified they were being recorded as part of an experiment. Hence, people questioned the validity and

usefulness of the experiment, jurors never gave consent, but the investigators defended themselves arguing that this information was really important and its importance justified secret observation.

Milgram's Research on obedience became the most "controversial and instructive case of problems of deception and consent." The experiment consisted of two people taken into the psychology laboratory to participate in a "memory experiment" (which was not the true experiment). One of them was to be the *learner*, the other one would be the *teacher*, and the authority figure of the real experiment would be the experimenter. The putative experiment was that the *teacher* should administer an electric shock to the *learner* every time he gave a wrong answer in a word-pair association (a range of shocks varying from 15 to 450 volts all labeled with verbal designators: from 'slight shock' all the way to 'XXX'). The *learner* was actually a disguised accomplice in the true experiment. So whenever the learner gave a wrong answer, the teacher was required by the authority figure to administer an electric shock, starting from the slightest one and going up in intensity. This is where the controversy begins. No actual shock was delivered to the disguised accomplice, but he would still act and verbalize discomfort from the putatively administered shocks. As the reactions of the accomplice turned worst, teachers would start questioning whether they should administer the next discharge. The experimenter, the authority figure, would adamantly answer "yes" and order to go on with the experiment. This would put the *teacher* in the stressful position of either following instructions from authority figures or stop inflicting pain to the *learner*.

Humphrey's Tea-Party experiment and Zimbardo's experiment are also as illustrative of all of this. These four experiments set the basis in order for informed consent to be taken seriously in codes of ethical research. The debate in behavioral sciences grew over the decades and it faced the same ethical problems that medicine

---

5   Ibid, p. 160.

had to face when dealing with this subject, the contradiction of an autonomy framework that respects disclosure of information with a beneficence model which focuses on the search for information. Not surprisingly, all the debate never reached a satisfactory balance between those two principles, "and perhaps [there] never will be."

The first steps taken by the American Government in research ethics can be traced back to the National Institute of Health and the American Army. The NIH opened its doors in 1953, and its research operated from the beginning with self-imposed principles. Informed Consent was indeed one of the points these principles addressed, stating clearly what would constitute informed consent and what would not. Interestingly, "the wording made the subject a partner in the research" and besides medical consent, if required also specific consent to research participation. There was hope that these principles of research would inspire other institutions to follow the same road, sadly, this road was ignored.

In the year 1962 the US congress passes the "Drug Amendments of 1962." This amendment sought to change the "loopholes in testing and warning requirements" as argued by Senators of the US Congress, so it contained "revolutionary instructions for new federal regulations, including provisions governing consent." For the first time in American history a provision required researchers to inform subjects about the experimental drugs being tested and to receive their consent prior to research (the only exception was if researchers though it would be against the best interests of the subject).

Following the events of World War II, the NIH grew to become the most important biomedical research center in America. This growth brought attention over the moral issues of the research undertaken at this center; it also brought general concern "about federal responsibility to protect the public interest and to monitor the massive sums expended by NIH." Hence some radical changes overtook the center in years to come. After a series of historical, institutional and political events, an Institutional Guide was issued governing matters of institutional reviews, informed consent requirements and matters particular to social and behavioral research, this guide was called the *Institutional Guide to DHEW [how it was called then, now Department of Health and Human Services] Policy on Protection of Human Subjects*. In this guide, informed consent was defined as "the agreement obtained from a subject, or from his authorized representative, to the subject's participation in an activity." This guide would eventually—after much discussion over controversial cases and the need to control and protect research subjects—evolve into "formal regulations" which would now rule the whole DHEW. Also at the time, the American Congress passed the National Research Act creating the National Commission for the Protection of Human Subjects of Biomedical and Behavioral Research, which was charged with the duty to recommend ethical guidelines "for the conduct of research involving human subjects to the secretary of DHEW, the Congress, and the President." Out of the deliberations, the commission outlined a schema of basic ethical principles and the subjects to which they apply:

-The Principle of Respect for Autonomy applies to Guidelines for Informed Consent.

-The Principle of Beneficence applies to guidelines for Risk-Benefit Assessment

-The Principle of Justice applies to guidelines for Selection of Subjects.

This would prove to be a sort of general strategy with which problems of research ethics and consent would be confronted applying basic principles of deliberation. In the case of informed consent, more than ever before, this commission made clear that the justification for informed consent was respect for autonomy, which is also the underlying principle. It was also understood that informed consent had three necessary conditions: information, comprehension and voluntariness.

Readings

Faden, Ruth R. and Beauchamp, Tom L., *A History and Theory of Informed Consent*, Oxford University Press, 1986: **274–286**.

Practical Scenarios

Instructions for Analysis:

1. Explain, in general terms, why the case is morally relevant and controversial.
2. Identify the central moral issue. Justify.
3. Identify and explain the main facts to be considered in your analysis.
4. Identify and explain the principles and theories useful in analyzing the case. Justify why those principles and theories are relevant in the case. Specify conflicts between them.
5. Identify and raise arguments to support the conflicting options/decisions/actions that are evident in the case (Specifications and balancing of rules are necessary at this stage).
6. Identify and weigh alternative courses of action and then decide. Justify your decision. Answer the question(s) posed by the author as part of your conclusion.

Scenario 1

The Burned Woman

A woman named Irma suffering breast cancer needed radiation following a radical mastectomy. She suffered terrible radiation burns, after which she sued her doctor, Dr. Brown, for the injury. One of the counts was that she had not consented to the risk of the radiation burn.

Dr. Brown defended himself claiming therapeutic privilege. He did not deny that he had failed to tell Irma about the risk of the burns. Often physicians in this position claim that such information might disturb the patient; perhaps even irrationally lead her to refuse consent to the needed treatment.

Question

Was Dr. Brown's decision morally right? Justify your answer.

Scenario 2

Please, Get the Consent Now!

You are doing a surgical rotation and the chart review demonstrates that the patient never signed the appropriate consent for the surgery. Your attending tells you that he had a long conversation with the patient who absolutely wants the surgery done. You are told to get his signature on the consent. When you tell the surgical resident that the patient had enough sedation to make you question his ability to sign the consent he tells you to take and guide the patient's hand if necessary to get the consent signed and in the medical record.[6]

Question

What should the physician do in this case? Why?

Scenario 3

Everybody Followed the Rules But Pop Black Died

William Black, a fifty-five-year-old homeless man, lived with his friends Bobby Tunkins and Lala Wigfall under the scaffolding at 113th Street and Amsterdam Avenue in Manhattan, just across the street from

---

6 Adapted from Taylor, Carol, *Health Care Ethics Course*, Georgetown University School of Medicine, AY 2010-2011.

St. Luke's Hospital. They made their living scavenging cans and bottles and collecting the deposit money. A good day would bring in ten dollars and keep them stocked with beer and wine.

Pop, as his friends called him, was born in Baltimore, the son of a steelworker. As an adult he held various jobs, and he was married, with two children. In the mid-1970s he became unemployed, started drinking, an had some trouble with the law. His marriage broke up. In 1977 he moved to New York to work in a factory with his younger brother. In 1980 the factory closed. Life went downhill for Pop Black after that, and by the late eighties he was living on the streets.

On the morning of October 17, 1994, Mr. Black was making his rounds collecting cans when he complained of feeling achy and began to cough up blood. By late that afternoon he was too sick to move, so Mr. Tunkins left him sitting on a sidewalk grate and went across the street to the hospital to get help. There he was informed that hospital policy prevented any doctors or nurses from leaving the emergency room. "That would be counterproductive to the mission of the ER, confusing and a waste of time," a hospital spokesperson later said. Tunkins was told to call 911. An ambulance responded about seven minutes later.

At this point stories conflict. Tunkins believes that Black was delirious and did not know where he was or what he was saying. The EMS technicians believed that Black was lucid and reported that he refused medical assistance. They left him where he was. "We don't have a mechanism in place to force someone to go to the hospital," an EMS official said later. "He was an RMA—refused medical attention."

Shortly after seven o'clock the next morning Mr. Tunkins and Ms. Wigfall found Pop Black unconscious and called EMS again. After some delay the ambulance crew arrived and pronounced him dead at 7:37 A.M. But they still did not pick him up; other arms of the city bureaucracy are in charge of that. Normally a dead body on the street is removed as quickly as possible in New York City. However, that morning was a busy one and Pop Black lay on the sidewalk in death for four hours, as he had done for the final fifteen hours of his life. "The thing about William," his brother told a reporter from the New York Times, "was that he fell from grace." Just so. However, his autonomy, his right to RMA, was respected to the end.[7]

Question

Was Pop Black's autonomy respected? Justify your arguments

---

7 Extracted from Gaylin, William; Jennings, Bruce, *The Perversion of Autonomy. Coercion and Constraints in a Liberal Society*, Georgetown University Press, 2003.

A History and Theory of Informed Consent

Ruth R. Faden and Tom L. Beauchamp

C overed by the account of autonomous action in Chapter 7, we now turn to analysis of the concepts of informed consent and competence. We argue that "informed consent" has two distinct senses or general uses. In the first sense, an informed consent is a special kind of autonomous action: an autonomous authorization by a patient or subject. The second sense of "informed consent" is analyzable in terms of rules governing informed consent in public policy and institutional contexts.

The policy dimensions of this second sense of informed consent require that attention also be paid to the concept of competence, especially the competence to consent. Competence is analyzed in later parts of the chapter in terms of criteria of autonomous *persons*, as distinct from autonomous *actions*. Judgments of competence, we argue, primarily serve a gatekeeper function by identifying persons from whom it is appropriate to obtain informed consents.

Two Concepts of Informed Consent

Legal, philosophical, regulatory, medical, and psychological literatures have generally discussed informed consent in terms of its "elements." The following elements have been identified as the concept's analytical components:[1]

1. *Disclosure*
2. *Comprehension*
3. *Voluntariness*
4. *Competence*
5. *Consent*

The fifth element is labeled "consent" in only a few analyses. Some commentators omit it entirely as an element; others prefer to call this element *decision*,[2] and still others prefer to emphasize *shared decisionmaking* or *collaboration*[3] as a substitute for the consent of a patient or subject. Whatever the precise formulation, the fifth element refers to the final stage in the act of giving an informed consent.

Disagreements such as those over the proper label for "consent" are minor, and there is otherwise more agreement than disagreement over the appropriateness of these five elements. Indeed, there may be more consensus on this analysis of informed consent into its elements than on any other topic in the literature on informed consent. These elements are also extensively used in this literature as the conditions in a *definition* of informed consent—or, as some prefer to say, as the conditions in a definition of *valid* consent.[4] According to this mode of definition, X is an informed consent if and only if some of the elements 1–5 above are conditions that are satisfied in the circumstances. Precisely which of the five elements is used varies from theory to theory. Transformation of all five elements into a definition of informed consent yields the following:

> Action X is an informed consent by person P to intervention I if and only if:
> 1. P receives a thorough *disclosure* regarding I,
> 2. P *comprehends* the disclosure,
> 3. P acts *voluntarily* in performing X,
> 4. P is *competent* to perform X, and
> 5. P *consents* to I.

Although this schema is at first glance an attractive definition of informed consent, and one that is faithful to the uses of the term in such practical contexts as clinical medicine and law, the list of conditions in this analysis is biased by the special concerns of medical convention and malpractice law. Conditions 1–5 are less suitable as conditions in a conceptual analysis or definition of informed consent than as a list of the elements of informed consent as they have emerged in institutional or regulatory settings in which consent requirements appear in policies. This approach to the definition of informed consent also unjustifiably escalates into prominence the special orientations of both medicine and law toward *disclosure* and *responsibility* for patients and subjects.

To take but one instance of the kind of bias at work in this form of definition, the U.S. Supreme Court in *Planned Parenthood of Central*

Missouri v. *Danforth* found cause to reflect on the meaning of "informed consent": "One might well wonder ... what 'informed consent' of a patient is ... [We] are content to accept, *as the meaning*, the giving of information to the patient as to just what would be done and as to its consequences."[5] This definition is strikingly similar to definitions provided by physicians in the national survey discussed in Chapter 3 (see pp. 98–99), where the focus was also exclusively on disclosure. Yet, this is a profoundly inadequate conception of the general *meaning* of "informed consent," one tainted by an implicit assumption of medical authority and by an unrelieved legal focus on the theory of liability, which delineates not a meaning but a *duty*.

There is nothing about the nature of an informed consent per se that requires disclosure as a necessary condition, and certainly nothing that would *orient* its *meaning* around disclosure. A person otherwise knowledgeable about a proposed intervention—a physician undergoing a procedure, for example—could give a well informed consent without any disclosure whatever.[6] Other conditions in the above list of conditions are not necessary for similar reasons. For example, consider element 4, competence: Some persons who are *legally* incompetent (which is often the referent of element 4) may give informed consents, and in some instances *psychologically* incompetent persons (also often the referent of element 4) may be able to do so. We return to this problem in the final section of this chapter.

The transformation of the above five-fold set of elements into a definition of informed consent thus raises as many problems and confusions as it offers insights. There is no necessary association between these elements and logical conditions. That is, there is no necessary connection between an analytical listing of the hallmark characteristics of informed consent and the logically necessary and sufficient conditions of informed consent that govern its meaning. Neither is there a necessary association between the *logical conditions* of informed consent and *normative requirements* (duties and the like) governing the obtaining of consent, although the two have often been uncritically conflated.[7] To assert that some condition—for example, voluntariness—*must* be present could be either a *normative* claim or could be a purely *logical* (conceptual) claim.[8] Our task in the following pages is the purely logical one of providing a conceptual analysis of informed consent.

Analyzing Informed Consent

What, then, is an informed consent? This question about the logical conditions of informed consent should be approached in the same spirit as the treatment of the logical conditions of autonomous action in Chapter 7. Answering this question is complicated because there are two common, entrenched, and starkly different meanings of "informed consent." That is, the term is analyzable in two profoundly different ways—not because of mere subtle differences of connotation that appear in different contexts, but because two different *conceptions* of informed consent have emerged from the histories traced in Chapters 3 through 6 and are still at work, however unnoticed, in literature on the subject.

In one sense, which we label *sense*$_1$, "informed consent" is analyzable as a particular kind of action by individual patients and subjects: an autonomous authorization. In the second sense, *sense*$_2$, informed consent is analyzable in terms of the web of cultural and policy rules and requirements of consent that collectively form the social practice of informed consent in institutional contexts where *groups* of patients and subjects must be treated in accordance with rules, policies, and standard practices. Here, informed consents are not always *autonomous* acts, nor are they always in any meaningful respect *authorizations*.

In analyzing these two concepts—sense$_1$, and sense$_2$—we will rely more on our theory of autonomous action (in Chapter 7) and our historical

analyses of informed consent (see Chapters 3 through 6) than on either ordinary language subtleties of the term "informed consent" or on beliefs pervasive in society about consent in medical settings. We have already noted how physicians interpreted the term "informed consent" in a recent survey. In that same survey, the responses from a sample of the American public were even more discouraging. When asked "What does the term informed consent mean to you?", one of the most popular answers from the public was that informed consent means that patients agree to treatment by letting the doctor do whatever is "necessary," "best," or "whatever he sees fit." Twenty-one percent of respondents said that they have no understanding of the term.[9] Such responses form an inadequate basis for a conceptual analysis of informed consent as that notion has emerged in modern medicine and research. The settings for the actual practice of obtaining consents also provide an unreliable basis, because the implicit understanding is often that "informed consent" means no more than the empty formality, as health professionals sometimes put it, of "consenting the patient"—that is, obtaining a signature on a consent form.[10]

With these cautions in mind, we can turn to more controlled methods of analyzing these two concepts of informed consent that rely only in part on their historical foundations.

Sense$_1$: Informed Consent as Autonomous Authorization

Just as choices, consents, and refusals are species of the larger category of *actions*, so informed consents and informed refusals are, in sense$_1$, species of the larger category of *autonomous* actions. However, it is mistaken to say that informed consent in this sense is *synonymous* with autonomous choice (or action). It is likewise wrong to hold that the conditions of informed consent are identical to the conditions of autonomous choice (or action). An informed consent is a specific kind of autonomous choice (or action), an autonomous authorization by patients or subjects.

Jon Waltz and T.W. Scheuneman, in an influential early article (discussed in Chapter 4), define informed consent in terms of two elements or conditions: "the dual elements of *awareness* and *assent.*" They require in addition that there be an "absence of such duress" as would render the assent "inoperative."[11] Their proposal is apparently that informed consent should be analyzed as an uncoerced willingness to undergo a procedure regarding which the patient or subject has adequate information (predominantly, in their analysis, through a disclosure of risks and consequences). On the basis of the information the assent occurs. This analysis is a foray in the right direction. The term "assent" is a synonym for one general meaning of "consent," and "awareness" points to the "informed" component; to assent is to agree with or acquiesce in an opinion or to comply with an arrangement. This strikes close to what occurs in giving an informed consent.

However, the idea of an informed consent suggests that a patient or subject does more than express agreement with, acquiesce in, yield to, or comply with an arrangement or a proposal. He or she actively *authorizes* the proposal in the act of consent.[12] John may *assent* to a treatment plan without authorizing it. The assent may be a mere submission to the doctor's authoritative order, in which case John does not call on his *own* authority in order to give permission, and thus does not authorize the plan. Instead, he acts like a child who submits, yields, or assents to the school principal's spanking and in no way gives permission for or authorizes the spanking. Just as the child merely submits to an authority in a system where the lines of authority are quite clear, so often do patients.

Accordingly, an informed consent in sense$_1$ should be defined as follows: An informed consent is an autonomous action by a subject or a patient that authorizes a professional either to involve the subject in research or to initiate a medical plan for the patient (or both). Following the analysis of *substantial* autonomy in Chapter 7, we can whittle down this definition by saying that an informed consent in sense$_1$ is given if a patient or subject with (1) substantial understanding and (2) in substantial absence of control by others (3) intentionally (4) authorizes a professional (to do I).

It follows analytically from our analysis in Chapter 7 that all substantially autonomous acts satisfy conditions 1–3; but it does not follow from that analysis alone that all such acts satisfy 4. The fourth condition, then, is what distinguishes informed consent as one *kind* of autonomous action. (Note also that the definition restricts the kinds of authorization to medical and research contexts.) A person whose act satisfies conditions 1–3 but who refuses an intervention gives an *informed refusal*. The conditions of this latter kind of action are identical to 1–4 above, except that the fourth condition is the converse, a nonauthorization or refusal to authorize.

The Problem of Shared Decisionmaking. This analysis of informed consent in sense$_1$ is deliberately silent on the question of how the authorizer and the agent(s) being authorized *arrive at an agreement* about the performance of "I." Recent commentators on informed consent in clinical medicine, notably Jay Katz and the President's Commission (see Chapter 3), have tended to equate the idea of informed consent with a model of "shared decisionmaking" between doctor and patient. The President's Commission titles the first chapter of its report on informed consent in the patient–practitioner relationship "Informed Consent as Active, Shared Decision Making," while in Katz's work "the idea of informed consent" and "mutual decisionmaking" are treated as virtually synonymous terms.[13]

There is of course an historical relationship in clinical medicine between medical decisionmaking and informed consent. The emergence of the legal doctrine of informed consent was instrumental in drawing attention to issues of decisionmaking as well as authority in the doctor–patient relationship. Nevertheless, it is a confusion to treat informed consent and shared decisionmaking as anything like *synonymous*. For one thing, informed consent is not restricted to clinical medicine. It is a term that applies equally to biomedical and behavioral research contexts where a model of shared decisionmaking is frequently inappropriate. Even in clinical contexts, the social and psychological dynamics involved in selecting medical interventions should be distinguished from the patient's *authorization*.

In Chapter 9 we endorse Katz's view that effective communication between professional and patient or subject is often instrumental in obtaining informed consents (sense$_1$), but we resist his conviction that the idea of informed consent entails that the patient and physician "share decisionmaking," or "reason together," or reach a consensus about what is in the patient's best interest. This is a manipulation of the concept from a too singular and defined moral perspective on the practice of medicine that is in effect a moral program for changing the practice. Although the patient and physician *may* reach a decision together, they need not. It is the essence of informed consent in sense$_1$ only that the patient or subject *authorizes autonomously;* it is a matter of indifference where or how the proposal being authorized originates.

For example, one might advocate a model of shared decisionmaking for the doctor-patient relationship without simultaneously advocating that every medical procedure requires the consent of patients. Even relationships characterized by an ample slice of shared decision-making, mutual trust, and respect would and should permit many decisions about routine and low-risk aspects of the patient's medical treatment to remain the exclusive province of the physician, and thus some decisions are likely always to remain subject exclusively to the physician's authorization. Moreover, in the uncommon situation, a patient could autonomously authorize the physician to make *all* decisions about medical treatment, thus giving his or her informed consent to an arrangement that scarcely resembles the sharing of decisionmaking between doctor and patient.[14]

Authorization. Because authorization is central to our account of informed consent in sense$_1$, it seems appropriate that we provide an analysis of the notion of authorization. Because to do so with thoroughness would require its own volume, our analysis must be brief: In authorizing, one both assumes responsibility for what one has authorized and transfers to another one's authority to implement it. There is no informed consent unless one *understands* these features of the act and *intends* to perform that act. That is, one must understand that one is assuming responsibility and warranting another to proceed.

To say that one assumes responsibility does not quite locate the essence of the matter, however, because a *transfer* of responsibility as well as of authority also occurs. One's authorization gives another both permission to proceed and the responsibility for proceeding. Depending on the social circumstances, X's having authorized Y to do I generally signifies either that X and Y *share* responsibility for the consequences of I or that the responsibility is entirely X's (assuming, of course, that Y executes I in a non-negligent and responsible fashion). Thus, the crucial element in an authorization is that the person who authorizes uses whatever right, power, or control he or she possesses in the situation to endow another with the right to act. In so doing, the authorizer assumes some responsibility for the actions taken by the other person. Here one could either authorize *broadly* so that a person can act in accordance with general guidelines, or *narrowly* so as to authorize only a particular, carefully circumscribed procedure.

Sense$_2$: Informed Consent as Effective Consent

By contrast to sense$_1$, sense$_2$, or *effective* consent, is a policy-oriented sense whose conditions are not derivable solely from analyses of autonomy and authorization, or even from broad notions of respect for autonomy. "Informed consent" in this second sense does not refer to *autonomous* authorization, but to a legally or institutionally *effective* (sometimes misleadingly called *valid*) authorization from a patient or a subject. Such an authorization is "effective" because it has been obtained through procedures that satisfy the rules and requirements defining a specific institutional practice in health care or in research.

We saw in Chapters 3 through 6 that the social and legal practice of requiring professionals to obtain informed consent emerged in institutional contexts, where conformity to operative rules was and still is the sole necessary and sufficient condition of informed consent. Any consent is an informed consent in sense$_2$ if it satisfies whatever operative rules apply to the practice of informed consent. Sense$_2$ requirements for informed consent typically do not focus on the autonomy of the act of giving consent (as sense$_1$ does), but rather on regulating the behavior of the *consent-seeker* and on establishing *procedures and rules* for the context of consent. Such requirements of professional behavior and procedure are obviously more readily monitored and enforced by institutions.

However, because formal institutional rules such as federal regulations and hospital policies govern whether an act of authorizing is effective, a patient or subject can autonomously authorize an intervention, and so give an informed consent in sense$_1$, and yet *not effectively authorize* that intervention in sense$_2$.

Consider the following example. Carol and Martie are nineteen-year-old, identical twins attending the same university. Martie was born with multiple birth defects, and has only one kidney. When both sisters are involved in an automobile accident, Carol is not badly hurt, but her sister is seriously injured. It is quickly determined that Martie desperately needs a kidney transplant. After detailed discussions with the transplant team and with friends, Carol consents to be the donor. There is no question that Carol's authorization of the transplant surgery is substantially autonomous. She is well informed and has long anticipated being in just such a circumstance. She has had ample opportunity over the years to consider what she would do were she faced with such a decision. Unfortunately, Carol's parents, who were in Nepal at the time of the accident, do not approve of her decision. Furious that they were not consulted, they decide to sue the transplant team and the hospital for having performed an unauthorized surgery on their minor daughter. (In this state the legal age to consent to surgical procedures is twenty-one.)

According to our analysis, Carol gave her informed consent in sense$_1$ to the surgery, but she did not give her informed consent in sense$_2$. That is, she autonomously authorized the transplant and thereby gave an informed consent in sense$_1$ but did not give a consent that was effective under the operative legal and institutional policy, which in this case required that the person consenting be a legally authorized agent. Examples of other policies that can define sense$_2$ informed consent (but not sense$_1$) include rules that consent be witnessed by an auditor or that there be a one-day waiting period between solicitation of consent and implementation of the intervention in order for the person's authorization to be effective. Such rules can and do vary, both within the United States by jurisdiction and institution, and across the countries of the world.[15]

Medical and research codes, as well as case law and federal regulations, have developed models of informed consent that are delineated entirely in a sense$_2$ format, although they have sometimes attempted to justify the rules by appeal to something like sense$_1$. For example, disclosure conditions for informed consent are central to the history of "informed consent" in sense$_2$, because disclosure has traditionally been a *necessary* condition of effective informed consent (and sometimes a *sufficient* condition!). The *Salgo* court spoke of a "full disclosure of facts" as *"necessary* to an informed consent," and the U.S. Supreme Court defined "informed consent" *entirely* in terms of disclosure.[16] The legal doctrine of informed consent, as examined in Chapters 2 and 4, is primarily a law of disclosure; satisfaction of disclosure rules virtually consumes "informed consent" in law.[17] This should come as no surprise, because the legal system needs a generally applicable informed consent mechanism by which injury and responsibility can be readily and fairly assessed in court. These disclosure requirements in the legal and regulatory contexts are not conditions of "informed consent" in sense$_1$; indeed disclosure may be entirely irrelevant to giving an informed consent in sense$_1$. If a person has an adequate *understanding* of relevant information without benefit of a disclosure, then, as we saw earlier, it makes no difference whether someone *disclosed* that information.

Other sense$_2$ rules besides those of disclosure have been enforced. These include rules requiring evidence of adequate comprehension of information and the aforementioned rules requiring the presence of auditor witnesses and mandatory waiting periods. Sense$_2$ informed consent requirements generally take the form of rules focusing on disclosure, comprehension, the minimization of potentially controlling influences, and competence. Examples of such sense$_2$ requirements can be found in the Federal Regulations discussed in Chapter 6. The last subsection of the 1966 FDA Regulations, for instance, provides the following formal definition of informed consent:

> 'Consent' or 'informed consent' *means* that the person involved has legal capacity to give consent, is so situated as to be able to exercise free power of choice, and is provided with a *fair* explanation of all material information concerning

the administration of the investigation drug, or his possible use as a control, as to enable him to make an understanding decision as to his willingness to receive said investigational drug. This latter element *requires* that before the acceptance of an affirmative decision by such person the investigator should make known to him. ... [a long list of items to be disclosed follows][18]

This definition was adapted by FDA officials from parts of the Declaration of Helsinki and the Nuremberg Code. The first principle of the Nuremberg Code requires "voluntary consent," the meaning of which is explicated as follows:

> This *means* that the person involved should have legal capacity to give consent; should be so situated as to be able to exercise free power of choice. ... and should have sufficient knowledge and comprehension of the elements of the subject matter involved as to enable him to make an understanding and enlightened decision. This latter element *requires* that before the acceptance of an affirmative decision by the experimental subject there should be made known to him. ... [a long list follows][19]

In the subsequent 1971 "Institutional Guide to DHEW Policy on Protection of Human Subjects"—the "Yellow Book"—the following abbreviated definition is provided:

> Informed consent *is* the agreement obtained from a subject, or from his authorized representative, to the subject's participation in an activity.
>
> The basic elements of informed consent are ... [a list of six types of *disclosure* to be made follows][20]

The above definitions of the term "informed consent" express the present-day mainstream conception in the federal government of the United States. They are also typical of international documents and state regulations, which all reflect a sense$_2$ orientation. These documents derive from some conviction—perhaps based on a social consensus—about the requirements or practices needed to enable effective authorizations in the special set of circumstances found in institutions dedicated to health care and research.

Although most formal definitions of informed consent in sense$_2$ have been forged from contexts of public policy and law, definitions of informed consent rooted more in moral theory than in law or public policy can also fall into the sense$_2$ class. The following legally-indebted definition—offered by Albert Jonsen, Mark Siegler, and William Winslade and designed for the teaching of medical ethics in medical schools and health care institutions—is illustrative:

> Informed consent is defined as the willing and uncoerced acceptance of a medical intervention by a patient after adequate disclosure by the physician of the nature of the intervention, its risks and benefits, as well as of alternatives with their risks and benefits.[21]

The Relationship Between Sense$_1$ and Sense$_2$

A sense$_1$ "informed consent" can fail to be an informed consent in sense$_2$ by a lack of conformity to applicable rules and requirements. Similarly, an informed consent in sense$_2$ may not be an informed consent in sense$_1$. The rules and requirements that determine sense$_2$ consents need not result in autonomous authorizations at all in order to qualify as informed consents. For example, under a North Carolina statute a signed consent form *constitutes* "valid consent" (informed consent in sense$_2$) so long as a reasonable person would have understood the information in its disclosed form, even if the patient in fact did not understand; moreover, if the patient had not been informed at all, but a reasonable person would have consented if informed, then the patient's "uninformed" consent is valid.[22]

Such peculiarities in informed consent law have led Jay Katz to argue that the legal doctrine of "informed consent" bears a "name" that "promises much more than its construction in case law has delivered." He has argued insightfully that the courts have, in effect, imposed a mere duty to warn on physicians, an obligation confined to risk disclosures and statements of proposed interventions. He maintains that "This judicially imposed obligation must be distinguished from the *idea* of informed consent, namely, that patients have a decisive role to play in the medical decisionmaking process. The idea of informed consent, though alluded to also in case law, cannot be implemented, as courts have attempted, by only expanding the disclosure requirements." By their actions and declarations, Katz believes, the courts have made informed consent a "cruel hoax" and have allowed "the idea of informed consent ... to wither on the vine."[23]

The most plausible interpretation of Katz's contentions is through the sense$_1$/sense$_2$ distinction. If a physician obtains a consent under the courts' criteria, then an informed consent (sense$_2$) has been obtained. But it does not follow that the courts are using the *right* standards, or *sufficiently rigorous* standards in light of a stricter autonomy-based model—or "idea" as Katz puts it—of informed consent (sense$_1$).[24] If Katz is correct that the courts have made a mockery of informed consent and of its moral justification in respect for autonomy, then of course his criticisms are thoroughly justified. At the same time, it should be recognized that people can proffer legally or institutionally effective authorizations under prevailing rules even if they fall far short of the standards implicit in sense$_1$.[25]

Sense$_1$ as a Model for Sense$_2$. Despite the differences between sense$_1$ and sense$_2$, a definition of informed consent need not fall into one or the other class of definitions. It may conform to both. Many definitions of informed consent in policy contexts reflect at least a strong and definite reliance on informed consent in sense$_1$. Although the conditions of sense$_1$ are not logically necessary conditions for sense$_2$, we take it as morally axiomatic that they *ought* to serve— and in fact have served—as the benchmark or model against which the moral adequacy of a definition framed for sense$_2$ purposes is to be evaluated. This position is, roughly speaking, Katz's position.

A defense of the moral viewpoint that policies governing informed consent in sense$_2$ *should* be formulated to conform to the standards of informed consent in sense$_1$ is not hard to express. We have argued in earlier chapters that the goal of informed consent in medical care and in research—that is, the purpose behind the obligation to obtain informed consents—is to enable potential subjects and patients to make autonomous decisions about whether to grant or refuse authorization for medical and research interventions. Accordingly, embedded in the reason for having the social institution of informed consent is the idea that institutional requirements for informed consent in sense$_2$ *should* be intended to maximize the likelihood that the conditions of informed consent in sense$_1$ will be satisfied—although we did not claim in Chapters 3 through 6 that historically they *have always* been so intended.

How informed consent in sense$_1$ might function as a normative standard for informed consent in sense$_2$ deserves at least brief explication. First, there is no way to decide rationally that a set of consent requirements in sense$_2$ is morally acceptable only if at least some particular percentage of the authorizations that follow from them—60% or 70% or 80% or 100%—satisfy the conditions of informed consent in sense$_1$. However, a comparative, pragmatic justification can be offered: A set Y of consent requirements in sense$_2$ is morally preferable to any set Z if, all other things being equal, (1) Y results in more

informed consents (in sense$_1$) than Z, (2) Y results in fewer "false negatives$_2$"—that is, fewer informed consents in sense$_1$ will fail to meet the formal requirements of informed consent in sense$_2$— than Z, and (3) Y results in fewer "false positives" than Z—that is, fewer authorizations that are not substantially autonomous will meet its formal requirements as informed consents in sense$_2$.

Here we need to reintroduce the distinction (discussed at the end of Chapter 6) between requirements that *have* served in institutional and policy contexts and those that *should* be operative in such contexts. Our book is not the appropriate forum for discussing the precision with which the standards in sense$_2$ *should* conform to the conditions of sense$_1$ in order to have a morally adequate standard for sense$_2$, but this moral matter is so vital that it deserves at least brief attention.

A major problem at the policy level, where rules and requirements must be developed and applied in the aggregate, is the following: The obligations imposed to enable patients and subjects to make authorization decisions must be evaluated not only in terms of the demands of a set of abstract conditions of "true" or sense$_1$ informed consent, but also in terms of the impact of imposing such obligations or requirements on various institutions with their concrete concerns and priorities. One must take account of what is fair and reasonable to require of health care professionals and researchers, the effect of alternative consent requirements on efficiency and effectiveness in the delivery of health care and the advancement of science, and—particularly in medical care—the effect of requirements on the welfare of patients. Also relevant are considerations peculiar to the particular social context, such as proof, precedent, or liability theory in case law, or regulatory authority and due process in the development of federal regulations and IRB consent policies.

Moreover, at the sense$_2$ level, one must resolve not only which requirements will define effective consent; one must also settle on the rules stipulating the conditions under which effective consents must be obtained. In some cases, hard decisions must be made about whether requirements of informed consent (in sense$_2$) should be imposed at all, even though informed consent (in sense$_1$) *could* realistically and meaningfully be obtained in the circumstances and could serve as a model for institutional rules. For example, should there be any consent requirements in the cases of minimal risk medical procedures and research activities?

The problem of how to develop a morally acceptable set of requirements for informed consent in sense$_2$ recalls the discussion in Chapter 1 of the need to balance competing moral principles and obligations in implementing policy or institutional rules. This need to balance is not a problem for informed consent in sense$_1$, which is not policy oriented. Thus, it is possible to have a *morally acceptable* set of requirements for informed consent in sense$_2$ that deviates considerably from the conditions of informed consent in sense$_1$. However, the burden of moral proof rests with those who defend such deviations since the primary moral justification of the obligation to obtain informed consent is respect for autonomous action.

Beyond Health Care and Research. One potential objection to our analysis of informed consent—in both sense$_1$ and sense$_2$—is that it is too narrow: Why confine the concept of informed consent to *medical* procedures and *research* projects? A wide variety of consents have nothing to do with medicine or research. All classical contractarian political theories, for example, employ some notion of voluntary and informed consent as the essential basis of the legitimacy or validity of government: The people authorize by their free acts of consent that a government obtain sovereignty. Many commonplace actions also qualify as informed consents. For example, in one wedding ceremony, the bride and groom are explicitly asked to give their "informed consent to marry. ..." In short, informed consent in this first sense could be applied to autonomously authorizing appliance repairs, withdrawing money from a checking account, hiring an agent, and hundreds of other daily activities.

We do not deny, of course, that the concept of informed consent could be broadened to mean *any* authorization that is substantially autonomous. But we do deny that this is a plausible reading of what the term has meant in any significant document on the subject of informed consent. We noted from the outset that our analysis is to be consonant with the historical development of the concept of informed consent, as presented in Chapters 3 through 6. The meaning that emerges from this history is restricted to research and medical care. For example, in contexts other than medicine and research (contracts and leases, e.g.), where the idea of a consent that is informed has been put to some serious work, the language that is used is almost always something like "express written consent" rather than "informed consent."

Practical Purposes of Sense$_1$. In the remainder of this book we focus on the conditions of informed consent in sense$_1$. However, our objective is not to present an *ideal* model of informed consent. Quite the contrary. In delineating informed consent in sense$_1$ in terms of *substantial* rather than *full* autonomy, as in Chapter 7, we have already rejected the view that it is never possible to obtain "true" informed consents. Many circumstances in medical care and research permit substantially autonomous authorizations, and in many settings they are now obtained.

The conditions of informed consent in sense$_1$ can be used to serve two practical purposes. First, because informed consent in this sense is an evaluative standard for informed consent in sense$_2$, a more detailed analysis of sense$_1$ should make it easier for deliberative bodies such as courts, commissions, hospital ethics committees, professional organizations, and IRBs to assess the moral adequacy of requirements of informed consent in sense$_2$. Policy makers should be able to determine what existing sense$_2$ requirements accomplish, how well they accomplish it, and how to implement desirable changes. Second, the conditions elaborated in Chapters 9 and 10 provide a blueprint for situations in which it is appropriate or morally desirable to obtain substantially autonomous authorizations. A better understanding of informed consent in sense$_1$ is also useful, of course, for those who wish to *exceed* operative policy or legal requirements at the sense$_2$ level.

In Chapters 9 and 10 we analyze the demands of two conditions of informed consent in sense$_1$ in order to show what can be done to increase the likelihood that these conditions will be satisfied. We do not consider the problem of *competence* in either chapter. This may appear surprising in the face of the substantial attention and prominence given to standards of competence in informed consent literature. But Chapters 9 and 10 are exclusively about informed consent in sense$_1$ and

competence is not in any conventional respect a sense$_1$ problem. In sense$_1$, if a patient's consent is sufficiently autonomous, then it is irrelevant whether the person giving the authorization is competent in the light of some legal policy or psychiatric standard. However, this is not true of informed consent in sense$_2$, where competence has enjoyed a justifiably central role in specifying *from whom* consent may and must be solicited. One problem is who in the circumstance counts as a legitimate authority for the purpose of consent. Because these issues are frequently treated at the policy level almost exclusively as problems of competence, we turn in conclusion to a brief discussion of competence as it functions in sense$_2$ requirements.

5. Euthanasia

In his article "Dilemmas of Life and Death," Walton defines euthanasia as a "deliberate intervention undertaken with the express intention of ending a life so as to relieve intractable suffering." We can consider this definition as pointing out the meaning of active euthanasia. On the other hand, one definition of passive euthanasia describes two possible scenarios. The first refers to "withdrawing or withholding procedures, means or medications required to maintain life, and the second point out the process of alleviating pain and distress with the understanding that said procedures, means and medications may possible hasten death. The second definition of passive euthanasia describes a situation that lends itself to analysis through the doctrine of double effect, which is a form of ethical criterion used to analyze issues where one intends that an action they are taking be good (alleviating pain and suffering, for instance), but in bringing about that act they are simultaneously bringing about an act that would normally be avoided (killing a person). According to the double effect, if a situation like this is to be ethically sound the intention of the act must be to promote good; the good act must be either beneficial or morally neutral.

Physician-assisted suicide is another variation of euthanasia. It is defined as providing a patient with the knowledge and means to commit suicide without participating directly in the act. Although the physician does not technically commit the act, the actions taken by the physician are carried out with the intention of assisting the patient in ending his/her life. It seems that physician-assisted suicide and active euthanasia are ethically similar. The intention of both is to end the life of a patient, and the physician must actively assist the patient in order to bring either form to fruition. Hence, there would not be ethical distinction between actively providing their own hands versus actively providing the necessary information and means with which a patient can kill him/herself. The intention is to facilitate death. The ends result in death. The slight variation in the means by which this death occurs is insignificant, as both require action by the physician.

The term passive euthanasia does not actually describe euthanasia, and aligns itself more closely to palliative care. The first definition of passive euthanasia implies a negative action such as withholding futile life-extending procedures, withholding a ventilator, or discontinuing the provision of medication. Although some argue that these actions hasten death, withholding treatment and procedures only appears to hasten death because it ceases to provide the unnatural means that were prolonging of their life. Everything that lives will die, and allowing a person to naturally die because you have removed unnatural treatments could perfectly be considered as something different from euthanasia. Removing or withholding those same treatments from a healthy person would not result in their death. The second definition of passive euthanasia involves taking action, but the intention of these actions is to provide relief to a struggling patient which is more akin to palliative care that it is to euthanasia. Actions associated to the concept of passive euthanasia have the potential to accelerate a patient's decline towards death, but death is not a guaranteed result of these treatments as well as it is not necessarily the main purpose.

The conflicts found among the definitions of issues within euthanasia debates contribute a fair amount to unnecessary confusion regarding what exactly euthanasia entails. Euthanasia is the deliberate act of providing or administering medication or procedures to a dying person with the specific intention of ending his/her life. A more ethically comprehensive definition of euthanasia would account for the relief of suffering and account for the will of the patient. In bioethical terms, euthanasia would be the deliberate act of providing or administering medication or procedures to a dying person at his/her request with the specific intention to end his/her life so as to relieve that person from intractable suffering. Administering medication or a procedure which is purely intended to relieve intractable suffering without the purpose of ending patient's life should not be considered an act of euthanasia.

The fact of the matter is: the end of life is still spent living. It is a physician's duty to care for a patient as long as that care will have an impact on that patient's quality of life. The final moments of life can still involve emotions, sensations, pain, and consciousness, and so a physician's involvement in the process of dying is as relevant as their involvement with a patient during earlier stages of life. Certainly, death is a medical issue, and physicians should be allowed to involve themselves. But to what extent does bioethics allow? Should physicians be allowed to actively participate in shortening a patient's life upon request?

Readings

Rachels, James, "Active and Passive Euthanasia," in *New England Journal of Medicine*, Massachusetts Medical Society, 1975: **78–80.**

Nesbitt, Winston, "Is Killing No Worse Than Letting Die," in *Journal of Applied Philosophy*, Blackwell Publishing, 12: 1, 1995: **101–105.**

Practical Scenarios

Instructions for analysis:

1. Explain, in general terms, why the case is morally relevant and controversial.
2. Identify the central moral issue. Justify.
3. Identify and explain the main facts to be considered in your analysis.
4. Identify and explain the principles and theories useful in analyzing the case. Justify why those principles and theories are relevant in the case. Specify conflicts between them.
5. Identify and raise arguments to support the conflicting options/decisions/actions that are evident in the case (Specifications and balancing of rules are necessary at this stage).
6. Identify and weigh alternative courses of action and then decide. Justify your decision. Answer the question(s) posed by the author as part of your conclusion.

Scenario 1

The Smiths

Mr. Smith is an 82-year-old male in end stage multiple organ system failure. The clinical consensus is that it is time to withdraw from aggressive management and the attending approaches Mr. Smith's wife about writing a comfort measures only order and a decision to withdraw life-sustaining medical interventions. Mr. Smith has been determined to lack decision making capacity. Staff is undecided about Mrs. Smith's capacity. She has carefully avoided every effort to engage her reasoning about his plan of care. She repeatedly makes statements begging the staff not to let her husband die. "He can't die." "I can't live without him!" Tell me this isn't happening." The Smiths are childless.[1]

Question

Is in this case euthanasia morally permissible? Why?

Scenario 2

Terry Schiavo (Theresa Marie Schindler)

Terri Schiavo entered a vegetative state in 1990 for undetermined reasons, possibly related to her long-term, untreated bulimia. In this persistent vegetative state she remained the last fifteen years of her life. Both Schiavo's doctors and her court-appointed doctors expressed the opinion that there existed no hope of rehabilitation. Her husband, Michael Schiavo, contended that it was his wife's wish that she not be kept alive through unnatural, mechanical means.

More than twenty times the Schiavo case was heard in Florida courts. On all occasions the court ruled that the Terri's fate was under her husband's control, respecting the sanctity of marriage. Schiavo's parents, Bob and Mary Schindler, refused to accept this verdict, feeling that their daughter would somehow recover. Of this struggle, Schiavo's attorney George Felos told

the US District Court, "The real grievance is not they [the Schindlers] did not have a day in court, that they did not have due process. The real grievance is they disagree with the result."

In 2003, a court-appointed guardian for Schiavo wrote that during the protracted legal struggle, her parents had "voiced the disturbing belief that they would keep Theresa alive at any and all costs", even if that required amputation of her limbs. "As part of the hypothetical presented", the guardian's report stated, "Schindler family members stated that even if Theresa had told them of her intention to have artificial nutrition withdrawn, they would not do it."

On February 25, 2005, a Pinellas County judge ordered the removal of Terri Schiavo's feeding tube. Several appeals and federal government intervention followed, which included U.S. President George W. Bush returning to Washington D.C. to sign legislation designed to keep her alive. After all attempts at appeals through the federal court system upheld the original decision to remove the feeding tube, staff at the Pinellas Park hospice facility where Terri was being cared for disconnected the feeding tube on March 18, 2005, and she died on March 31, 2005.[2]

Question

Was Pinellas County judge's decision morally right? Justify your answer.

Scenario 3

Mary Wants to Die

Mary is an educated, articulate, wealthy and until recently, healthy 78 year old, single woman. She has lived a rich and full life and sees nothing but diminishment in her future with a life increasingly constricted to her apartment. She does have advanced osteoporosis. A recent fall resulted in a leg fracture. When she told someone that she wished she could just fall asleep and never wake up, her friend told her that she should just

---

1 Adapted from Taylor, Carol, *Health Care Ethics Course*, Georgetown University School of Medicine, AY 2010–2011.

2 Adapted from http://www.nndb.com/people/435/000026357/ (July 2013).

stop eating and drinking. Her friend works for hospice and Mary is now asking this hospice to care for her until she dies. The medical director has asked the hospice ethics committee to make a recommendation about the advisability of admitting Mary to the inpatient hospice unit so she can be cared for as she grows weaker. There are also questions about whether or not hospice physicians and nurses should start recommending *terminal dehydration to patients like Mary who want to be dead but who do not have life-sustaining treatments to stop.*[3]

Question

Should the hospice staff let Mary die? Why?

3   Adapted from Taylor, Carol, *Health Care Ethics Course,* Georgetown University School of Medicine, AY 2010–2011.

Active and Passive Euthanasia

James Rachels

Abstract

The traditional distinction between active and passive euthanasia requires critical analysis. The conventional doctrine is that there is such an important moral difference between the two that, although the latter is sometimes permissible, the former is always forbidden. This doctrine may be challenged for several reasons. First of all, active euthanasia is in many cases more humane than passive euthanasia. Secondly, the conventional doctrine leads to decisions concerning life and death on irrelevant grounds. Thirdly, the doctrine rests on a distinction between killing and letting die that itself has no moral importance. Fourthly, the most common arguments in favor of the doctrine are invalid. I therefore suggest that the American Medical Association policy statement that endorses this doctrine is unsound. (N Engl J Med 292:78-80, 1975)

The distinction between active and passive euthanasia is thought to be crucial for medical ethics. The idea is that it is permissible, at least in some cases, to withhold treatment and allow a patient to die, but it is never permissible to take any direct action designed to kill the patient. This doctrine seems to be accepted by most doctors, and it is endorsed in a statement adopted by the House of Delegates of the American Medical Association on December 4,1973:

> The intentional termination of the life of one human being by another—mercy killing—is contrary to that for which the medical profession stands and is contrary to the policy of the American Medical Association.
>
> The cessation of the employment of extraordinary means to prolong the life of the body when there is irrefutable evidence that biological death is imminent is the decision of the patient and/or his immediate family.

Address reprint requests to Mr. Rachels at the Department of Philosophy, University of Miami, P.O. Box 8054, Miami, FL 33124

The advice and judgment of the physician should be freely available to the patient and/or his immediate family.

However, a strong case can be made against this doctrine. In what follows I will set out some of the relevant arguments, and urge doctors to reconsider their views on this matter.

To begin with a familiar type of situation, a patient who is dying of incurable cancer of the throat is in terrible pain, which can no longer be satisfactorily alleviated. He is certain to die within a few days, even if present treatment is continued, but he does not want to go on living for those days since the pain is unbearable. So he asks the doctor for an end to it, and his family joins in the request.

Suppose the doctor agrees to withhold treatment, as the conventional doctrine says he may. The justification for his doing so is that the patient is in terrible agony, and since he is going to die anyway, it would be wrong to prolong his suffering needlessly. But now notice this. If one simply withholds treatment, it may take the patient longer to die, and so he may suffer more than he would if more direct action were taken and a lethal injection given. This fact provides strong reason for thinking that, once the initial decision not to prolong his agony has been made, active euthanasia is actually preferable to passive euthanasia, rather than the reverse. To say otherwise is to endorse the option that leads to more suffering rather than less, and is contrary to the humanitarian impulse that prompts the decision not to prolong his life in the first place.

Part of my point is that the process of being "allowed to die" can be relatively slow and painful, whereas being given a lethal injection is relatively quick and painless. Let me give a different sort of example. In the United States about one in 600 babies is born with Down's syndrome. Most of these babies are otherwise healthy—that is, with only the usual pediatric care, they will proceed to an otherwise normal infancy. Some, however, are born with congenital defects such as intestinal obstructions that require operations if they are to live. Sometimes, the parents and the doctor will decide not to operate, and let the infant die. Anthony Shaw describes what happens then:

> ... When surgery is denied [the doctor] must try to keep the infant from suffering while natural forces sap the baby's life away. As a surgeon whose natural inclination is to use the scalpel to fight off death, standing by and watching a salvageable baby die is the most emotionally exhausting experience I know. It is easy at a conference, in a theoretical discussion, to decide that such infants should be allowed to die. It is altogether different to stand by in the nursery and watch as dehydration and infection wither a tiny being over hours and days. This is a terrible ordeal for me and the hospital staff—much more so than for the parents who never set foot in the nursery.[1]

I can understand why some people are opposed to all euthanasia, and insist that such infants must be allowed to live. I think I can also understand why other people favor destroying these babies quickly and painlessly. But why should anyone favor letting "dehydration and infection wither a tiny being over hours and days?" The doctrine that says that a baby may be allowed to dehydrate and wither, but may not be given an injection that would end its life without suffering, seems so patently cruel as to require no further refutation. The strong language is not intended to offend, but only to put the point in the clearest possible way.

My second argument is that the conventional doctrine leads to decisions concerning life and death made on irrelevant grounds.

Consider again the case of the infants with Down's syndrome who need operations for

---

1 Shaw A: 'Doctor. Do We Have a Choice?' *The New York Times Magazine*. January 30, 1972, p 54.

congenital defects unrelated to the syndrome to live. Sometimes, there is no operation, and the baby dies, but when there is no such defect, the baby lives on. Now, an operation such as that to remove an intestinal obstruction is not prohibitively difficult. The reason why such operations are not performed in these cases is, clearly, that the child has Down's syndrome and the parents and doctor judge that because of that fact it is better for the child to die.

But notice that this situation is absurd, no matter what view one takes of the lives and potentials of such babies. If the life of such an infant is worth preserving, what does it matter if it needs a simple operation? Or, if one thinks it better that such a baby should not live on, what difference does it make that it happens to have an unobstructed intestinal tract? In either case, the matter of life and death is being decided on irrelevant grounds. It is the Down's syndrome, and not the intestines, that is the issue. The matter should be decided, if at all, on that basis, and not be allowed to depend on the essentially irrelevant question of whether the intestinal tract is blocked.

What makes this situation possible, of course, is the idea that when there is an intestinal blockage, one can "let the baby die," but when there is no such defect there is nothing that can be done, for one must not "kill" it. The fact that this idea leads to such results as deciding life or death on irrelevant grounds is another good reason why the doctrine should be rejected.

One reason why so many people think that there is an important moral difference between active and passive euthanasia is that they think killing someone is morally worse than letting someone die. But is it? Is killing, in itself, worse than letting die? To investigate this issue, two cases may be considered that are exactly alike except that one involves killing whereas the other involves letting someone die. Then, it can be asked whether this difference makes any difference to the moral assessments. It is important that the cases be exactly alike, except

for this one difference, since otherwise one cannot be confident that it is this difference and not some other that accounts for any variation in the assessments of the two cases. So, let us consider this pair of cases:

In the first, Smith stands to gain a large inheritance if anything should happen to his six-year-old cousin. One evening while the child is taking his bath, Smith sneaks into the bathroom and drowns the child, and then arranges things so that it will look like an accident.

In the second, Jones also stands to gain if anything should happen to his six-year-old cousin. Like Smith, Jones sneaks in planning to drown the child in his bath. However, just as he enters the bathroom Jones sees the child slip and hit his head, and fall face down in the water. Jones is delighted; he stands by, ready to push the child's head back under if it is necessary, but it is not necessary. With only a little thrashing about, the child drowns all by himself, "accidentally," as Jones watches and does nothing.

Now Smith killed the child, whereas Jones "merely" let the child die. That is the only difference between them. Did either man behave better, from a moral point of view? If the difference between killing and letting die were in itself a morally important matter, one should say that Jones's behavior was less reprehensible than Smith's. But does one really want to say that? I think not. In the first place, both men acted from the same motive, personal gain, and both had exactly the same end in view when they acted. It may be inferred from Smith's conduct that he is a bad man, although that judgment may be withdrawn or modified if certain further facts are learned about him—for example, that he is mentally deranged. But would not the very same thing be inferred about Jones from his conduct? And would not the same further considerations also be relevant to any modification of this judgment? Moreover, suppose Jones pleaded, in his own defense, "After all, I didn't do anything except just stand there and watch the child drown. I didn't kill him; I only let him die." Again, if letting die were in itself less bad than killing, this defense should have at least some weight. But it does not. Such a "defense" can only be regarded as a grotesque perversion of moral reasoning. Morally speaking, it is no defense at all.

Now, it may be pointed out, quite properly, that the cases of euthanasia with which doctors are concerned are not like this at all. They do not involve personal gain or the destruction of normal healthy children. Doctors are concerned only with cases in which the patient's life is of no further use to him, or in which the patient's life has become or will soon become a terrible burden. However, the point is the same in these cases: the bare difference between killing and letting die does not, in itself, make a moral difference. If a doctor lets a patient die, for humane reasons, he is in the same moral position as if he had given the patient a lethal injection for humane reasons. If his decision was wrong—if, for example, the patient's illness was in fact curable—the decision would be equally regrettable no matter which method was used to carry it out. And if the doctor's decision was the right one, the method used is not in itself important.

The AMA policy statement isolates the crucial issue very well; the crucial issue is "the intentional termination of the life of one human being by another." But after identifying this issue, and forbidding "mercy killing," the statement goes on to deny that the cessation of treatment is the intentional termination of a life. This is where the mistake comes in, for what is the cessation of treatment, in these circumstances, if it is not "the intentional termination of the life of one human being by another?" Of course it is exactly that, and if it were not, there would be no point to it.

Many people will find this judgment hard to accept. One reason, I think, is that it is very easy to conflate the question of whether killing is, in itself, worse than letting die, with the very different question of whether most actual cases of killing are more reprehensible than most actual cases of letting die. Most actual cases of killing are clearly terrible (think, for example,

of all the murders reported in the newspapers), and one hears of such cases every day. On the other hand, one hardly ever hears of a case of letting die, except for the actions of doctors who are motivated by humanitarian reasons. So one learns to think of killing in a much worse light than of letting die. But this does not mean that there is something about killing that makes it in itself worse than letting die, for it is not the bare difference between killing and letting die that makes the difference in these cases. Rather, the other factors—the murderer's motive of personal gain, for example, contrasted with the doctor's humanitarian motivation—account for different reactions to the different cases.

I have argued that killing is not in itself any worse than letting die; if my contention is right, it follows that active euthanasia is not any worse than passive euthanasia. What arguments can be given on the other side? The most common, I believe, is the following:

"The important difference between active and passive euthanasia is that, in passive euthanasia, the doctor does not do anything to bring about the patient's death. The doctor does nothing, and the patient dies of whatever ills already afflict him. In active euthanasia, however, the doctor does something to bring about the patient's death: he kills him. The doctor who gives the patient with cancer a lethal injection has himself caused his patient's death; whereas if he merely ceases treatment, the cancer is the cause of the death."

A number of points need to be made here. The first is that it is not exactly correct to say that in passive euthanasia the doctor does nothing, for he does do one thing that is very important: he lets the patient die. "Letting someone die" is certainly different, in some respects, from other types of action—mainly in that it is a kind of action that one may perform by way of not performing certain other actions. For example, one may let a patient die by way of not giving medication, just as one may insult someone by way of not shaking his hand. But for any purpose of moral assessment, it is a type of action nonetheless. The decision to let a patient die is subject to moral appraisal in the same way that a decision to kill him would be subject to moral appraisal: it may be assessed as wise or unwise, compassionate or sadistic, right or wrong. If a doctor deliberately let a patient die who was suffering from a routinely curable illness, the doctor would certainly be to blame for what he had done, just as he would be to blame if he had needlessly killed the patient. Charges against him would then be appropriate. If so, it would be no defense at all for him to insist that he didn't "do anything." He would have done something very serious indeed, for he let his patient die.

Fixing the cause of death may be very important from a legal point of view, for it may determine whether criminal charges are brought against the doctor. But I do not think that this notion can be used to show a moral difference between active and passive euthanasia. The reason why it is considered bad to be the cause of someone's death is that death is regarded as a great evil—and so it is. However, if it has been decided that euthanasia—even passive euthanasia—is desirable in a given case, it has also been decided that in this instance death is no greater an evil than the patient's continued existence. And if this is true, the usual reason for not wanting to be the cause of someone's death simply does not apply.

Finally, doctors may think that all of this is only of academic interest—the sort of thing that philosophers may worry about but that has no practical bearing on their own work. After all, doctors must be concerned about the legal consequences of what they do, and active euthanasia is clearly forbidden by the law. But even so, doctors should also be concerned with the fact that the law is forcing upon them a moral doctrine that may well be indefensible, and has a considerable effect on their practices. Of course, most doctors are not now in the position of being coerced in this matter, for they do not regard themselves as merely going along with what the law requires. Rather, in statements such as the AMA policy statement that I have quoted, they are endorsing this doctrine as a central point of medical ethics. In that statement, active euthanasia is condemned not merely as illegal but as "contrary to that for which the medical profession stands," whereas passive euthanasia is approved. However, the preceding considerations suggest that there is really no moral difference between the two, considered in themselves (there may be important moral differences in some cases in their *consequences*, but, as I pointed out, these differences may make active euthanasia, and not passive euthanasia, the morally preferable option). So, whereas doctors may have to discriminate between active and passive euthanasia to satisfy the law, they should not do any more than that. In particular, they should not give the distinction any added authority and weight by writing it into official statements of medical ethics

Is Killing No Worse Than Letting Die?

Winston Nesbitt

Abstract

Those who wish to refute the view that it is worse to kill than to let die sometimes produce examples of cases in which an agent lets someone die but would be generally agreed to be no less reprehensible than if he had killed. It is argued that the examples produced typically possess a feature which makes their use in this context illegitimate, and that when modified to remove this feature, they provide support for the view which they were designed to undermine.

I want in this paper to consider a kind of argument sometimes produced against the thesis that it is worse to kill someone (that is, to deliberately take action that results in another's death) than merely to allow someone to die (that is, deliberately to fail to take steps which were available and which would have saved another's life). Let us, for brevity's sake, refer to this as the 'difference thesis', since it implies that there is a moral difference between killing and letting die.

One approach commonly taken by opponents of the difference thesis is to produce examples of cases in which an agent does not kill, but merely lets someone die, and yet would be generally agreed to be just as morally reprehensible as if he had killed. This kind of appeal to common intuitions might seem an unsatisfactory way of approaching the issue. It has been argued [1] that what stance one takes concerning the difference thesis will depend on the ethical theory one holds, so that we cannot decide what stance is correct independently of deciding what is the correct moral theory. I do not, however, wish to object to the approach in question on these grounds. It may be true that different moral theories dictate different stances concerning the different thesis, so that a theoretically satisfactory defence or refutation of the thesis requires a satisfactory defence of a theory which entails its soundness or unsoundness. However, the issue of its soundness or otherwise is a vital one in the attempt to

Winston Nesbitt, Department of Humanities, University of Tasmania at Launceston, PO Box 1214, Launceston, Tasmania 7250, Australia.

decide some pressing moral questions [2], and we cannot wait for a demonstration of the correct moral theory before taking up any kind of position with regard to it. Moreover, decisions on moral questions directly affecting practice are rarely derived from ethical first principles, but are usually based at some level on common intuitions, and it is arguable that at least where the question is one of public policy, this is as it should be.

2

It might seem at first glance a simple matter to show at least that common moral intuitions favour the difference thesis. Compare, to take an example of John Ladd's [3], the case in which I push someone who I know cannot swim into a river, thereby killing her, with that in which I come across someone drowning and fail to rescue her, although I am able to do so, thereby letting her die. Wouldn't most of us agree that my behaviour is morally worse in the first case?

However, it would be generally agreed by those involved in the debate that nothing of importance for our issue, not even concerning common opinion, can be learned through considering such an example. As Ladd points out, without being told any more about the cases mentioned, we are inclined to assume that there are other morally relevant differences between them, because there usually would be. We assume, for example, some malicious motive in the case of killing, but perhaps only fear or indifference in the case of failing to save. James Rachels and Michael Tooley, both of whom argue against the difference thesis, make similar points [4], as does Raziel Abelson, in a paper defending the thesis [5]. Tooley, for example, notes that as well as differences in motives, there are also certain other morally relevant differences between typical acts of killing and typical acts of failing to save which may make us judge them differently. Typically, saving someone requires

more effort than refraining from killing someone. Again, an act of killing necessarily results in someone's death, but an act of failing to save does not—someone else may come to the rescue. Factors such as these, it is suggested, may account for our tendency to judge failure to save (i.e., letting die) less harshly than killing. Tooley concludes that if one wishes to appeal to intuitions here, 'one must be careful to confine one's attention to pairs of cases that do not differ in these, or other significant respects' [6].

Accordingly, efforts are made by opponents of the difference thesis to produce pairs of cases which do not differ in morally significant respects (other than in one being a case of killing while the other is a case of letting die or failing to save). In fact, at least the major part of the case mounted by Rachels and Tooley against the difference thesis consists of the production of such examples. It is suggested that when we compare a case of killing with one which differs from it *only* in being a case of letting die, we will agree that either agent is as culpable as the other; and this is then taken to show that any inclination we ordinarily have to think killing worse than letting die is attributable to our tending, illegitimately, to think of typical cases of killing and of letting die, which differ in other morally relevant respects. I want now to examine the kind of example usually produced in these contexts.

3

I will begin with the examples produced by James Rachels in the article mentioned earlier, which is fast becoming one of the most frequently reprinted articles in the area [7]. Although the article has been the subject of a good deal of discussion, as far as I know the points which I will make concerning it have not been previously made. Rachels asks us to compare the following two cases. The first is that of Smith, who will gain a large inheritance should his six-year-old nephew die. With this in mind, Smith one evening sneaks into the bathroom where his nephew is taking a bath, and drowns him. The other case, that of Jones, is identical, except that as Jones is about to drown his nephew, the child slips, hits his head, and falls, face down and unconscious, into the bath water. Jones, delighted at his good fortune, watches as his nephew drowns.

Rachels assumes that we will readily agree that Smith, who kills his nephew, is no worse, morally speaking, than Jones, who merely lets his nephew die. Do we really want to say, he asks, that either behaves better from the moral point of view than the other? It would, he suggests, be a 'grotesque perversion of moral reasoning' for Jones to argue, 'After all, I didn't do anything except just stand and watch the child drown. I didn't kill him; I only let him die'. [8] Yet, Rachels says, if letting die were in itself less bad than killing, this defence would carry some weight.

There is little doubt that Rachels is correct in taking it that we will agree that Smith behaves no worse in his examples than does Jones. Before we are persuaded by this that killing someone is in itself morally no worse than letting someone die, though, we need to consider the examples more closely. We concede that Jones, who merely let his nephew die, is just as reprehensible as Smith, who killed his nephew. Let us ask, however, just what is the ground of our judgement of the agent in each case. In the case of Smith, this seems to be adequately captured by saying that Smith drowned his nephew for motives of personal gain. But can we say that the grounds on which we judge Jones to be reprehensible, and just as reprehensible as Smith, are that he let his nephew drown for motives of personal gain? I suggest not—for this neglects to mention a crucial fact about Jones, namely that he was fully prepared to kill his nephew, and would have done so had it proved necessary. It would be generally accepted, I think, quite independently of the present debate, that someone who is fully prepared to perform a reprehensible action, in the expectation of certain

circumstances, but does not do so because the expected circumstances do not eventuate, is just as reprehensible as someone who actually performs that action in those circumstances. Now this alone is sufficient to account for our judging Jones as harshly as Smith. He was fully prepared to do what Smith did, and would have done so if circumstances had not turned out differently from those in Smith's case. Thus, though we may agree that he is just as reprehensible as Smith, this cannot be taken as showing that his letting his nephew die is as reprehensible as Smith's killing his nephew—for we would have judged him just as harshly, given what he was prepared to do, even if he had not let his nephew die. To make this clear, suppose that we modify Jones' story along the following lines—as before, he sneaks into the bathroom while his nephew is bathing, with the intention of drowning the child in his bath. This time, however, just before he can seize the child, *he* slips and hits his head on the bath, knocking himself unconscious. By the time he regains consciousness, the child, unaware of his intentions, has called his parents, and the opportunity is gone. Here, Jones neither kills his nephew *nor* lets him die—yet I think it would be agreed that given his preparedness to kill the child for personal gain, he is as reprehensible as Smith.

The examples produced by Michael Tooley, in the book referred to earlier, suffer the same defect as those produced by Rachels. Tooley asks us to consider the following pair of scenarios, as it happens also featuring Smith and Jones. In the first, Jones is about to shoot Smith when he sees that Smith will be killed by a bomb unless Jones warns him, as he easily can. Jones does not warn him, and he is killed by the bomb—i.e., Jones lets Smith die. In the other, Jones wants Smith dead, and shoots him—i.e., he kills Smith.

Tooley elsewhere [9] produces this further example: two sons are looking forward to the death of their wealthy father, and decide independently to poison him. One puts poison in his father's whiskey, and is discovered doing so by the other, who was just about to do the same. The latter then allows his father to drink the poisoned whiskey, and refrains from giving him the antidote, which he happens to possess.

Tooley is confident that we will agree that in each pair of cases, the agent who kills is morally no worse than the one who lets die. It will be clear, however, that his examples are open to criticisms parallel to those just produced against Rachels. To take first the case where Jones is saved the trouble of killing Smith by the fortunate circumstance of a bomb's being about to explode near the latter: it is true that we judge Jones to be just as reprehensible as if he had killed Smith, but since he was fully prepared to kill him had he not been saved the trouble by the bomb, we would make the same judgement even if he had neither killed Smith nor let him die (even if, say, no bomb had been present, but Smith suffered a massive and timely heart attack). As for the example of the like-minded sons, here too the son who didn't kill was prepared to do so, and given this, would be as reprehensible as the other even if he had not let his father die (if, say, he did not happen to possess the antidote, and so was powerless to save him).

Let us try to spell out more clearly just where the examples produced by Rachels and Tooley fail. What both writers overlook is that what determines whether someone is reprehensible or not is not simply what he in fact does, but what he is prepared to do, perhaps as revealed by what he in fact does. Thus, while Rachels is correct in taking it that we will be inclined to judge Smith and Jones in his examples equally harshly, this is not surprising, since both are judged reprehensible for precisely the same reason, namely that they were fully prepared to kill for motives of personal gain. The same, of course, is true of Tooley's examples. In each example he gives of an agent who lets another die, the agent is fully prepared to kill (though in the event, he is spared the necessity). In their efforts to ensure that the members of each pair of cases they produce do not differ in any morally relevant respect (except that one is a case

of killing and the other of letting die), Rachels and Tooley make them *too* similar—not only do Rachels' Smith and Jones, for example, have identical motives, but both are guilty of the same moral offence.

4

Given the foregoing account of the failings of the examples produced by Rachels and Tooley, what modifications do they require if they are to be legitimately used to gauge our attitudes towards killing and letting die, respectively? Let us again concentrate on Rachels' examples. Clearly, if his argument is to avoid the defect pointed out, we must stipulate that though Jones was prepared to let his nephew die once he saw that this would happen unless he intervened, he was not prepared to kill the child. The story will now go something like this: Jones stands to gain considerably from his nephew's death, as before, but he is not prepared to kill him for this reason. However, he happens to be on hand when his nephew slips, hits his head, and falls face down in the bath. Remembering that he will profit from the child's death, he allows him to drown. We need, however, to make a further stipulation, regarding the explanation of Jones's not being prepared to kill his nephew. It cannot be that he fears untoward consequences for himself, such as detection and punishment, or that he is too lazy to choose such an active course, or that the idea simply had not occurred to him. I think it would be common ground in the debate that if the only explanation of his not being prepared to kill his nephew was one of these kinds, he would be morally no better than Smith, who differed only in being more daring, or more energetic, whether or not fate then happened to offer him the opportunity to let his nephew die instead. In that case, we must suppose that the reason Jones is prepared to let his nephew die, but not to kill him, is a moral one—not intervening to save the child, he holds, is one thing, but actually bringing about his death is another, and altogether beyond the pale.

I suggest, then, that the case with which we must compare that of Smith is this: Jones happens to be on hand when his nephew slips, hits his head, and falls unconscious into his bath water. It is clear to Jones that the child will drown if he does not intervene. He remembers that the child's death would be greatly to his advantage, and does not intervene. Though he is prepared to let the child die however, and in fact does so, he would not have been prepared to kill him, because, as he might put it, wicked though he is, he draws the line at killing for gain.

I am not entirely sure what the general opinion would be here as to the relative reprehensibility of Smith and Jones. I can only report my own, which is that Smith's behaviour is indeed morally worse than that of Jones. What I do want to insist on, however, is that, for the reasons I have given, we cannot take our reactions to the examples provided by Rachels and Tooley as an indication of our intuitions concerning the relative heinousness of killing and of letting die.

So far, we have restricted ourselves to discussion of common intuitions on our question, and made no attempt to argue for any particular answer. I will conclude by pointing out that, given the fairly common view that the *raison d'être* of morality is to make it possible for people to live together in reasonable peace and security, it is not difficult to provide a rationale for the intuition that in our modified version of Rachels' examples, Jones is less reprehensible than Smith. For it is clearly preferable to have Jones-like persons around rather than Smith-like ones. We are not threatened by the former—such a person will not save me if my life should be in danger, but in this he is no more dangerous than an incapacitated person, or for that matter, a rock or tree (in fact he may be better, for he *might* save me as long as he doesn't think he will profit from my death). Smith-like persons, however, *are* a threat—if such a person should come to believe that she will benefit sufficiently from my death, then not only must I expect no

help from her if my life happens to be in danger, but I must fear positive attempts on my life. In that case, given the view mentioned of the point of morality, people prepared to behave as Smith does are clearly of greater concern from the moral point of view than those prepared only to behave as Jones does; which is to say that killing is indeed morally worse than letting die.

Notes

1. See, for example, JOHN CHANDLER (1990) Killing and letting die—putting the debate in context, *Australasian Journal of Philosophy* 68, no. 4, 1990, pp. 420–431.

2. It underlies, or is often claimed to underlie, for example, the Roman Catholic position on certain issues in the abortion debate, and the view that while 'passive' euthanasia may sometimes be permissible, 'active' euthanasia never is. It also seems involved in the common view that even if it is wrong to fail to give aid to the starving of the world, thereby letting them die, it is not as wrong as dropping bombs on them, thereby killing them.

3. JOHN LADD (1985) Positive and negative euthanasia in JAMES E. WHITE (ed.), *Contemporary Moral Problems* (St Paul, West Publishing Co), pp. 58–68.

4. JAMES RACHELS (1979) Active and passive euthanasia in JAMES RACHELS (ed.), *Moral Problems* (NY, Harper and Row), pp. 490–497; MICHAEL TOOLEY (1983) *Abortion and Infanticide* (Oxford, Clarendon Press), pp. 187–188.

5. RAZIEL ABELSON (1982) There is a moral difference, in RAZIEL ABELSON and MARIE-LOUISE FRIQUEGNON (eds.), *Ethics for Modern Life* (New York, St Martin's Press), pp. 73–83.

6. TOOLEY, *op. cit.*, p. 189.

7. Apart from the anthology cited in footnote 4, it appears, for example, in JAMES E. WHITE (ed.) (1991) *Contemporary Moral Problems* (St Paul, West Publishing Co), pp. 103–107; BONNIE STEINBOCK (ed.) (1980) *Killing and Letting*

Die (Englewood Cliffs, NJ, Prentice-Hall), pp. 63–68; Tom L. Beauchamp and Leroy Walters (eds.) (1982) *Contemporary Issues in Bioethics* (Belmont, Wadsworth Publishing Co), pp. 313–316; Robert F. Weir (ed.) (1986) *Ethical Issues in Death and Dying* (NY, Columbia University Press), pp. 249–256; Ronald Munson (ed.) (1992) *Interventions and Reflections* (Belmont, Wadsworth Publishing Co), pp. 163–166; John Arras and Nancy Rhoden (eds.) (1989) *Ethical Issues in Modern Medicine* (Calif. Mayfield Publishing Co) pp. 241–244; and in Thomas A. Mappes and Jane S. Zembaty (eds.) (1977) *Social Ethics* (NY, McGraw-Hill), pp. 62–66.

8. Rachels, *op. cit.*, p. 494.

9. (1980) An irrelevant consideration: killing and letting die, in Bonnie Steinbock (ed.), *Killing and Letting Die* (Englewood Cliffs, NJ, Prentice-Hall), pp. 56–62.

6. Enhancement, Genetic Manipulation and Human Research

Also known as "Genetic Engineering" or "Genetic Modification," this concept refers to the direct human manipulation of the genome of any kind of organism (humans, animals, plants).

Genetic Manipulation involves the introduction of recombinant DNA (rDNA). This technology uses enzymes to cut and paste together DNA sequences of interest. The recombined DNA sequences can be placed into vehicles called vectors that ferry the DNA into a suitable host cell where it can be copied into synthetic genes in order to give an organism a desired phenotype.

When genetic material from another species is added to the host organism, we can call it a "transgenic" organism; when genetic material is added from the same species we can call it "cisgenic."

This technology allows a wide range of possibilities, especially when applied to humans. By modifying our inherited genetic information we can prevent genetic diseases, enhance intelligence and health, enable infertile parents to have children genetically related to them, reduce the social costs of genetic diseases, and benefit the human gene pool by promoting good genes and eradicating bad genes, among other uses.

These reasons are presented by supporters of Genetic Manipulation.

On the contrary, detractors respond that so-cial injustices might be created by cloning since modifying only some individuals would promote another form of discrimination. There are also concerns related to Health-Care resources which could be better spent on other areas, and medical dangers associated with the practice of genetic engineering.

Related to genetic engineering we have another, more precise concept:

Genetic Enhancement: Generally understood as the use of genetic engineering aimed at "improving the quality of the human genome." This contrasts with "Genetic Therapy" which entails using genetic engineering for "fixing" defective genes or inserting "corrected" genes as a means of therapy or repair. However, there is no clear scientific consensus about the difference.

Genetic Enhancement is directly related to the so-called "Eugenics" movement—from Greek Eu (good or well) with added suffix genēs (born, generation)—which has been one of the most controversial scientific subjects of the past century. The term was first coined by Sir Francis Galton in 1883 to describe deliberate efforts to control human reproduction (analogous to the deliberate reproduction used in agricultural sciences in those years) and its benefits. Since then, the rise of Nazism and their appropriation of the term, related to those infamous experiments they justified as "research," have given eugenics a negative connotation. Decades later, the human genome project, which started during the 1990's and ended in 2003, gave new life to the eugenics movement, as people started recognizing its potential for beneficial therapies used autonomously by individuals. The main aim of New Eugenics is then to improve the lifetime of future individuals who would otherwise face genetic deficiencies and/or disadvantages.

As with any technological development, ethical issues arise: Who should decide which are and which are not desirable eugenic goals? Should this power change future human beings and shape them as we see fit? Will the differences created be fair? Who should get access to enhancement of their genes? Does enhancement necessarily mean improvement?

Cloning can also be considered as a type of enhancement.

Cloning: From the Greek word *klon* (twig), cloning has different possible definitions. It can be defined as a means of asexual reproduction, in which there is no need of meiosis and fertilization (both are basic processes of sexual reproduction).

Another definition is the "transplantation of a nucleus from a cell into an ovum." This transplantation process removes chromosomal genetic information from an oocyte and fertilizes it with a diploid cell. This process is carried out instead of fertilizing a haploid oocyte with a haploid sperm. The most common and broad definition of cloning, however, is simply "making a genetic copy." That genetic identity does not necessarily equal phenotypic identity, due to epigenetic or environmental effects or to mutation in nuclear chromosomes or mitochondria.

There are numerous procedures used to clone mammals but two are by far the most common: making identical copies of embryos from embryonic cells and creating embryos with identical nuclear DNA from cells of embryos, fetuses, young animals and adult cells.

Cloning technology is not only applied to produce more offspring but also to obtain basic biological information useful elsewhere, such as research on birth defects, cancer and other diseases.

Among the most relevant applications of cloning we can find: making genetic copies of outstanding agricultural animals; enhancing transgenic technology; and therapeutic cloning to produce tissue and organ replacements for humans.

Due to the large myriad of possibilities that cloning technology presents, there are several related ethical issues to consider. Debate is abundant. On one hand, supporters of cloning assert that this technology, once perfected, will be of great assistance to humans. Their arguments concern cloning's benefits to the quality of human life. According to them, this is a solid moral impetus for cloning's development. On the other hand, in the eyes of church officials, a created life would have a diminished inherent value.

Other new and morally controversial possibilities raised by biotechnology are:

Stem cells: Embryonic stem cells were first grown in culture in 1998 by James Thomson at the University of Wisconsin. He reported to the journal Science that "such human embryonic stem cells formed a wide variety of recognizable tissue when planted into mice."

There are two major types of stem cells: embryonic stem-cells, isolated from the inner cell mass of blastocysts, and adult stem-cells, found in several tissues. In a developing embryo, stem cells can differentiate into specialized cells but also maintain normal turnover of regenerative organs, such as blood, skin, or intestinal tissues. When discovered, they attracted immediate attention from the scientific community because of their ability to diversify into different and specialized cell types. Also, they can self-renew to produce even more stem-cells, and seem to be able to trigger cell regeneration and colonize damaged tissue, by repairing in situ. These features are promising for patients with Alzheimer, spinal cord injuries, stroke, burns, heart disease, diabetes, osteoarthritis, and rheumatoid arthritis.

Such technology also entails diverse ethical concerns which have raised controversial and important objections. Many of these relate to the way stem cells are obtained (currently, they are obtained from adults, umbilical cord blood and fetal and embryonic tissue). General consensus is that embryos are the best source of stem cells for therapeutic purposes. However, this consensus is subject to change as research continues and ethical questions increase: Should embryos or fetuses be deliberately produced as a means of obtaining stem cells? Who gives consent when using embryonic or fetal tissue? (Certainly fetuses cannot consent). Should we desire, given the chance, immortality? How does that affect our conception of human nature?

Transgenics: According to the Encyclopedia of Genetics, transgenic organisms are "species in which the genome has been modified by the insertion of genes obtained from another species." During the late 1970's and 1980's "scientists invented procedures for combining the DNA of species as distantly related as plant and animals." These procedures are similar to gene therapy since both change cells for specific purposes.

The goal of transgenesis is to create a whole new modified living organism by incorporating genes from other species into all cells of the mature organism, including germ cells, so it can transfer the new genetic information when it reproduces.

The first transgenic transformation was performed in 1978 when yeast cells were transformed with the insertion of foreign DNA. Soon after, in 1979, mouse cells would be modified by the same process.

Transgenic plants cells prove to be of greater difficulty because they have thick cell walls in addition to cell membranes. Processes used to modify plants like "microinjection" and "biolistics" are slower and harder to perform. Nevertheless, a wide variety of transgenic plants have been designed for agricultural use; these we know as genetically modified food. A slowly ripening tomato was the first of these types of food to be marketed. Then corn, cotton, soybeans and potatoes were genetically enhanced and other crops would soon be genetically transformed and introduced into the market.

The global community has also criticized Transgenesis because it implies manipulation of life, hidden health risks, cruel violations of animal rights, and environmental risks. All of these issues and many others pose ethical quandaries that have been attended to by philosophers, scientists and bioethicists.

Bioinformatics: With biotechnology and semiconductor developments, scientists are now able to create "micro laboratories" that perform thousands of chemical reactions simultaneously, as a silicon chip performs computations, using systems of biologically derived molecules (some biochips can be electronic), such as DNA and proteins, to perform a computer's task: storing, retrieving, and processing data. Organic technology allows us to store and process information more efficiently through "the application of recombinant DNA technology to the development of specific products and procedures." Genetic engineering has made possible the emulation of computer processes without the use of silicon-based chips, which would begets a bright future for the informatics world. And although the development of this technology is at the moment rudimentary, scientists are already imagining possible uses for biological computing's vast potential.

Bioinformatics could be defined as a branch of technology that focuses on data storage and usage in biotechnology. Advances bring new information that needs to be processed, stored and made available for future reference. Thus, bioinformatics plays an important role "in relation to research and infrastructure for biotechnology."

Once again, this potential is not exempt from moral scrutiny. The most important of questions is the following: What do we use this technology for and why?

These new techniques have opened new horizons for biotechnology but also present new challenges for bioethics. All biotechnological achievements mean new possibilities of therapy but also imply a voracious appetite for enhancement, an appetite to realize in practice all that is possible in theory. Complex issues, such as commercial eugenics, genetic discrimination and bioterrorism, among others, are no longer fiction. Biotechnology has a double face; it presents at once benefit and burden. This ambiguity refutes its alleged neutrality. The teleology of biotechnological development promises improvements in the physical human condition yet risks subsuming moral prudence to a fascination for biotechnological commodities.

Readings

Glannon, Walter, "Genetic Enhancement," in Glannon, Walter, *Genes and Future People: Philosophical Issues in Human Genetics*, Westview Press, 2011: 94–101.

Sandel, Michael J., "The Case Against Perfection: What's Wrong with Designer Children, Bionic Athletes, and Genetic Engineering," in *The Atlantic Monthly*, (April 2004): 51–62.

Resnik, David B., "The Moral Significance of the Therapy-Enhancement Distinction in Human Genetics," in *Cambridge Quarterly of Healthcare Ethics* 9: 3 (Summer 2000): 365–377.

Hellman, Samuel; Hellman, Deborah S., "Of Mice but Not Men: Problems of the Randomized Clinical Trial," in The New England Journal of Medicine, 324, no. 22, Massachusetts Medical Society, 1991: 1585–1589.

Marquis, Don, "How to Resolve and Ethical Dilemma Concerning Randomized Clinical Trials," in The New England Journal of Medicine, 341, no. 9, Massachusetts Medical Society, 1991: 691–693.

Purdy, Laura M., "Genetics and Reproductive Risk: Can Having Children Be Immoral?" in Purdy, Laura, *Reproducing Persons: Issues in Feminist Bioethics*, Ithaca, NY: Cornell University Press, 1996: 39–49.

McMahan, Jeff, "The Morality of Screening for Disability," in *Ethics, Law and Moral Philosophy of Reproductive Biomedicine*, vol. 10, supp. 1, March 2005: 129–132.

Practical Scenarios

Instructions for analysis:

1. Explain, in general terms, why the case is morally relevant and controversial.
2. Identify the central moral issue. Justify.
3. Identify and explain the main facts to be considered in your analysis.
4. Identify and explain the principles and theories useful in analyzing the case. Justify why those principles and theories are relevant in the case. Specify conflicts between them.
5. Identify and raise arguments to support the conflicting options/decisions/actions that are evident in the case (Specifications and balancing of rules are necessary at this stage).
6. Identify and weigh alternative courses of action and then decide. Justify your decision. Answer the question(s) posed by the author as part of your conclusion.

Scenario 1

The Tuskegee Study

This study can be considered as one of the most determinant milestones in the emergence of bioethics since it implied several systematic violations of basic ethical principles and it also tacitly involved the consideration of diverse classes of human beings by denying and neglecting the dignity and most elemental rights of some of them by virtue of their racial, economic and social condition. Evidently, the members of National Commission and later Beauchamp and Childress in their seminal book Principles of Biomedical Ethics took into consideration this case, among others, to conceive their vision of bioethics, its main goals, tasks and theoretical guidelines. For this reason, it is important that readers know, even if in a synoptic way, what actually happened. The facts were, more or less, as follows.

In 1932, before penicillin was fully developed, treatments for syphilis were both very ineffective and also dangerous because of its toxicity. At that time, there were no scientific parameters to accurately determine whether the possible benefits of the treatments could justify the risks associated with them. Thus, it was impossible to recognize the natural history of the disease, and science lacked relevant information to develop appropriate therapies. It was thought that the solution to the problem was in knowing the natural progression of syphilis; that is, to know what would happen to people infected with it, from the initial stages to the fatal end.

Thus, that same year the American Public Health Service began a clinical investigation that would extend for 40 years, and would become known worldwide as "The Tuskegee Syphilis Experiment." The purposes of the study seemed plausible. However, the procedure chosen to implement it was very controversial, and it has since become the subject of many moral sanctions. The experiment was to study the spontaneous evolution of syphilis in 399 African American subjects, inhabitants of the town of Tuskegee, Maicon County, Alabama, who were apparently duped by scientists into believing that they only had "bad blood" and should be treated sooner. Most of these subjects had a latent syphilis, namely, a secondary syphilis. Therefore, most of them were in the early latent stage. These 399 subjects

were never divided into "treatment" or "no treatment" groups. They were all there simply to be studied. Aditionally, a control group was comprised of 201 disease-free individuals. These subjects were observed until 1936, probably due to lack of funds or perhaps because researchers were by then only interested in the "bad blood" group.

It is important to stress that the Tuskegee experiment was not a scientific research properly. There was an evident lack of scientific method while the experiment was carried out. There were several notorious gaps and inconsistencies in the experiment. Physicians returned only after few years the study had started. Visits were not always documented. There was a hiatus between 1939 and 1948 where no protocols were extended, and no visits were documented. Moreover, between 1963 and 1970 there was not any visit to the experimental subjects either. Except the nurse, Eunice Rivers, nobody remained with the subjects. The experiment was quite irregular and was carried out with very sloppy procedures.

The reasons for these inconsistencies were the absolute irresponsibility and scientific blindness of the physicians in charge, and the total obscurity of the experiment's purposes. In this scientific "initiative," the American Public Health Service got help from the Tuskegee Institute and together started calling for subjects.

Everyone who wanted to be attended just had to meet a nurse at a specific place, date and hour in order to be transported "to the Tuskegee Hospital for the free treatment." The letter did not alert about any perils and risks for the subjects' health and stressed the study was free of charge. Indeed, the letter finished as follows: "REMEMBER THIS IS YOUR LAST CHANCE FOR SPECIAL FREE TREATMENT. BE SURE TO MEET THE NURSE." It was signed, "Macon County Health Department."

The letter produced the expected results and the experiment started being carried out. It lasted for 40 years, and even after penicillin was determined to be an effective treatment for syphilis in 1943 the experiment continued without any modifications.

In July 26 of 1972, an investigative report written by Jean Heller of the Associated Press uncovered the experiment and caused its termination. By then, 28 of the 399 subjects had died of syphilis, and an additional 100 had died of various complications as a result of not treating the disease. Furthermore, 19 children contracted syphilis during their period of gestation.[1]

Question

Which bioethical principles were violated during the study and why?

Scenario 2

Inoculating Cancer Cells into Human Bodies

During the summer of 1963, Chester M. Southam and Deogracias B. Custodio together injected live, cultured cancer cells into the bodies of 22 debilitated patients at the Jewish Chronic Disease Hospital (JCDH) in Brooklyn, New York. Custodio, a Philippine-born, unlicensed medical resident at JCDH, was participating in a medical experiment designed by Southam, a distinguished physician-researcher at the Sloan-Kettering Institute in New York City, and associate professor of medicine at Cornell University Medical College. The purpose of the research was to determine whether the previously established immune deficiency of cancer patients was caused by their cancer or, alternatively, by their debilitated condition. Southam thus looked to a group of noncancerous but highly debilitated elderly patients who might bear out his guiding hypothesis that cancer, not old age, was the cause of the previously witnessed immune deficiency. Importantly, he believed on the basis of long experience that the injection of cultured cancer cells posed no risk to these patients, and that all of the cells would eventually be rejected by their immune systems. Although Southam's professional credentials were impeccable, and although his work was deemed by his peers to be of the utmost scientific importance, the JCDH experiment soon erupted in a major public controversy. Critics denounced Southam's methods as

being comparable to those of the Nazi physicians tried at Nuremburg, whereas his defenders countered that he was a distinguished physician-researcher, and by all accounts an honorable man, who merely had the bad luck to be caught in the shifting rip tides of history.[2]

Question

Do you think this experiment was ethically justifiable? Why?

Scenario 3

The Test Tube Baby

A Colorado couple used genetic tests to create a test tube baby that would have the exact type of cells desperately needed to save their 6-year-old daughter, doctors said yesterday. The case represents the first time a couple is known to have screened their embryos before implanting one in the mother's womb for the purpose of saving the life of sibling. The test tube baby, named Adam, was born in Denver on August 29. Doctors collected cells from his umbilical cord, a painless procedure, and on September 26 infused them into his sister Molly's circulatory system. The girl is recuperating in a Minneapolis hospital, and within about a week doctors should know whether the procedure was successful.

Whether or not the transplant works, doctors and ethicists said, the procedure is both a promising and worrisome harbinger of where scientific advances are taking human reproduction in the near future—at least for those who can afford to take the path. On the one hand, experts said, that the future will be one in which the power of genetics and embryo cell research will lead to novel therapies for incurable diseases. On the other hand, the new work also points to a future in which parents will have unprecedented options to

1 Adapted from Valdes, Erick, *Bioethical Principlism. Origins, Foundations and Problems*, Germany, VDM Verlag Dr. Muller, 2012.

2 Extracted from Arras, John D., "The Jewish Chronic Disease Hospital Case" in Emanuel, Ezekiel J. *et al.*, *The Oxford Textbook of Clinical Research Ethics*, Oxford University Press, 2008.

choose the traits of their children, for whatever practical or capricious reason they may have.[3]

Question

Is it morally permissible that parents have unlimited autonomy in making decisions about what type of children they want? Why?

Scenario 4

The Death of Jesse Gelsinger

Between 1997 and 1999, Jesse Gelsinger, 18, and 17 other subjects participated in the clinical protocol "Recombinant Adenovirus Gene Transfer in Adults With Partial Ornithine Transcarbamylase Deficiency." Dr. James M. Wilson was a coinvestigator and sponsor of the research. His main collaborators were Steven E. Raper, a surgeon at the University of Pennsylvania, who was the principal investigator, and Mark L. Batshaw of the Children's National Medical Center in Washington, DC., who was the coprincipal investigator.

The adenovirus-derived vector contained a functional OTC gene. The vector was rendered incapable of replicating by the deletion of two adenoviral genes; it was designed to be safer than earlier versions of the vector. The purpose of the research was to determine a safe dose of recombinant adenovirus to serve as a treatment for adults with partial OTC.

The protocol called for groups of three or four participants to be assigned to one six dosing regimens; each group received a progressively higher dose of the vector, with adjustment for their body weight.

About 18 hours following infusion of the adenovirus vector, Gelsinger developed altered mental status and jaundice—neither of which had been seen in the first 127 study participants. He subsequently developed the systemic inflammatory response syndrome, disseminated intravascular coagulation and multiple organ system failure, and the acute respiratory distress syndrome. Gelsinger died on September 17, 1999, 98 hours following gene transfer.[4]

Question

What are the limits of science (if any) in researching with humans subjects? Can Gelsinger's death be morally justified? Provide rational and impartial arguments.

---

3   Adapted from The Washington Post, October 3, 2000, A1, 14.

4   Extracted and adapted from Steinbrook, Robert, "The Gelsinger Case" in Emanuel, Ezekiel J. et al., The Oxford Textbook of Clinical Research Ethics, Oxford University Press, 2008.

Genetic Enhancement

Walter Glannon

Gene therapy must be distinguished from genetic enhancement. The first is an intervention aimed at treating disease and restoring physical and mental functions and capacities to an adequate baseline. The second is an intervention aimed at improving functions and capacities that already are adequate. Genetic enhancement augments functions and capacities "that without intervention would be considered entirely normal."[24] Its goal is to "amplify 'normal' genes in order to make them better."[25] In chapter 1, I cited Norman Daniels's definitions of health and disease as well as what the notion of just health care entailed. This involved maintaining or restoring mental and physical functions at or to normal levels, which was necessary to ensure fair equality of opportunity for all citizens. Insofar as this aim defines the goal of medicine, genetic enhancement falls outside this goal. Furthermore, insofar as this type of intervention is not part of the goal of medicine and has no place in a just health care system, there are no medical or moral reasons for genetically enhancing normal human functions and capacities.

Some have argued that it is mistaken to think that a clear line of demarcation can be drawn between treatment and enhancement, since certain forms of enhancement are employed to prevent disease. Leroy Walters and Julie Gage Palmer refer to the immune system as an example to make this point:

In current medical practice, the best example of a widely accepted health-related physical enhancement is immunization against infectious disease.

With immunizations against diseases like polio and hepatitis B, what we are saying is in effect, "The immune system that we inherited from our parents may not be adequate to ward off certain viruses if we are exposed to them." Therefore, we will enhance the capabilities of our immune system by priming it to fight against these viruses.

From the current practice of immunizations against particular diseases, it would seem to be only a small step to try to enhance the general function of the immune system by genetic means. ... In our view, the genetic enhancement of the immune system would be morally justifiable if this kind of enhancement assisted in preventing disease and did not cause offsetting harms to the people treated by the technique.[26]

Nevertheless, because the goal of the technique would be to prevent disease, it would not, strictly speaking, be enhancement, at least not in terms of the definitions given at the outset of this section. Genetically intervening in the immune system as described by Walters and Palmer is a means of maintaining it in proper working order so that it will be better able to ward off pathogens posing a threat to the organism as a whole. Thus, it is misleading to call this intervention "enhancement." When we consider what is normal human functioning, we refer to the whole human organism consisting of immune, endocrine, nervous, cardiovascular, and other systems, not to these systems understood as isolated parts. The normal functioning in question here pertains to the ability of the immune system to protect the organism from infectious agents and thus ensure its survival. Any preventive genetic intervention in this system would be designed to maintain the normal functions of the organism, not to restore them or raise them above the norm. It would be neither therapy nor enhancement but instead a form of maintenance. Therefore, the alleged ambiguity surrounding what Walters and Palmer call "enhancing" the immune system does not impugn the distinction between treatment and enhancement.

If enhancement could make adequately functioning bodily systems function even better, then presumably there would be no limit to the extent to which bodily functions can be enhanced. Yet, beyond a certain point, heightened immune sensitivity to infectious agents can lead to an overly aggressive response, resulting in autoimmune disease that can damage healthy cells, tissues, and organs. In fact, there would be a limit to the beneficial effects of genetic intervention in the immune system, a limit beyond which the equilibrium between humoral and cellular response mechanisms would be disturbed.[27] If

any intervention ensured that the equilibrium of the immune system was maintained in proper working order, then it would be inappropriate to consider it as a form of enhancement.

To further support the treatment-enhancement distinction, consider a nongenetic intervention, the use of a bisphosphonate such as alendronate sodium. Its purpose is to prevent postmenopausal women from developing osteoporosis, or to rebuild bone in women or men who already have osteoporosis. Some might claim that, because it can increase bone density, it is a form of enhancement. But its more general purpose is to prevent bone fractures and thus maintain proper bone function so that one can have normal mobility and avoid the morbidity resulting from fractures. In terms of the functioning of the entire organism, therefore, it would be more accurate to consider the use of bisphosphonates as prevention, treatment, or maintenance rather than enhancement.

Some might raise a different question. Suppose that the parents of a child much shorter than the norm for his age persuaded a physician to give him growth hormone injections in order to increase his height. Suppose further that the child's shortness was not due to an iatrogenic cause, such as radiation to treat a brain tumor. Would this be treatment or enhancement? The question that should be asked regarding this issue is not whether the child's height is normal for his age group. Rather, the question should be whether his condition implies something less than normal physical functioning, such that he would have fewer opportunities for achievement and a decent minimum level of well-being over his lifetime. Diminutive stature alone does not necessarily imply that one's functioning is or will be so limited as to restrict one's opportunities for achievement. Of course, being short might limit one's opportunities if one wanted to become a professional basketball player. But most of us are quite flexible when it comes to formulating and carrying out life plans. Robert Reich, the treasury secretary in President Clinton's first administration, is just one example of how one can achieve very much in life despite diminutive stature. If a child's stature significantly limited his functioning and opportunities, then growth-hormone injections should be considered therapeutic treatment. If his stature were not so limiting, then the injections should be considered enhancement.

Admittedly, there is gray area near the baseline of adequate functioning where it may be difficult to distinguish between treatment and enhancement. Accordingly, we should construe the baseline loosely or thickly enough to allow for some minor deviation above or below what would be considered normal functioning. An intervention for a condition near the baseline that would raise one's functioning clearly above the critical level should be considered an enhancement. An intervention for a condition making one's functioning fall clearly below the baseline, with the aim of raising one's functioning to the critical level, should be considered a treatment. For example, an athlete with a hemoglobin level slightly below the norm for people his age and mildly anemic may want to raise that level significantly in order to be more competitive in his sport. To the extent that his actual hemoglobin level does not interfere with his ordinary physical functioning, an intervention to significantly raise that level would be an instance of enhancement. In contrast, for a child who has severe thalassemia and severe anemia, with the risk of bone abnormalities and heart failure, an intervention to correct the disorder would be an instance of treatment.

The main moral concern about genetic enhancement of physical and mental traits is that it would give some people an unfair advantage over others with respect to competitive goods like beauty, sociability, and intelligence. Unlike the cognitively disabled individual considered earlier, we can assume that their mental states would not be so different and that they would retain their identity. Enhancement would be unfair because only those who could afford the technology would have access to it, and many people are financially worse off than others

through no fault of their own. Insofar as the possession of these goods gives some people an advantage over others in careers, income, and social status, the competitive nature of these goods suggests that there would be no limit to the benefits that improvements to physical and mental capacities would yield to those fortunate enough to avail themselves of the technology. This is altogether different from the example of immune-system enhancement. There would be no diminishing marginal value in the degree of competitive advantage that one could have over others for the social goods in question and presumably no limit to the value of enhancing the physical and mental capacities that would give one this advantage. Not having access to the technology that could manipulate genetic traits in such a way as to enhance these capacities would put one at a competitive disadvantage relative to others who would have access to it.

Advancing an argument similar to the one used by those who reject the treatment-enhancement distinction, one might hold that competitive goods collapse the categorical distinction between correcting deficient capacities and improving normal ones. This is because competitive goods are continuous, coming in degrees, and therefore the capacities that enable one to achieve these goods cannot be thought of as either normal or deficient.[28] Nevertheless, to the extent that any form of genetic intervention is motivated by the medical and moral aim to enable people to have adequate mental and physical functioning and fair equality of opportunity for a decent minimum level of well-being, the goods in question are not *competitive* but *basic*. In other words, the aim of any medical intervention by genetic means is to make people better off than they were before by raising or restoring them to an absolute baseline of normal physical and mental functioning, not to make them comparatively better off than others. Competitive goods above the baseline may be continuous; but the basic goods that enable someone to reach or remain at the baseline are not. Given that these two types of goods are distinct, and that they result from the distinct aims and practices of enhancement and treatment, we can affirm that enhancement and treatment can and should be treated separately. We can uphold the claim that the purpose of any genetic intervention should be to treat people's abnormal functions and restore them to a normal level, not to enhance those functions that already are normal.

As I have mentioned, genetic enhancement that gave some people an advantage over others in possessing competitive goods would entail considerable unfairness. A likely scenario would be one in which parents paid to use expensive genetic technology to raise the cognitive ability or improve the physical beauty of their children. This would give them an advantage over other children with whom they would compete for education, careers, and income. Children of parents who could not afford to pay for the technology would be at a comparative disadvantage. Even if the goods in question fell above the normal functional baseline, one still could maintain that such an advantage would be unfair. It would depend on people's ability to pay, and inequalities in income are unfair to the extent that they result from some factors beyond people's control.

We could not appeal to the notion of a genetic lottery to resolve the problem of fairness regarding genetic enhancement. For, as I argued in the last section, such a lottery is better suited to meeting people's needs than their preferences, and enhancements correspond to people's preferences. Moreover, a lottery might only exacerbate the problem by reinforcing the perception of unfairness, depending on how losers in the lottery interpreted the fact that others won merely as a result of a random selection. One suggestion for resolving the fairness problem (short of banning the use of the technology altogether) would be to make genetic enhancement available to all. Of course, how this system could be financed is a question that admits of no easy answer. But the more important substantive point is that universal access to genetic enhancement would not be

a solution. Indeed, the upshot of such access would provide a reason for prohibiting it.

Universal availability of genetic enhancement would mean that many competitive goods some people had over others would be canceled out collectively. The idea of a competitive advantage gradually would erode, and there would be more equality among people in their possession of goods. There would not be complete equality, however. Differing parental attitudes toward such goods as education could mean differences in the extent to which cognitive enhancement was utilized. Some parents would be more selective than others in sending their children to better schools or arranging for private tutors. So, there still would be some inequality in the general outcome of the enhancement. But quite apart from this, the process of neutralizing competitive goods could end up being self-defeating on a collective level.[29] More specifically, one probable side-effect of boosting children's mental capacity on a broad scale would be some brain damage resulting in cognitive and affective impairment in some of the children who received the genetic enhancement. The net social cost of using the technology would outweigh any social advantage of everyone using it. If no one is made better off than others in their possession of social goods, but some people are made worse off than they were before in terms of their mental functioning, then the net social disadvantage would provide a reason for prohibiting collective genetic enhancement.

There is another moral aspect of enhancement that should be considered. I have maintained that inequalities above the baseline of normal physical and mental functioning are of no great moral importance and may be neutral on the question of fairness. Although equality and fairness are closely related, one does not necessarily imply the other. Again, fairness pertains to meeting people's needs. Once these needs have been met, inequalities in the possession of goods relating to preferences are not so morally significant. Thus, if the idea of an absolute baseline implies that people's basic physical and mental needs have been met, and if people who are comparatively better or worse off than others all have functioning at or above the baseline, then any inequalities in functioning above this level should not matter very much morally. If this is plausible, then it seems to follow that there would be nothing unfair and hence nothing morally objectionable about enhancements that made some people better off than others above the baseline. Nevertheless, this could undermine our belief in the importance of the fundamental equality of all people, regardless of how well off they are in absolute terms. Equality is one of the social bases of self-respect, which is essential for social harmony and stability.[30] Allowing inequalities in access to and possession of competitive goods at any level of functioning or welfare might erode this basis and the ideas of harmony and stability that rest on it. Although it would be difficult to measure, this type of social cost resulting from genetic enhancement could constitute another reason for prohibiting it.

Yet, suppose that we could manipulate certain genes to enhance our noncompetitive virtuous traits, such as altruism, generosity, and compassion.[31] Surely, these would contribute to a stable, well-ordered society and preserve the principle of fair equality of opportunity. Nothing in this program would be incompatible with the goal of medicine as the prevention and treatment of disease. But it would threaten the individual autonomy essential to us as moral agents who can be candidates for praise and blame, punishment and reward. What confers moral worth on our actions, and indeed on ourselves as agents, is our capacity to cultivate certain dispositions leading to actions. This cultivation involves the exercise of practical reason and a process of critical self-reflection, whereby we modify, eliminate, or reinforce dispositions and thereby come to identity with them as our own. Autonomy consists precisely in this process of reflection and identification. It is the capacity for reflective self-control that enables us to take responsibility for our mental states and

the actions that issue from them. Given the importance of autonomy, it would be preferable to have fewer virtuous dispositions that we can identify with as our own than to have more virtuous dispositions implanted in us through genetic enhancement. These would threaten to undermine our moral agency because they would derive from an external source.[32] Even if our genes could be manipulated in such a way that our behavior always conformed to an algorithm for the morally correct course of action in every situation, it is unlikely that we would want it. Most of us would rather make autonomous choices that turned out not to lead to the best courses of action. This is because of the intrinsic importance of autonomy and the moral growth and maturity that come with making our own choices under uncertainty. The dispositions with which we come to identify, imperfect as they may be, are what make us autonomous and responsible moral agents. Enhancing these mental states through artificial means external to our own exercise of practical reason and our own process of identification would undermine our autonomy by making them alien to us.

In sum, there are four reasons why genetic enhancement would be morally objectionable. First, it would give an unfair advantage to some people over others because some would be able to pay for expensive enhancement procedures while others would not. Second, if we tried to remedy the first problem by making genetic enhancement universally accessible, then it would be collectively self-defeating. Although much competitive unfairness at the individual level would be canceled out at the collective level, there would be the unacceptable social cost of some people suffering from adverse cognitive or emotional effects of the enhancement. Third, inequalities resulting from enhancements above the baseline of normal physical and mental functioning could threaten to undermine the conviction in the fundamental importance of equality as one of the bases of self-respect, and in turn social solidarity and stability. Fourth, enhancement of noncompetitive dispositions would threaten to undermine the autonomy and moral agency essential to us as persons.

Negative and Positive Eugenics: Is There a Slippery Slope?

The two forms of genetic intervention that I have been discussing in this chapter could be characterized as eugenics, defined as "the use of science applied to the qualitative and quantitative improvement of the human genome."[33] "Eugenics" is almost universally regarded as a dirty word, owing largely to its association with the evil practice of human experimentation in Nazi Germany and the widespread sterilization of certain groups of people in the United States and Canada, earlier in the twentieth century.[34] One cannot help but attribute some eugenic aspects to genethical questions about the number and sort of people who should exist. But there is a broader conception of eugenics (literally "good creation" in Greek) that need not have the repugnant connotation of improving the human species.

The purpose of terminating an embryo with a mutation that would cause a disease, or of giving gene therapy to someone with a disease, is not to improve the human genome or the human species but instead to prevent or treat disease in identifiable people. The purpose is not the impersonal one of increasing the quantity and quality of types of experiences, but instead the person-affecting one of preventing harm to and benefiting people who have or would have to experience the symptoms associated with severe disease. Accordingly, while retaining a broad genethical focus, we should distinguish between positive and negative eugenics. The first type is motivated by the perfectionist ideal of improving the human species, whereas the second is motivated by the beneficent ideal of health promotion through disease prevention and treatment.

To the extent that the aim of gene therapy is to prevent or control disease, and that the aim of genetic enhancement is to improve people's already normal traits and capacities, these two forms of genetic intervention correspond to negative and positive forms of eugenics.

Forms of eugenics not involving direct genetic intervention have been practiced since antiquity. In Plato's *Republic* and *Laws*, for example, an ideal society would encourage "judicious matings," meaning that mating between members of the ruling and mercantile classes would be discouraged. Only those people most likely to produce the "best" offspring were encouraged to mate, especially within the ruling class. This example of positive eugenics is morally objectionable because it involves discrimination on the basis of social class. By the same token, however, many people today select mates with whom they believe they will have children with favorable physical and intellectual traits, giving them a competitive advantage over others for social goods. This is also a version of positive eugenics, even though it does not involve genetic intervention. Nor would most people acknowledge it as such.

Selecting a specific mate in order to have children with specific traits and capacities by itself is not morally objectionable to the extent that it is not part of a state-sponsored program, does not involve any coercion, and does not give an unfair advantage to some people over others in having children. Although this practice may seem objectionable to some because it is motivated to have children with more than just normal physical and mental functioning, it could be defended on moral grounds. For, in the natural process of reproduction, it cannot be predicted precisely which traits a child will have, given the parents' genetic profile alone. Epigenesis and the incomplete penetrance of genotypes largely account for this uncertainty. On the other hand, genetically intervening to produce a child with specific traits and capacities might be objectionable because it could largely shape the child's fate and cast doubt on her autonomy and responsibility for the good she achieves in her life.

An example of negative eugenics without genetic intervention would be if a person from one race married a person from another race with the intention of not passing on any deleterious mutations and diseases to offspring. According to the "consanguinity coefficient," the more similar the genotypes of two people are, the more likely they will produce offspring with deleterious genes causing or predisposing them to certain diseases. Conversely, the more different the two genotypes are, the less likely they will pass on deleterious genes to their offspring. Thus, if a Caucasian woman were to marry an Asian man, and both believed that their different genotypes meant a higher probability of passing on normal genes to their children, then they could be said to practice negative eugenics. They would want to ensure that any of their children did not have a high risk of inheriting mutations that would likely result in disease. Unlike the example of positive eugenics given above, there would be nothing morally objectionable about this practice because the parents' intention would be to reduce the risk of disease in their children and thereby prevent them from harm.

Similar reasoning applies to the case of a rabbi who advises a man and woman who are Orthodox Ashkenazi Jews and carriers of the Tay-Sachs allele not to marry, or else not to have children. Provided that the rabbi's advice was not coercive and the couple made a voluntary, informed decision, this too would be a morally defensible form of negative eugenics. It would aim at preventing harm by eliminating the risk of having a child with Tay-Sachs disease.

It might be more appropriate to call this last preventive strategy a form of *euphenics*, a beneficial manipulation of environmental factors to prevent or treat diseases.[35] Better education and nutrition would be more effective ways of achieving this goal in the general population. Still, genetic testing for the presence of mutations making people susceptible to various diseases can be part of a general euphenics program. Knowing the symptoms and genetic cause of a disease may enable us to devise treatments

that can control its symptoms. Again, the best-known disorder fitting this description is PKU. Restricting an affected child's dietary intake of phenylalanine can neutralize the harmful effects of this disorder and ensure a life without severe mental retardation. In addition, people with sickle-cell anemia can avoid morbidity by taking penicillin, and those with alpha-thalassemia may be cured by bone-marrow transplantation. The social environment can play an important role as well. I already have pointed out that the severity of schizophrenia can be controlled to some extent by familial and social support of those who have the disorder. Despite differences of definition, ultimately the goal of both negative eugenics and euphenics is the same—health promotion through prevention and treatment of disease.

As in the distinction between gene therapy and genetic enhancement, the main distinction between negative and positive eugenics is that the first is based on the principle of beneficence and the second on the principle of perfectionism. In gene therapy, the goal is to benefit people by restoring or raising them to adequate physical and mental functioning and giving them opportunities to achieve a decent minimum level of lifetime well-being. In genetic enhancement, the goal is to give additional benefits to people who already have adequate functioning, perfecting their traits and capacities and giving them an advantage over others in competing for social goods. In the first case, we are morally obligated to create people *without* certain traits, or to remove these traits once they exist. But we are obligated to do this only if the traits in question cause severe disease and disability and severely restrict people's opportunities. In the second case, we are morally obligated to create people *with* certain traits, or to add them to existing people in order to raise their functioning and increase their opportunities above the norm for persons. But how can we be so sure that negative eugenics will not evolve into positive eugenics? Is there not a slippery slope here?

Bernard Williams notes that the slippery-slope argument "is often applied to matters of medical practice. If X is allowed, the argument goes, then there will be a natural progression to Y."[36] For present purposes, we can take X to represent gene therapy and negative eugenics, and Y to represent genetic enhancement and positive eugenics. The natural progression from X, with the ostensible aim of raising or restoring people's functioning to a normal level, to Y leads to the "horrible result" of positive eugenics at the bottom of the slope.[37] Presumably, what makes the eugenic slope slippery is that once we get on the negative side, we cannot get off and fall on to the positive side. The point of the argument is that we should not get on the slope to begin with. Negative eugenics is not morally justifiable and should not be practiced, because it inevitably leads to the positive eugenics and the violations of human value and dignity that it entails.

Many invoke the slippery-slope argument to reject controversial practices in biotechnology. But if the argument is to serve as a ground for rejecting these practices, then it must be sound. True premises must entail the conclusion. Let us now examine the logical form of the argument as it is applied to eugenics and determine whether it is sound.

There are three different species of the slippery-slope argument: conceptual—relating to vagueness of terms; precedential—relating to the need to treat similar cases consistently; and causal—relating to the avoidance of the actions that will initiate a sequence of events leading to an undesirable result.[38] The classic or generic argument, the one most often advanced in discussions of biotechnology, includes aspects of all three species. First, defenders of the slippery-slope argument exploit any vagueness in the definition of terms. They claim that the difference between treatment and enhancement is vague, since many enhancements really are treatments,

and vice versa. Treatments and enhancements fall along a single continuum of medical interventions; the difference between them is one of degree rather than of kind. Second, they claim that, since treatments and enhancements involve only differences of degree, cases germane to one are assimilable to cases germane to the other. Consistency requires that we treat relevantly similar cases in the same way, and since cases of treatment and enhancement (negative and positive eugenics) are relevantly similar, cases of one are assimilable, or logically linked, to cases of the other. Third, they claim that, since treatment and enhancement are assimilable to each other, cases of one will cause cases of the other. This embodies the idea of the dangerous precedent. That is, case (a) may be prima facie acceptable, while cases (b), (c), and (n) are not. Yet, because (a) is relevantly similar and thus assimilable to (b), (c), and (n), doing (a) would set a dangerous precedent, as it would cause (b), (c), and (n). Therefore, (a) should not be permitted.[39]

Incorporating aspects of all three of the more particular arguments that I have just laid out, the logical form of the more general slippery-slope argument for the issue at hand looks something like this:

1. Case (a)—an instance of treatment, negative eugenics—is prima facie acceptable.
2. But cases (b), (c), ... and (n)—instances of enhancement, positive eugenics—are unacceptable.
3. Cases (a) through (n) are assimilable, as they differ from each other only in degree, falling along a continuum of cases of the same type.
4. Case (a), if permitted, will be a precedent for cases (b) through (n).
5. Permitting (a) will cause (b) through (n).
6. Therefore, case (a) should not be permitted.

The Case Against Perfection: What's Wrong with Designer Children, Bionic Athletes, and Genetic Engineering

Michael J. Sandel

reakthroughs in genetics present us with a promise and a predicament. The promise is that we may soon be able to treat and prevent a host of debilitating diseases. The predicament is that our newfound genetic knowledge may also enable us to manipulate our own nature—to enhance our muscles, memories, and moods; to choose the sex, height, and other genetic traits of our children; to make ourselves "better than well." When science moves faster than moral understanding, as it does today, men and women struggle to articulate their unease. In liberal societies they reach first for the language of autonomy, fairness, and individual rights. But this part of our moral vocabulary is ill equipped to address the hardest questions posed by genetic engineering. The genomic revolution has induced a kind of moral vertigo.

Consider cloning. The birth of Dolly the cloned sheep, in 1997, brought a torrent of concern about the prospect of cloned human beings. There are good medical reasons to worry. Most scientists agree that cloning is unsafe, likely to produce offspring with serious abnormalities. (Dolly recently died a premature death.) But suppose technology improved to the point where clones were at no greater risk than naturally conceived offspring. Would human cloning still be objectionable? Should our hesitation be moral as well as medical? What, exactly, is wrong with creating a child who is a genetic twin of one parent, or of an older sibling who has tragically died—or, for that matter, of an admired scientist, sports star, or celebrity?

Some say cloning is wrong because it violates the right to autonomy: by choosing a child's genetic makeup in advance, parents deny the child's right to an open future. A similar objection can be raised against any form of bioengineering that allows parents to select or reject genetic characteristics. According to this argument, genetic enhancements for musical talent, say, or athletic prowess, would point children toward particular choices, and so designer children would never be fully free.

At first glance the autonomy argument seems to capture what is troubling about human cloning and other forms of genetic engineering. It is not persuasive, for two reasons. First, it wrongly implies that absent a designing parent, children are free to choose their characteristics for themselves. But none of us chooses his genetic inheritance. The alternative to a cloned or genetically enhanced child is not one whose future is unbound by particular talents but one at the mercy of the genetic lottery.

Second, even if a concern for autonomy explains some of our worries about made-to-order children, it cannot explain our moral hesitation about people who seek genetic remedies or enhancements for themselves. Gene therapy on somatic (that is, nonreproductive) cells, such as muscle cells and brain cells, repairs or replaces defective genes. The moral quandary arises when people use such therapy not to cure a disease but to reach beyond health, to enhance their physical or cognitive capacities, to lift themselves above the norm.

Like cosmetic surgery, genetic enhancement employs medical means for nonmedical ends—ends unrelated to curing or preventing disease or repairing injury. But unlike cosmetic surgery, genetic enhancement is more than skin-deep. If we are ambivalent about surgery or Botox injections for sagging chins and furrowed brows, we are all the more troubled by genetic engineering for stronger bodies, sharper memories, greater intelligence, and happier moods. The question is whether we are right to be troubled, and if so, on what grounds.

In order to grapple with the ethics of enhancement, we need to confront questions largely lost from view—questions about the moral status of nature, and about the proper stance of human beings toward the given world. Since these questions verge on theology, modern philosophers and political theorists tend to shrink from them. But our new powers of biotechnology make them unavoidable. To see why this is so, consider four examples already on the horizon: muscle enhancement, memory enhancement, growth-hormone treatment, and reproductive technologies that enable parents to choose the sex and some genetic traits of their children. In each case what began as an attempt to treat a disease or prevent a genetic disorder now beckons as an instrument of improvement and consumer choice.

Muscles. Everyone would welcome a gene therapy to alleviate muscular dystrophy and to reverse the debilitating muscle loss that comes with old age. But what if the same therapy were used to improve athletic performance? Researchers have developed a synthetic gene that, when injected into the muscle cells of mice, prevents and even reverses natural muscle deterioration. The gene not only repairs wasted or injured muscles but also strengthens healthy ones. This success bodes well for human applications. H. Lee Sweeney, of the University of Pennsylvania, who leads the research, hopes his discovery will cure the immobility that afflicts the elderly. But Sweeney's bulked-up mice have already attracted the attention of athletes seeking a competitive edge. Although the therapy is not yet approved for human use, the prospect of genetically enhanced weight lifters, home-run sluggers, linebackers, and sprinters is easy to imagine. The widespread use of steroids and other performance-improving drugs in professional sports suggests that many athletes will be eager to avail themselves of genetic enhancement.

Suppose for the sake of argument that muscle-enhancing gene therapy, unlike steroids, turned out to be safe—or at least no riskier than a rigorous weight-training regimen. Would there be a reason to ban its use in sports? There is something unsettling about the image of genetically altered athletes lifting SUVs or hitting 650-foot home runs or running a three-minute mile. But what, exactly, is troubling about it? Is it simply that we find such superhuman spectacles too bizarre to contemplate? Or does our unease point to something of ethical significance?

It might be argued that a genetically enhanced athlete, like a drug-enhanced athlete, would have an unfair advantage over his unenhanced competitors. But the fairness argument against enhancement has a fatal flaw: it has always been the case that some athletes are better endowed genetically than others, and yet we do not consider this to undermine the fairness of competitive sports. From the standpoint of fairness, enhanced genetic differences would be no worse than natural ones, assuming they were safe and made available to all. If genetic enhancement in sports is morally objectionable, it must be for reasons other than fairness.

Memory. Genetic enhancement is possible for brains as well as brawn. In the mid-1990s scientists managed to manipulate a memory-linked gene in fruit flies, creating flies with photographic memories. More recently researchers have produced smart mice by inserting extra copies of a memory-related gene into mouse embryos. The altered mice learn more quickly and remember things longer than normal mice. The extra copies were programmed to remain active even in old age, and the improvement was passed on to offspring.

Human memory is more complicated, but biotech companies, including Memory Pharmaceuticals, are in hot pursuit of memory-enhancing drugs, or "cognition enhancers," for human beings. The obvious market for such drugs consists of those who suffer from Alzheimer's and other serious memory disorders. The companies also have their sights on a bigger market: the 81 million Americans over fifty, who are beginning to encounter the memory loss that comes naturally with age. A drug that reversed age-related memory loss would be a bonanza for the pharmaceutical industry: a Viagra for the brain. Such use would straddle the line between remedy and enhancement. Unlike a treatment for Alzheimer's, it would cure no disease; but insofar as it restored capacities a person once possessed, it would have a remedial aspect. It could also have purely nonmedical uses: for example, by a lawyer cramming to memorize facts for an upcoming trial, or by a business executive eager to learn Mandarin on the eve of his departure for Shanghai.

Some who worry about the ethics of cognitive enhancement point to the danger of creating two classes of human beings: those with access to enhancement technologies, and those who must make do with their natural capacities. And if the enhancements could be passed down the generations, the two classes might eventually become subspecies—the enhanced and the merely natural. But worry about access ignores the moral status of enhancement itself. Is the scenario troubling because the unenhanced poor would be denied the benefits of bioengineering, or because the enhanced affluent would somehow be dehumanized? As with muscles, so with memory: the fundamental question is not how to ensure equal access to enhancement but whether we should aspire to it in the first place.

Height. Pediatricians already struggle with the ethics of enhancement when confronted by parents who want to make their children taller. Since the 1980s human growth hormone has been approved for children with a hormone deficiency that makes them much shorter than average. But the treatment also increases the height of healthy children. Some parents of healthy children who are unhappy with their stature (typically boys) ask why it should make a difference whether a child is short because of a hormone deficiency or because his parents happen to be short. Whatever the cause, the social consequences are the same.

In the face of this argument some doctors began prescribing hormone treatments for children whose short stature was unrelated to any medical problem. By 1996 such "off-label" use accounted for 40 percent of human-growth-hormone prescriptions. Although it is legal to prescribe drugs for purposes not approved by the Food and Drug Administration, pharmaceutical companies cannot promote such use. Seeking to expand its market, Eli Lilly & Co. recently persuaded the FDA to approve its human growth hormone for healthy children whose projected adult height is in the bottom one percentile—under five feet three inches for boys and four feet eleven inches for girls. This concession raises a large question about the ethics of enhancement: If hormone treatments need not be limited to those with hormone deficiencies, why should they be available only to very short children? Why shouldn't all shorter-than-average children be able to seek treatment? And what about a child of average height who wants to be taller so that he can make the basketball team?

Some oppose height enhancement on the grounds that it is collectively self-defeating; as some become taller, others become shorter relative to the norm. Except in Lake Wobegon, not every child can be above average. As the unenhanced began to feel shorter, they, too, might seek treatment, leading to a hormonal arms race that left everyone worse off, especially those who couldn't afford to buy their way up from shortness.

But the arms-race objection is not decisive on its own. Like the fairness objection to bioengineered muscles and memory, it leaves unexamined the attitudes and dispositions that prompt the drive for enhancement. If we were bothered only by the injustice of adding shortness to the problems of the poor, we could remedy that unfairness by publicly subsidizing height enhancements. As for the relative height deprivation suffered by innocent bystanders, we could compensate them by taxing those who buy their way to greater height. The real question is whether we want to live in a society where parents feel compelled to spend a fortune to make perfectly healthy kids a few inches taller.

Sex selection. Perhaps the most inevitable nonmedical use of bioengineering is sex selection. For centuries parents have been trying to choose the sex of their children. Today biotech succeeds where folk remedies failed.

One technique for sex selection arose with prenatal tests using amniocentesis and ultrasound. These medical technologies were developed to detect genetic abnormalities such as spina bifida and Down syndrome. But they can also reveal the sex of the fetus—allowing for the abortion of a fetus of an undesired sex. Even among those who favor abortion rights, few advocate abortion simply because the parents do not want a girl. Nevertheless, in traditional societies with a powerful cultural preference for boys, this practice has become widespread.

Sex selection need not involve abortion, however. For couples undergoing *in vitro* fertilization (IVF), it is possible to choose the sex of the child before the fertilized egg is implanted in the womb. One method makes use of preimplantation genetic diagnosis (PGD), a procedure developed to screen for genetic diseases. Several eggs are fertilized in a petri dish and grown to the eight-cell stage (about three days). At that point the embryos are tested to determine their sex. Those of the desired sex are implanted; the others are typically discarded. Although few couples are likely to undergo the difficulty and expense of IVF simply to choose the sex of their child, embryo screening is a highly reliable means of sex selection. And as our genetic knowledge increases, it may be possible to use PGD to cull embryos carrying undesired genes, such as those associated with obesity, height, and skin color. The science-fiction movie *Gattaca* depicts a future in which parents routinely screen embryos for sex, height, immunity to disease, and even IQ. There is something troubling about the *Gattaca* scenario, but it is not easy to identify what exactly is wrong with screening embryos to choose the sex of our children.

One line of objection draws on arguments familiar from the abortion debate. Those who believe that an embryo is a person reject embryo screening for the same reasons they reject abortion. If an eight-cell embryo growing in a petri dish is morally equivalent to a fully developed human being, then discarding it is no better than aborting a fetus, and both practices are equivalent to infanticide. Whatever its merits, however, this "pro-life" objection is not an argument against sex selection as such.

The latest technology poses the question of sex selection unclouded by the matter of an embryo's moral status. The Genetics & IVF Institute, a for-profit infertility clinic in Fairfax, Virginia, now offers a sperm-sorting technique that makes it possible to choose the sex of one's child before it is conceived. X-bearing sperm, which produce girls, carry more DNA than Y-bearing sperm, which produce boys; a device called a flow cytometer can separate them. The process, called MicroSort, has a high rate of success.

If sex selection by sperm sorting is objectionable, it must be for reasons that go beyond the debate about the moral status of the embryo. One such reason is that sex selection is an instrument of sex discrimination—typically against girls, as illustrated by the chilling sex ratios in India and China. Some speculate that societies with substantially more men than women will be less stable, more violent, and more prone to crime or war. These are legitimate worries—but the sperm-sorting company has a clever way of addressing them. It offers MicroSort only to couples who want to choose the sex of a child for purposes of "family balancing." Those with more sons than daughters may choose a girl, and vice versa. But customers may not use the technology to stock up on children of the same sex, or even to choose the sex of their firstborn child. (So far the majority of MicroSort clients have chosen girls.) Under restrictions of this kind, do any ethical issues remain that should give us pause?

The case of MicroSort helps us isolate the moral objections that would persist if muscle-enhancement, memory-enhancement, and height-enhancement technologies were safe and available to all.

It is commonly said that genetic enhancements undermine our humanity by threatening our capacity to act freely, to succeed by our own efforts, and to consider ourselves responsible—worthy of praise or blame—for the things we do and for the way we are. It is one thing to hit seventy home runs as the result of disciplined training and effort, and something else, something less, to hit them with the help of steroids or genetically enhanced muscles. Of course, the roles of effort and enhancement will be a matter of degree. But as the role of enhancement increases, our admiration for the achievement fades—or, rather, our admiration for the achievement shifts from the player to his pharmacist. This suggests that our moral response to enhancement is a response to the diminished agency of the person whose achievement is enhanced.

Though there is much to be said for this argument, I do not think the main problem with enhancement and genetic engineering is that they undermine effort and erode human agency.

The deeper danger is that they represent a kind of hyperagency—a Promethean aspiration to remake nature, including human nature, to serve our purposes and satisfy our desires. The problem is not the drift to mechanism but the drive to mastery. And what the drive to mastery misses and may even destroy is an appreciation of the gifted character of human powers and achievements.

To acknowledge the giftedness of life is to recognize that our talents and powers are not wholly our own doing, despite the effort we expend to develop and to exercise them. It is also to recognize that not everything in the world is open to whatever use we may desire or devise. Appreciating the gifted quality of life constrains the Promethean project and conduces to a certain humility. It is in part a religious sensibility. But its resonance reaches beyond religion.

It is difficult to account for what we admire about human activity and achievement without drawing upon some version of this idea. Consider two types of athletic achievement. We appreciate players like Pete Rose, who are not blessed with great natural gifts but who manage, through striving, grit, and determination, to excel in their sport. But we also admire players like Joe DiMaggio, who display natural gifts with grace and effortlessness. Now, suppose we learned that both players took performance-enhancing drugs. Whose turn to drugs would we find more deeply disillusioning? Which aspect of the athletic ideal—effort or gift—would be more deeply offended?

Some might say effort: the problem with drugs is that they provide a shortcut, a way to win without striving. But striving is not the point of sports; excellence is. And excellence consists at least partly in the display of natural talents and gifts that are no doing of the athlete who possesses them. This is an uncomfortable fact for democratic societies. We want to believe that success, in sports and in life, is something we earn, not something we inherit. Natural gifts, and the admiration they inspire, embarrass the meritocratic faith; they cast doubt on the conviction that praise and rewards flow from effort alone. In the face of this embarrassment we inflate the moral significance of striving, and depreciate giftedness. This distortion can be seen, for example, in network-television coverage of the Olympics, which focuses less on the feats the athletes perform than on heartrending stories of the hardships they have overcome and the struggles they have waged to triumph over an injury or a difficult upbringing or political turmoil in their native land.

But effort isn't everything. No one believes that a mediocre basketball player who works and trains even harder than Michael Jordan deserves greater acclaim or a bigger contract. The real problem with genetically altered athletes is that they corrupt athletic competition as a human activity that honors the cultivation and display of natural talents. From this standpoint, enhancement can be seen as the ultimate expression of the ethic of effort and willfulness—a kind of high-tech striving. The ethic of willfulness and the biotechnological powers it now enlists are arrayed against the claims of giftedness.

The ethic of giftedness, under siege in sports, persists in the practice of parenting. But here, too, bioengineering and genetic enhancement threaten to dislodge it. To appreciate children as gifts is to accept them as they come, not as objects of our design or products of our will or instruments of our ambition. Parental love is not contingent on the talents and attributes a child happens to have. We choose our friends and spouses at least partly on the basis of qualities we find attractive. But we do not choose our children. Their qualities are unpredictable, and even the most conscientious parents cannot be held wholly responsible for the kind of children they have. That is why parenthood, more than other human relationships, teaches what the theologian William F. May calls an "openness to the unbidden."

May's resonant phrase helps us see that the deepest moral objection to enhancement lies less in the perfection it seeks than in the human disposition it expresses and promotes. The problem is not that parents usurp the autonomy of a child they design. The problem lies in the hubris of the designing parents, in their drive to master the mystery of birth. Even if this disposition did not make parents tyrants to their children, it would disfigure the relation between parent and child, and deprive the parent of the humility and enlarged human sympathies that an openness to the unbidden can cultivate.

To appreciate children as gifts or blessings is not, of course, to be passive in the face of illness or disease. Medical intervention to cure or prevent illness or restore the injured to health does not desecrate nature but honors it. Healing sickness or injury does not override a child's natural capacities but permits them to flourish.

Nor does the sense of life as a gift mean that parents must shrink from shaping and directing the development of their child. Just as athletes and artists have an obligation to cultivate their talents, so parents have an obligation to cultivate their children, to help them discover and develop their talents and gifts. As May points out, parents give their children two kinds of love: accepting love and transforming love. Accepting love affirms the being of the child, whereas transforming love seeks the well-being of the child. Each aspect corrects the excesses of the other, he writes: "Attachment becomes too quietistic if it slackens into mere acceptance of the child as he is." Parents have a duty to promote their children's excellence.

These days, however, overly ambitious parents are prone to get carried away with transforming love—promoting and demanding all manner of accomplishments from their children, seeking perfection. "Parents find it difficult to maintain an equilibrium between the two sides of love," May observes. "Accepting love, without transforming love, slides into indulgence and finally neglect. Transforming love, without accepting love, badgers and finally rejects." May finds in these competing impulses a parallel with modern science: it, too, engages us in beholding the given world, studying and savoring it, and also in molding the world, transforming and perfecting it.

The mandate to mold our children, to cultivate and improve them, complicates the case against enhancement. We usually admire parents who seek the best for their children, who spare no effort to help them achieve happiness and success. Some parents confer advantages on their children by enrolling them in expensive schools, hiring private tutors, sending them to tennis camp, providing them with piano lessons, ballet lessons, swimming lessons, SAT-prep courses, and so on. If it is permissible and even admirable for parents to help their children in these ways, why isn't it equally admirable for parents to use whatever genetic technologies may emerge (provided they are safe) to enhance their children's intelligence, musical ability, or athletic prowess?

The defenders of enhancement are right to this extent: improving children through genetic engineering is similar in spirit to the heavily managed, high-pressure child-rearing that is now common. But this similarity does not vindicate genetic enhancement. On the contrary, it highlights a problem with the trend toward hyperparenting. One conspicuous example of this trend is sports-crazed parents bent on making champions of their children. Another is the frenzied drive of overbearing parents to mold and manage their children's academic careers.

As the pressure for performance increases, so does the need to help distractible children concentrate on the task at hand. This may be why diagnoses of attention deficit and hyperactivity disorder have increased so sharply. Lawrence Diller, a pediatrician and the author of *Running on Ritalin*, estimates that five to six percent of American children under eighteen (a total of four to five million kids) are currently prescribed Ritalin, Adderall, and other stimulants, the treatment of choice for ADHD. (Stimulants counteract hyperactivity by making it easier to focus and sustain attention.) The number of Ritalin prescriptions for children and adolescents has tripled over the past decade, but not all users suffer from attention disorders or hyperactivity.

High school and college students have learned that prescription stimulants improve concentration for those with normal attention spans, and some buy or borrow their classmates' drugs to enhance their performance on the SAT or other exams. Since stimulants work for both medical and nonmedical purposes, they raise the same moral questions posed by other technologies of enhancement.

However those questions are resolved, the debate reveals the cultural distance we have traveled since the debate over marijuana, LSD, and other drugs a generation ago. Unlike the drugs of the 1960s and 1970s, Ritalin and Adderall are not for checking out but for buckling down, not for beholding the world and taking it in but for molding the world and fitting in. We used to speak of nonmedical drug use as "recreational." That term no longer applies. The steroids and stimulants that figure in the enhancement debate are not a source of recreation but a bid for compliance—a way of answering a competitive society's demand to improve our performance and perfect our nature. This demand for performance and perfection animates the impulse to rail against the given. It is the deepest source of the moral trouble with enhancement.

Some see a clear line between genetic enhancement and other ways that people seek improvement in their children and themselves. Genetic manipulation seems somehow worse—more intrusive, more sinister—than other ways of enhancing performance and seeking success. But morally speaking, the difference is less significant than it seems. Bioengineering gives us reason to question the low-tech, high-pressure child-rearing practices we commonly accept. The hyperparenting familiar in our time represents an anxious excess of mastery and dominion that misses the sense of life as a gift. This draws it disturbingly close to eugenics.

The shadow of eugenics hangs over today's debates about genetic engineering and enhancement. Critics of genetic engineering argue that human cloning, enhancement, and the quest for designer children are nothing more than "privatized" or "free-market" eugenics. Defenders of enhancement reply that genetic choices freely made are not really eugenic—at least not in the pejorative sense. To remove the coercion, they argue, is to remove the very thing that makes eugenic policies repugnant.

Sorting out the lesson of eugenics is another way of wrestling with the ethics of enhancement. The Nazis gave eugenics a bad name. But what, precisely, was wrong with it? Was the old eugenics objectionable only insofar as it was coercive? Or is there something inherently wrong with the resolve to deliberately design our progeny's traits?

James Watson, the biologist who, with Francis Crick, discovered the structure of DNA, sees nothing wrong with genetic engineering and enhancement, provided they are freely chosen rather than state-imposed. And yet Watson's language contains more than a whiff of the old eugenic sensibility. "If you really are stupid, I would call that a disease," he recently told *The Times* of London. "The lower 10 percent who really have difficulty, even in elementary school, what's the cause of it? A lot of people would like to say, 'Well, poverty, things like that.' It probably isn't. So I'd like to get rid of that, to help the lower 10 percent." A few years ago Watson stirred controversy by saying that if a gene for homosexuality were discovered, a woman should be free to abort a fetus that carried it. When his remark provoked an uproar, he replied that he was not singling out gays but asserting a principle: women should be free to abort fetuses for any reason of genetic preference—for example, if the child would be dyslexic, or lacking musical talent, or too short to play basketball.

Watson's scenarios are clearly objectionable to those for whom all abortion is an unspeakable crime. But for those who do not subscribe to the pro-life position, these scenarios raise a hard question: If it is morally troubling to contemplate abortion to avoid a gay child or a dyslexic one, doesn't this suggest that something is wrong with acting on any eugenic preference, even when no state coercion is involved?

Consider the market in eggs and sperm. The advent of artificial insemination allows prospective parents to shop for gametes with the genetic traits they desire in their offspring. It is a less predictable way to design children than cloning or pre-implantation genetic screening, but it offers a good example of a procreative practice in which the old eugenics meets the new consumerism. A few years ago some Ivy League newspapers ran an ad seeking an egg from a woman who was at least five feet ten inches tall and athletic, had no major family medical problems, and had a combined SAT score of 1400 or above. The ad offered $50,000 for an egg from a donor with these traits. More recently a Web site was launched claiming to auction eggs from fashion models whose photos appeared on the site, at starting bids of $15,000 to $150,000.

On what grounds, if any, is the egg market morally objectionable? Since no one is forced to buy or sell, it cannot be wrong for reasons of coercion. Some might worry that hefty prices would exploit poor women by presenting them with an offer they couldn't refuse. But the designer eggs that fetch the highest prices are likely to be sought from the privileged, not the poor. If the market for premium eggs gives us moral qualms, this, too, shows that concerns about eugenics are not put to rest by freedom of choice.

A tale of two sperm banks helps explain why. The Repository for Germinal Choice, one of America's first sperm banks, was not a commercial enterprise. It was opened in 1980 by Robert Graham, a philanthropist dedicated to improving the world's "germ plasm" and counteracting the rise of "retrograde humans." His plan was to collect the sperm of Nobel Prize-winning scientists and make it available to women of high intelligence, in hopes of breeding supersmart babies. But Graham had trouble persuading Nobel laureates to donate their sperm for his bizarre scheme, and so settled for sperm from young scientists of high promise. His sperm bank closed in 1999.

In contrast, California Cryobank, one of the world's leading sperm banks, is a for-profit company with no overt eugenic mission. Cappy Rothman, M.D., a co-founder of the firm, has nothing but disdain for Graham's eugenics, although the standards Cryobank imposes on the sperm it recruits are exacting. Cryobank has offices in Cambridge, Massachusetts, between Harvard and MIT, and in Palo Alto, California, near Stanford. It advertises for donors in campus newspapers (compensation up to $900 a month), and accepts less than five percent of the men who apply. Cryobank's marketing materials play up the prestigious source of its sperm. Its catalogue provides detailed information about the physical characteristics of each donor, along with his ethnic origin and college major. For an extra fee prospective customers can buy the results of a test that assesses the donor's temperament and character type. Rothman reports that Cryobank's ideal sperm donor is six feet tall, with brown eyes, blond hair, and dimples, and has a college degree—not because the company wants to propagate those traits, but because those are the traits his customers want: "If our customers wanted high school dropouts, we would give them high school dropouts."

Not everyone objects to marketing sperm. But anyone who is troubled by the eugenic aspect of the Nobel Prize sperm bank should be equally troubled by Cryobank, consumer-driven though it be. What, after all, is the moral difference between designing children according to an explicit eugenic purpose and designing children according to the dictates of the market? Whether the aim is to improve humanity's "germ plasm" or to cater to consumer preferences, both practices are eugenic insofar as both make children into products of deliberate design.

A number of political philosophers call for a new "liberal eugenics." They argue that a moral distinction can be drawn between the old eugenic policies and genetic enhancements that do not restrict the autonomy of the child. "While old-fashioned authoritarian eugenicists sought to produce citizens out of a single centrally designed mould," writes Nicholas Agar, "the distinguishing mark of the new liberal eugenics is

state neutrality." Government may not tell parents what sort of children to design, and parents may engineer in their children only those traits that improve their capacities without biasing their choice of life plans. A recent text on genetics and justice, written by the bioethicists Allen Buchanan, Dan W. Brock, Norman Daniels, and Daniel Wikler, offers a similar view. The "bad reputation of eugenics," they write, is due to practices that "might be avoidable in a future eugenic program." The problem with the old eugenics was that its burdens fell disproportionately on the weak and the poor, who were unjustly sterilized and segregated. But provided that the benefits and burdens of genetic improvement are fairly distributed, these bioethicists argue, eugenic measures are unobjectionable and may even be morally required.

The libertarian philosopher Robert Nozick proposed a "genetic supermarket" that would enable parents to order children by design without imposing a single design on the society as a whole: "This supermarket system has the great virtue that it involves no centralized decision fixing the future human type(s)."

Even the leading philosopher of American liberalism, John Rawls, in his classic A Theory of Justice (1971), offered a brief endorsement of noncoercive eugenics. Even in a society that agrees to share the benefits and burdens of the genetic lottery, it is "in the interest of each to have greater natural assets," Rawls wrote. "This enables him to pursue a preferred plan of life." The parties to the social contract "want to insure for their descendants the best genetic endowment (assuming their own to be fixed)." Eugenic policies are therefore not only permissible but required as a matter of justice. "Thus over time a society is to take steps at least to preserve the general level of natural abilities and to prevent the diffusion of serious defects."

But removing the coercion does not vindicate eugenics. The problem with eugenics and genetic engineering is that they represent the one-sided triumph of willfulness over giftedness, of dominion over reverence, of molding over beholding. Why, we may wonder, should we worry about this triumph? Why not shake off our unease about genetic enhancement as so much superstition? What would be lost if biotechnology dissolved our sense of giftedness?

From a religious standpoint the answer is clear: To believe that our talents and powers are wholly our own doing is to misunderstand our place in creation, to confuse our role with God's. Religion is not the only source of reasons to care about giftedness, however. The moral stakes can also be described in secular terms. If bioengineering made the myth of the "self-made man" come true, it would be difficult to view our talents as gifts for which we are indebted, rather than as achievements for which we are responsible. This would transform three key features of our moral landscape: humility, responsibility, and solidarity.

In a social world that prizes mastery and control, parenthood is a school for humility. That we care deeply about our children and yet cannot choose the kind we want teaches parents to be open to the unbidden. Such openness is a disposition worth affirming, not only within families but in the wider world as well. It invites us to abide the unexpected, to live with dissonance, to rein in the impulse to control. A *Gattaca*-like world in which parents became accustomed to specifying the sex and genetic traits of their children would be a world inhospitable to the unbidden, a gated community writ large. The awareness that our talents and abilities are not wholly our own doing restrains our tendency toward hubris.

Though some maintain that genetic enhancement erodes human agency by overriding effort, the real problem is the explosion, not the erosion, of responsibility. As humility gives way, responsibility expands to daunting proportions. We attribute less to chance and more to choice. Parents become responsible for choosing, or failing to choose, the right traits for their children. Athletes become responsible for acquiring, or failing to acquire, the talents that will help their teams win.

One of the blessings of seeing ourselves as creatures of nature, God, or fortune is that we are not wholly responsible for the way we are. The more we become masters of our genetic endowments, the greater the burden we bear for the talents we have and the way we perform. Today when a basketball player misses a rebound, his coach can blame him for being out of position. Tomorrow the coach may blame him for being too short. Even now the use of performance-enhancing drugs in professional sports is subtly transforming the expectations players have for one another; on some teams players who take the field free from amphetamines or other stimulants are criticized for "playing naked."

The more alive we are to the chanced nature of our lot, the more reason we have to share our fate with others. Consider insurance. Since people do not know whether or when various ills will befall them, they pool their risk by buying health insurance and life insurance. As life plays itself out, the healthy wind up subsidizing the unhealthy, and those who live to a ripe old age wind up subsidizing the families of those who die before their time. Even without a sense of mutual obligation, people pool their risks and resources and share one another's fate.

But insurance markets mimic solidarity only insofar as people do not know or control their own risk factors. Suppose genetic testing advanced to the point where it could reliably predict each person's medical future and life expectancy. Those confident of good health and long life would opt out of the pool, causing other people's premiums to skyrocket. The solidarity of insurance would disappear as those with good genes fled the actuarial company of those with bad ones.

The fear that insurance companies would use genetic data to assess risks and set premiums recently led the Senate to vote to prohibit genetic discrimination in health insurance. But the bigger danger, admittedly more speculative, is that genetic enhancement, if routinely practiced, would make it harder to foster the moral sentiments that social solidarity requires.

Why, after all, do the successful owe anything to the least-advantaged members of society? The best answer to this question leans heavily on the notion of giftedness. The natural talents that enable the successful to flourish are not their own doing but, rather, their good fortune—a result of the genetic lottery. If our genetic endowments are gifts, rather than achievements for which we can claim credit, it is a mistake and a conceit to assume that we are entitled to the full measure of the bounty they reap in a market economy. We therefore have an obligation to share this bounty with those who, through no fault of their own, lack comparable gifts.

A lively sense of the contingency of our gifts—a consciousness that none of us is wholly responsible for his or her success—saves a meritocratic society from sliding into the smug assumption that the rich are rich because they are more deserving than the poor. Without this, the successful would become even more likely than they are now to view themselves as self-made and self-sufficient, and hence wholly responsible for their success. Those at the bottom of society would be viewed not as disadvantaged, and thus worthy of a measure of compensation, but as simply unfit, and thus worthy of eugenic repair. The meritocracy, less chastened by chance, would become harder, less forgiving. As perfect genetic knowledge would end the simulacrum of solidarity in insurance markets, so perfect genetic control would erode the actual solidarity that arises when men and women reflect on the contingency of their talents and fortunes. hirty-five years ago Robert L. Sinsheimer, a molecular biologist at the California Institute of Technology, glimpsed the shape of things to come. In an article titled "The Prospect of Designed Genetic Change" he argued that freedom of choice would vindicate the new genetics, and set it apart from the discredited eugenics of old.

To implement the older eugenics ... would have required a massive social programme carried out over many generations. Such a programme could not have been initiated without the consent and co-operation of a major fraction of the population, and would have been continuously subject to social control. In contrast, the new eugenics could, at least in principle, be implemented on a quite individual basis, in one generation, and subject to no existing restrictions. According to Sinsheimer, the new eugenics would be voluntary rather than coerced, and also more humane. Rather than segregating and eliminating the unfit, it would improve them. "The old eugenics would have required a continual selection for breeding of the fit, and a culling of the unfit," he wrote. "The new eugenics would permit in principle the conversion of all the unfit to the highest genetic level."

Sinsheimer's paean to genetic engineering caught the heady, Promethean self-image of the age. He wrote hopefully of rescuing "the losers in that chromosomal lottery that so firmly channels our human destinies," including not only those born with genetic defects but also "the 50,000,000 'normal' Americans with an IQ of less than 90." But he also saw that something bigger than improving on nature's "mindless, age-old throw of dice" was at stake. Implicit in technologies of genetic intervention was a more exalted place for human beings in the cosmos. "As we enlarge man's freedom, we diminish his constraints and that which he must accept as given," he wrote. Copernicus and Darwin had "demoted man from his bright glory at the focal point of the universe," but the new biology would restore his central role. In the mirror of our genetic knowledge we would see ourselves as more than a link in the chain of evolution: "We can be the agent of transition to a whole new pitch of evolution. This is a cosmic event."

There is something appealing, even intoxicating, about a vision of human freedom unfettered by the given. It may even be the case that the allure of that vision played a part in summoning the genomic age into being. It is often assumed that the powers of enhancement we now possess arose as an inadvertent by-product of biomedical progress—the genetic revolution came, so to speak, to cure disease, and stayed to tempt us with the prospect of enhancing our performance, designing our children, and perfecting our nature. That may have the story backwards. It is more plausible to view genetic engineering as the ultimate expression of our resolve to see ourselves astride the world, the masters of our nature. But that promise of mastery is flawed. It threatens to banish our appreciation of life as a gift, and to leave us with nothing to affirm or behold outside our own will.

The Moral Significance of the Therapy-Enhancement Distinction in Human Genetics

David B. Resnik

Introduction

The therapy-enhancement distinction occupies a central place in contemporary discussions of human genetics and has been the subject of much debate.[1-7] At a recent conference on gene therapy policy, scientists predicted that within a few years researchers will develop techniques that can be used to enhance human traits.[8] In thinking about the morality of genetic interventions, many writers have defended somatic gene therapy,[9,10] and some have defended germ-line gene therapy,[11,12] but only a handful of writers defend genetic enhancement[13], or even give it a fair hearing.[14-16] The mere mention of genetic enhancement makes many people cringe and brings to mind the Nazi eugenics programs, Aldous Huxley's *Brave New World*, "The X-Files," or the recent movie "Gattaca." Although many people believe that gene therapy has morally legitimate medical uses,[17,18] others regard genetic enhancement as morally problematic or decidedly evil.[19-21]

The purpose of this essay is to examine the moral significance of the therapy-enhancement distinction in human genetics. Is genetic enhancement inherently unethical? Is genetic therapy inherently ethical? I will argue that the distinction does not mark a firm boundary between moral and immoral genetic interventions, and that genetic enhancement is not inherently immoral. To evaluate the acceptability of any particular genetic intervention, one needs to examine the relevant facts in light of moral principles. Some types of genetic therapy are morally acceptable while some types of genetic enhancement are unacceptable. In defending this view, I will discuss and evaluate several different ways of attempting to draw a solid moral line between therapy and enhancement.[22]

Somatic versus Germline Interventions

Before discussing the therapy-enhancement distinction, it is important that we understand another distinction that should inform our discussions, viz. the distinction between somatic and germline interventions.[23,24] Somatic interventions attempt to modify somatic cells, while germline interventions attempt to modify germ cells. The gene therapy clinical trials that have been performed thus far have been on somatic cells. If we combine these two distinctions, we obtain four types of genetic interventions:

Somatic genetic therapy (SGT)
Germline genetic therapy (GLGT)
Somatic genetic enhancement (SGE)
Germline genetic enhancement (GLGE)

While I accept the distinction between somatic and germline interventions, it is important to note that even interventions designed to affect somatic cells can also affect germ cells: current SGT trials carry a slight risk of altering germ cells.[25] Even so, one might argue that this is a morally significant distinction because somatic interventions usually affect only the patient, while germline interventions are likely to affect future generations.[26] In any case, the therapy-enhancement distinction encompasses somatic as well as germline interventions, and my discussion of this distinction will include both somatic as well as germline interventions.

The Concepts of Health and Disease

Perhaps the most popular way of thinking about the moral significance of the therapy-enhancement distinction is to argue that the aim of genetic therapy is to treat human diseases while the aim of genetic enhancement is to perform other kinds of interventions, such as altering or "improving" the human body.[27-29] Since genetic therapy serves morally legitimate goals, genetic therapy is morally acceptable; but since genetic enhancement serves morally questionable or illicit goals, genetic enhancement is not morally acceptable.[30-33] I suspect that many people view the distinction and its moral significance in precisely these terms. W. French Anderson states a clear case for the moral significance of genetic enhancement:

On medical and ethical grounds we should draw a line excluding any form of genetic engineering. We should not step over the line that delineates treatment from enhancement.[34]

However, this way of thinking of medical genetics makes at least two questionable assumptions: (1) that we have a clear and uncontroversial account of health and disease, and (2) that the goal of treating diseases is morally legitimate, while other goals are not. To examine these assumptions, we need to take a quick look at discussions about the concepts of health and disease.

The bioethics literature contains a thoughtful debate about the definitions of health and disease and it is not my aim to survey that terrain here.[35,36] However, I will distinguish between two basic approaches to the definition of health, a value-neutral (or descriptive) approach and a value-laden (or normative) one.[37] According to the value-neutral approach, health and disease are descriptive concepts that have an empirical, factual basis in human biology. Boorse defended one of the most influential descriptive approaches to health and disease: a diseased organism lacks the functional abilities of a normal member of its species.[38] To keep his approach value-neutral, Boorse interprets "normal" in statistical terms, i.e., "normal" = "typical." Daniels expands on Boorse's account of disease by suggesting that natural selection can provide an account of species-typical functions: functional abilities are traits that exist in populations because they have contributed to the reproduction and survival of organisms that possessed them.[39] Thus a human with healthy lungs has specific respiratory capacities that are normal in our species, and these capacities have been "designed" by natural selection. A human who lacks these capacities, such as someone with cystic fibrosis or emphysema, has a disease.

According to the value-laden approach, our concepts of health and disease are based on social, moral, and cultural norms. A healthy person is someone who falls within these norms; a diseased person deviates from them. Someone who deviates from species-typical functions could be considered healthy in a society that views that deviation as healthy: although schizophrenia has a biological basis, in some cultures schizophrenics are viewed as "gifted" or "sacred," while in other cultures they are viewed as "mentally ill." Likewise, some cultures view homosexuality as a disease, while others do not.[40-42]

Many different writers have tried to work out variants on these two basic approaches to health and disease, and some have tried to develop compromise views,[43,44] but suffice it to say that the first assumption mentioned above—i.e., that we have a clear and uncontroversial account of health and disease—is questionable.

Even if we lack an uncontroversial account of disease, we could still ask whether either of the two basic approaches would condemn genetic enhancement unconditionally. Consider the descriptive approach first. If statements about disease merely describe deviations from species-typical traits, does it follow that we may perform genetic interventions to treat diseases but not to enhance otherwise healthy people? Since we regard the concept of disease as descriptive, we cannot answer this question without making some normative assumptions. Saying that someone has a disease is like saying that he or she has red hair, is five feet tall, or was born in New York City. These descriptions of that person carry no normative import. Hence the descriptive account of disease, by itself, does not provide us with a way of drawing a solid moral line between therapy and enhancement. For this approach to disease to draw moral boundaries between therapy and enhancement, it needs to be supplemented by a normatively rich account of the rightness of therapy and wrongness of enhancement.

Perhaps the normative approach fairs better than the descriptive one. If we accept this view, it follows that therapy has some positive moral value, since therapy is an attempt to treat diseases, which are defined as traits or abilities that do not fall within social or cultural norms. If it is "bad" to have a disease, then we are morally justified in performing interventions that attempt to treat or prevent diseases, since these procedures impart "good" states of being. Thus this normative approach implies that therapy is morally right. But does it imply that enhancement is morally wrong? The answer to this question depends, in large part, on the scope of the concepts of health and disease. If we hold that the concept of health defines a set of traits and abilities that should be possessed by all members of society and that any deviations are diseases, then any intervention that results in a deviation from these norms would be viewed as immoral. Hence, enhancement would be inherently immoral. But this account of health and disease is way too broad; there must be some morally neutral traits and abilities. If there are no morally neutral traits and abilities, then any person that deviates from health norms is "sick." This view would leave very little room for individual variation, to say nothing of the freedom to choose to deviate from health norms. If we accept a narrower account of health and disease, then we will open up some room for morally acceptable deviations from health norms. But this interpretation implies that enhancement interventions could be morally acceptable, provided that they do not violate other moral norms, such as nonmaleficence, autonomy, utility, and so on. Enhancement would not be inherently wrong, on this view, but the rightness or wrongness of any enhancement procedure would depend on its various factual and normative aspects.

The upshot of this discussion is that neither of the two main approaches to health and disease provides us with solid moral boundaries between genetic enhancement and genetic therapy. One might suggest that we examine alternative approaches, but I doubt that other, more refined theories of health and disease will provide us with a way of drawing sharp moral boundaries between genetic enhancement and genetic therapy. Perhaps we should look at other ways of endowing the distinction with moral significance.

The Goals of Medicine

A slightly different approach to these issues asserts that genetic therapy is on solid moral ground because it promotes the goals of medicine, while genetic enhancement promotes other, morally questionable goals. But what are the goals of medicine? This is not an easy question to answer, since medicine seems to serve a variety of purposes, such as the treatment of disease, the prevention of disease, the promotion of human health and well-being, and the relief of suffering. Many of the so-called goals of medicine, such as the prevention of disease and the promotion of human health, may also be promoted by procedures that we would classify as forms of enhancement.[45] For example, some writers have suggested that we might be able to perform genetic interventions that enhance the human immune system by making it better able to fight diseases, including cancer.[46] Most people would accept the idea that providing children with immunizations against the measles, mumps, and rubella promotes the goals of medicine. If we accept the notion that ordinary, nongenetic enhancement of the immune system promotes the goals of medicine, then shouldn't we also agree that genetic enhancements of the immune system serve the same goals? And what about other forms of healthcare, such as rhinoplasty, liposuction, orthodontics, breast augmentation, hair removal, and hair transplants? If these cosmetic procedures serve medical goals, then cosmetic uses of genetic technology, such as somatic gene therapy for baldness, and germline gene therapy for straight teeth, would also seem to serve medical goals. Finally, consider the procedures that are designed to relieve suffering, such as pain control and anesthesia. If we can develop drugs to promote these goals, then why not develop genetic procedures to meet similar objectives? It is not beyond the realm of possibility that we could use genetic therapy to induce the body to produce endorphins. Many forms of enhancement may serve medical goals. Once again, the therapy-enhancement appears not to set any firm moral boundaries in genetic medicine.

One might attempt to avoid this problem by narrowly construing the goals of medicine: the goals of medicine are to treat and prevent diseases in human beings. Other uses of medical technology do not serve the goals of medicine. There are two problems with this response. First, it assumes that we agree on the goals of medicine and the definitions of health and disease. Second, even if we could agree that medicine's goals are to treat and prevent diseases and we can define "health" and "disease," why would it be immoral to use medical technology and science for nonmedical purposes? If a medical procedure, such as mastectomy, is developed for therapeutic purposes, what is wrong with using that procedure for "nonmedical" purposes, such as breast reduction surgery in men with overdeveloped breasts? Admittedly, there are many morally troubling nonmedical uses of medical science and technology, such as the use of steroids by athletes and the use of laxatives by anorexics, but these morally troubling uses of medicine are morally troubling because they violate various moral principles or values, such as fairness and nonmaleficence, not because they are nonmedical uses of medicine.

One might argue that those who use medical science and technology for nonmedical purposes violate medicine's professional norms, but this point only applies to those who consider themselves to be medical professionals. If a procedure violates medical norms, it is medically unethical, but this does not mean that the procedure is unethical outside of the context of medical care. For example, the American Medical Association holds that it is unethical for physicians to assist the state in executions, but this policy does not constitute an unconditional argument against capital punishment. To make the case against capital punishment, one must appeal to wider moral and political norms. Hence the goals of medicine also do not set a morally sharp dividing line between genetic therapy and enhancement.

Our Humanness

One might try to draw moral boundaries between genetic therapy and genetic enhancement by arguing that genetic enhancement is inherently immoral because it changes the human form. Genetic therapy only attempts to restore or safeguard our humanness, while enhancement changes those very features that make us human. Although GLGE and GLGT can more profoundly change human traits than SGE and SGT, both technologies can alter our humanness (or our humanity). To explore these issues in depth, we need to answer two questions: (1) What traits or abilities make us human? and (2) Why would it be wrong to change those traits or abilities? Philosophers have proposed answers to the first question ever since Aristotle defined man as "the rational animal." A thorough answer to the question of defining our humanness takes us way beyond the scope of this essay, but I will offer the reader a brief perspective.[47]

If we have learned anything from the abortion debate, we have learned that it is not at all easy to specify necessary and sufficient conditions for a thing to be human. Humanness is best understood as a cluster concept in that it can be equated with a list of characteristics but not with a set of necessary and sufficient conditions.[48] Some of these characteristics include:

a) physical traits and abilities, such an opposable thumb, bipedalism, etc.
b) psychosocial traits and abilities, such as cognition, language, emotional responses, sociality, etc.
c) phylogenetic traits, such as membership in the biological species Homo sapiens.

The beings that we call "'human" possess many of these traits and abilities, even though some humans have more of these traits and abilities than others. For example, a newborn and an adult have many of the same physical and phylogenetic traits and abilities, even though the adult has more psychosocial traits and abilities. For my purposes, I do not need to say which of these traits and abilities are more "central" to the concept of humanness, since I am not defending a definition that provides necessary or sufficient conditions.

The question I would like to explore in more depth concerns the wrongness of changing those traits that make us human. Would it be inherently wrong to alter the human form? This question presupposes the pragmatically prior question, Can we alter the human form? The answer to this question depends on two factors: (1) the definition of our humanness; and (2) our scientific and technological abilities. According to the definition I assume in this essay, it is possible to alter the human form, since the human form consists of a collection of physiological, psychosocial, and phylogenetic traits and abilities, which can be changed in principle.[49] Although we lacked the ability to change the traits that constitute our humanness at one time, advances in science and technology have given us the ability to change human traits. Since we have good reasons to believe that we can change our humanness, we can now ask whether we should do so.

Most moral theories, with the notable exception of the natural law approach, imply that there is nothing inherently wrong with changing the human form. For the purposes of this essay, I will not examine all of these moral theories here but will only briefly mention two very different perspectives on morality that reach similar conclusions. According to utilitarianism, an action or policy that alters our humanness could be morally right or it could be morally wrong, depending on the consequences of that action or policy. If genetic enhancement produces a greater balance of good/bad consequences, then enhancement would be morally acceptable. For example, genetic interventions that enhance the human immune system might be morally acceptable, but interventions that result in harmful mutations would be unacceptable.

Kantians would object to attempts to alter our humanness if those attempts violate human dignity and autonomy. Some, but not all, genetic interventions could threaten our dignity and autonomy. For example, using SGT to promote hair growth should pose no threat to human dignity and autonomy (if informed consent is not violated), but using GLGE to create a race of "slaves" or "freaks" would pose a dire threat to dignity and autonomy. The main point here is that most moral theories would hold that there is nothing inherently wrong with changing our humanness; the moral rightness or wrongness of such attempts depends on their relation to other moral concerns, such as utility, autonomy, natural rights, virtue, etc.[50]

However, the natural law approach to morality could be interpreted as implying that tampering with the human form is inherently wrong. This argument assumes that the human form has inherent worth and that any changes to that form defile or destroy its worth. The human form is morally sacred and should not be altered.[51] For example, one might hold that a great painting, such as the "Mona Lisa," has inherent worth and it should therefore be left as it is; to change the "Mona Lisa" is to destroy it. Or perhaps one might argue that it would be wrong to change the formula for "Coke" or the plot of "Hamlet." But what is inherently wrong with changing the human form?

One argument that changing the human form is inherently wrong is that natural selection has "designed" us to have specific traits, and that any attempt to change those traits would be a foolhardy and vain intervention in nature's wisdom. It has taken thousands of years of adaptation for the human species to evolve into its present form. How can we possibly improve on nature's perfection? We are more likely to make a major blunder or mistake with human genetic engineering than to make an important advance.[52] Human genetic engineering is likely to produce harmful mutations, gross abnormalities, Frankenstein monsters, etc.[53] There are two problems with this neo-Darwinian view. First, it

is Panglossian and naïve: natural selection is not perfect—nature makes mistakes all the time. We possess many traits, such as the appendix, that serve no useful function. There are some traits that we could add, such as enhancements to the immune system, that could be very useful. Though we should not underestimate nature's wisdom and our ignorance, it is simply false that nature has made us perfect with no room for change or improvement.[54] Second, the argument overestimates human ignorance and carelessness. The history of medical technology allows us to see that while we have had many failures in altering the human form, such as Nazi eugenics programs, we have also had some successes, such as artificial limbs and eyeglasses. Although we should exhibit extreme care, discretion, and circumspection in all genetic interventions, not all changes we make in the human form will result in natural disasters.

A second argument approaches the issue from a theological perspective. According to this view, God, not natural selection, has designed us to have specific traits. Hence any human attempt to change those traits would be a foolish (and arrogant) challenge to God's wisdom. Those who attempt to "play God" by changing human nature commit the mortal sin of hubris. One obvious difficulty with this argument is that it is not likely to convince nonbelievers, but let us set aside that problem and engage in some speculative theology. The question we need to ask in response to this argument is, Would God not want us to change human traits? Changes we can now make to human traits could promote human welfare and justice. Why would God allow us to have this power and not use it? Of course, God would not want us to use our power to increase human suffering or injustice, but why would He not want us to use this power for good purposes? Although several well-known theologians have taken a strong stance against human genetic engineering,[55] religious denominations are not united in their opposition to genetic engineering.[56] For example, the National Council of Churches adopted a resolution that the effort to use genetics to improve on nature is not inherently wrong, and the Council later stated that God has given men and women powers of cocreation, though these powers should be used with care.[57,58]

Regardless of whether one accepts the views of a particular church, it is not at all clear that a theologically based natural law theory provides us with good reasons for thinking that it is inherently wrong to change the human form. One could accept a theologically based approach to morality that leaves some room for human beings to alter the human form, provided that we exhibit wisdom, care, and restraint in changing our form.[59] Some changes (e.g., those that result in suffering or injustice) are morally wrong, but other changes (e.g., those that promote happiness or justice) are morally acceptable.

The Rights of the Unborn

Another way of arguing that at least some forms of genetic enhancement are inherently wrong is to claim that GLGE and GLGT violate the rights of unborn children.[60] These procedures are often said to violate the rights of unborn children because they:

a) are experimental procedures that violate the informed consent of unborn children;[61]

b) deny unborn children the right to have a germline that has not been genetically manipulated;[62] or

c) deny unborn children a right to an open future.[63]

All of these arguments make the morally controversial assumption that unborn children have rights. I will not challenge this assertion here.[64] Even if one assumes that unborn children have rights, it still does not follow that GLGE or GLGT violate those rights.

Let's consider (a) first. GLGT and GLGE do not violate the unborn child's right to informed consent because this right can be exercised by competent adults acting in the child's best interests. We allow proxy consent as a legitimate way of exercising informed consent for many procedures that can profoundly affect the welfare of children, such as fetal surgery and experimental surgery on newborns to repair congenital defects. If it makes sense to use proxy consent in these kinds of experiments, then it should also make sense to use proxy consent for other types of experiments, such as GLGT or GLGE, provided that these experiments can be shown to be in the best interests of unborn children.[65]

(B) is a very esoteric position. What kind of right is the "right to have a genome that has not been genetically manipulated"? Most writers conceive of rights in terms of interests: rights function to protect the interests of individuals.[66] Interests are needs and benefits that most people require to have a fulfilling life, such as freedom, health, education, self-esteem, and so on. So do unborn children have an interest in being born with a genome that has not been manipulated? If such an interest exists, then it is highly unusual and certainly not universal. Children whose parents hold specific religious or philosophical doctrines that forbid germline manipulation may have an interest in being born with an unadulterated genome, but other children will not have this interest. For most children, being born with a genome that predisposes them to health and a wide range of opportunities is more important than being born with a genome that has not been manipulated.

This bring us to argument (c). A right to an "open future" is a right to make one's own choices and life plans on reaching adulthood.[67] Parents who excessively impose their own choices, values, and life plans on their children may violate this right. For example, parents who decide to have a son castrated in order to make sure that he becomes a good singer close off many choices and plans that he could have made as an adult, e.g., having children through natural means. The right to an open future is by no means an unusual or esoteric right, since almost all children have the interests that this right protects, e.g., freedom of choice, freedom of opportunity, etc. But even if we admit this much, does it follow that GLGT or GLGE constitute an inherent violation of this right? I don't think so. While some uses of genetic technology could be regarded as an overbearing imposition of parental values on children, other uses of GLGT and GLGE may augment a child's right to an open future. If parents use GLGE to enhance a child's immune system, then they could be increasing his opportunities to an open future by helping him fight diseases, which can limit opportunities. On the other hand, parents who attempt to produce an eight-foot-tall child in order to make her into a basketball player probably are violating her right to an open future by imposing their choices on her life.

However, there is not a sharp distinction between violating a child's right to an open future and being a responsible parent.[68] We readily accept the idea that parents should try to raise children who are healthy, intelligent, responsible, and happy, and we endorse various parental attempts to promote these values, such as private education, athletics, SAT preparation, and so on. Parents that act in the best interests of the children and have hope for their future are simply being good parents. But when does this healthy and responsible concern for a child's future interfere with the child's right to choose his own values and life plans? This is not an easy question to answer. In any case, this quandary supports my claim that GLGT and GLGE do not inherently violate a child's right to an open future. Some uses of these technologies might have this effect; others might not. The upshot of this section is that we have once again debunked several arguments that might be construed as proving that genetic enhancement is inherently wrong. It may be wrong under some circumstances, but not in others.

Eugenics

Some have attacked GLGT and GLGE on the grounds that they constitute a form of eugenics, an attempt to control the human gene pool.[69] Is eugenics inherently wrong? To understand this question, we can distinguish between positive and negative eugenics: positive eugenics attempts to increase the number of favorable or desirable genes in the human gene pool, while negative eugenics attempts to reduce the number of undesirable or harmful genes, e.g., genes that cause genetic diseases. We should also distinguish between state-sponsored and parental eugenics: under state-sponsored eugenics programs the government attempts to control the human gene pool; in parental eugenics parents exert control over the gene pool through their reproductive choices.[70]

Parental eugenics occurs every time people select mates or sperm or egg donors. Most people do not find this kind of eugenics to be as troubling as the state-sponsored eugenics programs envisioned by Aldous Huxley or implemented by Nazi Germany. Indeed, one might argue that this kind of eugenics is a morally acceptable exercise of parental rights.[71] Moreover, most parents do not make their reproductive choices with the sole aim of controlling the human gene pool; any effects these choices have on the gene pool are unintended consequences of parental actions. As long as we accept the idea that parents should be allowed to make some choices that affect the composition of the human gene pool, then parental eugenics is not inherently wrong.

But what about state-sponsored eugenics? One might argue that state-sponsored eugenics programs, such as involuntary sterilization of the mentally disabled or mandatory genetic screening, are morally wrong because they:

a) constitute unjustifiable violations of individual liberty and privacy;
b) are a form of genetic discrimination;

c) can have adverse evolutionary consequences by reducing genetic diversity; and

d) can lead us down a slippery slope toward increased racial and ethnic hatred, bias, and genocide.

Although these arguments do not prove that all forms of state-sponsored eugenics are morally wrong, they place a strong burden of proof on those who defend these programs. It is not my aim to explore state-sponsored eugenics in depth here.[72] However, even if we assume that state-sponsored eugenics is inherently wrong, this still only proves that some forms are GLGE or GLGT are inherently wrong. There is nothing inherently wrong with parental choices to use GLGE or GLGT to help children achieve health, freedom, and other values. Thus arguments that appeal to our concerns about eugenics do not prove that genetic enhancement is inherently wrong. Some forms of genetic enhancement, e.g., state-sponsored eugenics, are wrong, others are not.

Conclusion: The Significance of the Distinction

Two decades ago, James Rachels challenged the moral significance of the active-passive euthanasia distinction in a widely anthologized essay.[73] This paper has attempted to perform a similar debunking of the therapy-enhancement distinction in human genetics. It has considered and rejected a variety of different ways of arguing that the therapy-enhancement distinction in human genetics marks a solid, moral boundary. Genetic enhancement is not inherently immoral nor is genetic therapy inherently moral. Some forms of enhancement are immoral, others are not; likewise, some types of therapy are immoral, others are not. The implication of this view is that we should not use the therapy-enhancement

distinction as our moral compass in human genetics. In evaluating the ethical aspects of any particular genetic intervention, we should ask not whether it is therapy or enhancement but whether the intervention poses significant risks, offers significant benefits, violates or promotes human dignity, is just or unjust, and so on.

Having said this much, I think some forms of enhancement can be morally justified, provided that they can be shown to be safe and effective. For example, using genetic technology to protect people against diseases could be justified on the grounds that it benefits patients. I think one can even justify the use of genetics for cosmetic purposes in terms of benefits to patients. We can also view some forms of genetic therapy as unacceptable (at present) because they pose unjustifiable risks to patients or future generations. For example, all forms of GLGT and some types of SGT, such as a procedure for fighting cancer at the genetic level, are too risky, given our current scientific and technical limitations. In any case, the moral assessment of these procedures depends on considerations of probable benefits and harms (as well as other moral qualities), not on their classification as "therapy" or "enhancement."

So what is the significance of the therapy-enhancement distinction? What role should it play in thinking about the ethics of human genetics? Can it guide public policy? The most I can say in favor of the distinction is that it defines moral zones without any sharp boundaries. The significance of the distinction may lie in its ability to address our fears and hopes: we hope that genetic therapy will help us treat diseases and improve human health, but we fear that genetic enhancement will lead us down a slippery slope toward a variety of undesirable consequences, such as discrimination, bias, eugenics, injustice, biomedical harms, and so on.[74] Genetic enhancement will probably always dwell in shadow of the slippery slope argument, while genetic therapy will probably always bask in the glory of modern medicine. Our hopes and fears may or may not be warranted; only time will tell. In the meantime, even if the therapy-enhancement distinction does not draw any solid moral boundaries, we need to be aware of the distinction in public dialogues about genetics. In these dialogues, it may be useful to address the fears of enhancement and the hopes of therapy while attempting to grapple with the realities of the genetic revolution.

Notes

1. Juengst E. Can enhancement be distinguished from prevention in genetic medicine? *Journal of Medicine and Philosophy* 1997;22:125-42.

2. Holtug N. Altering humans—the case for and against human gene therapy. *Cambridge Quarterly of Healthcare Ethics* 1997;6:157-74.

3. Berger E, Gert B. Genetic disorders and the ethical status of germ-line gene therapy. *Journal of Medicine and Philosophy* 1991;16:667-83.

4. Anderson W. Human gene therapy: scientific and ethical considerations. *Journal of Medicine and Philosophy* 1985;10:275-91.

5. Anderson W. Human gene therapy: why draw a line? *Journal of Medicine and Philosophy* 1989;14:81-93.

6. Anderson W. Genetics and human malleability. *Hastings Center Report* 1990;20(1): 21-4.

7. McGee G. *The Perfect Baby*. Lanham, Md.: Rowman and Littlefield, 1997.

8. Vogel G. Genetic enhancement: from science fiction to ethics quandary. *Science* 1997;277:1753-4.

9. See note 4, Anderson 1985.

10. Fowler G, Juengst, E, and Zimmerman B. Germ-line gene therapy and the clinical ethos of medical genetics. *Theoretical Medicine* 1989;19:151-7.

11. See note 3, Berger, Gert 1991.

12. Zimmerman B. Human germ-line gene therapy: the case for its development and use. *Journal of Medicine and Philosophy* 1991; 16:593-612.

13. Glover J. *What Sort of People Should There Be?* New York: Penguin Books, 1984.

14. See note 7, McGee 1997.

15. Resnik D. Debunking the slippery slope argument against human germ line gene therapy. *Journal of Medicine and Philosophy* 1993;19:23-40.

16. Resnik D. Genetic engineering and social justice: a Rawlsian approach. *Social Theory and Practice* 1997;23(3):427-48.

17. See note 3, Berger, Gert 1991.

18. See note 4, Anderson 1985.

19. See note 6, Anderson 1990.

20. Rifkin J. *Algeny*. New York: Viking Press, 1983.

21. Ramsey P. *Fabricated Man: The Ethics of Genetic Control*. New Haven: Yale University Press, 1970.

22. It is not my aim in this essay to argue that there is no distinction between therapy and enhancement; I am only attempting to question the moral significance of the distinction. If it turns out that there is not a tenable distinction between therapy and enhancement, so much the worse for the moral significance of this distinction. For the purpose of this essay I will define "enhancement" as a medical intervention that has goals other than therapeutic ones. There may be many types of enhancement on this view. Some forms of enhancement, such as a circumcision, can have therapeutic aims as well, e.g., preventing urinary tract infections. Some forms of therapy, such a heart transplantation, could have enhancement effects, e.g., a person could acquire an above average heart. Some interventions, such as preventative medicine, could straddle the line between enhancement and therapy. For further discussion, see note 1, Juengst 1997.

23. See note 4, Anderson 1985.

24. Suzuki D, Knudtson P. *Genethics*. Cambridge, Mass.: Harvard University Press, 1989.

25. Resnik D, Langer P, Steinkraus H. *Human Germ-line Gene Therapy: Scientific, Ethical, and Political Issues*. Austin, Texas: RG Landes, 1999.

26. See note 24, Suzuki, Knudtson 1989.

27. See note 5, Anderson 1989.

28. See note 6, Anderson 1990.

29. Baird P. Altering human genes: social, ethical, and legal implications. *Perspectives in Biology and Medicine* 1994;37:566-75.

30. In the current debate in bioethics, several writers have attempted to use the concepts of health and disease to distinguish between genetic therapy and genetic enhancement.

31. See note 1, Juengst 1997.

32. See note 3, Berger, Gert 1991.

33. See note 5, Anderson 1989.

34. See note 6, Anderson 1990:24.

35. Caplan A. The concepts of health, illness, and disease. In: Veatch R, ed. *Medical Ethics*, 2nd ed. Sudbury, Mass.: Jones and Bartlett, 1997:57-74.

36. Khushf G. Expanding the horizon of reflection on health and disease. *Journal of Medicine and Philosophy* 1995;1-4.

37. Some writers distinguish between relativist and nonrelativist accounts; some others distinguish between biological and social accounts. But the basic insight is the same: the concepts of health and disease are normative or descriptive.

38. Boorse C. Health as a theoretical concept. *Philosophy of Science* 1977;44:542-73.

39. Daniels N. *Just Health Care*. Cambridge: Cambridge University Press, 1985.

40. Sigerist H. *Civilization and Disease*. Chicago: University of Chicago Press, 1943.

41. Pellegrino, ED, Thomasma, DC. *For the Patient's Good*. New York: Oxford University Press, 1988.

42. For an overview of the normative approach, see Caplan A. *Moral Matters*. New York: John Wiley and Sons, 1995.

43. Culver C, Gert B. *Philosophy in Medicine*. New York: Oxford University Press, 1982.

44. Lennox J. Health as an objective value. *Journal of Medicine and Philosophy* 1995;20:501-11.

45. See note 44, Lennox 1995.

46. Culver K. The current status of gene therapy research. *The Genetic Resource* 1993;7:5-10.

47. See note 25, Resnik, Langer, Steinkraus 1999.

48. English J. Abortion and the concept of a person. *Canadian Journal of Philosophy* 1975;5(2):233-43.

49. It is possible to define "human" in such a way that it is logically impossible to change our humanness. If we stipulate that possession of single property is a necessary and sufficient condition for being human, then any changes we make in that property would result in people that are not human. For example, we can define "triangle" "three-sided object." If me make an object that has four sides, it is not an altered triangle; it is not a triangle at all. For a definition of humanness that would seem to imply that it is difficult (though not impossible) to alter our humanness, see Anderson W. Genetic engineering and our humanness. *Human Gene Therapy* 1994;5:755-60.

50. See note 25, Resnik, Langer, Steinkrauss 1999.

51. For the purposes of this essay, I will not attribute this view to any particular author, since I think it deserves consideration on its own merit. For writers who come close to defending this view, see note 8, Vogel 1997, as well as Kass L. *Toward a More Natural Science*. New York: Free Press, 1985.

52. See note 20, Rifkin 1983.

53. These arguments do not address genetic enhancement per se, since they also apply to GLGT and they do not apply to SGT or SGE.

54. See note 25, Resnik, Langer, Steinkrauss 1999.

55. See note 21, Ramsey 1970.

56. Cole-Turner, R. Genes, religion, and society: the developing views of the churches. *Science and Engineering Ethics* 1997;3(3):273-88.

57. National Council of Churches. *Human Life and the New Genetics*. New York: National Council of Churches of Christ in the U.S.A., 1980.

58. National Council of Churches. *Genetic Engineering: Social and Ethical Consequences*. New York: National Council of Churches of Christ in the U.S.A., 1983.

59. Peters, T. *Playing God?: Genetic Determinism and Human Freedom*. New York: Routledge, 1997.

60. For further discussion see Buchanan A, Brock D. *Deciding for Others*. Cambridge: Cambridge University Press, 1989.

61. Lappé, M. Ethical issues in manipulating the human germ line. *Journal of Medicine and Philosophy* 1991;16:621-39.

62. Commission of the European Community. *Adopting a Specific Research and Technological Development Programme in the Field of Health*. Brussels: Commission of the European Community, 1989.

63. Davis D. Genetic dilemmas and the child's right to an open future. *Hastings Center Report* 1997;27(2):7-15.

64. These arguments do not constitute an objection to SGT or SGE.

65. See note 25, Resnik, Langer, Steinkrauss 1999.

66. Feinberg J. *Social Philosophy*. Englewood Cliffs, N.J.: Prentice-Hall, 1973.

67. Feinberg J. The child's right to an open future. In: Aiken W and Lafollette H, eds. *Whose Child? Children's Rights, Parental Authority, and State Power*. Totowa, N.J.: Littlefield, Adam, 1980:124-53.

68. See note 7, McGee 1997.

69. For further discussion of eugenics, see Paul D. *Controlling Human Heredity: 1865 to the Present*. Atlantic Highlands, N.J.: Humanities Press International, 1995.

70. Kitcher P. *The Lives to Come*. New York: Simon and Schuster, 1997.

71. Robertson J. *Children of Choice*. Princeton, N.J.: Princeton University Press, 1994.

72. For further discussion, see Parens E. Taking behavioral genetics seriously. *Hastings Center Report* 1996;26(4):13-8.

73. Rachels J. Active and passive euthanasia. *New England Journal of Medicine* 1975;292(2): 78-80.

74. See note 15, Resnik 1993.

Of Mice But Not Men: Problems of the Randomized Clinical Trial

Samuel Hellman and Deborah S. Hellman

As medicine has become increasingly scientific and less accepting of unsupported opinion or proof by anecdote, the randomized controlled clinical trial has become the standard technique for changing diagnostic or therapeutic methods. The use of this technique creates an ethical dilemma.[1,2] Researchers participating in such studies are required to modify their ethical commitments to individual patients and do serious damage to the concept of the physician as a practicing, empathetic professional who is primarily concerned with each patient as an individual. Researchers using a randomized clinical trial can be described as physician-scientists, a term that expresses the tension between the two roles. The physician, by entering into a relationship with an individual patient, assumes certain obligations, including the commitment always to act in the patient's best interests. As Leon Kass has rightly maintained, "the physician must produce unswervingly the virtues of loyalty and fidelity to his patient."[3] Though the ethical requirements of this relationship have been modified by legal obligations to report wounds of a suspicious nature and certain infectious diseases, these obligations in no way conflict with the central ethical obligation to act in the best interests of the patient medically. Instead, certain nonmedical interests of the patient are preempted by other social concerns.

The role of the scientist is quite different. The clinical scientist is concerned with answering questions—i.e., determining the validity of formally constructed hypotheses. Such scientific information, it is presumed, will benefit humanity in general. The clinical scientist's role has been well described by Dr. Anthony Fauci, director of the National Institute of Allergy and Infectious Diseases, who states the goals of the randomized clinical trial in these words: "It's not to deliver therapy. It's to answer a scientific question so that the drug can be available for everybody once you've established safety and efficacy."[4] The demands of such a study can conflict in a number of ways with the physician's duty to minister to patients. The study may create a false dichotomy in the physician's

PROSPECTIVE authors should consult "Information for Authors," which appears in the first issue of each month and may be obtained from the *Journal* office.

opinions: according to the premise of the randomized clinical trial, the physician may only know or not know whether a proposed course of treatment represents an improvement; no middle position is permitted. What the physician thinks, suspects, believes, or has a hunch about is assigned to the "not knowing" category, because knowing is defined on the basis of an arbitrary but accepted statistical test performed in a randomized clinical trial. Thus, little credence is given to information gained beforehand in other ways or to information accrued during the trial but without the required statistical degree of assurance that a difference is not due to chance. The randomized clinical trial also prevents the treatment technique from being modified on the basis of the growing knowledge of the physicians during their participation in the trial. Moreover, it limits access to the data as they are collected until specific milestones are achieved. This prevents physicians from profiting not only from their individual experience, but also from the collective experience of the other participants.

The randomized clinical trial requires doctors to act simultaneously as physicians and as scientists. This puts them in a difficult and sometimes untenable ethical position. The conflicting moral demands arising from the use of the randomized clinical trial reflect the classic conflict between rights-based moral theories and utilitarian ones. The first of these, which depend on the moral theory of Immanuel Kant (and seen more recently in neo-Kantian philosophers, such as John Rawls[5]), asserts that human beings, by virtue of their unique capacity for rational thought, are bearers of dignity. As such, they ought not to be treated merely as means to an end; rather, they must always be treated as ends in themselves. Utilitarianism, by contrast, defines what is right as the greatest good for the greatest number—that is, as social utility. This view, articulated by Jeremy Bentham and John Stuart Mill, requires that pleasures (understood broadly, to include such pleasures as health and well-being) and pains be added together. The morally correct act is the act that produces the most pleasure and the least pain overall.

A classic objection to the utilitarian position is that according to that theory, the distribution of pleasures and pains is of no moral consequence. This element of the theory severely restricts physicians from being utilitarians, or at least from following the theory's dictates. Physicians must care very deeply about the distribution of pain and pleasure, for they have entered into a relationship with one or a number of individual patients. They cannot be indifferent to whether it is these patients or others that suffer for the general benefit of society. Even though society might gain from the suffering of a few, and even though the doctor might believe that such a benefit is worth a given patient's suffering (i.e., that utilitarianism is right in the particular case), the ethical obligation created by the covenant between doctor and patient requires the doctor to see the interests of the individual patient as primary and compelling. In essence, the doctor–patient relationship requires doctors to see their patients as bearers of rights who cannot be merely used for the greater good of humanity.

As Fauci has suggested,[4] the randomized clinical trial routinely asks physicians to sacrifice the interests of their particular patients for the sake of the study and that of the information that it will make available for the benefit of society. This practice is ethically problematic. Consider first the initial formulation of a trial. In particular, consider the case of a disease for which there is no satisfactory therapy—for example, advanced cancer or the acquired immunodeficiency syndrome (AIDS). A new agent that promises more effectiveness is the subject of the study. The control group must be given either an unsatisfactory treatment or a placebo. Even though the therapeutic value of the new agent is unproved, if physicians think that it has promise, are they acting in the best interests of their patients in allowing them to be randomly assigned to the control group? Is persisting in such an assignment consistent with the specific commitments taken on in the doctor–patient relationship? As a result of interactions with patients with AIDS and their advocates, Merigan[6] recently suggested modifications in the design of clinical trials that attempt to deal with the unsatisfactory treatment given to the control group. The view of such activists has been expressed by Rebecca Pringle Smith of Community Research Initiative in New York: "Even if you have a supply of compliant martyrs, trials must have some ethical validity."[4]

If the physician has no opinion about whether the new treatment is acceptable, then random assignment is ethically acceptable, but such lack of enthusiasm for the new treatment does not augur well for either the patient or the study. Alternatively, the treatment may show promise of beneficial results but also present a risk of undesirable complications. When the physician believes that the severity and likelihood of harm and good are evenly balanced, randomization

may be ethically acceptable. If the physician has no preference for either treatment (is in a state of equipoise[7,8]), then randomization is acceptable. If, however, he or she believes that the new treatment may be either more or less successful or more or less toxic, the use of randomization is not consistent with fidelity to the patient.

The argument usually used to justify randomization is that it provides, in essence, a critique of the usefulness of the physician's beliefs and opinions, those that have not yet been validated by a randomized clinical trial. As the argument goes, these not-yet-validated beliefs are as likely to be wrong as right. Although physicians are ethically required to provide their patients with the best available treatment, there simply is no best treatment yet known.

The reply to this argument takes two forms. First, and most important, even if this view of the reliability of a physician's opinions is accurate, the ethical constraints of an individual doctor's relationship with a particular patient require the doctor to provide individual care. Although physicians must take pains to make clear the speculative nature of their views, they cannot withhold these views from the patient. The patient asks from the doctor both knowledge and judgment. The relationship established between them rightfully allows patients to ask for the judgment of their particular physicians, not merely that of the medical profession in general. Second, it may not be true, in fact, that the not-yet-validated beliefs of physicians are as likely to be wrong as right. The greater certainty obtained with a randomized clinical trial is beneficial, but that does not mean that a lesser degree of certainty is without value. Physicians can acquire knowledge through methods other than the randomized clinical trial. Such knowledge, acquired over time and less formally than is required in a randomized clinical trial, may be of great value to a patient.

Even if it is ethically acceptable to begin a study, one often forms an opinion during its course—especially in studies that are impossible to conduct in a truly double-blinded fashion—that makes it ethically problematic to continue. The inability to remain blinded usually occurs in studies of cancer or AIDS, for example, because the therapy is associated by nature with serious side effects. Trials attempt to restrict the physician's access to the data in order to prevent such unblinding. Such restrictions should make physicians eschew the trial, since their ability to act in the patient's best interests will be limited. Even supporters of randomized clinical trials, such as Merigan, agree that interim findings should be presented to patients to ensure that no one receives what seems an inferior treatment.[6] Once physicians have formed a view about the new treatment, can they continue randomization? If random assignment is stopped, the study may be lost and the participation of the previous patients wasted. However, if physicians continue the randomization when they have a definite opinion about the efficacy of the experimental drug, they are not acting in accordance with the requirements of the doctor–patient relationship. Furthermore, as their opinion becomes more firm, stopping the randomization may not be enough. Physicians may be ethically required to treat the patients formerly placed in the control group with the therapy that now seems probably effective. To do so would be faithful to the obligations created by the doctor–patient relationship, but it would destroy the study.

To resolve this dilemma, one might suggest that the patient has abrogated the rights implicit in a doctor–patient relationship by signing an informed-consent form. We argue that such rights cannot be waived or abrogated. They are inalienable. The right to be treated as an individual deserving the physician's best judgment and care, rather than to be used as a means to determine the best treatment for others, is inherent in every person. This right, based on the concept of dignity, cannot be waived. What of altruism, then? Is it not the patient's right to make a sacrifice for the general good? This question must be considered from both positions—that of the patient and that of the

physician. Although patients may decide to waive this right, it is not consistent with the role of a physician to ask that they do so. In asking, the doctor acts as a scientist instead. The physician's role here is to propose what he or she believes is best medically for the specific patient, not to suggest participation in a study from which the patient cannot gain. Because the opportunity to help future patients is of potential value to a patient, some would say physicians should not deny it. Although this point has merit, it offers so many opportunities for abuse that we are extremely uncomfortable about accepting it. The responsibilities of physicians are much clearer; they are to minister to the current patient.

Moreover, even if patients could waive this right, it is questionable whether those with terminal illness would be truly able to give voluntary informed consent. Such patients are extremely dependent on both their physicians and the health care system. Aware of this dependence, physicians must not ask for consent, for in such cases the very asking breaches the doctor–patient relationship. Anxious to please their physicians, patients may have difficulty refusing to participate in the trial the physicians describe. The patients may perceive their refusal as damaging to the relationship, whether or not it is so. Such perceptions of coercion affect the decision. Informed-consent forms are difficult to understand, especially for patients under the stress of serious illness for which there is no satisfactory treatment. The forms are usually lengthy, somewhat legalistic, complicated, and confusing, and they hardly bespeak the compassion expected of the medical profession. It is important to remember that those who have studied the doctor–patient relationship have emphasized its empathetic nature.

> [The] relationship between doctor and patient partakes of a peculiar intimacy. It presupposes on the part of the physician not only knowledge of his fellow men but sympathy. ...

This aspect of the practice of medicine has been designated as the art; yet I wonder whether it should not, most properly, be called the essence.[9]

How is such a view of the relationship consonant with random assignment and informed consent? The Physician's Oath of the World Medical Association affirms the primacy of the deontologic view of patients' rights: "Concern for the interests of the subject must always prevail over the interests of science and society."[10]

Furthermore, a single study is often not considered sufficient. Before a new form of therapy is generally accepted, confirmatory trials must be conducted. How can one conduct such trials ethically unless one is convinced that the first trial was in error? The ethical problems we have discussed are only exacerbated when a completed randomized clinical trial indicates that a given treatment is preferable. Even if the physician believes the initial trial was in error, the physician must indicate to the patient the full results of that trial.

The most common reply to the ethical arguments has been that the alternative is to return to the physician's intuition, to anecdotes, or to both as the basis of medical opinion. We all accept the dangers of such a practice. The argument states that we must therefore accept randomized, controlled clinical trials regardless of their ethical problems because of the great social benefit they make possible, and we salve our conscience with the knowledge that informed consent has been given. This returns us to the conflict between patients' rights and social utility. Some would argue that this tension can be resolved by placing a relative value on each. If the patient's right that is being compromised is not a fundamental right and the social gain is very great, then the study might be justified. When the right is fundamental, however, no amount of social gain, or almost none, will justify its sacrifice. Consider, for example, the experiments on humans done by physicians under the Nazi regime. All would agree that these

are unacceptable regardless of the value of the scientific information gained. Some people go so far as to say that no use should be made of the results of those experiments because of the clearly unethical manner in which the data were collected. This extreme example may not seem relevant, but we believe that in its hyperbole it clarifies the fallacy of a utilitarian approach to the physician's relationship with the patient. To consider the utilitarian gain is consistent neither with the physician's role nor with the patient's rights.

It is fallacious to suggest that only the randomized clinical trial can provide valid information or that all information acquired by this technique is valid. Such experimental methods are intended to reduce error and bias and therefore reduce the uncertainty of the result. Uncertainty cannot be eliminated, however. The scientific method is based on increasing probabilities and increasingly refined approximations of truth.[11] Although the randomized clinical trial contributes to these ends, it is neither unique nor perfect. Other techniques may also be useful.[12]

Randomized trials often place physicians in the ethically intolerable position of choosing between the good of the patient and that of society. We urge that such situations be avoided and that other techniques of acquiring clinical information be adopted. For example, concerning trials of treatments for AIDS, Byar et al.[13] have said that "some traditional approaches to the clinical-trials process may be unnecessarily rigid and unsuitable for this disease." In this case, AIDS is not what is so different; rather, the difference is in the presence of AIDS activists, articulate spokespersons for the ethical problems created by the application of the randomized clinical trial to terminal illnesses. Such arguments are equally applicable to advanced cancer and other serious illnesses. Byar et al. agree that there are even circumstances in which uncontrolled clinical trials may be justified: when there is no effective treatment to use as a control, when the prognosis is uniformly poor, and when there is a reasonable expectation of benefit without excessive toxicity. These conditions are usually found in clinical trials of advanced cancer.

The purpose of the randomized clinical trial is to avoid the problems of observer bias and patient selection. It seems to us that techniques might be developed to deal with these issues in other ways. Randomized clinical trials deal with them in a cumbersome and heavy-handed manner, by requiring large numbers of patients in the hope that random assignment will balance the heterogeneous distribution of patients into the different groups. By observing known characteristics of patients, such as age and sex, and distributing them equally between groups, it is thought that unknown factors important in determining outcomes will also be distributed equally. Surely, other techniques can be developed to deal with both observer bias and patient selection. Prospective studies without randomization, but with the evaluation of patients by uninvolved third parties, should remove observer bias. Similar methods have been suggested by Royall.[12] Prospective matched-pair analysis, in which patients are treated in a manner consistent with their physician's views, ought to help ensure equivalence between the groups and thus mitigate the effect of patient selection, at least with regard to known covariates. With regard to unknown covariates, the security would rest, as in randomized trials, in the enrollment of large numbers of patients and in confirmatory studies. This method would not pose ethical difficulties, since patients would receive the treatment recommended by their physician. They would be included in the study by independent observers matching patients with respect to known characteristics, a process that would not affect patient care and that could be performed independently any number of times.

This brief discussion of alternatives to randomized clinical trials is sketchy and incomplete. We wish only to point out that there may be satisfactory alternatives, not to describe and evaluate them completely. Even if randomized clinical trials were much better than any alternative, however, the ethical dilemmas they present may put their use at variance with the primary obligations of the physician. In this regard, Angell cautions, "If this commitment to the patient is attenuated, even for so good a cause as benefits to future patients, the implicit assumptions of the doctor–patient relationship are violated."[14] The risk of such attenuation by the randomized trial is great. The AIDS activists have brought this dramatically to the attention of the academic medical community. Techniques appropriate to the laboratory may not be applicable to humans. We must develop and use alternative methods for acquiring clinical knowledge.

University of Chicago
Chicago, IL 60637-1470
SAMUEL HELLMAN, M.D.

Harvard University
Cambridge, MA 02138
DEBORAH S. HELLMAN, M.A.

References

1. Hellman S. Randomized clinical trials and the doctor–patient relationship: an ethical dilemma. Cancer Clin Trials 1979; 2: **189–93.**
2. *Idem.* A doctor's dilemma: the doctor–patient relationship in clinical investigation. In: Proceedings of the Fourth National Conference on Human Values and Cancer, New York, March 15–17, 1984. New York: American Cancer Society, 1984: **144–6.**
3. Kass LR. Toward a more natural science: biology and human affairs. New York: Free Press, 1985: **196.**
4. Palca J. AIDS drug trials enter new age. Science 1989; 246: **19–21.**

5. Rawls J. A theory of justice. Cambridge, Mass.: Belknap Press of Harvard University Press. 1971: **183-92, 446–52.**

6. Merigan TC. You *can* teach an old dog new tricks—how AIDS trials are pioneering new strategies. N Engl J Med 1990; 323: **1341–3.**

7. Freedman B. Equipoise and the ethics of clinical research. N Engl J Med 1987; 317: **141–5.**

8. Singer PA, Lantos JD, Whitington PF, Broelsch CE, Siegler M. Equipoise and the ethics of segmental liver transplantation. Clin Res 1988; 36: **539–45.**

9. Longcope WT. Methods and medicine. Bull Johns Hopkins Hosp 1932; 50: **4–20.**

10. Report on medical ethics. World Med Assoc Bull 1949; 1: **109, 111.**

11. Popper K. The problem of induction. In: Miller D, ed. Popper selections. Princeton, N.J.: Princeton University Press, 1985: **101–17.**

12. Royall RM. Ethics and statistics in randomized clinical trials. Stat Sci 1991; 6(1): **52–62.**

13. Byar DP, Schoenfeld DA, Green SB, et al. Design considerations for AIDS trials. N Engl J Med 1990; 323: **1343–8.**

14. Angell M. Patients' preferences in randomized clinical trials. N Engl J Med 1984; 310: **1385–7.**

How to Resolve an Ethical Dilemma Concerning Randomized Clinical Trials

Don Marquis

A n apparent ethical dilemma arises when physicians consider enrolling their patients in randomized clinical trials. Suppose that a randomized clinical trial comparing two treatments is in progress, and a physician has an opinion about which treatment is better. The physician has a duty to promote the patient's best medical interests and therefore seems to be obliged to advise the patient to receive the treatment that the physician prefers. This duty creates a barrier to the enrollment of patients in randomized clinical trials.[1-10] Two strategies are often used to resolve the dilemma in favor of enrolling patients in clinical trials.

The "Either You Know Which Is Better or You Don't" Strategy

According to one strategy, physicians should not recommend one treatment over another if they do not really know which one is better, and they do not really know which treatment is better in the absence of data from randomized clinical trials.[11] Data from uncontrolled studies are often influenced by the desire on both the investigator's part and the patient's part to obtain positive results.[12] Journal editors are more likely to publish reports of studies with positive results than reports of studies with negative results.[13] A treatment recommendation based on weaker evidence than that obtained from a randomized clinical trial is like a recommendation based on a mere hunch or an idiosyncratic preference.[14] Thus, according to this argument, in the absence of data from a randomized clinical trial, evidence that provides an adequate basis for recommending a treatment rarely exists, and the enrollment dilemma is based on a mistake.

This strategy for resolving the dilemma is simplistic. It assumes that evidence available to physicians can be only one of two kinds: gold-standard evidence or worthless prejudice. But clinical judgments may be based on evidence of intermediate quality, including physicians'

I am indebted to Erin Fitz-Gerald, Nina Ainslie, Stephen Williamson, Sarah Taylor, Jerry Menikoff, Don Hatton, and Ron Stephens for their criticisms.

experience with their own patients, their conversations with colleagues concerning their colleagues' experience, their evaluation of the results of nonrandomized studies reported in the literature, their judgment about the mechanism of action of one or both treatments, or their view of the natural history of a given disease. Evidence need not be conclusive to be valuable; it need not be definitive to be suggestive. Because all good physicians allow evidence of intermediate quality to influence their professional judgment when a relevant randomized clinical trial is not being conducted, it is unreasonable to claim that such evidence has no worth when a relevant randomized clinical trial is being conducted. Therefore, the "either you know which is better or you don't" strategy for dealing with the enrollment dilemma is not persuasive.

Adopting a Less Strict Therapeutic Obligation

The dilemma about enrolling patients in randomized clinical trials is generated by the claim that a physician has a strict therapeutic obligation to inform the patients of the physician's treatment preference, even when the preference is based on evidence that is not of the highest quality. The dilemma could be resolved if the physician's therapeutic obligation were less strict. This strategy was developed by Freedman.[14,15] He argued that the standard for determining whether a physician has engaged in medical malpractice or committed some other violation punishable by a professional disciplinary body is the standard of good practice as determined by a consensus of the medical community. There is no consensus about which of two treatments being compared in a randomized clinical trial is superior. (Otherwise, why conduct the trial?) Therefore, enrolling a patient in the trial does not violate the physician's

therapeutic obligation to the patient, regardless of the physician's treatment preference. In addition, a patient who consults a physician with a preference for treatment A could have consulted a physician who preferred treatment B. Therefore, enrolling a patient in a randomized clinical trial in order to be randomly assigned (perhaps) to treatment B does not make such a patient worse off than he or she would otherwise have been.

Despite these points, compelling arguments for the stricter interpretation of therapeutic obligation remain. In the first place, consider what physicians expect when they seek professional advice from their malpractice attorneys, their tax advisors, or for that matter, their own physicians. Surely they expect—and believe they have a right to expect—not merely minimally competent advice, but the best professional judgments of the professionals they have chosen to consult. In the second place, patients choose physicians in order to obtain medical advice that is, in the judgment of those physicians, the best available. If physicians do not provide such advice, then they tacitly deceive their patients, unless they disclose to their patients that they are not bound by this strict therapeutic obligation. Physicians should adopt the strict therapeutic obligation.

A Resolution

The clash between a strict therapeutic obligation and a less strict one is only apparent. On the one hand, the less strict therapeutic obligation is supported by the argument that it is morally permissible to offer to enroll a patient in a randomized clinical trial. On the other hand, the strict therapeutic obligation is supported by the arguments concerning treatment recommendations. Recommending is different from offering to enroll. A recognition of this difference provides the basis for a solution to the dilemma.

Suppose that a randomized clinical trial is being conducted to compare treatments A and B and that a physician prefers A and informs the patient of this preference. All physicians have an obligation to obtain their patients' informed consent to treatment. A physician has respected this right only if he or she explains to the patient the risks and benefits of reasonable alternatives to the recommended treatment and offers the patient an opportunity to choose an alternative, if that is feasible. Either treatment B or enrollment in the trial comparing A and B is a reasonable alternative to treatment A, because presumably, A is not known to be superior to B. Indeed, there is some evidence that enrollment in a randomized clinical trial is a superior therapeutic alternative when a trial is available.[16] Respect for a patient's values is a central purpose of informed consent. A particular patient may place a greater value on participation in a study that will contribute to medical progress and to the well-being of patients in the future than on the unproved advantages of following the physician's recommendation. Therefore, a physician can both recommend a treatment and ask whether the patient is willing to enroll in the randomized clinical trial.

This resolution is based on the recognition that there can be evidence of the superiority of a treatment that falls short of the gold standard for evidence but is better than worthless. It also takes into account the good arguments for the view that physicians have a strict obligation to recommend the best treatment on the basis of their professional judgment, even when the recommendation is based on evidence that falls short of the gold standard. Nevertheless, because all physicians have an obligation to take informed consent seriously, because respect for informed consent entails offering a patient the reasonable alternatives to the recommended treatment, and because enrollment in an appropriate randomized clinical trial is often a reasonable therapeutic option, one could argue that offering a patient the opportunity to be enrolled in a clinical trial is not only morally permissible

but, in many cases, also morally obligatory, if a relevant trial is being conducted and if enrollment in it is feasible. Taking informed consent seriously resolves the dilemma about whether to enroll patients in randomized clinical trials.

Is this analysis clinically realistic? Some may argue that if clinicians inform their patients that they prefer treatment A, then few of their patients will consent to participate in a trial comparing A with B. Furthermore, many clinicians may be unwilling to invest the time necessary to explain the option of enrollment in a trial, particularly if it seems unlikely that a patient, knowing the physician's preference for one of the treatments, will choose to participate in the trial.

On the other hand, in recent years the public has been exposed to a barrage of medical information and misinformation. Explaining to patients the difference between solid scientific evidence of the merits of a treatment and weaker evidence of its merits is worthwhile, whether or not a relevant randomized clinical trial is being conducted. When a relevant trial is being conducted, offering the patient enrollment in the trial should not impose on the physician a large, additional burden of explanation. Physicians can promote enrollment by explaining that their preference is based only on limited evidence, which may or may not be reliable. They can also explain that data from randomized clinical trials have often shown that the initial studies of new treatments were overly optimistic.[17]

In addition, using this informed-consent strategy to resolve the enrollment dilemma may not be morally optional. My analysis is based on two important obligations of physicians. The first is the strict obligation to recommend the treatment that is, in the physician's professional judgment, the best choice for the patient. The second is the obligation to obtain the patient's informed consent to the recommended treatment. The duty of obtaining informed consent implies that the physician is obligated to offer the patient the opportunity to enroll in a clinical trial when one is available, even if the physician has a treatment preference. The physician owes this duty to the individual patient, not simply to future patients who may benefit from advances in medical knowledge. Thus, the informed-consent strategy for resolving the dilemma about enrolling patients in randomized clinical trials leads to the conclusion that physicians have a greater duty to offer their patients enrollment in trials than has previously been realized. A strict, thoroughly defensible, therapeutic obligation need not interfere with the conduct of randomized clinical trials.

Don Marquis, Ph.D.
University of Kansas
Lawrence, KS 66045

I am indebted to Erin Fitz-Gerald, Nina Ainslie, Stephen Williamson, Sarah Taylor, Jerry Menikoff, Don Hatton, and Ron Stephens for their criticisms.

References

1. Chalmers TC. The ethics of randomization as a decision-making technique and the problem of informed consent. Report of the 14th conference $$ directors, June 3-4, 1967. Bethes-$$ 87–93.
2. $$ operative clinical trials. Ann N Y Acad Sci 1970;169: **487–95.**
3. Kolata GB. Clinical trials: methods and ethics are debated. Science 1977;198: **1127–31.**
4. Wikler D. Ethical considerations in randomized clinical trials. Semin Oncol 1981;8: **437–41.**
5. Schafer A. The ethics of the randomized clinical trial. N Engl J Med 1982;307: **719–24.**
6. Marquis D. Leaving therapy to chance. Hastings Cent Rep 1983;13: **40–7.**
7. Gifford R. The conflict between randomized clinical trials and the therapeutic obligation. J Med Philos 1986;11: **347–66.**
8. Hellman S, Hellman DS. Of mice but not men: problems of the randomized clinical trial. N Engl J Med 1991;324: **1585–9.**
9. Gifford R. Community equipoise and the ethics of randomized clinical trials. Bioethics 1995;9: **127–48.**
10. Markman M. Ethical difficulties with randomized clinical trials involving cancer patients: examples from the field of gynecologic oncology. J Clin Ethics 1992;3: **193–5.**
11. Spodick DH. Ethics of the randomized clinical trial. N Engl J Med 1983;308: **343.**
12. Passamani E. Clinical trials—are they ethical? N Engl J Med 1991; 324: **1589–92.**
13. Altman L. Negative results: a positive viewpoint. New York Times. April 29, 1986: **B6.**
14. Freedman B. Equipoise and the ethics of clinical research. N Engl J Med 1987;317: **141–5.**
15. *Idem.* A response to a purported ethical difficulty with randomized clinical trials involving cancer patients. J Clin Ethics 1992;3: **231–4.**
16. Davis S, Wright PW, Schulman SF, et al. Participants in prospective, randomized clinical trials for resected non-small cell lung cancer have improved survival compared with nonparticipants in such trials. Cancer 1985; 56: **1710–8.**
17. Sacks H, Chalmers TC, Smith H Jr. Randomized versus historical controls for clinical trials. Am J Med 1982; 72: **233–40.**

Genetics and Reproductive Risk: Can Having Children Be Immoral?

Laura M. Purdy

I s it morally permissible for me to have children? A decision to procreate is surely one of the most significant decisions a person can make. So it would seem that it ought not be made without some moral soul searching.

There are many reasons why one might hesitate to bring children into this world if one is concerned about their welfare. Some are rather general, such as the deteriorating environment or the prospect of poverty. Others have a narrower focus, such as continuing civil war in one's country or the lack of essential social support for childrearing in the United States. Still others may be relevant only to individuals at risk of passing harmful diseases to their offspring.

There are many causes of misery in this world, and most of them are unrelated to genetic disease. In the general scheme of things, human misery is most efficiently reduced by concentrating on noxious social and political arrangements. Nonetheless, we should not ignore preventable harm just because it is confined to a relatively small corner of life. So the question arises, Can it be wrong to have a child because of genetic risk factors?[1]

Unsurprisingly, most of the debate about this issue has focused on prenatal screening and abortion: much useful information about a given fetus can be made available by recourse to prenatal testing. This fact has meant that moral questions about reproduction have become entwined with abortion politics, to the detriment of both. The abortion connection has made it especially difficult to think about whether it is wrong to prevent a child from coming into being, because doing so might involve what many people see as wrongful killing; yet there is no necessary link between the two. Clearly, the

---

[1] I focus on genetic considerations, although with the advent of AIDS the scope of the general question here could be expanded. There are two reasons for sticking to this relatively narrow formulation. One is that dealing with a smaller chunk of the problem may help us to think more clearly, while realizing that some conclusions may nonetheless be relevant to the larger problem. The other is the peculiar capacity of some genetic problems to affect ever more individuals in the future.

This essay is loosely based on "Genetic Diseases: Can Having Children Be Immoral?" originally published in *Genetics Now*, ed. John L. Buckley (Washington, D.C.: University Press of America, 1978), and subsequently anthologized in a number of medical ethics texts. Thanks to Thomas Mappes and David DeGrazia for their helpful suggestions about updating the article.

existence of genetically compromised children can be prevented not only by aborting already existing fetuses but also by preventing conception in the first place.

Worse yet, many discussions simply assume a particular view of abortion without recognizing other possible positions and the difference they make in how people understand the issues. For example, those who object to aborting fetuses with genetic problems often argue that doing so would undermine our conviction that all humans are in some important sense equal.[2] However, this position rests on the assumption that conception marks the point at which humans are endowed with a right to life. So aborting fetuses with genetic problems looks morally the same as killing "imperfect" people without their consent.

This position raises two separate issues. One pertains to the legitimacy of different views on abortion. Despite the conviction of many abortion activists to the contrary, I believe that ethically respectable views can be found on different sides of the debate, including one that sees fetuses as developing humans without any serious moral claim on continued life. There is no space here to address the details, and doing so would be once again to fall into the trap of letting the abortion question swallow up all others. However, opponents of abortion need to face the fact that many thoughtful individuals do *not* see fetuses as moral persons. It follows that their reasoning process, and hence the implications of their decisions, are radically different from those envisioned by opponents of prenatal screening and abortion. So where the latter see genetic abortion as murdering people who just don't measure up, the former see it as a way to prevent the development of persons who are more likely to live miserable lives, a position consistent with a worldview that values persons equally and holds that each deserves a high-quality life. Some of those who object to genetic abortion

appear to be oblivious to these psychological and logical facts. It follows that the night-mare scenarios they paint for us are beside the point: many people simply do not share the assumptions that make them plausible.

How are these points relevant to my discussion? My primary concern here is to argue that conception can sometimes be morally wrong on grounds of genetic risk, although this judgment will not apply to those who accept the moral legitimacy of abortion and are willing to employ prenatal screening and selective abortion. If my case is solid, then those who oppose abortion must be especially careful not to conceive in certain cases, as they are, of course, free to follow their conscience about abortion. Those like myself who do not see abortion as murder have more ways to prevent birth.

Huntington's Disease

There is always some possibility that reproduction will result in a child with a serious disease or handicap. Genetic counselors can help individuals determine whether they are at unusual risk and, as the Human Genome Project rolls on, their knowledge will increase by quantum leaps. As this knowledge becomes available, I believe we ought to use it to determine whether possible children are at risk *before* they are conceived.

In this chapter I want to defend the thesis that it is morally wrong to reproduce when we know there is a high risk of transmitting a serious disease or defect. This thesis holds that some reproductive acts are wrong, and my argument puts the burden of proof on those who disagree with it to show why its conclusions can be overridden. Hence it denies that people should be free to reproduce mindless of the consequences.[3] However, as moral argument, it

---

2 For example, see Leon Kass, "Implications of Prenatal Diagnosis for the Human Right to Life," in *Ethical Issues in Human Genetics*, ed. Bruce Hilton et al. (New York: Plenum, 1973).

3 This is, of course, a very broad thesis. I defend an even broader version in Chapter 2, "Loving Future People."

should be taken as a proposal for further debate and discussion. It is not, by itself, an argument in favor of legal prohibitions of reproduction.[4]

There is a huge range of genetic diseases. Some are quickly lethal; others kill more slowly, if at all. Some are mainly physical, some mainly mental; others impair both kinds of function. Some interfere tremendously with normal functioning, others less. Some are painful, some are not. There seems to be considerable agreement that rapidly lethal diseases, especially those, such as Tay-Sachs, accompanied by painful deterioration, should be prevented even at the cost of abortion. Conversely, there seems to be substantial agreement that relatively trivial problems, especially cosmetic ones, would not be legitimate grounds for abortion.[5] In short, there are cases ranging from low risk of mild disease or disability to high risk of serious disease or disability. Although it is difficult to decide where the duty to refrain from procreation becomes compelling, I believe that there are some clear cases. I have chosen to focus on Huntington's disease to illustrate the kinds of concrete issues such decisions entail. However,

the arguments are also relevant to many other genetic diseases.[6]

The symptoms of Huntington's disease usually begin between the ages of thirty and fifty:

> Onset is insidious. Personality changes (obstinacy, moodiness, lack of initiative) frequently antedate or accompany the involuntary choreic movements. These usually appear first in the face, neck, and arms, and are jerky, irregular, and stretching in character. Contradictions of the facial muscles result in grimaces; those of the respiratory muscles, lips, and tongue lead to hesitating, explosive speech. Irregular movements of the trunk are present; the gait is shuffling and dancing. Tendon reflexes are increased. ... Some patients display a fatuous euphoria; others are spiteful, irascible, destructive, and violent. Paranoid reactions are common. Poverty of thought and impairment of attention, memory, and judgment occur. As the disease progresses, walking becomes impossible, swallowing difficult, and dementia profound. Suicide is not uncommon.[7]

The illness lasts about fifteen years, terminating in death.

Huntington's disease is an autosomal dominant disease, meaning it is caused by a single defective gene located on a non-sex chromosome. It is passed from one generation to the next via affected individuals. Each child of such an

---

4 Why would we want to resist legal enforcement of every moral conclusion? First, legal action has many costs, costs not necessarily worth paying in particular cases. Second, legal enforcement tends to take the matter out of the realm of debate and treat it as settled. But in many cases, especially where mores or technology are rapidly evolving, we don't want that to happen. Third, legal enforcement would undermine individual freedom and decision-making capacity. In some cases, the ends envisioned are important enough to warrant putting up with these disadvantages.

5 Those who do not see fetuses as moral persons with a right to life may nonetheless hold that abortion is justifiable in these cases. I argue at some length elsewhere that lesser defects can cause great suffering. Once we are clear that there is nothing discriminatory about failing to conceive particular possible individuals, it makes sense, other things being equal, to avoid the prospect of such pain if we can. Naturally, other things rarely are equal. In the first place, many problems go undiscovered until a baby is born. Second, there are often substantial costs associated with screening programs. Third, although women should be encouraged to consider the moral dimensions of routine pregnancy, we do not want it to be so fraught with tension that it becomes a miserable experience. (See Chapter 2, "Loving Future People.")

6 It should be noted that failing to conceive a single individual can affect many lives: in 1916, 962 cases could be traced from six seventeenth-century arrivals in America. See Gordon Rattray Taylor, *The Biological Time Bomb* (New York: Penguin, 1968), p. 176.

7 *The Merck Manual* (Rahway, N.J.: Merck, 1972), pp. 1363,1346. We now know that the age of onset and severity of the disease are related to the number of abnormal replications of the glutamine code on the abnormal gene. See Andrew Revkin, "Hunting Down Huntington's," *Discover* (December 1993): 108.

affected person has a 50 percent risk of inheriting the gene and thus of eventually developing the disease, even if he or she was born before the parent's disease was evident.[8]

Until recently, Huntington's disease was especially problematic because most affected individuals did not know whether they had the gene for the disease until well into their childbearing years. So they had to decide about childbearing before knowing whether they could transmit the disease or not. If, in time, they did not develop symptoms of the disease, then their children could know they were not at risk for the disease. If unfortunately they did develop symptoms, then each of their children could know there was a 50 percent chance that they, too, had inherited the gene. In both cases, the children faced a period of prolonged anxiety as to whether they would develop the disease. Then, in the 1980s, thanks in part to an energetic campaign by Nancy Wexler, a genetic marker was found that, in certain circumstances, could tell people with a relatively high degree of probability whether or not they had the gene for the disease.[9] Finally, in March 1993, the defective gene itself was discovered.[10] Now individuals can find out whether they carry the gene for the disease, and prenatal screening can tell us whether a given fetus has inherited it. These technological developments change the moral scene substantially.

How serious are the risks involved in Huntington's disease? Geneticists often think a 10 percent risk is high.[11] But risk assessment also depends on what is at stake: the worse the possible outcome, the more undesirable an otherwise small risk seems. In medicine, as elsewhere, people may regard the same result quite differently. But for devastating diseases such as Huntington's this part of the judgment should be unproblematic: no one wants a loved one to suffer in this way.[12]

There may still be considerable disagreement about the acceptability of a given risk. So it would be difficult in many circumstances to say how we should respond to a particular risk. Nevertheless, there are good grounds for a conservative approach, for it is reasonable to take special precautions to avoid very bad consequences, even if the risk is small. But the possible consequences here *are* very bad: a child who may inherit Huntington's disease has a much greater than average chance of being subjected to severe and prolonged suffering. And it is one thing to risk one's own welfare, but quite another to do so for others and without their consent.

Is this judgment about Huntington's disease really defensible? People appear to have quite different opinions. Optimists argue that a child born into a family afflicted with Huntington's disease has a reasonable chance of living a satisfactory life. After all, even children born of an afflicted parent still have a 50 percent chance of escaping the disease. And even if afflicted themselves, such people will probably enjoy some thirty years of healthy life before symptoms appear. It is also possible, although not at all likely, that some might not mind the symptoms caused by the disease. Optimists can point to diseased persons who have lived fruitful lives, as well as those who seem genuinely glad to be alive. One is Rick Donohue, a sufferer from the Joseph family disease: "You know, if my mom hadn't had me, I wouldn't be here for the life I have had. So there is a good possibility I will have children."[13] Optimists therefore conclude

8 Hymie Gordon, "Genetic Counseling," *JAMA* 217, no. 9 (August 30,1971): 1346.
9 See Revkin, "Hunting Down Huntington's," 99-108.
10 "Gene for Huntington's Disease Discovered," *Human Genome News* 5, no. 1 (May 1993): 5.
11 Charles Smith, Susan Holloway, and Alan E. H. Emery, "Individuals at Risk in Families—Genetic Disease," *Journal of Medical Genetics* 8 (1971): 453.

12 To try to separate the issue of the gravity of the disease from the existence of a given individual, compare this situation with how we would assess a parent who neglected to vaccinate an existing child against a hypothetical viral version of Huntington's.
13 *The New York Times*, September 30, 1975, p. 1. The Joseph family disease is similar to Huntington's disease except that symptoms start appearing in the twenties. Rick

that it would be a shame if these persons had not lived.

Pessimists concede some of these facts but take a less sanguine view of them. They think a 50 percent risk of serious disease such as Huntington's is appallingly high. They suspect that many children born into afflicted families are liable to spend their youth in dreadful anticipation and fear of the disease. They expect that the disease, if it appears, will be perceived as a tragic and painful end to a blighted life. They point out that Rick Donohue is still young and has not experienced the full horror of his sickness. It is also well-known that some young persons have such a dilated sense of time that they can hardly envision themselves at thirty or forty, so the prospect of pain at that age is unreal to them.[14]

More empirical research on the psychology and life history of suffers and potential sufferers is clearly needed to decide whether optimists or pessimists have a more accurate picture of the experiences of individuals at risk. But given that some will surely realize pessimists' worst fears, it seems unfair to conclude that the pleasures of those who deal best with the situation simply cancel out the suffering of those others when that suffering could be avoided altogether.

I think that these points indicate that the morality of procreation in such situations demands further investigation. I propose to do this by looking first at the position of the possible child, then at that of the potential parent.

Possible Children and Potential Parents

The first task in treating the problem from the child's point of view is to find a way of referring to possible future offspring without seeming to confer some sort of morally significant existence on them. I follow the convention of calling children who might be born in the future but who are not now conceived "possible" children, offspring, individuals, or persons.

Now, what claims about children or possible children are relevant to the morality of childbearing in the circumstances being considered? Of primary importance is the judgment that we ought to try to provide every child with something like a minimally satisfying life. I am not altogether sure how best to formulate this standard, but I want clearly to reject the view that it is morally permissible to conceive individuals so long as we do not expect them to be so miserable that they wish they were dead.[15] I believe that this kind of moral minimalism is thoroughly unsatisfactory and that not many people would really want to live in a world where it was the prevailing standard. Its lure is that it puts few demands on us, but its price is the scant attention it pays to human well-being.

How might the judgment that we have a duty to try to provide a minimally satisfying life for our children be justified? It could, I think, be derived fairly straightforwardly from either utilitarian or contractarian theories of justice, although there is no space here for discussion of the details. The net result of such analysis would be to conclude that neglecting this duty would create unnecessary unhappiness or unfair disadvantage for some persons.

Of course, this line of reasoning confronts us with the need to spell out what is meant by "minimally satisfying" and what a standard based on this concept would require of us.

Donohue was in his early twenties at the time he made this statement.

14   I have talked to college students who believe that they will have lived fully and be ready to die at those ages. It is astonishing how one's perspective changes over time and how ages that one once associated with senility and physical collapse come to seem the prime of human life.

---

15   The view I am rejecting has been forcefully articulated by Derek Parfit, *Reasons and Persons* (Oxford: Clarendon, 1984). For more discussion, see Chapter 2, "Loving Future People."

Conceptions of a minimally satisfying life vary tremendously among societies and also within them. *De rigeur* in some circles are private music lessons and trips to Europe, whereas in others providing eight years of schooling is a major accomplishment. But there is no need to consider this complication at length here because we are concerned only with health as a prerequisite for a minimally satisfying life. Thus, as we draw out what such a standard might require of us, it seems reasonable to retreat to the more limited claim that parents should try to ensure something like normal health for their children. It might be thought that even this moderate claim is unsatisfactory as in some places debilitating conditions are the norm, but one could circumvent this objection by saying that parents ought to try to provide for their children health normal for that culture, even though it may be inadequate if measured by some outside standard.[16] This conservative position would still justify efforts to avoid the birth of children at risk for Huntington's disease and other serious genetic diseases in virtually all societies.[17]

This view is reinforced by the following considerations. Given that possible children do not presently exist as actual individuals, they do not have a right to be brought into existence, and hence no one is maltreated by measures to avoid the conception of a possible person. Therefore, the conservative course that avoids the conception of those who would not be expected to enjoy a minimally satisfying life is at present the only fair course of action. The alternative is a laissez-faire approach that brings into existence the lucky, but only at the expense of the unlucky. Notice that attempting to avoid the creation of the unlucky does not necessarily lead to *fewer* people being brought into being; the question boils down to taking steps to bring those with better prospects into existence, instead of those with worse ones.

I have so far argued that if people with Huntington's disease are unlikely to live minimally satisfying lives, then those who might pass it on should not have genetically related children. This is consonant with the principle that the greater the danger of serious problems, the stronger the duty to avoid them. But this principle is in conflict with what people think of as the right to reproduce. How might one decide which should take precedence?

Expecting people to forego having genetically related children might seem to demand too great a sacrifice of them. But before reaching that conclusion we need to ask what is really at stake. One reason for wanting children is to experience family life, including love, companionship, watching kids grow, sharing their pains and triumphs, and helping to form members of the next generation. Other reasons emphasize the validation of parents as individuals within a continuous family line, children as a source of immortality, or perhaps even the gratification of producing partial replicas of oneself. Children may also be desired in an effort to prove that one is an adult, to try to cement a marriage, or to benefit parents economically.

Are there alternative ways of satisfying these desires? Adoption or new reproductive technologies can fulfill many of them without passing on known genetic defects. Sperm replacement has been available for many years via artificial insemination by donor. More recently, egg donation, sometimes in combination with contract pregnancy,[18] has been used to provide eggs for women who prefer not to use their own. Eventually it may be possible to clone individual humans, although that now seems a long way

---

16   I have some qualms about this response, because I fear that some human groups are so badly off that it might still be wrong for them to procreate, even if that would mean great changes in their cultures. But this is a complicated issue that needs to be investigated on its own.

17   Again, a troubling exception might be the isolated Venezuelan group Nancy Wexler found, where, because of inbreeding, a large proportion of the population is affected by Huntington's. See Revkin, "Hunting Down Huntington's."

18   Or surrogacy, as it has been popularly known. I think that "contract pregnancy" is more accurate and more respectful of women. Eggs can be provided either by a woman who also gestates the fetus or by a third party.

off. All of these approaches to avoiding the use of particular genetic material are controversial and have generated much debate. I believe that tenable moral versions of each do exist.[19]

None of these methods permits people to extend both genetic lines or realize the desire for immortality or for children who resemble both parents; nor is it clear that such alternatives will necessarily succeed in proving that one is an adult, cementing a marriage, or providing economic benefits. Yet, many people feel these desires strongly. Now, I am sympathetic to William James's dictum regarding desires: "Take any demand, however slight, which any creature, however weak, may make. Ought it not, for its own sole sake be satisfied? If not, prove why not."[20] Thus a world where more desires are satisfied is generally better than one where fewer are. However, not all desires can be legitimately satisfied, because as James suggests, there may be good reasons, such as the conflict of duty and desire, why some should be overruled.

Fortunately, further scrutiny of the situation reveals that there are good reasons why people should attempt with appropriate social support to talk themselves out of the desires in question or to consider novel ways of fulfilling them. Wanting to see the genetic line continued is not particularly rational when it brings a sinister legacy of illness and death. The desire for immortality cannot really be satisfied anyway, and people need to face the fact that what really matters is how they behave in their own lifetimes. And finally, the desire for children who

physically resemble one is understandable, but basically narcissistic, and its fulfillment cannot be guaranteed even by normal reproduction. There are other ways of proving one is an adult, and other ways of cementing marriages—and children don't necessarily do either. Children, especially prematurely ill children, may not provide the expected economic benefits anyway. Nongenetically related children may also provide benefits similar to those that would have been provided by genetically related ones, and expected economic benefit is, in many cases, a morally questionable reason for having children.

Before the advent of reliable genetic testing, the options of people in Huntington's families were cruelly limited. On the one hand, they could have children, but at the risk of eventual crippling illness and death for them. On the other, they could refrain from childbearing, sparing their possible children from significant risk of inheriting this disease, perhaps frustrating intense desires to procreate—only to discover, in some cases, that their sacrifice was unnecessary because they did not develop the disease. Or they could attempt to adopt or try new reproductive approaches.

Reliable genetic testing has opened up new possibilities. Those at risk who wish to have children can get tested. If they test positive, they know their possible children are at risk. Those who are opposed to abortion must be especially careful to avoid conception if they are to behave responsibly. Those not opposed to abortion can responsibly conceive children, but only if they are willing to test each fetus and abort those who carry the gene. If individuals at risk test negative, they are home free.

What about those who cannot face the test for themselves? They can do prenatal testing and abort fetuses who carry the defective gene. A clearly positive test also implies that the parent is affected, although negative tests do not rule out that possibility. Prenatal testing can thus bring knowledge that enables one to avoid passing the disease to others, but only, in some cases, at the cost of coming to know

19 The most powerful objections to new reproductive technologies and arrangements concern possible bad consequences for women. However, I do not think that the arguments against them on these grounds have yet shown the dangers to be as great as some believe. So although it is perhaps true that new reproductive technologies and arrangements should not be used lightly, avoiding the conceptions discussed here is well worth the risk. For a series of viewpoints on this issue, including my own "Another Look at Contract Pregnancy" (Chapter 12), see Helen B. Holmes, *Issues in Reproductive Technology I: An Anthology* (New York: Garland, 1992).

20 William James, *Essays in Pragmatism*, ed. A. Castell (New York: Hafner, 1948), p. 73.

with certainty that one will indeed develop the disease. This situation raises with peculiar force the question of whether parental responsibility requires people to get tested.

Some people think that we should recognize a right "not to know." It seems to me that such a right could be defended only where ignorance does not put others at serious risk. So if people are prepared to forego genetically related children, they need not get tested. But if they want genetically related children, then they must do whatever is necessary to ensure that affected babies are not the result. There is, after all, something inconsistent about the claim that one has a right to be shielded from the truth, even if the price is to risk inflicting on one's children the same dread disease one cannot even face in oneself.

In sum, until we can be assured that Huntington's disease does not prevent people from living a minimally satisfying life, individuals at risk for the disease have a moral duty to try not to bring affected babies into this world. There are now enough options available so that this duty needn't frustrate their reasonable desires. Society has a corresponding duty to facilitate moral behavior on the part of individuals. Such support ranges from the narrow and concrete (such as making sure that medical testing and counseling is available to all) to the more general social environment that guarantees that all pregnancies are voluntary, that pronatalism is eradicated, and that women are treated with respect regardless of the reproductive options they choose.

The Morality of Screening for Disability

Jeff McMahan

Abstract

Many people object to preimplantation or prenatal screening for disability on the grounds that it is discriminatory, has pernicious effects on the lives of existing disabled people, expresses a hurtful view of disabled people, and reduces human diversity, I argue that if these objections are held to be strong enough to show that screening is wrong, they must also imply the permissibility of causing oneself to have a disabled rather than a non-disabled child. Indeed, those who object to screening on these grounds and also claim that it is not worse to be disabled than not to be, seem to be committed to accepting the permissibility of deliberately causing disabling prenatal injury, even for frivolous reasons, If we cannot accept these implications, we cannot accept that the objections to screening show that it is wrong.

Keywords

disability, ethics, prenatal injury, screening

My topic is the morality of using screening technologies to enable potential parents to avoid having a disabled child. The relevant techniques include preconception genetic and non-genetic testing of potential parents, preimplantation genetic diagnosis (PGD), and prenatal screening with the option of abortion. Many people use these techniques and are grateful to have them. Others, however, object to their use, even when abortion is not an issue. The most common objections can be grouped into four basic types.

First, the opponents of screening and selection urge that these practices are perniciously discriminatory, in that their aim is to rid the world of people of a certain type, people who have increasingly come to share a sense of collective identity and solidarity. Some might even argue that for society to endorse and support screening for disability is analogous to promoting efforts to prevent the births of people of a particular racial group.

Jeff McMahan is Professor of Philosophy at Rutgers University, New Brunswick, NJ, USA. He was educated at Oxford and Cambridge and is the author of *The Ethics of Killing: Problems at the Margins of Life*, published in 2002 by Oxford University Press. He is presently working on a sequel provisionally called *The Ethics of Killing: Self-Defense, War, and Punishment.* This too will be published by OUP in the Oxford Ethics Series, edited by Derek Parfit.

Department of Philosophy, Rutgers University, 26 Nichol Avenue, New Brunswick, NJ 08901–2882, USA Correspondence: e-mail: JMcMahan@Princeton.edu

Second, the practices of screening and selection are not just detrimental to the disabled as a group but may also be harmful to individual disabled people in various ways. They may, for example, reinforce or seem to legitimize forms of discrimination against existing disabled people. And, if effective, they also reduce the *number* of disabled people, thereby making each disabled person a bit more unusual and a bit more isolated. The reduction in numbers may. in addition, diminish the visibility and political power of disabled people generally.

Third, it is often held that a reduction in the number of disabled people would have an adverse effect on human diversity. To eliminate the disabled would be to eliminate a type of human being who makes a unique contribution to the world. For the disabled themselves, and indeed their mere presence among the rest of us, teach valuable lessons about respect for difference, about the nobility of achievement in the face of grave obstacles, and even about the value of life and what makes a life worth living.

Fourth, it is often held that practices of screening and selection express a view of disabled people that is hurtful to existing disabled people. Efforts to prevent disabled people from existing are said to express such views as that disabled people ought not to exist, that it is bad if disabled people exist, or at least worse than if normal people exist, that disabled people are not worth the burdens they impose on their parents and on the wider society, and so on. Screening and selection, in other words, seem to say to existing disabled people: 'The rest of us are trying to prevent the existence of other people like you'.

One can respond to these objections to screening and selection, as some of the speakers at this conference have done, by appealing to rights of individual liberty. One could grant that the practices are objectionable for the reasons given but argue that those reasons are overridden by rights to reproductive freedom and by the benefits to those who are able to exercise those rights. But I want to advance a reason

for scepticism about the force of the objections themselves.

The objections do of course express serious and legitimate concerns, concerns that must be addressed in appropriate ways. But I will argue that they're insufficiently strong to show that screening and selection are wrong or should be prohibited. For if they were taken to show that, they would also have implications beyond the practices of screening and selection. They would also imply the permissibility of certain types of action that most people believe are impermissible.

Consider this hypothetical example: Suppose there is a drug that has a complex set of effects. It is an aphrodisiac that enhances a woman's pleasure during sexual intercourse. But it also increases fertility by inducing ovulation. If ovulation has recently occurred naturally, this drug causes the destruction of the egg that is present in one of the fallopian tubes but also causes a new and different egg to be released from the ovaries. In addition, however, it has a very high probability of damaging the new egg in a way that will cause any child conceived through the fertilization of that egg to be disabled. The disability caused by the drug is, let us suppose, one that many potential parents seek to avoid through screening. But it is also, like virtually all disabilities, not so bad as to make life not worth living. Suppose that a woman takes this drug primarily to increase her pleasure but also with the thought that it may increase the probability of conception—for she wants to have a child. She is aware that the drug is likely to cause her to have a disabled child but she is eager for pleasure and reflects that it might be rather nice to have a child who might be more dependent than children usually are. Although she does not know it. she has in fact just ovulated naturally so the drug destroys and replaces the egg that was already present but also damages the new egg, thereby causing the child she conceives to be disabled.

Note that because the drug causes the woman's ovaries to release a new egg, the disabled child she conceives is a different individual from the child she would have had if she hadn't taken the drug.

Many people think that this woman's action is morally wrong. It is wrong to cause the existence of a disabled child rather than a child without a disability, just for the sake of one's own sexual pleasure. There are, of course, some who think that rights to reproductive freedom make it permissible to choose to have a disabled child just as they also make it permissible to try to avoid having a disabled child. But most of us do not share that view. Most of us think that if it would be wrong to cause an already born child to become disabled, and if it would be wrong to cause a future child to be disabled through the infliction of prenatal injury, it should also be wrong to cause a disabled child to exist rather than a child without a disability.

There are of course differences. Whether they are morally significant and if so to what extent, are matters to which I will return shortly. For the moment, the important point to notice is that if the arguments I cited earlier show that screening and selection are wrong, they should also show that the action of the woman who takes the aphrodisiac is permissible. This is because if it is morally *mandatory* to *allow* oneself to have a disabled child rather than to try, through screening, to have a child who would not be disabled, then it must be at least *permissible* to *cause* oneself to have a disabled rather than a non-disabled child.

Let me try to explain this in greater detail. If it is wrong for the woman to take the aphrodisiac, that must be because there is a moral objection to voluntarily having a disabled child—an objection that's strong enough to make it wrong to cause oneself, by otherwise permissible means, to have a disabled rather than a non-disabled child. But if there is such an objection, it must surely be strong enough to make it at least permissible for people to try. by morally acceptable means, to avoid having a disabled child and to have a non-disabled child instead, and to make it impermissible for others to prevent them from making this attempt.

Yet the critics of screening believe not only that it is wrong for people to try to avoid having a disabled child and to have a non-disabled child instead, but even that it is permissible for others to prevent them from having a non-disabled rather than a disabled child. It would be inconsistent for these critics to condemn the woman in this example for causing herself to have a disabled rather than a non-disabled child and to condemn those who try to cause themselves *not* to have a disabled rather than a non-disabled child.

The crucial premise here is that if it would be morally objectionable to try to *prevent* a certain outcome, and permissible to deprive people of the means of preventing that outcome, then it ought to be permissible to *cause* that outcome, provided one does so by otherwise permissible means.

Note also that if we were to assert publicly that it would be wrong for this woman to do what would cause her to have a disabled child rather than a non-disabled child, or if we were to attempt to prevent her from taking the drug—for example, by making the drug illegal on the ground that il causes 'birth defects'—our action would be vulnerable to the same objections that opponents of screening and selection urge against those practices.

If, for example, we were publicly to state the reasons why it would be objectionable for the woman to take the drug—that the disabled child's life might be likely to contain more hardship and less good than the life of a non-disabled child, that provision for the disabled child's special needs would involve greater social costs, and so on—the evaluations of disability and of disabled people that might be thought to be implicit in these claims could be deeply hurtful to existing disabled people, and if we were to prevent this woman and others from being able to take the drug, this would reduce the number of disabled people relative to the number there would otherwise have been, thereby threatening the collective identity and political power of existing disabled people.

In short, the arguments of the opponents of screening seem to imply not only that it would be permissible for the woman to take the aphrodisiac, thereby causing herself to have a disabled child, but also that it would be wrong even to voice objections to her action.

Some opponents of screening and selection may be willing to accept these implications. They might argue that there are relevant differences between causing oneself to have a disabled child rather than a different non-disabled child and causing an existing individual to be disabled. For example, in the latter case but not the former, there is a victim, someone for whom one's act is worse. So there are objections to causing an existing individual to be disabled that do not apply to merely causing a disabled person to exist, and to assert these objections merely expresses the view that it can be worse to be disabled than not to be, which seems unobjectionable, since it does not imply any view of disabled people themselves. Screening and selection, by contrast, are held to express a pernicious and degrading view of disabled people.

Thus, opponents of screening and selection typically think that they can draw the line between action by a woman that may cause her to conceive a child who will be disabled and. for example, action taken by a pregnant woman that injures her fetus, causing it to be disabled when it otherwise would not have been. But in fact many people, especially among the disabled themselves, contend that it is no worse to be disabled than not to be. They claim that disabilities are 'neutral' traits. So, for example. Harriet McBryde Johnson (2003), a disabled lawyer, emphatically repudiates the 'unexamined assumption that disabled people are inherently "worse off", that we "suffer", that we have lesser "prospects of a happy life"'.

The view that it is not bad to be disabled, apart from any ill effects caused by social discrimination, would be very difficult to sustain if it implied that to cause a person to become disabled would not harm that person, or that it is irrational to be averse to becoming disabled. But

in fact those who claim that it is not bad in itself to *be* disabled can accept without inconsistency that it can be bad to *become* disabled. They can appeal to the *transition costs*. It is bad to become disabled because this can involve loss and discontinuity, requiring that one abandon certain goals and projects and adapt to the pursuit of different ones instead. It is these effects thai make it rational to fear becoming disabled and they are a major part of the explanation of why it is wrong to cause someone to become disabled. The other major part is that the causation of disability involves a violation of the victim's autonomy.

But notice that these considerations do not count against causing disability through prenatal injury. For congenital disability does not have transition costs, and fetuses are not autonomous.

It seems, therefore, that opponents of screening and selection who also claim that it is not worse to be disabled have no basis for objecting to the infliction of prenatal injury that causes congenital disability. Moreover, to object to the infliction of disabling prenatal injury or to enact measures to prevent it would seem to express a negative view of disability and perhaps of the disabled themselves, At a minimum, it expresses the view that it is bad to be disabled, or at least worse than not to be disabled. And, if effective, efforts to prevent disabling prenatal injury would have other effects comparable to those of prohibiting or restricting screening for disability and selection, such as reducing the number of disabled people who would be born, thereby also threatening the sense of collective identity and solidarity among the disabled as well as diminishing their visibility and political power. Finally, prevention of prenatal injury would also threaten human diversity. It would deprive those who would have had contact with the person if he had been disabled of the unique benefits that disabled people offer to others.

So for those opponents of selection who also hold that it is not a harm or misfortune to be disabled, it seems that there are not only no reasons to object to the infliction of disabling prenatal injury but even positive reasons not to object to it and not to try to prevent it.

Suppose there were an aphrodisiac that would greatly enhance a woman's pleasure during sex but would, if taken during pregnancy, injure the fetus in a way that would cause it to be congenitally severely disabled. Those who oppose screening and selection for the reasons I cited earlier and who also hold that it is not bad in itself to be disabled are logically committed by their own arguments to accept that it would be permissible for a pregnant woman to take this aphrodisiac just to increase her own pleasure, and they are further committed to accept that it would be wrong to try to prevent the woman from taking the aphrodisiac or even to criticize her for doing so.

If we think that these conclusions are mistaken, which they surely are. we must reject some part of the case against screening and selection.

I will conclude by briefly suggesting a more positive way of addressing the concerns of those who oppose screening and selection. My sense is that the chief worry of those opposed to screening and selection has to do with the expressive effects of these practices. The worry is, as I noted earlier, that these practices give social expression to a negative view of disabled people, thereby reinforcing other forms of discrimination against them.

But notice that it is usually only people who have not had a disabled child who are averse to doing so. Those people who actually have a disabled child tend overwhelmingly to be glad that they had the particular child they had. If any child they might have had would have been disabled, they tend to prefer having had their actual disabled child to having had no child at all. If they could have had a non-disabled child but it would have been a different child, they tend to prefer their actual disabled child. Of course, what they would usually most prefer is that their actual child had not been disabled. But it is almost invariably the case that any action that would have enabled them to avoid having a disabled child would have caused them to have a different child. When the parents appreciate this fact, they cease to wish that anything had been different in the past, and focus their hopes on the possibility of a cure.

In short, most people who currently have or have had a disabled child in the past do not regret having done so. They are, instead, glad to have had their actual child and frequently testify to the special joy and illumination afforded by being bound to a disabled child. This very different evaluation of having a disabled child by those who actually have experience of it is no less rational and no less authoritative than the evaluation that many people make prospectively that it would be bad or worse to have a disabled child.

We could therefore try to offset any negative expressive effects of screening and selection by giving public expression to these different and equally valid evaluations. I do not have any suggestions for how we might do this. That's a matter for specialists in public policy, not philosophers. But the crucial point is that it would be morally and strategically better for disabled people and their advocates to focus their efforts on positive proposals of this sort rather than to stigmatize and to seek to restrict or suppress practices such as screening and selection. By crusading against screening and selection, they risk making themselves appear to the wider public as fanatics bent on imposing harmful restrictions on others. That would certainly not serve the cause of obtaining justice for the disabled.

Reference

Johnson HM 2003 Unspeakable conversations. *New York Times Magazine* 16 February 2003, p.79.

Received 10 November 2004; refereed and accepted 10 November 2004.

Credits

President's Council on Bioethics, Selection from: "Biotechnology and the Pursuit of Happiness," *Beyond Therapy: Biotechnology and the Pursuit of Happiness*, pp. 1–20. Copyright in the Public Domain.

Fritz Jahr, "Bio-Ethics, 1927," *Fritz Jahr and the Foundations of Global Bioethics: The Future of Integrative Bioethics*, ed. Amir Muzur and Hans-Martin Sass, pp. 1-4. Copyright © 2012 by LIT Verlag. Reprinted with permission.

Fritz Jahr, "Animal Protection and Ethics, 1928," *Fritz Jahr and the Foundations of Global Bioethics: The Future of Integrative Bioethics*, ed. Amir Muzur and Hans-Martin Sass, pp. 9–12. Copyright © 2012 by LIT Verlag. Reprinted with permission.

Fritz Jahr, "Three Studies on the Fifth Commandment, 1934," *Fritz Jahr and the Foundations of Global Bioethics: The Future of Integrative Bioethics*, ed. Amir Muzur and Hans-Martin Sass, pp. 31–35. Copyright © 2012 by LIT Verlag. Reprinted with permission.

Van Rensselaer Potter, "Human Survival," *Global Bioethics: Building on the Leopold Legacy*, pp. 31–55. Copyright © 1988 by Michigan State University Press. Reprinted with permission.

The Belmont Report: Copyright in the Public Domain.

Tom L. Beauchamp, "The Origins and Evolution of the Belmont Report," *Belmont Revisited: Ethical Principles for Research with Human Subjects*, ed. James F. Childress, Eric M. Meslin, and Harold T. Shapiro, pp. 12–25. Copyright © 2005 by Georgetown University Press. Reprinted with permission.

Aristotle, The Basic Works of Aristotle, ed. Richard McKeon, pp. 952–964, 1022–1036. Copyright © 2001 by Random House, Inc. Reprinted with permission.

Immanuel Kant, *Fundamental Principles of the Metaphysics of Ethics*, trans. Thomas Kingsmill Abbott. Copyright in the Public Domain. John Stuart Mill, "What Utilitarianism Is," Utilitarianism. Copyright in the Public Domain.

Hans Jonas, "The Altered Nature of Human Action," *The Imperative of Responsibility: In Search of an Ethics for the Technological Age*, pp. 1–24. Copyright © 1983 by University of Chicago Press. Reprinted with permission.

Tom L. Beauchamp and James F. Childress, "Moral Norms," *Principles of Biomedical Ethics*, pp. 1–25. Copyright © 2008 by Oxford University Press. Reprinted with permission.

Bernard Gert, Charles M. Culver, and K. Danner Clouser, "Principlism," *Bioethics: A Return to Fundamentals*, pp. 71–92. Copyright © 1997 by Oxford University Press. Reprinted with permission.

Daniel Callahan, "Individual Good and Common Good: A Communitarian Approach to Bioethics," *The Roots of Bioethics: Health, Progress, Technology,*

Death, pp. 50–61. Copyright © 2012 by Oxford University Press. Reprinted with permission.

Tom L. Beauchamp and James F. Childress, *Principles of Biomedical Ethics*, pp. 101–108. Copyright © 2008 by Oxford University Press. Reprinted with permission.

Tom L. Beauchamp and James F. Childress, *Principles of Biomedical Ethics*, pp. 150–156. Copyright © 2008 by Oxford University Press. Reprinted with permission.

Tom L. Beauchamp and James F. Childress, *Principles of Biomedical Ethics*, pp. 202–209. Copyright © 2008 by Oxford University Press. Reprinted with permission.

Tom L. Beauchamp and James F. Childress, *Principles of Biomedical Ethics*, pp. 249–258. Copyright © 2008 by Oxford University Press. Reprinted with permission.

John-Stewart Gordon, Oliver Rauprich, and Jochen Vollmann, "Applying the Four-Principle Approach," *Bioethics*, no. 25, issue 6, pp. 293–300. Copyright © 2011 by John Wiley & Sons, Inc. Reprinted with permission.

Tom L. Beauchamp, "Making Principlism Practical: A Commentary on Gordon, Rauprich, and Vollmann," *Bioethics*, no. 25, issue 6, pp. 301–303. Copyright © 2011 by John Wiley & Sons, Inc. Reprinted with permission.

Alan H. Goldman, "Refutation of Medical Paternalism," *The Moral Foundations of Professional Ethics*, pp. 173–195. Copyright © 1980 by Rowman & Littlefield Publishers, Inc. Reprinted with permission.

Terrence F. Ackerman, "Why Doctors Should Intervene," *Hastings Center Report*, vol. 12, issue 4, pp. 14–17. Copyright © 1982 by John Wiley & Sons, Inc. Reprinted with permission.

Immanuel Kant, "On a Supposed Right to Lie from Altruistic Motives," *Critique of Practical Reason and Other Works on the Theory of Ethics*, trans. Thomas Kingsmill Abbott. Copyright in the Public Domain.

David C. Thomasma, "Telling the Truth to Patients: A Clinical Ethics Exploration," *Cambridge Quarterly of Healthcare Ethics*, vol. 3, no. 3, pp. 375–382. Copyright © 1994 by Cambridge University Press. Reprinted with permission.

Mark Siegler, "Confidentiality in Medicine-A Decrepit Concept," *The New England Journal of Medicine*, vol. 307, no. 24, pp. 1518–1521. Copyright © 1982 by Massachusetts Medical Society. Reprinted with permission.

Howard Brody, "Medical Futility: A Useful Concept?" *Medical Futility and the Evaluation of Life-Sustaining Intervention*, ed. Marjorie B. Zucker and Howard D. Zucker, pp. 1–14. Copyright © 1997 by Cambridge University Press. Reprinted with permission.

William Prip and Anna Moretti, "Medical Futility: A Legal Perspective," *Medical Futility and the Evaluation of Life-Sustaining Intervention*, ed. Marjorie B. Zucker and Howard D. Zucker, pp. 136–154. Copyright © 1997 by Cambridge University Press. Reprinted with permission.

Ruth R. Faden and Tom L. Beauchamp, *A History and Theory of Informed Consent*, pp. 274–287. Copyright © 1986 by Oxford University Press. Reprinted with permission.

James Rachels, "Active and Passive Euthanasia," *New England Journal of Medicine*, vol. 292, no. 2, pp. 78–80. Copyright © 1975 by Massachusetts Medical Society. Reprinted with permission.

Winston Nesbitt, "Is Killing No Worse Than Letting Die?" *Journal of Applied Philosophy*, vol. 12, issue 1, pp. 101–106. Copyright © 1995 by John Wiley & Sons, Inc. Reprinted with permission.

Walter Glannon, "Genetic Enhancement," *Genes and Future People: Philosophical Issues in Human Genetics*, pp. 94–105. Copyright © 2001 by Perseus Books Group. Reprinted with permission.

Michael J. Sandel, "The Case Against Perfection: What's Wrong with Designer Children, Bionic Athletes, and Genetic Engineering," *The Atlantic Monthly*, vol. 293, no. 3, pp. 51-62. Copyright © 2004 by Michael J. Sandel. Reprinted with permission.

David B. Resnik, "The Moral Significance of the Therapy-Enhancement Distinction in Human Genetics," *Cambridge Quarterly of Healthcare Ethics*, vol. 9, issue 3, pp. 365–377. Copyright © 2000 by Cambridge University Press. Reprinted with permission.

Samuel Hellman and Deborah S. Hellman, "Of Mice but Not Men: Problems of the Randomized